W9-DHX-952

67 C

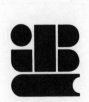

Health Insurance in Practice

William A. Glaser

Health Insurance in Practice

INTERNATIONAL VARIATIONS IN FINANCING, BENEFITS, AND PROBLEMS

Jossey-Bass Publishers

San Francisco • Oxford • 1991

HEALTH INSURANCE IN PRACTICE
International Variations in Financing, Benefits, and Problems
by William A. Glaser

Copyright © 1991 by: Jossey-Bass Inc., Publishers
350 Sansome Street
San Francisco, California 94104

&

Jossey-Bass Limited
Headington Hill Hall
Oxford OX3 0BW

HD
7101
G54
1991

Library of Congress Cataloging-in-Publication Data

Glaser, William A.
   Health insurance in practice : international variations in financing, benefits, and problems / William A. Glaser.
      p.   cm.—(The Jossey-Bass health series)
   Includes bibliographical references.
   Includes index.
   ISBN 1-55542-373-6
   1. Insurance, Health.   2. Medicine, State.   I. Title.
II. Series.
   [DNLM: 1. Financing, Organized—economics.   2. Insurance Benefits.
3. Insurance Health.   W 100 G548h]
   HD7101.G54   1991
   368.3—dc20
   DNLM/DLC
for Library of Congress   91-7035
                                                                                 CIP

Manufactured in the United States of America

JACKET DESIGN BY WILLI BAUM

FIRST EDITION

Code 9168

The Jossey-Bass Health Series

Contents

Contents

For our friends,
Gwen Gentile, M.D.,
and
Donald Helbig, M.D.

Preface

The United States has serious difficulties in health care. Many persons lack financial coverage and services. Those with insurance protection often find it incomplete and must pay much additional cash. Costs cannot be controlled. Doctors and other providers are beset by complicated rules, burdensome paperwork, and disputes.

The United States appears unable to solve these problems. But all other developed countries have nationwide financing arrangements that either solve these problems or prevent them from arising in the first place. This book describes how other countries have taken voluntary and private health insurance—the method long used in the United States—and transformed it into stable systems of social protection for their entire populations. (The principal countries with these arrangements are Germany, France, the Netherlands, Belgium, and Switzerland.) The book describes these statutory health insurance systems in detail and contrasts them with the private and chaotic health sector of the United States on the one hand and, on the other, with the fully governmentalized arrangements ("socialized medicine") in a few other countries (such as Great Britain). The book concentrates on the countries with various mixes of social insurance and private insurance—that is, where subscribers pay premiums or payroll taxes into a fund that pays their health care bills—since these arrangements are plausible models for reform in the United States. I do not focus on the countries with government takeovers of the providers (as in Great Britain) or full public financing of health services (as in Canada), since the United States is unlikely to emulate them.

The book describes how countries with statutory health insurance solve the unavoidable difficulties in health care finance. Governments and insurance carriers respond in many different ways in capping total expenditures, controlling the reimbursement of providers, shifting some costs to patients, increasing payroll taxes, transferring money from other social security accounts and from the government Treasury, and so on. Costs must be controlled without cutting coverage and benefits, since they are guaranteed—universal entitlement was, after all, the reason for having statutory health insurance in the first place. Every country encounters other issues, as well, such as the administration of complex systems, the coverage of the many new and expensive technologies, and the method of adding long-term-care benefits.

The book is not a plea on behalf of statutory health insurance. Rather, it describes the gradual universalization of statutory health insurance in many countries, the advantages and disadvantages of the alternatives, the difficulties and remedies in cost containment and administration, and its replacement by national health services in a few countries. For a specialist in cross-national research like myself, it is more interesting if countries differ rather than if they adopt the same model. Some countries may pay a heavy price—like the United States today—but that is their prerogative.

Research Methods

As in all my previous research projects, my evidence consists primarily of interviews with administrators and health care researchers in Europe and the United States, supplemented by the administrative and research literature. I focused on social security, statutory health insurance, and private voluntary health insurance during my visits to France, West Germany, Belgium, the Netherlands, Switzerland, Italy, Spain, and Great Britain during 1986 and 1987. Over the two years, I spent one or two months in each country and made a few follow-up visits during 1990. I describe my research methods in Appendix B. This research project about health insurance financing built upon my previous field research about insurance reimbursement of doctors and hospitals during the 1960s, 1970s, and early 1980s.

Audience and Applications

Because health insurance is such an important topic, specialized books have been written about each country's methods as textbooks for courses. This book has a broader perspective and generalizes about the methods common to all developed countries rather than enumerating details about each one. Teachers and students of public policy and administration who examine their own country in depth can use this book to understand their arrangements in wider perspective, as well as identify the particular and the universal features of their forms of health insurance. Many countries now have scholars who analyze "the modern welfare state" using books about the history and current status of social security generally. This book provides the most complete overview of the health insurance component of social security.

Another audience is the policymakers in each country who search for the solutions to their own problems and look for possible answers elsewhere. This lessons-from-abroad form of comparative analysis has become common in European social security and in European health care finance, and this book informs Western Europeans about the institutions and processes of all their neighbors. Interest in harmonizing health and social security has increased steadily in recent years as the European economy unifies. Lessons from abroad suddenly were sought throughout Eastern Europe when the Communist systems—including their national health services—collapsed. In manuscript, this book has already been studied by Eastern Europeans seeking to establish new statutory health insurance arrangements.

A large potential audience for such lessons is in the United States. America has attempted to cover its population and finance its insurance by private voluntary methods, but these have failed. The research project yielding this book began as a collection of lessons from Europe for the reform of American health insurance, supported by a research grant from the United States government. A long special report and several papers from this project have circulated within the executive and legislative branches in Washington and among policy analysts elsewhere in America. Each chapter in this book ends with specific lessons for the United States. The final chapter describes a possible mode of statutory health insurance for the United States that emulates other developed countries. Paralyzed by the complexity of the subject and by a profusion of unworkable proposals, American analysts and policymakers should profit by these new suggestions—"new" only in the American forum, since they have long operated successfully in other developed countries.

Overview of the Contents

Chapter One summarizes the basic forms of health care financing and the principal characteristics of health insurance systems. It orients the reader to the many topics that follow. Chapter Two contrasts the philosophy of private insurance and the philosophy of social protection that underlies statutory health insurance in all developed countries. Chapter Three summarizes the historic expansion of coverage before and after the private and particularistic insurance arrangements were expanded by government intervention into universal and well-funded programs. This and later chapters conclude with estimates of the effects on services, utilization, and the health of the population—in Chapter Three, the effects of expanding coverage on access and health in contrast to the gaps that characterize the United States.

Chapter Four describes the organization and management of health insurance carriers in the different types of developed country—those with universal obligatory health insurance (such as France, Germany, Belgium, and Holland), those with publicly subsidized and regulated universal insurance (such as Switzerland), and the one predominantly private system (the United States). The chapter describes the role of private health insurance in countries with national health services (such as Great Britain and Spain) and those with full public financing (such as Canada). The chapter also describes relations between associations of health insurance carriers and government, as well as the relation between statutory health insurance and the social security system at large. Additional details about health insurance structures in each country appear in Appendix A.

Chapters Five through Nine summarize how statutory and private health insurance are financed and how governments and the managers of carriers make financial decisions. Chapter Five describes the various forms of social security payroll taxes and explains how some of this money reaches the subscribers' carriers. Payroll taxes—the staple of social security financing—are suspected of drawbacks, and Chapter Six reports attempts to remedy or replace them. Chapter Seven summarizes flat-rate premium systems used primarily in private health insurance but also in some statutory arrangements. It also describes the effects of competition on premiums. In order to redistribute finances and cover the heavier users who pay less, several countries have government subsidies (Chapter Eight) and interfund transfers (Chapter Nine).

Chapters Ten through Sixteen set forth the principal benefits and their variations among countries, the relations between carriers and providers, the carriers' payment of the providers, and methods of deciding reimbursement rates and ground rules. The topics are physician services (Chapter Ten), hospital care (Chapter Eleven), pharmaceutical drugs (Chapter Twelve), dentistry (Chapter Thirteen), and mental health care (Chapter Fourteen). Chapter Fifteen describes the tentative beginnings and novel financing arrangements for long-term care of the elderly. Chapter Sixteen explains how health professionals, government, and carriers decide to add new acute-care benefits.

Chapter Seventeen summarizes the methods of containing costs in health insurance and the performance of each method in practice. All countries with statutory health insurance have developed machinery to decide on expenditure targets and have crafted a set of instruments to enforce them. This chapter explains why the United States alone is unable to control health care costs and why it cannot do so under present arrangements.

Chapter Eighteen summarizes the principal effects of statutory universal health insurance on services, utilization, and health. It explains why statutory health insurance failed in some countries, where health care was then taken over by government. The chapter summarizes recent proposals for reform of statutory health insurance and explains why—in light of the recent success in stabilizing these accounts—major revisions are unlikely.

Chapter Nineteen describes a design for statutory health insurance that follows European precedents and might be enacted in the United States. I do not argue that America must adopt it, since such a conviction would bias the entire book. But the scenario is an option that can solve the enormous problems facing the country—if Americans seriously want to improve their situation. The favorite American proposals—mandating wider employer-paid coverage, creating complete Treasury-based public financing of the Canadian type, and creating more categorical programs—cannot be enacted by Congress and cannot be administered efficiently.

The book is organized by topic and does not describe individual countries at length. Many books and articles already describe the individual countries. Appendix A presents brief factual descriptions.

Acknowledgments

The research was supported by Grant No. 5 RO1 HSO5255, National Center for Health Services Research, U.S. Department of Health and Human Services.

For their reading of my preliminary report and final book manuscript, I am indebted to George A. Silver, Alis Valencia, Brian Abel-Smith, Odin W. Anderson, Carole Dillard, James K. Hutchinson, Jos Kesenne, Bryan R. Luce, Ira Raskin, Steven S. Sharfstein, Linda Siegenthaler, Robert Sigmond, Milton I. Roemer, and Albert Wertheimer. Xenia Lisanevich and Don Yoder contributed exceptional editorial help. As in all my research, I relied on the libraries of Columbia University.

For expert typing of all manuscripts, I am grateful to Dorothy Mullen, Sharon Swint, Kelly Owen, and Charlotte Fisher.

New York City   William A. Glaser
August 1991

The Author

William A. Glaser is professor of health services management at the New School for Social Research in New York. He received his B.A. degree (1948) from New York University in political science and his M.A. (1949) and Ph.D. (1952) degrees from Harvard University, also in political science.

His main research activities have been in cross-national comparative research about health services, government, and other topics. His books on comparative health care include *Paying the Doctor* (1970), *Social Settings and Medical Organization* (1970), *Health Insurance Bargaining* (1978), and *Paying the Hospital* (1987). From other cross-national research, he has written *The Brain Drain* (1978). From research about American government, he has written *Public Opinion and Congressional Elections* (1962) and *Pretrial Discovery and the Adversary System* (1968). In his many research projects, Glaser has prepared reports advising government agencies and private organizations.

From 1956 to 1982, Glaser was a senior research associate at Columbia University.

Health Insurance in Practice

PART ONE

Understanding
Health Insurance

The first four chapters give an overview of the basic features of health insurance that vary among countries and lie at the heart of controversies. Chapter One is designed to orient the reader to the many topics that will be examined in detail throughout the book. It gives brief highlights of cross-national variations in sources of payment, the role of government, coverage of population groups, benefits, types of carrier, methods of reimbursement, and relations between carriers and providers. The chapter clarifies the difference between health insurance and other methods of managing and reimbursing services, such as national health systems and full public financing.

Chapter Two summarizes the philosophies underlying social security and private commercial insurance, a distinction manifested in the fundamental institutional differences between European statutory health insurance and the American approach. The chapter describes how social insurance and private insurance coexist in the same societies.

Chapter Three describes the evolution of obligatory social insurance in all countries and shows how the United States tries to promote alternative private methods to achieve the same ends. The chapter describes how mixed public/private arrangements leave gaps in coverage and problems of access for some persons.

Chapter Four presents the organization of health insurance in the countries with comprehensive programs. It examines the relationship between the carriers and the entire social security system. The chapter also summarizes the organization of the private companies who supplement mainstream social insurance in some countries and who are the principal financial administrators in a few.

CHAPTER 1

Financial Systems:
An International Overview

──────────────── **Summary** ────────────────

Every developed country except the United States has extensive organized methods of paying for health care. Most have statutory health insurance systems in which the private insurance funds gain many new members throughout the population, administer money collected by requirement from subscribers and employers, and pay the health care providers—all according to laws. A few countries have national health services, a system in which government owns, manages, and fully finances health care for all citizens.

    Insurance carriers have many forms and perform many functions, according to the dominant financing system in that country. They are the principal financial administrators in countries with statutory health insurance and in America's private market. They provide supplementary coverage in countries with national health services. This book describes the wide variety of forms of insurance in developed countries.

    Many Americans think that the only alternative to their private and unorganized system is full governmental domination. But reality is very different. Government only enacts frameworks, converts insurance premiums into social security taxes, and contains costs. The insurance carriers and health care providers remain private and autonomous.

Sources of Payment for Health Services

Several methods can raise and distribute money for health care. One alone or several in combination may be used to finance a particular transaction for one person. The mix of arrangements varies among countries.

Insurance Fund. In this case, a pool of money is created by many subscribers who pay regular contributions. The subscriber is entitled to full benefits whenever he needs medical care.[1] Benefits usually are not related to the size of individual contributions, since the fund is a method of pooling small contributions to cover occasional large losses by a few.

Membership in "private" insurance funds is voluntary, and public regulations are few. "Social" insurance funds are based on an obligatory membership by entire social classes; their sizes and revenues are large, and government extensively regulates their organization, subscription rates, benefits, and accounts. This book focuses on the forms of social and private insurance in health.

Prepaid Savings. In this system, an individual can deposit contributions in an account—regularly or occasionally, at the same or varying rates—and can draw upon it to cover future medical costs. The account is earmarked for him alone, and any unused balance passes to his heirs. Common in pension financing, the method now is considered in several countries (particularly the United States) to pay for long-term health care in old age.

Government. When a country has this arrangement, the annual budget of the national or provincial government covers the bulk of health services for the population. General tax revenue—derived from personal income taxes, business income taxes, value-added taxes, sales taxes, and the like—is pooled in the Treasury and pays for the entire government budget. No taxes are earmarked for health alone. In one version, the Ministry of Health operates hospitals, employs doctors, and provides other services; their capital costs, operating costs, and wages ultimately come from general revenue. Examples are countries with national health services, such as Great Britain, Sweden, and Eastern Europe.[2] Or the providers can remain private and the Ministry pays them for each service rendered, as in Canada.[3]

Eligibility for benefits is not overtly related to paying taxes. The law defines eligibility, and usually all inhabitants are covered. In practice, though, all have paid some form of income, consumption, or sales taxes. Since this book focuses on social and private insurance, it does not examine systems with full public financing.

Charitable Funds. Private charities—usually associated with churches—were once a principal source of financing of health care in Europe and North America. They are still important, although recently they have been eclipsed by growing expenditure through insurance funds and government budgets. As in the case of hospitals, the providers' managers seek large charitable donations by a few rich persons, a constant stream of smaller donations from the general public, or both. Charities today may still operate, pay capital costs, and cover much of the operating costs of large installations such as hospitals and nursing homes. Or they may contribute to the capital and operating costs of special units, such as programs mixing clinical research and patient care in teaching hospitals. Countries without statutory social insurance and without general government funding, such as the United States, still depend heavily on philanthropy.

Cash Payments by the Patient. Once small health charges—for ambulatory visits to doctors, pharmaceuticals, and so forth—were usually paid out-of-pocket in all countries. Insurance and government financing were intended to eliminate point-of-service payment, so that access would not be discouraged and the poor would not be burdened.

Cash payments survive more or less in all countries. Some comprehensive social insurance programs—as in France—are intentionally designed to divide all costs between the carriers and the patients. Some benefits that might be wasted—such as pharmaceutical drugs—require user charges in almost every country. In a few nations, such as the United States, the insurance system is voluntary and incomplete, many people are uninsured and underinsured, and many must pay personally. Since no country covers all benefits by social insurance and government financing, the patient must personally pay for the omitted benefits, such as dentistry or nursing home care.

The Role of Government

Obligatory Insurance. Since the late nineteenth century, most European national governments have enacted laws requiring certain occupations to join sickness funds, levying payroll taxes on their workers and employers, and requiring the sickness funds to provide benefits to the workers and their dependents. Certain occupations were successively added to obligatory coverage. Each new occupation was required to pay payroll taxes, and the sickness funds steadily grew. The national government administers the agencies for collecting the money and distributing it to the sickness funds.[4]

In federal systems of government, either the national or provincial governments may enact such obligatory social insurance laws. Usually—as in Germany—the national government takes the lead, and the provinces enact compatible implementing legislation. Leaving coverage and ground rules entirely to the discretion of the provinces would result in excessive diversity.

Conditional Grants. Instead of requiring citizens to join and pay premiums, government may encourage voluntary enrollment by subsidizing the sickness funds. Instead of compelling the sickness funds to follow rules, government may set grant conditions with the same effects. Switzerland, for example, thereby achieves considerable nationwide uniformity in the operation of health insurance despite the absence of a national mandatory law and despite a diversity among the cantons' insurance laws.

Regulation of Private Insurance. Every country regulates nonprofit and for-profit insurance in health and all other lines. The purpose is to protect consumers against fraud, profiteering, and bankruptcy of carriers. As well, regulation prevents predatory and ruinous competition among carriers.

Every country with obligatory social health insurance also has private health insurance for the voluntarily insured and for extra benefits beyond those of the statutory system. Therefore, every country has two channels of regulation and financial monitoring—one over the social insurance carriers and the other over the private health insurance companies. In the United States, with its small social insurance sector (Medicare), most health insurance is administered by private companies and is monitored by their regulators in state government.

Coverage of the Population

Statutory. During the late nineteenth and early twentieth centuries, every obligatory social insurance system began with blue-collar workers in factories, mines, and similar settings. Their wives and children were included then or soon after. Later amendments successively added white-collar workers, service workers, farmers, self-employed businessmen, other employees, and their dependents. Finally, pensioners and the unemployed were required to join sickness funds.

In several countries, such as France and Belgium, all categories of the population were eventually added, so that coverage became complete. In others, such as Germany and Holland, persons over a certain income level (regardless of occupation) or persons in certain jobs were not required to join. In these countries, between 10 and 30 percent of the populations were free to choose voluntary membership in the official sickness funds, purchase of private commercial insurance, or self-insurance.

The United States has never enacted statutory health insurance on an occupation-by-occupation basis, since it has assumed that the entire population will be covered by private insurance purchased by employers or other groups based on the workplace. Instead, the United States enacted health insurance as part of the Social Security system for retired persons over the age of sixty-five. Everyone else must obtain private insurance or public welfare. Thus, the Americans reversed the usual sequence in starting and spreading obligatory coverage.

Private. During the first decades of statutory health insurance, the population is divided among the obligatorily covered blue-collar workers, the privately covered affluent elites, and the uninsured. The uncovered, particularly the farmers and farm workers, are undertreated and their regions are underprovided. Eventually all uninsured are covered by the statutory system.

The elites may be required to join the official system too, as in France and Belgium, and often they resist. They do so because their social security taxes exceed their private premiums for the financial benefit of the total system and because they lose discretion to shop for the most suitable benefit package. Often a political compromise is created for the self-employed, managers, civil servants, and other elites, so that their private carriers are fiscal intermediaries under the official system, and these persons can purchase thinner cover for lower premiums.

Even when substantial fractions of the population are not required to join statutory health insurance, as in Holland (up to the 1990s) and Germany, everyone buys private cover voluntarily in preference to assuming the risks personally. Health insurance is considered part of normal living. In some countries, such as Switzerland, every voluntary subscriber is induced to join by government subsidies to the carriers. As a result, the coverage of the population has steadily increased even when obligatory membership is not universal.

The only exception is the United States. The mixture of voluntary group insurance, voluntary individual insurance, and Medicare seemed to expand coverage steadily until well into the 1970s. However, coverage then decreased because the group market crumbled.

Ownership of Carriers

Mutual Assistance Funds. Before the enactment of national health insurance laws, most carriers in all countries were consumer cooperatives, often associated with the labor movement. They were governed by the trade union or by a board elected by the subscribers. Examples were the *mutualités* and *sociétés mutuelles* of Belgium and France and the *Innungskrankenkassen* and *Betriebskrankenkassen* of Germany. These mutual assistance funds continued as the carriers under statutory health insurance.

Many private commercial insurance firms selling all lines—particularly life and health—are nonprofit consumer cooperatives, that is, "mutual insurance companies." They have the predominant market share in private health insurance in nearly all countries. At times they remain as carriers under the statutory schemes. In Switzerland, for example, they receive government subsidies, conform to statutory conditions, and enroll most of the population.

Government. In some countries, conservative governments take the financial administration away from the mutual assistance funds in order to free the statutory health insurance system from political domination by the trade unions and political parties of the Left, in order to increase the voice of the taxpaying employers, and in order to improve financial management. The new sickness funds are autonomous public corporations governed by boards representing workers and employers and monitored by the Ministries of Social Affairs and Finance. They are usually run by professional managers. They are not line departments of the Ministries.

In Fascist countries, such as Italy under Mussolini and Spain under Franco, health insurance administration was transferred from the mutual assistance funds to special public funds led by the political party and dedicated to the policy of national unity. After the governments became democratized, the public funds survived under nonpartisan and professional management.

Mixed arrangements are possible. American Medicare has governmental funds (the Hospital Insurance Trust Fund and the Supplemental Medical Insurance Trust Fund) to enroll subscribers, collect payroll taxes and premiums, and monitor total spending. The claims are collected, screened, and paid by nonprofit and for-profit insurance carriers under contract with the government.

Stockholders. Many private insurance companies—particularly specialists in property and casualty lines—are owned by stockholders. Or they are part of syndicates owned by stockholders. They retain some profits and distribute shares to the owners, whereas the mutual insurance companies refund profits to policyholders in the form of dividends.

A few stock companies sell health insurance in the private market—often in order to complete portfolios of the customers who buy other lines. But stock companies usually avoid even the private market in health, since the field is unpredictable, expensive in administration, and prone to deficits. The stock companies usually are not the fiscal intermediaries in social insurance, since they cannot earn profits, are deprived of underwriting discretion, and are monitored closely by government.

Sources of Funds

Premiums. Under private health insurance contracts, the subscribers pay premiums to the carriers in return for coverage. The premium might be a general rate averaged across all subscribers and designed to cover the average cost of claims (a "community rate"). Or it might vary by the age, sex, occupation, and other characteristics of the subscriber, calculated to cover the costs of the claims from that class (a "graduated" or "step" rate). Or it might vary by the age of enrollment of the subscriber, remaining the same throughout his life except for general underwriting adjustments for all policyholders and calculated to cover the expected lifetime costs of each age class (a "level" or "age-of-entry" rate). Since premiums are set by the carrier according to its business aims, experience, and underwriting methodology, they vary among carriers despite comparable portfolios.

The national health insurance statute may not completely transfer rate setting to government. The sickness funds may continue to set their own rates, as in Germany and Switzerland. To ensure that the rates are not excessively high or excessively low, they are regulated by the government agency that monitors the annual accounts and products of the sickness funds.

Payroll Taxes. Statutory health insurance laws usually integrate health financing into the social security taxation system. As in the pension, disability, workers' compensation, and other programs, a percentage of each worker's wages and each employer's payroll is earmarked for each worker's sickness fund. The self-employed are taxed a percentage of their earnings. The rates for all social security programs are recommended each year by the Ministries of Finance and Social Affairs, are approved by the Prime Minister and Cabinet, and are enacted by the Parliament.

If certain groups are required to participate but are not employed, the Parliament levies special taxes that are percentages of income. Examples are a percentage of the elderly person's pension and a percentage of the unemployed person's benefit check.

Subsidies. Sickness funds run deficits because bad risks incur high costs (but contribute little) and the healthy employed subscribers do not pay enough over their costs. Some governments subsidize the sickness funds from national or provincial Treasuries.

Transfers Among Funds. If government provides no subsidies or low ones, it may require transfers from carriers with surpluses to those with chronic deficits. The health insurance system is therefore treated as a financial unit, even if it is a mosaic of distinct organizations.

Associations of sickness funds may arrange such transfers among their own members in order to stave off bankruptcies and government intervention, as in Germany.

Special Taxes. In a few countries, particularly France, the Parliament levies excise taxes on products that damage health and cause high medical costs, such as alcohol and tobacco. The entire revenue goes to the sickness funds.

Paying the Benefits

A variety of arrangements are possible in compensating the insurance subscriber for his loss or in providing the eligible beneficiary with his benefit.

Cash Benefits. The carrier pays a fixed amount of cash to the subscriber. The exact sum varies by risk, is specified by the contract, and is paid when the loss occurs. The carrier requires some proof of the event. The payment is not explicitly reserved for paying for this loss alone, but that is the intent of the policy. The payment covers part of the loss at least indirectly, since it goes into the subscriber's cash pool, which is unexpectedly diminished by loss of normal revenue or by the need to pay bills. Such insurance is common for:

☐ Invalidity payments to workers who suffer loss of wages, extra expenses at home, or both.
☐ Invalidity payments to employers who suffer loss of revenue when fewer workers report or who must hire additional replacements while invalids stay on the payroll.
☐ Patients with certain medical care expenses. They pay doctors, hospitals,

pharmacists, and others and receive "cash benefits" or "indemnity pay-ments" from their carriers. There is no relation between the provider's charge and the carrier's indemnity schedule. The provider need only certify that the patient has received care, and the patient collects the cash payment from the carrier. These arrangements are found in insurance policies for extra benefits and are rarely used in mainstream medical care benefits for the entire pop-ulation. The United States is the only country that regularly uses the indem-nity method in many basic medical care policies.

Direct Service. The carrier provides medical care to the subscriber. The sickness fund owns and operates polyclinics, hospitals, testing laboratories, and pharmacies. It employs doctors, nurses, dentists, pharmacists, and others on full-time or part-time salaries. Subscribers' premiums cover all operating costs of the system. When the subscriber needs care, he uses the carrier's facility and em-ployees, usually without additional point-of-service payments. A century ago, this was a common form of medical care insurance in Europe and America. It survives today only in Spain, in Israel, in American HMOs, and in several de-veloping countries.

Scheduled Benefits: Service Benefits or Reimbursement. The carrier pays the medical care providers' bills when the carrier's subscribers obtain care. Sub-scribers' premiums to the carrier create the pool to cover all bills and adminis-trative costs. This is now the most common form of medical care insurance in developed countries. The two methods of paying providers are the following:

☐ *"Service benefits," called* tiers payant *in French.* Usually the provider bills the carrier and the carrier pays the provider. For physician and hospital services, the patient usually pays nothing, although recently some countries have added cost sharing. Partial patient cost sharing has long been common for dentistry, drugs, prostheses, and certain other bills. Service benefits are the most common form of medical care insurance.

☐ *"Cash benefits," called* tiers garant *in French.* The provider bills the sub-scriber, the subscriber pays the provider, and the subscriber recovers in whole or in large part from the carrier. This method is disappearing in practice: today, many providers and carriers agree to substitute direct billing. (The traditional reimbursement steps are made meaningless when patients delay paying the provider and first collect the reimbursement from the carrier as if they had already paid the provider.) Cash benefit systems almost always involve patient cost sharing, since carriers usually do not reimburse the bills in full. Unlike an indemnity payment system, the provider's fees and the carrier's reimbursement are closely related, often by means of a fee schedule.

In theory, any method of financing—traditional insurance, prepayment, or social insurance—might be consistent with any benefit structure. But in practice, definite connections exist. Commercial insurers usually offer fixed cash payments for each risk (according to an indemnity schedule), since they seek to predict costs accurately, maintain profits, avoid unexpected deficits, keep premiums low and competitive, and avoid troublesome arguments with health care providers. Since social insurance is associated with a social policy to help the needy, it usually offers service benefits, full coverage of providers' costs, and little cost sharing by patients. Even before a country enacts a universal statute that redistributes money, some insurance carriers with wide voluntary membership may try to perform the social functions of service benefits and generous reimbursement, supported by high community-wide rates. (An example is America's Blue Cross and Blue Shield.)

Relations with Health Care Providers

Reimbursement of the Patient. If the traditional cash benefit system is retained, the sickness fund has no direct and continuous relations with providers. Doctors prize their independence and argue there is no reason for them to discuss medical practice and fees with sickness funds. As evidence justifying claims for reimbursement, patients submit receipts for doctors' services to the sickness funds. The carriers pay according to an indemnity schedule, and doctors claim the right to charge whatever they like, according to each doctor's eminence and each patient's ability to pay.

This method survives in private health insurance long after it is challenged in social insurance. Such patients are affluent enough to cover providers' extrabilling. Private health insurance is designed to help subscribers pay for the exceptionally expensive specialists and private clinics.

Eventually a showdown occurs in social insurance between the government and sickness funds on the one hand and the medical association on the other. The social security system cannot keep raising payroll taxes to keep pace with physicians' charges so that subscribers are reimbursed in full. If the sickness funds are capped and subscribers must pay steadily higher extra-billing by the doctors, the taxpayers complain they are not getting their money's worth and government finance officers complain about perversion of a public service. Eventually a compromise is framed, whereby the medical association and the sickness funds regularly negotiate contracts, fee schedules, and prices that are legally binding or voluntarily accepted by all the doctors. The reimbursement method of claims administration may survive, but the system works like service benefits.

Direct Payment. In all countries with statutory health insurance, sickness funds pay hospitals directly. In most countries, they pay office doctors directly, according to a fee schedule ("relative values scale") and prices ("conversion factors") negotiated regularly between the sickness funds and medical association and (in most cases) automatically approved by government.

Hospital and doctors therefore deal constantly with the sickness funds.

Doctors send their claims to the carriers and receive their payments. Doctors' claim forms are subject to utilization review and second opinions by the sickness funds' control doctors.

Employment. Before the enactment of statutory health insurance, some mutual assistance funds hired their own doctors. Subscribers patronized these doctors without paying extra fees. They were not reimbursed if they went to other doctors. The physicians usually could treat other patients, unless the sickness fund had enough members to occupy their "panel doctors" full time. When these sickness funds became carriers under statutory health insurance—as in Germany, in France (1928-1945), and in Great Britain (1911-1948)—they delivered care through their panels. A few sickness funds, as in France, created their own health centers, pharmacies, and hospitals, thereby offering them without cost sharing to their own members and at higher fees with cost sharing to other insured patients.

Closed panels were eliminated in all countries, since the medical profession did not wish to be employees of the laymen running sickness funds and since all doctors needed access to all patients in order to earn their livelihood. All national health insurance laws eventually guaranteed the subscriber's free choice of primary doctor, and they guaranteed all doctors' right to practice and to be reimbursed under insurance. Some laws explicitly forbade the official carriers to employ doctors and to operate health centers. Private insurance firms could operate such facilities—for example, the French mutual assistance funds continued to operate them after being replaced as the official carriers in 1945—but the subscribers under social insurance cannot be locked into them.

Since the United States has never enacted statutory health insurance for the general population, it still has health insurance carriers that employ their own doctors and operate their own health centers and hospitals. The subscriber pays for their salaries and operating costs, he can use them with little or no cost sharing, and he is not reimbursed if he patronizes other providers. They are called "staff-model" or "group-model" health maintenance organizations (HMOs). The one American social insurance program (Medicare) offers to pay the annual subscription fees for any beneficiary who wishes to join. The HMOs are simply one of the many competing insurance and provider arrangements allowed to proliferate in America's free health care market. Few doctors create them. Few subscribers—whether young or Medicare beneficiaries—join them.

Notes

The notes in this book contain many sources with statistical and other evidence supporting statements in the text. The study generalizes about comparative health care financing institutions and processes and belongs to comparative public administration. Including a host of statistical statements and tables would make the book prolix in style, excessive in length, and unwieldy in size. Moreover, as we shall see, the raw statistics about health care financing are uneven in quality, are not comparable across countries in format, and contain too few breakdowns for all the topics in this book. But the reader wishing such heterogeneous numerical evidence can find it in the sources cited throughout in the notes.

1. Since English has no generally accepted (and convenient) pronoun that means "either he or she," throughout the book I use "he" in the traditional generic impersonal sense—that is, referring to any male or female person.

2. Excellent descriptions are in Victor W. Sidel and Ruth Sidel, *A Healthy State,* 2nd ed. (New York: Pantheon Books, 1983).

3. Anne Crichton and David Hsu, *Canada's Health Care System: Its Funding and Organization* (Ottawa: Canadian Hospital Association Press, 1990); and Robert G. Evans, *Strained Mercy: The Economics of Canadian Health Care* (Toronto: Butterworths, 1984).

4. National health insurance systems are described in Alan Maynard, *Health Care in the European Community* (London: Croom Helm, 1975); Brian Abel-Smith (ed.), *Eurocare* (Basel: Health Service Consultants, 1984); Jan Blanpain and others, *National Health Insurance and Health Resources* (Cambridge: Harvard University Press, 1978); and *Eurohealth Handbook* (New York: Robert S. First, annual).

CHAPTER 2

Health Insurance
and Social Solidarity

————————————— Summary —————————————

Modern health care financing abroad is based on the philosophy and politics of social solidarity, not on the techniques of private insurance, despite the widespread use of the words "health insurance." The details vary among countries, but a common feature is redistributive financing: a large number of people are taxed in order to cover the costs of those who use health care services, even though the high payers are often low users and the high users are often low payers.

"Health insurance" originated in the mutual aid societies created centuries ago by craftsmen and urban workmen. At first, each member paid into a fund and the benefits were replacement earnings during illness, burial expenses, and help to widows and orphans. Some funds hired doctors to treat sick members. Each person paid to protect his friends and colleagues; each could claim the benefits if he suffered. During the nineteenth and twentieth centuries, the mutual protection societies expanded from their local and collegial origins, included more workers of different ranks in the covered industries, and grew throughout each country. Government solved problems of income security and health care access by requiring universal membership and imposing payroll taxes on workers and employers. Social solidarity and redistributive financing began on a small scale among friends but became universal and nationwide. Health insurance became an integral part of social security.

"Insurance" implies a person's self-centered calculations to protect himself against loss. A self-centered insurance company creates pools to spread risks, so it can market policies, bear the risks, and earn profits. But "insurance" in this form is designed to avoid exceptionally risky persons, not to protect them at a loss for a social good.

Some insurance-like features can be found in Europe. These techniques are used for insuring extra benefits. In a few countries (such as Germany) private insurance methods apply to a small market not covered by the obligatory system, but this formerly common situation is now rare. Once a system of social solidarity and redistributive financing is established for an entire country, it cannot be unscrambled in favor of voluntary private insurance. Populations become accustomed to thinking of health insurance as part of social security, and few want to change.

The United States alone tries to cover its population by means of a competitive private market. Even in prosperous times, adverse selection by subscribers burdens some carriers, preferred-risk selection by carriers leaves bad risks uncovered, financing is not redistributive, and public charity remains. During economic downturns, many citizens lose coverage and most carriers are underfunded.

The Nature of Insurance

Insurance is a social arrangement to reduce the risk of a serious loss through cooperation of many similarly situated persons or organizations. Each individual can lose much if the event strikes, but he cannot predict its occurrence. An insurance carrier pools the many comparable individuals, calculates the value of each type of loss, calculates the proportion of members of that class suffering the loss each year, and converts that proportion into a probability for each individual. All subscribers contribute to the fund covering losses by paying a fractional share each year.[1]

The risk must be "insurable" according to several criteria, some inherent in the original conception of insurance, some required by modern methods:[2]

☐ A large number of persons face the same risk:
  • Modern mathematical methods can then calculate the probability of occurrence for each class of persons and the appropriate premium to keep the pool solvent with a reasonable safety margin.
  • Subscribers can join and quit while the pool survives.
  • An individual can bring a unique risk to an underwriter, who calculates his individual probability of loss and negotiates the premium he pays a syndicate of investors. But this case is rare in the modern insurance industry, particularly in health.
☐ The loss can be priced exactly. The underwriter can calculate an accurate premium. The subscriber accepts the payment as final. The insurer can confirm that the loss has actually occurred and can be held liable for the claim.
☐ The occurrence of the loss is a random probability:
  • It is not certain to occur to everyone. If someone wishes to cushion the unpleasant results of an inevitable loss, he cannot call upon an insurance pool but must use other mechanisms, such as savings.

- A person cannot collect the cash benefit by generating the loss himself. Such fraud would bankrupt the carrier and reduce the other subscribers' cover.
- If the loss occurs to too many subscribers at the same time, the pool can be bankrupted.

☐ The loss must be reasonable:

- If it is extremely expensive, it can be covered provided that it does not occur often and the insurance/reinsurance pool is large. Otherwise, premiums will become high and unmarketable, or the pool becomes insolvent.
- Trivial losses are not covered. The administration of such claims is too expensive.

The original image of insurance depicts a private voluntary business relationship. Persons and organizations buy insurance to protect themselves against their own losses. Since they are self-interested, they wish to pay the lowest possible premiums calculated for their own risks and losses. The insurance carrier and its investors also have a self-interest: if they maximize premiums and minimize losses, they earn high profits and pay their staffs and sales agents generously. Subscribers are expected to shop among carriers for the best offer, the individual may bargain with one carrier to shape the final contract, the subscriber may decide that assuming the risk through self-insurance is best for him, and each carrier has the right to refuse bad risks.

The economy of health is quite varied. Acute ambulatory medical care, hospitalization, drugs, dentistry, and long-term care all involve different forms of service and different financial transactions. Although health care financing is often called "health insurance," financing arrangements other than classic insurance are common. Some health risks fit the foregoing criteria of insurability, but many do not.[3]

Small and Recurrent Losses

Insurance is supposed to be designed and purchased for the large and uncertain losses, not for the small and frequent ones. The individual person or organization is supposed to pay the small frequent losses from current revenue, as part of the cost of living or cost of business.[4] This policy has two advantages: each individual will pay for his own costs and preferences and will not overpay for the benefit of others; all will save the extra costs ("loadings") to administer the insurance or prepayment system.

Therefore, a question when designing insurance for certain types of benefit for certain types of subscriber is whether their losses are small and frequent or large, serious, rare, and unpredictable. If they face small and predictable costs, there are better financing methods—such as personal budgeting and savings—than paid-in-full insurance.[5]

Prepayment

If a loss is certain to occur eventually, an individual or organization may self-insure by means of a personal savings fund. The savings arrangement can be formalized. The individual or organization may create a special fund in a bank or other savings institution; public policy may encourage the device through tax exemptions or subsidies; and the subscriber can use the fund whenever the need arises. The prepaid fund is individual. The subscriber can use up to its total for his expenses but no more; if health care costs are less than the total, he (or his heirs) can claim the balance. Such individual prepayment accounts have long been common for private pensions in all countries, and one now hears proposals for their use for acute health care (in the United States) and for long-term care (in many countries).

Another form of prepayment places providers slightly "at risk" and therefore has some insurance-like features. A large number of subscribers pay equal "capitation rates" to the provider. All will need some services, but they cannot predict the volumes, types, and times. The provider must operate each year within the total revenue from the capitation rates by setting them high enough, recruiting enough subscribers, working efficiently, and rejecting bad risks. The prepayment method has been used by Britain's nonprofit hospitals before the National Health Service[6] and by groups of physicians at various times in Europe and the United States.[7]

Social Solidarity vs. Individual Responsibility

Traditional insurance reasoning is individualistic: the subscriber (whether a person or an organization) buys a policy covering his own risks, the premium is calculated actuarially to cover the probability of his loss, and a premium table gives him the option of paying higher premiums for higher monetary compensation. The insurer reduces risks for himself by placing comparable subscribers in the same premium class, and the revenue pool is enough to cover all payments for loss. Each member of the class is equally likely to overpay or underpay premiums in relation to recovery for a loss. Although an insurance company would like to overcharge subscribers, it is restrained by the probability that competing companies can take away subscribers by offering actuarially accurate premiums for the same coverage. Some health insurance in developed countries today resembles this model of rational calculation by self-serving individuals and organizations, but most coverage does not now and never has.

Modern health insurance evolved out of collective arrangements among craftsmen and workers that originated many centuries ago.[8] European guilds regulated affairs of each occupation. Eventually they added financial relief for their members and for their deceased members' widows and orphans. Instead of letting the sick, the widows, and the orphans depend on the charity of the local government and the church, each guild protected its own members. The craftsmen received invalidity cash payments when they could not work; the widows received funeral expenses and death benefits.

Guilds could raise only small amounts of money from their members, and the benefits were low. Revenue methods varied among guilds, and some were richer than others. Most required flat rates, such as a standard initiation fee and an annual subscription fee; others charged each member for each product he sold, thereby collecting more from the richer members. The watchword in all these groups was social solidarity: the resources of the guild were pooled to help the unfortunate members and their bereaved families. The payers did not get benefits at the time of their payment, since they could still work; the beneficiaries did not pay premiums at the time of need. All payers faced the same risk and were equally likely to need benefits. Outsiders did not receive benefits from the guild.

In addition to the guilds, which organized individual occupations, there were mutual aid societies that combined members from several similar occupations. They did not regulate economic activity—as the guilds did—but they provided the same social benefits.[9] Similar arrangements were created among the industrial workers of the nineteenth century. They too needed invalidity payments; their widows and children also needed funeral expenses and death benefits if the worker died. Mutual aid societies within individual plants and towns were created by trade unions, political parties, employers, and churches. To make benefits more reliable, money had to be collected more systematically; every member paid a predictable subscription fee, and some employers contributed administrative help and cash. In order to collect more money, higher payments were eventually sought from the better-paid workers. The arrangement was based on social solidarity: all workers in the plan were expected to join and pay; all members were eligible for standard benefits regardless of variations in contribution due to length of membership and income level; retired members might receive pensions even when they no longer contributed. Nonmembers were not covered.

Instead of making only the traditional invalidity cash payments, all mutual aid societies in nineteenth-century and early twentieth-century Europe eventually tried to cure members by providing medical care. They contracted with office doctors or employed their own. A few created polyclinics and pharmacies. Social solidarity was greatly extended. Instead of getting only fixed invalidity payments, the ill workers also got unlimited medical services at the society's expense. Thus, the healthy wage-earner paid to treat others. Societies subsequently extended the care to the workers' wives, the workers' children, and retirees, thereby greatly increasing costs and the active members' premiums. Any variations in contributions were based on workers' incomes, usually not on family size or medical risk. To cover the costs of the underpayers, unmarried members and heads of small families paid into the fund more than they drew out.[10]

The national health insurance laws beginning in the 1880s in Germany made social solidarity official policy and eventually spread it to entire populations.[11] The mutual aid societies were designated the official carriers. All members of certain occupations were required to join sickness funds. Revenue came from payroll taxes, a percentage of the worker's wage matched more or less by the employer. Since the payroll tax was a fixed percentage, the better-paid workers contributed more. Payroll taxes did not vary by family size. The same basic medical care benefits were available to all workers and (usually) all dependents, regardless of contributions. (Invalidity payments differed in logic, since often they were a fraction of the worker's wage.) The laws added more groups to basic coverage steadily throughout the twentieth century until now, when virtually entire populations are obligatory members.

Statutory "social insurance" in health and other sectors overrode methods of evaluating and underwriting insurable risks under traditional insurance. Following are its essential features:

☐ The statute identifies large classes of persons who must be covered and (often) other large classes who can choose coverage. All carriers recognized under the law must accept all eligible applicants.
☐ Usually the same premium—either a percentage of earnings or a fixed amount—is collected from every household regardless of risk. This book will describe some exceptions, usually benefiting vulnerable subscribers.
☐ All subscribers are fully entitled to all benefits.
☐ Carriers cannot ask supplements from subscribers presenting greater health risks. Usually carriers cannot ask supplements from subscribers with larger households.
☐ While government presses carriers to control costs, unavoidable deficits are covered by government subsidies. Carriers are not allowed to go bankrupt and leave subscribers unprotected.

The pooling of risks in traditional insurance enables some persons to benefit more than they pay and causes others to pay more than they regain. This outcome for individuals is the inevitable result of pooling risks: some suffer smaller losses than the average subscriber; others experience higher losses. The mutual aid societies, on the other hand, openly told their members that they were mechanisms enabling the better-off members of an occupational or religious community to help the less fortunate. The numbers of overpayers and underpayers bound by statutory social solidarity increased and the redistribution of money grew:

Pay more than costs of their utilization	*Draw more from the funds than their payments*
Higher wage-earners	Lower wage-earners
Self-employed (in some but not all countries)	Disabled temporarily or permanently
Single persons	Retired
Small families	Large families
Young	Old

The redistributive effects of social insurance can be found in every country. They can be traced, for example, in the voluminous research about morbidity and utilization in the general regime of France, which levies payroll taxes on all employed workers and salaried managers in France, without an income ceiling. The higher the wage, the higher the payment into the sickness funds. Morbidity is inverse to income: the lower classes have more illnesses and injuries. As social class rises, per capita use and costs of health services under the universal health insurance program stay approximately the same or decline. From the payroll tax revenue, the system earns profits from the richer and uses them to cover the losses from the poorer. (The rich spend more than the poor in purchases of specialists' services, dentistry, and some other forms of health care, but they cover these items from personal cash and private health insurance, not from the redistributive statutory system for basic services.)[12]

Social solidarity permeates basic health insurance throughout Europe, as will be evident throughout my analysis of specific topics in this volume. Since social solidarity involves the systematic redistribution of resources from the better-off to the less fortunate, it is altogether different from the pooling of randomly occurring risks under insurance. Healthier persons are not allowed to opt out of the general scheme, form their own class, and pay low actuarial premiums. For the general scheme, premiums are set and benefits are distributed under a social policy. In some countries all members of certain occupations or residents of certain areas are assigned automatically to certain sickness funds, and the carriers cannot compete for their affiliation by offering lower premiums or more generous benefits.

The Place of True Insurance

Some traditional insurance methods survive in modern-day European health care financing—for example, in the extra benefits not provided by the statutory programs. Such benefits include private fees for the chief of service in the hospital, private hospital rooms, and the full out-of-pocket payments not covered by the basic social insurance. The individual or the entire family buys a policy from the sickness fund or a private insurance company. The carrier may offer a variety of policies with different benefits and with varying premiums calculated to cover the actuarial costs of the benefits to the company. Some companies offer a choice: the subscriber may buy cheaper policies and share more of the costs of care. For these private policies, the carrier may charge according to a premium table based on age and sex (if the policy is individual) or size of family (if the policy is for a family). Some carriers sell private policies to groups (such as clubs or the managements of business firms) and the actuaries calculate an "experience rate" based on the actual recent costs of each group.

No European country can provide a true test of the comparative performance of social insurance and private insurance, because of the current division of the markets: social insurance covers nearly entire populations for basic benefits; private insurance just covers extra benefits. One might seek to examine the two markets in Holland, but they were never comparable: before the reforms of the 1990s, 70 percent under a certain income ceiling had statutory and obligatory insurance; 30 percent above the income ceiling had private, voluntary, and individually varied policies.[13] The system, however, undermined Holland's deep faith in social solidarity. The private insurers preferred good risks, the private firms gathered profits, and the sickness funds suffered deficits. The expensive risks—usually older persons—were priced out of the private market and accepted their guaranteed right to social insurance. The sickness funds during the 1980s forced the private companies to cover these transfers by equalization payments (described in Chapter Nine). The national government intervened in 1986 by requiring the private carriers to keep their pensioners at affordable premiums, thereby obliging them to practice social solidarity. Finally, the law was amended to make statutory health insurance universal. Distinctions between sickness funds and private carriers disappeared, all collected the same payroll taxes to pay for the same basic benefits, and each person could choose any social or private carrier.

The American Market

The United States remains the only developed country that relies on traditional insurance for the basic health care protection of most of its population. The country never followed Europe and never enacted statutory health insurance, and the private insurance industry stepped into the breach. Problems resulted, however, particularly in recent years. The inevitable outcomes of competition and the economic tactics of the carriers produce the difficulties of financing and coverage that social solidarity and universal social insurance are designed to eliminate.

For many years, many Blue Cross/Blue Shield Plans throughout the country behaved like social insurance carriers. They accepted all risks all year round or during open enrollment periods. In their market for individual policies, they charged all persons identical community rates calculated to break even across all risks. Much of the American population was covered by group contracts between employers and Blue Cross/Blue Shield, and the rates yielded extra cash to defray the costs of groups and individuals whose costs significantly exceeded their premiums.[14]

Commercial insurance companies then entered the markets by offering lower rates to the younger individual subscribers and lower experience rates to the groups. In order to keep market share, the Blues throughout the country have reluctantly moved toward age-graded rate structures for individuals, experience rates with rebates of surplus to groups, and exclusion clauses for poor health risks.[15] Where community rates are still preserved—as in several Northeastern states—the state governments must intervene by guaranteeing the Blues extra cash through discounts from hospital charges.

The American Social Security system was designed during the 1930s by a generation of economists steeped in the ideology of social solidarity and expert in the techniques of redistributive financing.[16] By the 1970s, policy analysis in health care financing had been captured by proponents of the opposite view-point: neoclassical economists who believed in free markets, competition, mini-mization of insurance coverage, and purchase of any insurance by each beneficiary at the lowest possible price.[17] No voices were raised against reduction of coverage by employers, the resistance to community rates by individuals, and the compet-itive price cutting by carriers. By the 1980s, the United States had become what Holland had avoided: a case study in the adverse social consequences of self-centered individualistic purchases. Increasing numbers of the poor, the workers, and the less healthy lacked coverage, as the next chapter reports. Instead of earn-ing extra money to cover the poor and the bad risks, many Blue Cross/Blue Shield Plans and many commercial insurance companies repeatedly lost money on health insurance and had to cut benefits.[18]

In such a private health insurance system, public charity from general rev-enue is retained to help the indigent. (It disappears when a country enacts uni-versal statutory health insurance.) During a short period in the mid-1960s when the United States government toyed with new social policies, it enacted Medicaid. But without a strong and continuing public dedication to social solidarity, Med-icaid has always been vulnerable to budget cutbacks and provider fraud. For go-vernment officials, the policy priority for Medicaid has always been cost containment rather than humanitarian service delivery. Instead of the universal coverage and mainstream benefits of a socially solidary program, Medicaid never has covered all the poor, individual states often have reduced coverage, and Me-dicaid has never delivered the same care as that received by the privately insured.[19] Medicaid has often been a favorite guinea pig for the policy theorists' faith in the benefits of competitive private markets. Providers would get contracts to care for the poor not by guaranteeing the highest quality but by offering the lowest prices. The clear signal was the state government's disinterest in protecting the poor. Providers have commonly responded by underserving and profiteering.[20]

Americans are so devoted to competitive markets—because of ideology and the pressures from smaller insurers—that they have institutionalized them in the health insurance for the national government's civil servants. (In other countries, public employees receive either statutory health insurance or a special package with standard benefits and standard premiums.) The Federal Employee Health Benefits Program (FEHBP) provides yet another illustration of the adverse selec-tion and premium spiral that result when competitive private markets allow subscribers a choice between high-coverage/high-premium policies and low-coverage/low-premium plans. The older and less healthy pick the policies with more complete coverage despite the higher premiums; the younger and healthier pick the policies with lower premiums and higher deductibles. As costs and premiums rise steadily for the high-option plans, their healthier subscribers then transfer to low-option alternatives. The only brake on adverse selection and the premium spiral is inertia: some better risks retain the high-option plan because of habit or extreme aversion to risk.[21] (Faced with these inescapable trends on a national scale, Dutch policymakers finally eliminated the private market and universalized statutory health insurance.)

The Mirage of Privatization

Enthusiasm for social solidarity led to a great expansion of benefits and coverage in Europe after World War II. When economies turned down in the 1970s and 1980s, the systems were saddled with high expenditures, high taxes, and much trouble in government budgeting. As this book will show, every country now tries to control payments to providers: social solidarity is supposed to benefit the public, not produce waste and windfalls for providers. In nearly every country, a few limits are placed on benefits. [22]

Occasionally one hears a call to scrap the social protection systems in favor of a privatized insurance market. [23] But no policymaker in any European country seriously proposes such a measure. Rather, as this book will show, financial policymakers in statutory health insurance and social security are trying to make the established systems more efficient. In a few cases subscribers and patients are given more choices. But the established health insurance and social security systems are not cut or privatized, since no population would agree.

As social security grew, its financing of benefits soon became "pay-as-you-go." The first beneficiaries were paid for by the current taxpayers. Thereafter, all current payments were used to cover expenditures. An individual's payments did not go into a fund earmarked for his exclusive use. Only a small reserve was maintained. Social insurance systems collecting obligatory taxes from everyone can use pay-as-you-go financing, while private voluntary insurance must maintain individual earmarked accounts or establish a large reserve. Health insurance is inherently close to a full pay-as-you-go system: current income goes out quickly to cover current bills of members of the risk pool. Social insurance also uses pay-as-you-go for pensions, which might otherwise be based on lifetime savings reserved for the benefit of each individual.

Once a complete social security system has become a mature pay-as-you-go arrangement, it cannot be reorganized into a method of individual capitalized accounts. All those currently receiving pensions and other benefits would continue receiving them, and this would necessitate a continuation of payroll taxes on the economically active and their employers into pay-as-you-go accounts. New enrollees would have to pay a second set of payroll taxes and voluntary premiums to build up their own future individually earmarked entitlements in the capitalized system. As the rest of this book will show, modern economies now have difficulty paying for one set of payroll taxes, much less two. [24]

Even though social security systems—once they become completely financed according to social solidarity—cannot be unscrambled into systems of individual capitalized accounts, hybrid arrangements are possible. Several countries now have two-tier pension systems:

☐ *Basic pension:* statutory, obligatory, and universal coverage; payroll taxes on workers and employers; pensions only slightly related to earnings history and prior contributions; fixed rules for the payroll taxes and the benefits.

☐ *Supplementary pension:* financed by payments into an individual account; pension related to prior contributions and earnings history; may be negotiated by each individual with a carrier or negotiated collectively between a trade union and an employer; creation of a supplementary pension system within each industry may be voluntary or (as in France) required by law; its economic soundness may be regulated (as in the United States), but the terms are left to the participants.

The trend in social security may be toward two-tier arrangements in pensions and other sectors.[25] The same might be possible in health: a basic benefit package paid for by payroll taxes would cover everyone; other benefits would be assigned to a second package flexible in both details and financing; the two accounts would be kept separate.[26] Already in several countries, the upper-income groups covered by statutory health insurance voluntarily buy extra private policies for supplementary benefits.

Implications for the United States

Health care financing in all other developed countries is permeated by the philosophy of social solidarity, while such financing in the United States is permeated by conflicting philosophies and organizational instability. As a result, other developed countries have universal coverage, universal access, highly redistributive financing, and little cost sharing by the poor. The United States has a mosaic of categorical programs depending heavily on voluntary participation and appeal to self-interest. American arrangements cover and pay for many persons. But there remain gaps: incomplete coverage, barriers to access by some, different services for rich and poor, a confusing system of finance, and much out-of-pocket payment. By now it is obvious that—if full coverage and mainstream medicine are desired for all—the only solution is a comprehensive law explicitly recognizing the premise of social solidarity.

One can debate whether American public policy should be based on individual self-reliance or on social solidarity. America has always been different, the society of entrepreneurs and rebels, and its present health care financing could just as well continue. But Americans at least should be fully aware of how different they are, the ideological roots of the difference, and the price they pay in health services.[27] If they want universal access and mainstream benefits for all, they cannot achieve them with individualistic ideologies and practices. If they remain committed to individualism, self-reliance, and competition, the inevitable result will continue to be a diverse, unstable, and controversial health care system. Other developed countries have opted to retain individualism and competition in other economic sectors; health, however, is regarded as a different market.

At times, such as the 1930s and 1960s, it appears as if the United States will adopt the ideology and institutions of social solidarity and extend them to health care coverage and financing. But at other times, such as the 1920s and 1980s, the government-of-the-day preaches individual self-gratification, and the business interests with extra cash eliminate private redistributive arrangements. During the 1980s, for example, competition in the private insurance market has produced a trend from community rates to age-graduated rates barely able to cover actuarial costs. Large employers insist on premium rebate clauses in group insurance contracts or they self-insure, so the insurance companies cannot use any profits to cover deficits from poor risks; small employers resist offering any health insurance for their workers, let alone agreeing to pay community rates that yield the carriers extra cash. Both large and small employers self-finance any employee health care costs in large part to evade state premium taxes designed to finance pools for the uninsured.

The fundamental differences in ideology and practice between the United States and other developed countries are barriers to mutual appreciation. Many American policymakers and health administrators do not realize that they are exceptions to a worldwide trend and imagine that foreign health care finance resembles their own. Therefore, they are not interested in any lessons from abroad. Europeans, however, are well aware that American health care lacks social insurance and depends on private financing. European scholars and journalists often describe the incomplete access and coverage of the poor in the United States.[28] These shortcomings contribute to the decline of America's reputation. Americans may answer that they are always ready to enact special ("categorical") programs to provide sufficient care for the truly needy who cannot pay. But every European country—even those with capitalist economies and conservative governments—now assumes that health financing must be universal, standardized, and redistributive.

Notes

1. Insurance is a worldwide industry, and individual companies often enter other national markets. Basic conceptions of insurance, as well as fundamental actuarial methods, are universal. For example, compare the leading textbooks, such as Robert I. Mehr and Emerson Cammack, *Principles of Insurance*, 7th ed. (Homewood, Ill.: Irwin, 1980); Henri Loubergé, *Economie et finance d'assurance et de la réassurance* (Paris: Dalloz, 1981); and Dieter Farny and others (ed.), *Handbuch der Versicherung* (Karlsruhe: Verlag Versicherungswirtschaft, 1987). The world's insurance experts meet every few years to share new developments at the International Congress of Actuaries. While technical methods are identical, each country's social security system and insurance industry may use them in different ways, as this book will show. The similarity in methods and diversity in applications are evident in Hans Georg Timmer (ed.), *Technischen Methoden der privaten Krankenversicherung in Europa: Marktverhältnisse und Wesensmerk-*

male der Versicherungstechnik (Karlsruhe: Verlag Versicherungswirtschaft, 1990).

2. The criteria for insurability appear in many sources, such as Baruch Berliner, *Limits of Insurability of Risks* (Englewood Cliffs, N.J.: Prentice-Hall, 1982), and Willi Berghoff, "Untersuchungen über die Dynamik der Krankenversicherungsgrundlagen," *Mitteilungen der Vereinigung Schweizerischer Versicherungsmathematiker*, vol. 72, no. 2 (1972), pp. 5–35.

3. The difficulty in fitting health risks to the rigorous definition of insurability is summarized in Duncan R. MacIntyre, *Voluntary Health Insurance and Rate Making* (Ithaca: Cornell University Press, 1962), pp. 21–26; in A. Ceci, "Riesgo de enfermedad: contingencias a cubrirse mediante seguro o mediante asistencia," in International Social Security Association, *Les problèmes actuariels et statistiques de la Sécurité sociale* (Geneva: Editions Internationales, 1957), vol. 1, pp. 123–145; in Kenneth J. Arrow, "Uncertainty and the Welfare Economics of Medical Care," *American Economic Review*, vol. 53, no. 5 (Dec. 1963), pp. 961–967; and in the subsequent essays in *American Economic Review*, vol. 55, no. 1 (March 1965), pp. 140–158.

4. Mehr and Cammack, *Principles of Insurance* (see note 1, above), pp. 498–499.

5. See the analysis of pharmaceutical and dental insurance in R. G. Evans and M. F. Williamson, *Extending Canadian Health Insurance: Options for Pharmacare and Denticare* (Toronto: Ontario Economic Council and University of Toronto Press, 1978), pp. 47–53, 120–121, 219–220, 227–228.

6. William A. Glaser, *Paying the Hospital* (San Francisco: Jossey-Bass, 1987), pp. 63–65.

7. I. M. Rubinow, *Standards of Health Insurance* (New York: Henry Holt, 1916), chaps. 5 and 15, app. II; and George Rosen, "Contract or Lodge Practice and Its Influence on Medical Attitudes to Health Insurance," *American Journal of Public Health*, vol. 67, no. 4 (April 1977), pp. 374–378.

8. The ideological reasons why all developed countries have adopted social protection policies are summarized in Kenneth E. Boulding, *Principles of Economic Policy* (Englewood Cliffs, N.J.: Prentice-Hall, 1958), chap. 10. The evolution of the ideology of social solidarity and its effects on French public policy are traced in J.E.S. Hayward, "Solidarity: The Social History of an Idea in Nineteenth Century France," *International Review of Social History*, vol. IV, pt. 2 (1959), pp. 261–284.

9. For descriptions of the financial benefits and social services of the guilds, see Jean Bennet, *La Mutualité Française des origines à la Révolution de 1789* (Paris: Coopérative d'Information et d'Edition Mutualiste, 1981); George Clune, *The Medieval Gild System* (Dublin: Browne and Nolem, 1943); and Rudolf Wissell, *Des Alten Handwerks Recht und Gewohnheit* (Berlin: Verlag Ernst Wasmuth, 1929), vol. 1, pp. 400–411. I am also indebted to personal communications from Sylvia Thrupp.

10. Many histories of the modern mutual benefit funds have been pub-

lished, such as Jean Bennet, *La Mutualité Française à travers sept siècles d'histoire* (Paris: Coopérative d'Information et d'Edition Mutualiste, 1975); Rudolf Rezsohazy, *Histoire du mouvement mutualiste chrétien en Belgique* (Brussels: Aux Editions Erasme, 1957); and Horst Peters, *Die Geschichte der Sozialen Versicherung*, 3rd ed. (Sankt Augustin: Asgard Verlag, 1978).

11. Peter A. Köhler and Hans F. Zacher (eds.), *The Evolution of Social Insurance 1881-1981* (London: Frances Pinter, 1982); and Henri Hatzfeld, *Du paupérisme à la Sécurité sociale* (Paris: Librairie Armand Colin, 1971). In many countries—France, Holland, Great Britain, and others—wars were followed by great expansion of coverage and benefits. The wars were led by governments of national unity, which pledged such improvements if the workers fought for victory. See Richard M. Titmuss, *Essays on "The Welfare State"* (London: Allen & Unwin, 1958), chap. 4.

12. Thérèse Lecomte, *Evolution de la morbidité déclarée: France 1970-1980* (Paris: Centre de Recherche pour l'Etude et l'Observation des Conditions de Vie, 1983), chap. 5; Silvie LeRoux, *Les inégalités devant la santé* (Paris: La Documentation Française, 1985); Andrée Mizrahi and others, *Medical Care, Morbidity and Costs* (Oxford: Pergamon Press, 1983), pp. 88-91, 160-161; Andrée and Arié Mizrahi, *Evolution à long terme des disparités des dépenses médicales: France 1960-1970-1980* (Paris: Centre de Recherche d'Etude et de Documentation en Economie de la Santé, 1986), pp. 19-25, 62-70; and papers at a conference on social inequalities in health problems and services, conducted by the European Regional Office, World Health Organization, 1984.

13. The two Dutch markets are described in G. W. de Wit, *De financiering van ziektekostenverzekeringen* (Rotterdam: Nationale-Nederlanden, 1986).

14. Odin Anderson, *Blue Cross Since 1929: Accountability and the Public Trust* (Cambridge, Mass.: Ballinger, 1975).

15. The trend is still under way at present. It varies among the seventy-six Blue Cross/Blue Shield Plans and has not yet entirely duplicated the underwriting and rate-setting methods of the insurance companies. See *Health Insurance: Comparing Blue Cross and Blue Shield Plans with Commercial Insurers* (Washington: General Accounting Office, 1986); and *AIDS and Health Insurance* (Washington: Health Program, Office of Technology Assessment, 1988), pp. 11-30. The Blues deviated from pure community rating in the 1950s, when the commercial insurers first entered their group and nongroup markets, according to MacIntyre, *Voluntary Health Insurance and Rate-Making* (see note 3, above), chap. 7.

16. Edwin E. Witte, *The Development of the Social Security Act* (Madison: University of Wisconsin Press, 1963); and Martha Derthick, *Policymaking for Social Security* (Washington: Brookings Institution, 1970), especially pt. 2.

17. Martin Feldstein, *Hospital Costs and Health Insurance* (Cambridge: Harvard University Press, 1981), pt. 2; Mark V. Pauly (ed.), *National Health Insurance: What Now, What Later, What Never?* (Washington: American Enterprise Institute for Public Policy Research, 1980), pt. 3 and Rita Ricardo-

Campbell, *The Economics and Politics of Health* (Chapel Hill: University of North Carolina Press, 1982), passim, especially pp. 329–340.

18. For an overview of the industry during the tumultous 1980s, see *Health Insurance and the Uninsured: Background Data and Analysis* (Washington: Congressional Research Service, Library of Congress, 1988), chaps. 2, 4. Its poor financial performance is summarized in "Accident and Health Premiums," an annual report published every December in *Best's Review: Life/Health Insurance Edition*; and Paul J. Kenkel, "Losses Send Blues Scrambling,," *Modern Healthcare*, vol. 18, no. 27 (July 1, 1988), pp. 14–19.

19. Robert Stevens and Rosemary Stevens, *Welfare Medicine in America* (New York: Free Press, 1974); and Stephen M. Davidson, *Medicaid Decisions: A Systematic Analysis of the Cost Problem* (Cambridge, Mass.: Ballinger, 1980).

20. Zachary Dyckman and others, *Competitive Bidding for Health Services* (Baltimore: Office of Research and Demonstrations, Health Care Financing Administration, U.S. Department of Health and Human Services, 1986). Pages 12–16 describe the euphoric design and the scandal-ridden implementation of the Medicaid scheme in Arizona.

21. The design of FEHBP and its problems of adverse selection are described in William M. Mercer, Inc., *Review of the Federal Employees Health Benefits Program* (Washington: Government Printing Office, 1982), a report to the Committee on Post Office and Civil Service, House of Representatives, 97th Cong., 2nd Sess., Committee Print No. 97-8. The forces causing and counteracting a premium spiral are summarized in Michael Spence, "Product Differentiation and Performance in Insurance Markets," *Journal of Public Economics,* vol. 10 (Oct. 1978), pp. 427–447; and James A. Schuttinga and others, "Health Plan Selection in the Federal Employees Health Benefits Program," *Journal of Health Politics, Policy and Law,* vol. 10, no. 1 (Spring 1985), pp. 119–139. Spence predicts government intervention to stabilize any multiple-choice insurance market when adverse selection and premium spirals get out of control.

22. Jean-Pierre Dumont, *L'impact de la crise économique sur les systèmes de protection sociale* (Geneva: International Social Security Association, 1981); and Vladimir Rys, "Developments and Trends in Social Security 1984–1986: Report of the Secretary General," *International Social Security Review,* vol. 39, no. 4 (1986), pp. 375–460.

23. For two European critiques of statutory health insurance, see Jörg Finsinger and others, "Some Observations on Greater Competition in the German Health Insurance System from a U.S. Perspective," *Managerial and Decision Economics,* vol. 7, no. 3 (Sept. 1986), pp. 152–162; and Frans F. H. Rutten and Wynand P.M.M. van de Ven, "Concurrentie en ziektekostenverzekering," in J. H. Hagen (ed.), *Concurrentie in de Nederlandse gezondheidszorg* (Lochem: Uitgeversmaatschappij de Tijdstroom, 1985), pp. 54–91. For a British critique of a national health service, see Arthur Seldon, *The Litmus Papers* (London: Centre for Policy Studies, 1980). A British rebuttal is in A. J. Culyer, "The Withering

of the Welfare State? Whither the Welfare State?" (Vancouver: Department of Economics, University of British Columbia, 1986).

24. The impossibility of shifting to an individually capitalized system as a solution to France's chronic social security problems is explained in Commission des Comptes de la Sécurité Sociale, *Rapport de décembre 1985* (Paris: Ministère des Affaires Sociales et de la Solidarité Nationale, 1985), pp. 152–154.

25. For a good summary of France's intricate two-tier pension system, see Jean-François Chadelat and Gérard Pellissier, *Les retraites des Français* (Paris: La Documentation Française, 1986). Several two-tier arrangements are described in *Conjugating Public and Private: The Case of Pensions* (Geneva: International Social Security Association, 1987).

26. Such a two-tier health insurance system was recommended for Holland by the Commissie Structuur en Financiering Gezondheidszorg (W. Dekker and others), *Bereidheid tot verandering* (The Hague: Distributiecentrum Overheidspublikaties, 1987). A modified version—more benefits in the obligatory tier and fewer in the voluntary tier—will be implemented during the 1990s, according to *Werken aan zorgvernieuwing: Actieprogramma van het beleid voor de zorgsector in de jaren negentig* (Rijswijk: Ministerie van Welzijn, Volksgezondheid en Cultuur, 1988), Tweede Kamer, zitting 1989–90, 21,545, nos. 1–2, pp. 50–71.

27. Why the ideology and institutions of social solidarity became firmly rooted in continental Europe but not in the Anglo-Saxon countries (such as the United States) is explained in Douglas E. Ashford, "The British and French Social Security Systems: Welfare States by Intent and Default," in Douglas E. Ashford (ed.), *Nationalizing Social Security in Europe and America* (Greenwich, Conn.: JAI Press, 1986), pp. 245–270.

28. After living several years in the United States, a Belgian physician notes the absence of social solidarity in the financing and provision of American health services: Jean-Pierre De Landtsheer, "Organisation du système de santé aux Etats-Unis," *Les cahiers du GERM*, vol. 22, no. 200 (March 1987), pp. 45–47. For an insightful comparison of how Americans and Europeans define "poverty" and other "needs" as a prelude to designing their contrasting social policies, see Sweden's Walter Korpi, "Approaches to the Study of Poverty in the United States: Critical Notes from a European Perspective," in Vincent T. Covello (ed.), *Poverty and Public Policy* (Boston: G. K. Hall, 1980), pp. 287–314. When the Americans enact social benefit programs, according to an experienced British observer, they administer them in a less efficient and more grudging manner than the Europeans do: T. E. Chester, "America—A Reluctant Welfare State?" *National Westminster Bank Review*, Jan. 1971, pp. 32–47.

CHAPTER 3

Coverage and Access

──────────────────────── Summary ────────────────────────

Every European country has steadily expanded access, usually by successively adding new groups to obligatory health insurance. If some groups—usually elites—are not covered, they insure voluntarily. An important motive for universal coverage is social solidarity: the better-off pay into the sickness funds to cover the costs of heavier users. When expensive nonpayers are added, government often covers the deficits with subsidies.

Statutory health insurance began with the industrial workers who had participated in the private and voluntary stage. The new laws obliged membership by all workers in those categories throughout the country and required all workers and their employers to pay social security taxes. This policy established a firm organizational and financial basis. Other groups were added from time to time: white-collar workers, managers, and farmers. The self-employed were added, often over their opposition, resulting in compromises that limited their taxes and gave them special regimes.

The retired and unemployed were eventually kept in the mainstream social insurance program, thereby eliminating the need for charitable services run by government. Since the retired and unemployed can afford to pay their carriers less than their actuarial costs, the employed subscribers must pay more, thereby necessitating redistributive financing beyond traditional insurance calculations. Some countries have complicated organization and financing, since some occupations have the political leverage to limit their taxes.

A completely private voluntary insurance system leaves a substantial fraction of the population uncovered, as American experience demonstrates. Some of the poor must be helped by public welfare, a traditional method that disappears under universal statutory health insurance. In private voluntary systems, coverage declines during economic downtowns. Lack of coverage hinders access to primary care and harms the health of the poor.

Universal coverage with full benefits ensures prompt access for all. It improves health, particularly because of the prompt and widespread use of primary care. The system also guarantees generous financing for hospitals and doctors. Bad debts disappear.

Historical Development

Before the enactment of statutory health insurance by European national governments, each country had numerous private and public programs. Many occupations and social groups organized self-help societies: the most energetic craftsmen had guilds and mutual aid societies providing cash benefits, and they added health services during the nineteenth century; the most militant industrial workers (miners, railwaymen, metalworkers) organized unions, and the unions created sickness funds; to prevent the working class from falling entirely under socialist leadership, the Catholic Church organized rival unions and sickness funds. Some local governments and private reformers organized mutual aid societies for their inhabitants. Doctors in some countries (such as Holland) organized prepayment arrangements with lists of local residents.

Other arrangements existed simultaneously. For centuries, the very poor relied on churches and municipal welfare offices to provide free inpatient care and to pay for outpatient services. On the other hand, private insurance companies during the late nineteenth and twentieth centuries sold cash benefit policies to the rich and the self-employed.

The principal national laws mandating health insurance were enacted between 1883 and 1915, but a few countries (such as France and Holland) waited until later. The laws are constantly updated by amendments and regulations. In every country, the first national statute covers all blue-collar occupations that already had health insurance because of their own efforts, the help of employers, or the laws of local governments. Then other occupations are added in subsequent amendments by the national Parliament:

- [ ] White-collar workers
- [ ] Managers with higher incomes
- [ ] Farmers
- [ ] Farm workers
- [ ] Self-employed shopkeepers, craftsmen, and professionals
- [ ] Pensioners
- [ ] Unemployed

Most civil servants already have health benefits. In some countries, they keep their special programs; in others, they are added to the general regime.

During the twentieth century, several countries solved problems of incomplete coverage and inadequate financing by enacting full public funding of health care from general revenue and governmental management of hospitals—namely, Great Britain, Eastern Europe, Scandinavia, and (without government ownership) Canada. Every person automatically had full benefits by right, regardless of his employment and payment of taxes. Municipal welfare offices no longer paid for anyone's medical care.

During the 1950s and 1960s, the political Left and the Center in all other developed countries desired the same result. But the doctors, the voluntary associations that owned the hospitals, the sickness fund managers, the businessmen, and the political Right opposed "socialized medicine." The political compromise was to extend national health insurance to include everyone else—farmers, farm workers, the pensioners, and the unemployed—even if they could pay only very low payroll taxes or none at all. The rich and the self-employed also had to be added in order to bring more revenue into the sickness funds.

The universal obligatory health insurance outcomes of the 1970s and 1980s are conducted according to more pronounced methods of social solidarity than ever before. (Some details appear later in this book.) Employed persons and their employers pay steadily higher payroll taxes, resulting from increases in the rates and increases in the income ceilings. Their payments far exceed their utilization. Growing numbers of elderly and disabled generate a large fraction of the sickness funds' expenditures, but they contribute very little. Some sickness funds have such unfavorable dependency ratios that government subsidizes them or transfers money from social security regimes with extra cash (such as family allowances). No country's national health insurance law enables anyone in the obligatory categories to opt out: the departing persons would be the better-paid and healthier young, and their loss would accentuate the financial imbalance in the sickness funds.

Coverage at Present

Table 3.1 shows the approximate proportions of the population covered for basic acute-care health insurance in the five principal countries of my field research around 1987. Formerly, several occupational groups had the option of joining the statutory sickness funds voluntarily. The self-employed, professionals, and white-collar workers, for example, could choose between the statutory carriers and private insurance companies. Many picked the sickness funds because—as a result of public subsidies or other advantages—these carriers' rates were lower or their benefits were higher than those of the private health insurance arrangements. The recent trend is to eliminate the option: nearly entire populations are obligatorily enrolled in sickness funds. In those countries where compulsory coverage is not yet universal, the voluntary premiums for the sickness funds are now so high and the private carriers have become so active that the voluntarily insured select the private companies.

Table 3.1. Extent and Forms of Insurance Coverage in Western Europe.

Basic coverage	France	West Germany	Holland	Belgium	Switz-erland
Sickness funds					
Obligatory by law	98 %	77 %	51 %	98 %	25 %
Voluntary	—	12	19	1	71
Private insurance companies	1.5	9	30	1	2
Not insured	0.5	2	0.1	0+	2
	100 %	100 %	100 %	100 %	100 %
(Total population in millions)	(53)	(61)	(14)	(10)	(6.4)

Source: Data extracted from statistical reports listed in Appendix A.

Until 1986, some 20 percent of the members of Dutch sickness funds were voluntary, but a law temporarily changed the rules: thereafter everyone under a certain income was assigned to sickness funds; everyone over the ceiling had to use private carriers; the private companies had to keep their pensioners and could no longer force them to seek "voluntary" enrollment in the sickness funds. The new system implemented after 1990 eliminated voluntary choice of coverage: all upper-income persons would have to sign up for a minimum package—although, like everyone else now, they would still have free choice of private carriers.[1]

Considerable numbers of persons in each country buy supplementary insurance either from their sickness funds or from private carriers. The largest market is in France: perhaps as much as 70 percent of the population now belongs to the nonprofit *mutuelles,* partly because these carriers appeal to the ideology of social solidarity and partly because they cover the obligatory cost sharing under the main health insurance. The precise number of extra policies is not accurately recorded in Europe, since carriers are legally obligated to report only enrollment in the statutory health insurance. In the growing and competitive markets for supplementary health insurance, many companies guard their sales figures.

In basic coverage, every subscriber and (usually) all his immediate dependents have identical benefits. Before the enactment of obligatory coverage, the sickness funds usually provided invalidity and medical coverage only for the workers. The wife and children were covered only if the sickness fund had extra cash (usually only if the worker paid extra premiums). During the first decades of statutory health insurance, this pattern continued.[2] Eventually the payroll taxes rose in order to cover the entire family. Today the original arrangement survives only in Switzerland.

If some occupations have special regimes, they might lack certain benefits. For example, in some countries the self-employed do not receive invalidity payments from their special sickness funds, but they do receive all other benefits.

More often the variations refer to cost sharing between patients and carriers; the patients have the standard benefits from their special sickness fund but must pay more or less out-of-pocket than the majority of persons under the general regime.

The Politics of Expansion

When statutory health insurance is first enacted, it is confined to the "natural" constituency that first organized it voluntarily and seeks legislation and tax collection to strengthen it—namely, the blue-collar workers. The trade unions dominate the social insurance funds and the legislative politics, even when the employers come to pay most of the payroll taxes and even when governing boards become *paritaire* (equal representation from trade unions and employers).

From the start, the few white-collar employees in each workplace with sickness funds were automatically included. Not until the mid-twentieth century did the white-collar workers become a large share of the labor force and acquire their own lifestyles. But in most countries, they have been frozen into the basic sickness funds. The last exception is Germany, where such workers over an earnings ceiling can switch to other carriers, thereby worsening the finances of the basic sickness funds.

After the blue-collar and white-collar workers were covered in the original design of national health insurance, adding further occupations created political controversies and financial difficulties. These were fought over at various times after World War II. Following were the principal sectors.

Farmers and Farm Workers. These groups previously had very little private health insurance or protection against work accidents. Since they had little purchasing power, few doctors practiced in rural areas and the hospitals were primitive. When farmers and farm workers were hospitalized, the social welfare offices of the communes had to bear much of the cost. The rural population had lower utilization and worse health than the city-dwellers.

Statutory and obligatory health insurance had long been in place to solve the access and financing problems for the urban workers. But the farmers and farm workers did not fit the social insurance model so easily:

☐   Their incomes were lower. The yield from payroll taxes could not cover the medical costs that had been inflated by decades of urban pricing, technological advance, and medical wage increases.

☐   The self-employed farmers claimed that their incomes were too low to cover their own costs, let alone a share of payroll taxes for the farm workers.

☐   The self-employed farmers customarily concealed their incomes from tax collectors.

☐   The rural population had worse health and potentially higher costs than the city-dwellers.

☐ If a statutory health insurance system had cost sharing (as in France), the farmers and farm workers said they could not afford it.

The agricultural interest groups generally fought inclusion in the general regime, since it would impose on them full payroll taxes, standard benefits, and full cost sharing by patients. In some countries, the political struggle over the program delayed its resolution for many years. (Germany, for example, did not enact statutory health insurance for the complete farming sector until 1972, nearly a century after the law for the workers.)[3] The concessions to the farmer and farm workers include:

☐ In some countries (such as France and Germany) a special regime governed primarily by representatives from agricultural interest groups and monitored by the Ministry of Agriculture.
☐ Lower premiums than in the general regime.
☐ Lower cost sharing by patients than in the general regime.
☐ Subsidies by the national government to cover the excess costs of the retired and the farm workers. Help for the retired farmers and miners are the only government subsidies provided in the otherwise completely self-financed insurance system of Germany.

These concessions are part of the series of income supports, tax concessions, subsidies, and beneficial regulations granted by European governments to their politically powerful farmers.

Self-Employed. Small businessmen, craftsmen, and self-employed professionals bought private pensions, private health insurance, and private property insurance long before World War II. A substantial share of the private insurance industry depended on this business.

Just after World War II, several governments sought to enact a universal social security system based on social solidarity and highly redistributive financing. Since the self-employed were richer than the rest of the population, their financial contributions were indispensable. Great Britain's National Health Service (NHS) automatically included the self-employed without singling them out and without arousing them to resist the entire enterprise: the self-employed and everyone else paid progressive income taxes into the general Treasury, rather than new taxes earmarked for the NHS alone; the Ministry of Health got a share of the total expenditure budget; and the self-employed were eligible for the standard benefits.

But when the French social security planning commission in 1945 proposed that the self-employed be included in the new general regime, the self-employed resisted. Politically conservative and personally individualistic, they opposed the ideology of social solidarity. As high earners of income and low users of health services, they did not wish to see their money diverted to benefit the workers and the poor. They wanted to keep personal earnings-related pensions. In health, they wanted to keep the option of sliding premium scales that allowed them to choose cheaper policies with higher cost sharing.

Chapter Four describes how the self-employed in France were able to keep a separate regime with a different structure of pensions and health insurance.[4] A few other countries have special regimes too. Another arrangement is Belgium's: the self-employed have a different package of payroll taxes and benefits, but they can join any of the regular sickness funds. Therefore, every Belgian *mutualité* must keep two accounts: one for its self-employed members, one for everyone else. One reason for all these concessions has been the political leverage of the self-employed with conservative political parties: the ground rules for the inclusion of the self-employed must be enacted by a (usually coalition) Cabinet and by Parliament. Another reason has been the need to persuade the self-employed to cooperate: if the premiums are too high, they will understate their incomes, harming tax collections in general revenue as well as in social security.[5]

The special arrangements for the self-employed include the following elements:

☐ If there is a separate management or a completely independent fund, the governing council is drawn from representatives of interest groups of the self-employed and none from trade unions.

☐ If the payroll tax (premium) rate is a proportion of income, it is less than the total collected from both worker and employer in the regime for the employed.

☐ The arrangement for the self-employed has an income ceiling upon which the tax rate is levied, but the general regime has no ceiling or a higher one.

☐ The arrangement for the self-employed may have an income floor: persons earning less are exempt. But the general regime applies to all low-income workers.

☐ The person has free choice of carrier. *Mutualités* and private health insurance companies are able to prosper.

The foregoing are the exceptional rules when the self-employed are required to accept coverage under statutory health insurance. In addition, there are some qualifications to obligatory coverage:

☐ *By income level.* Only the lowest-income self-employed are required to join in Germany. Most can insure voluntarily or self-insure, exactly as they have done for a century. They can choose among the basic sickness funds (*Krankenkassen*), the elite sickness funds (*Ersatzkassen*), and private insurance companies. Much of the competition among carriers in the health insurance market is over the self-employed. (Holland had such a voluntary and competitive market for upper-income persons until the 1990s.)

☐ *By benefits.* The Belgian self-employed are required to insure only for "heavy risks," that is, inpatient hospitalization and high specialist bills. Their compulsory premiums are designed only to cover these risks. They can buy voluntary insurance for the "lighter risks," and nearly all are persuaded by their *mutualités* to buy this coverage.

The self-employed's successful resistance to social solidarity has created structural and financial problems for the larger systems of health insurance and social security in Europe. Every social security and statutory health insurance system is complicated and difficult to understand, in large part because of the special arrangements for the self-employed. Since the lower premium rates and the lower income ceiling eliminate any overpayments beyond the self-employed's costs, no extra cash is available to help the less affluent. Some critics argue that the self-employed, therefore, have been relieved of the fiscal contribution to social security expected from higher-income groups.[6]

Retired. Originally, sickness funds protected only the workers who were contributing premiums. Within each country and across different countries, sickness funds varied in coverage of their retired and permanently disabled members. In the spirit of social solidarity, some funds continued to cover their retirees, for low or no premiums, provided that these persons had been full subscribers for many years. Many funds could not afford retirees' high costs, however, so they confined coverage to the active workers and their dependents, and the retirees had to depend on the social welfare offices of the communes. When the retirees were hospitalized, the public hospital recovered very little in fees and had to depend on operating subsidies from government. The retirees had to pass a means test for public assistance.[7]

After World War II—in Germany, as early as 1941—all countries added retirees to statutory health insurance. The legislative dates and the financial mechanisms varied. Some countries (such as Germany and Holland) enacted special programs and procedures for the aged.[8] Others (such as France) merely provided that the pensioners remain covered, either under the general regime or under their previous sickness funds. Subsidies from the national government's tax-supported Treasury became common, since the retirees were not covered by employer-paid payroll taxes and their costs were high. In a few countries (such as France, Germany, and Holland) regular procedures were established for transfers or money from sickness funds with extra cash to funds with many pensioners. In a few countries (such as Germany and Switzerland), the pension funds paid health insurance premiums on behalf of the pensioners. After many years of low or no premiums, the elderly during the late 1970s and 1980s were required to pay premiums deducted from their pension checks.

The elderly retain statutory health insurance but are no longer covered by any other social security program. Since they are retired, they no longer need unemployment, work-accident, or disability insurance. They no longer pay into the pension program but instead take money out. Coverage of the elderly has produced great administrative complications and financial burdens for statutory health insurance in every country. The details are analyzed in later chapters of this book.

Poor and Unemployed. The social welfare offices of communes and churches provided cash, housing services, and health services for centuries in both cities and rural areas. National and regional governments helped the local governments with cash. These programs were substantial until the elderly were added to statutory health insurance. Some retirees are still helped today if their pensions are too low to cover the premiums and cost sharing.

Mere poverty does not automatically necessitate medical help from the welfare office. Earners of very low incomes are nearly always covered by statutory health insurance and are entitled to full benefits equal to those of the highest earners. (The welfare office is called upon for income supplements, no longer payments to health providers.) The persons lacking health insurance coverage are the completely unemployed. After statutory health insurance was extended to all workers and farmers, there seemed to be no more problem, since unemployment rates in postwar Europe were very low. Unexpectedly, the economy of every country declined during the late 1970s, unemployment increased, and millions of people in each country were no longer covered. They no longer had employers to contribute payroll taxes, and they lacked the cash for voluntary premiums.

Coverage was already in place in Germany and Holland, where the obligatory health insurance laws for some time had continued to cover those persons who had lost covered jobs. The assumption was that unemployment was temporary. A variety of methods helped the sickness funds keep these members without full payroll taxes. France and Holland subsidized the sickness funds as the recession deepened and the financial burden to the carriers worsened. A few countries collected premiums from the agency that administered unemployment insurance. A few began to collect premiums from the unemployed themselves.

By now the elderly, the unemployed, and the poor are covered by statutory health insurance by a variety of government subsidies and personal premiums. The welfare programs of the communes have saved money and diminished in size. Now they pay for the cost sharing by the very poor and pay for home health services for the elderly and disabled.[9]

Voluntary Choice of Insurance

The trend has been toward universal coverage through statutory health insurance or a national health service. This approach fulfills several goals, such as implementing social solidarity, protecting the nation's "human capital," and providing generous financing for providers. During the late 1970s in the United States and more recently in Europe—as reported in Chapter Two—devotees of free markets criticized all insurance arrangements other than direct purchase by subscribers. The buyer would then determine his preferred tradeoff between premium and coverage. He might even decide to assume the risk entirely and buy other goods and services. The insurance and health industries would become more competitive, more cost-conscious, and more efficient.

Practice. Very few countries still have a substantial voluntary market where citizens might behave in the foregoing manner. Real people in all countries appear extremely "risk-averse" in health. Since most people are fully covered by statutory health insurance, almost everyone else buys the same thing voluntarily. In fact, the rich—who are lower users—insure themselves even more than the rest of the population by buying supplementary policies for extra benefits.

Most of the Swiss population can save premiums by self-insuring, but almost no one does. However, the Swiss cannot choose among variable packages of benefits and premiums: the national law provides subsidies for any sickness fund offering a basic benefit package and requiring a certain level of cost sharing; every carrier offers that standard policy; and almost no one selects the option of self-insurance.

The Netherlands once was the only country where a more calculating Economic Man might have been found in health insurance. Until the 1990s, the upper classes were never covered by statutory health insurance. They made each other calculation-wise by discussing coverage and premiums among themselves on social occasions. The insurance industry taught them to calculate risks and premiums by publicizing many arrangements. None of the voluntarily insured could depend on the standard packages and standard premiums of the statutory sickness funds, since they had to buy in the private market. Therefore, many Dutch delighted in buying—and often revising—policies with higher deductibles and lower premiums. But this was the limit of their choice. Almost nobody in Holland abstained from buying some form of health insurance; almost nobody self-insured completely.

Self-centered insurance, as Chapter Two explained, contradicts the redistributive practices of social solidarity. If the rich buy only the insurance to cover their own risks, their surplus cash cannot be used to pay for the poor, the elderly, and the sick. If the bulk of the population and the rich buy from different carriers in two separate markets, the social insurance market will face deficits while the private market will be profitable. To remedy this imbalance temporarily, Holland equalized by means of the interfund transfers described in Chapter Nine. To prevent its recurrence permanently, Holland universalized statutory health insurance and its financing by payroll taxes during the 1990s.

Sliding Scales. In a few countries, one hears serious proposals to vary the premiums and cost sharing in statutory health insurance. Subscribers could opt for lower premiums in return for a higher deductible. The method is spreading in Swiss supplementary insurance for extra benefits, and some recommend that Swiss law allow such options in statutory insurance. The change would not reduce or eliminate entitlement to the basic benefits but would merely make the coinsurance rates a free consumer/carrier agreement, rather than a standard clause in the government's law. No one would lose access under insurance by opting to pay no premiums, since most Swiss are free to make their choice now, and almost none do.

On the other hand, the Dutch private market long offered this option, and many persons took it. Anyone could pay lower premiums by forgoing coverage for general practice. But this step did not reduce access, since the subscribers had enough cash to pay for general practice out-of-pocket. In fact, some subscribers profited from the option: if their employers gave cash allowances for purchase of health insurance, the employees could pocket the savings. In 1983, 28 percent of the privately insured had no coverage for general practice and 42 percent had partial coverage.[10] This option may be offered to all the Dutch under universal statutory health insurance during the 1990s, but it may be feasible only for the supplementary package and its variable premiums. In no country do the payroll taxes earmarked for social insurance allow for sliding scales or rebates; rather, they are the mechanisms for redistributive financing.

Coverage in America's Private Market

The United States retains the mixture of diverse private arrangements that once characterized every developed country. A European health insurance law establishes full coverage for a social class and expands it subsequently to other social classes. The law guarantees full and standardized benefits for each class and sets adequate financing. Since Medicare was enacted by the national government, the United States has provided such general coverage and standardized benefits only for persons over the age of sixty-five. Consequently no other social group has ever been fully protected, and accurate statistical estimates of coverage have rarely been possible. Even when many persons have been insured—during certain periods since World War II, for example—their benefits have been diverse and changeable. Once a national health insurance law has been enacted, no one in the covered categories can lose protection, but America occasionally has experienced reductions in coverage.[11]

The American system—like any predominantly private voluntary method—has always left a substantial fraction of the population without any coverage at all, let alone incomplete coverage. In 1959, at least 28 percent of the civilian population had no coverage of any sort and 6 percent in addition had only hospital coverage.[12] The high-water mark of coverage should have been reached around 1977; the economy was prosperous, employers were still offering generous plans to workers and dependents, individuals could afford individual policies, Medicare covered everyone over sixty-five, and Medicaid covered many of the indigent. Nevertheless, 12.3 percent of the entire population and 13.7 percent of those younger than sixty-five had no third-party coverage of any sort—not even Medicaid. The distribution by age and other characteristics appears in Table 3.2.

Table 3.2. Percentage of American Population Without Insurance Coverage.

Population groups	1977	1987
Total	18.3	20.8
Age		
Less than 6	27.0	30.2
6–17	22.2	
6–18		25.9
18–24	28.6	
19–24		35.7
25–54	16.7	19.4
55–64	14.0	16.3
65+	0.1	1.3
Sex		
Male	17.8	20.8
Female	18.7	20.6
Race		
White	13.7	14.8
Black	36.2	39.2
Hispanic	38.0	46.1

Sources: Unpublished and corrected data from the National Center for Health Services Research. Preliminary reports are Judith A. Kasper and others, "Who Are the Uninsured?" (Washington: National Center for Health Services Research, 1980), and Pamela Farley Short and others, "A Profile of Uninsured Americans" (Washington: National Center for Health Services and Research, 1989).

I include persons relying on Medicaid in the table's figures, since Medicaid is public assistance and not genuine insurance.[13]

The economic recession and cost containment of the 1980s are widely thought to have reduced American health insurance coverage suddenly and drastically. Fewer companies were said to offer group plans. Workers and dependents were expected to contribute premiums and therefore could withdraw from coverage. Part-time and temporary employment without fringe benefits grew. The facts—summarized in Table 3.2—show that the proportion of uninsured rose, particularly among young men, children, and nonwhites. A voluminous literature and public debate suddenly discovered the "problems of the uninsured," implying that the successful American system had unexpectedly and greatly deteriorated. But the clamor was misleading: American methods have always fallen far short of complete coverage. Some of the apparent deterioration of coverage was due to the higher birth rates of minority groups that had never been covered, and some was due not to the insurance system itself but to cutbacks in Medicaid. (Among persons younger than sixty-five, 6.7 percent were on Medicaid in 1977 and 5.9 percent in 1987.)

The starting point for coverage in America is employer group contracts, but not all workers and their dependents are covered today. The lower the social status of the industry, the lower the worker's income, the fewer the hours of work, and the smaller his employer, the less likely the worker and his family are to have any insurance coverage. (Since the family has a breadwinner—however badly paid—it is not eligible for Medicaid.) Table 3.3 shows coverage rates for the employed in 1987 and their dependents. The unemployed—an additional source of low coverage—are not included in these figures.

Curing the problem of the uninsured would require changing the system. One reform would be universal statutory health insurance like the methods described in this book. Another remedy would be a categorical program funded by general revenue, such as expansion of Medicaid to cover all the uninsured. But public assistance is unlikely: after its first years, Medicaid has been frequently cut back. A few meaningless reforms were enacted, such as a requirement that em-

Table 3.3. Health Insurance Coverage of Workers and Their Families in 1987.

Characteristics of principal employed adult in household	Percentage with employer group coverage	Percentage uninsured
Status		
Full-time worker	81.9	12.7
Part-time worker	59.7	24.1
Self-employed	54.7	22.9
Industry		
Mining	86.9	10.0
Manufacturing	85.9	10.3
Transportation, communications	85.4	10.4
Financial service, insurance	84.3	8.3
Professional service	80.3	10.5
Public administration, military	77.2	7.1
Sales	68.3	21.4
Repair service	66.8	21.6
Entertainment	60.6	30.2
Construction	60.6	30.6
Personal service	52.5	31.5
Agriculture, forestry, fishery	40.7	29.6
Number of employees in firm		
More than 500	89.4	6.1
101 to 500	88.3	7.1
26 to 100	82.4	12.3
10 to 25	74.0	17.8
Less than 10	56.5	26.3
Hourly wage of worker		
Over $15.00	91.3	5.1
$10.01–$15.00	90.3	6.6
$5.01–$10.00	78.5	14.6
$3.51–$5.00	56.3	30.4
$3.50 or less	53.9	30.1

Note: I have omitted from each line the percentage who bought some sort of individual or family policy.

Source: Data extracted from Pamela Farley Short and others, "A Profile of Uninsured Americans" (Washington: National Center for Health Services Research, 1989).

ployers keep discharged workers in their groups upon payment of actuarial premiums. A few states created pools to pay hospitals' bad debts, where the revenue for the pools came from taxes on hospital bills or health insurance premiums; the taxes were passed on to the remaining insurance subscribers, thereby giving employees and individuals incentives to abandon their coverage.

The Bush administration's only proposal to date has been voluntary enrollment in Medicaid by the uninsured upon payment of premiums. Instead of enacting an effective remedy, the national and state governments published numerous and repetitious monographs describing the magnitude and causes of lack of coverage, study commissions enumerated all the policy options, legislative committees held hearings, economists and policy analysts obtained research grants and published reports.[14] But—since any significant reform would require national government leadership, coherent decisions, and new public spending—virtually nothing has been done.

Effects on Utilization and Health

What difference does it make? If people have no health insurance coverage, do they use health services less often or in different ways? Does lower access or different forms of utilization affect the health of all the uninsured or that of particular persons?

Does medical care improve health? Clearly the expansion of statutory health insurance in coverage and benefits has greatly expanded and improved the services of hospitals and physicians and has greatly increased their use by the public. Even though some skeptics argue that public health has accomplished much more than clinical care, the services have improved everybody's health.[15]

The United States is the only developed country now that can demonstrate the effects of an extensive lack of insurance coverage. In every other developed country, coverage is universal (Table 3.1), access is therefore universal, and any differentials in use within the country are due to administrative variations among the carriers and benefit packages. (The variations and their results will be discussed later in this book.) Current comparisons between countries with statutory health insurance and the United States show higher utilization abroad. Initial and (particularly) repeat visits to office doctors are more common in Germany than in the United States, for example, because statutory health insurance has long guaranteed access, patients need not share costs at the point of service, and German doctors have developed a corresponding style of practice.[16]

Utilization and Morbidity. In most developed countries, the substantial expansion of statutory coverage occurred long ago. In only a few cases can the results be measured historically—namely, where a major sector has been added during the era of full statistical reporting. This evidence shows that introduction of widespread coverage increases utilization, directs money into the geographical area and social sector, improves the supply of providers, and narrows the gaps in morbidity. A documented example is the introducton and expansion of health insurance in agriculture in France.[17]

When the United States had limited insurance coverage years ago, utilization of services was low. As coverage expanded across the population, use of health services steadily increased.[18] Enactment of the national government's one statutory scheme (Medicare) in 1965 provided complete and generous coverage to an entire social category (persons sixty-five and over) in place of the limited private enrollments with thinner benefits. Very quickly, utilization broadened: more of the elderly were hospitalized, their care was more technically advanced and more expensive, their stays were longer, physician inpatient care increased, office visits with doctors replaced home visits, and patients paid less out-of-pocket. Utilization increased most noticeably among the least advantaged categories with the lowest rates of private coverage, that is, those over seventy-five and the blacks.[19] Since the national government's actuaries had not realized the magnitude and severity of the unexpressed demand when this population lacked any health insurance, they greatly underestimated the increase in utilization, service intensity, and costs during the first years of Medicare.[20]

For every American group under the age of sixty-five, one can compare the insured and uninsured today. In every social category, the uninsured use health services less than the insured. The reason is not voluntary adverse selection of insurance: within each self-reported health status, the uninsured use fewer services. Lower utilization is most pronounced among the poor and among minority groups. Office visits to doctors are particularly likely to suffer among the uninsured; when they seek help, many substitute visits to hospital emergency rooms— at higher costs to the system.[21] (Even if uninsured persons have Medicaid, their office visits to doctors do not become "normal" in number, since most physicians refuse to accept them.)[22]

Important clinical effects result. If someone has been uninsured or on Medicaid for a long time, he is unlikely to have a primary care physician. The poor and nonwhite without insurance are particularly unlikely to have a regular doctor. The poor and nonwhite have a number of problems that call for special attention, such as adolescent pregnancy, substance abuse and poor nutrition by young unmarried mothers, premature births, and low-birthweight babies. The United States has more premature births and more disabling illness among neonates than any other developed country. Recent research shows that premature births and neonatal illnesses are particularly high among the uninsured and Medicaid enrollees. The mothers did not receive regular prenatal care because they did not have the mainstream health insurance essential for acceptance by a primary care doctor.[23]

The flurry of publications about prenatal and neonatal health problems of the uninsured implied that the defect in American health care finance was new. But like the gaps in American coverage, it was an old and chronic fact that had never been recognized. For decades, Americans had been aware that infant mortality was higher in the United States than in other developed countries,[24] and they had searched fruitlessly for explanations.[25] The reasons then were the same as now: the uninsured did not have primary care, and primary care was essential for perinatal health. Modern hospital technology had merely changed the problem—it reduced infant mortality and unintentionally generated growing problems of neonatal disability—but the absence of insurance coverage for prenatal care remained the same.

Lack of insurance coverage results in lower access and use of primary care for adults as well, particularly among the poor and minority groups. But these classes have higher-than-average health needs. The only exception to their pattern of lower utilization is visits to the hospital emergency room: since the uninsured adults do not have family doctors, they use emergency rooms more often than the insured do.[26]

A universal and egalitarian financing method opens access but does not automatically equalize utilization. In some countries, the upper classes navigate the system more successfully than the lower classes do, and the former have higher per capita costs. In other countries, the lower classes—with the help of their newly acquired and fully reimbursed family doctor—become higher users. But utilization never correlates simply with social class, since the self-employed are usually lower users, whether their health insurance is private or statutory.[27]

Effects on Services. Health insurance pays providers. As coverage expands, every country has widened its market and increased its spending for hospitals, doctors, drugs, and other covered services. A perfect correlation does not exist between the rise in spending and the spread of coverage, because other forces also govern cost increases. Coverage by European statutory health insurance expanded most between the end of World War II and 1970, for example, but costs rose fastest during the 1970s.[28] Health care wages and service intensity—two principal determinants of aggregate health costs—rose faster after 1970 than before.

One might expect the adoption of statutory health insurance to reshape services, but the relationship is never so simple, since many other variables operate. For example, one might expect more doctors to practice in rural areas: private insurance was thin there, and the new statutory insurance guarantees full fees for treating the residents. Therefore, one might expect a wider geographical distribution of doctors in countries with statutory health insurance than in the United States. But such hypotheses exaggerate the pecuniary motives of doctors. Physicians—particularly specialists—gravitate to the cities in all countries in large part because of lifestyle choices, the availability of clinical facilities, and opportunities for a more interesting practice.[29] Even if insurance is thinner in rural areas and small towns, American doctors—like those in Europe—can earn very high incomes there. While rural doctors earn lower gross incomes than urban doctors in the United States, their practice costs are lower, their net incomes approach those of urban doctors, their living costs are lower, and therefore they rank as top earners in their communities.[30]

If a health insurance system—whether private or statutory—covers certain

social classes and not others, the services used by the former will be developed
more than those used by the latter, or the two sets of services will develop in
different styles. Between 1911 and 1948, for example, Great Britain had a statutory
National Health Insurance that covered only general practice for the working
class. Specialists were paid by out-of-pockets assisted by private health insurance,
and the clientele was middle and upper class. As a result, specialty care and the
nonprofit hospitals were underfunded and clustered in the cities with patients
capable of paying, such as London and Liverpool. National Health Insurance
was not merely expanded but was replaced by the National Health Service because the postwar Labour Government thought that only government management and Treasury financing could expand the hospitals and specialty services
and could spread them extensively across the country.[31]

In like manner, the structure of coverage is one of several reasons for the
universal division between general practice and specialization in the American
medical profession. Employer group coverage began as an alliance with Blue
Cross, a prepayment system for the American hospital industry. Group contracts
added Blue Shield but—like the private medical care insurance bought by the
middle class—it started by paying only for technical procedures performed in
hospitals. Ambulatory care by internists and general practitioners (GPs) was
added only after several decades. By then, the American medical profession had
responded to the financing signals—and to other causes—by specializing in large
numbers. The American medical profession might have become reoriented toward primary care if American health insurance had suddenly become universal
and covered at full fees the population most needing primary care: the poor, the
low-paid workers, and minority groups. But that has never happened. Medicaid
has unintentionally reinforced the hospital-centered and technical orientation of
American health care financing by failing to create a primary care market and
subsidizing self-referrals to the hospital.

In contrast, European health insurance began with primary care, now
covers it generally for entire populations, and added hospital coverage only at
later stages. In every European country with statutory health insurance, general
practitioners are at least half the medical profession, whereas GPs and "specialists
in family medicine" together are fewer than one-sixth of all American doctors.[32]

Implications for the United States

Universal Obligatory Coverage. Every developed country takes universal
coverage for granted, primarily through obligatory health insurance but also
through voluntary coverage by the nonobligatory minority. Whether under obligatory or voluntary arrangements, everyone has access and the ancient issues of
means tests and finding cash have been forgotten. The United States is the only
developed country where the problem of finding a reimbursement system for
someone still exists.

The speculation by economists about operating insurance markets through tradeoffs between prices and coverage is rarely observed in practice. Populations want universal and thorough coverage, providers want guaranteed payment, and government's laws help them. Voluntary markets usually result in equally generous coverage, with only healthy and prosperous people—as in the now defunct Dutch private market—consciously selecting cheaper policies and fewer benefits. This should be no surprise to Americans, since whenever research about insurance moves from the classroom blackboard to the real world, whenever one studies American consumers with the intelligence and cash to make rational choices, the results are overinsurance and adverse selection of the more thorough coverage.[33]

Universal coverage—whether under statutory health insurance or a national health service—eliminates all eligibility questions. Providers know that every inhabitant is covered: the only administrative issue is which carrier should get the bill. Even when not everyone is obligatorily insured, providers know that the uncovered can pay (since they are the wealthier) and have voluntary insurance. This situation avoids all the American administrative complexities of establishing which third parties (sometimes several) cover each patient and finding the money (usually through belated cost shifting) to cover the bad debts.

Understanding One's Own Coverage. Because American health insurance lacks standard rules and is fluid, few Americans understand the details of their benefits, aside from the simple fact of some sort of third-party coverage.[34] Some patients receive denials or partial reimbursements, while others have better luck. Only the carrier's computer keeps track of each individual's entitlements. Insurance rules are often manipulated to improve prospects of reimbursement—for example, many American contracts refuse to cover preventive services, so doctors insert false acute diagnoses to help patients get paid.[35] In order to generalize about the benefits for the American population's numerous group and individual contracts, a vast interview survey of the population is necessary, but the resulting report is likely to be so intricate as to be incomprehensible.[36] Uncertainty about benefits is as much a problem as lack of any coverage.

In contrast, a national health insurance law not only makes clear who is covered but also enables each person to know in advance his benefits and cost-sharing obligations. Even when some occupations have different rules and regimes, the variations are limited and everyone in each broad occupational category shares the same entitlements. The rules remain stable and comprehensible.

Special Regimes and Special Groups. If the United States ever enacts universal statutory health insurance, Americans should not expect the result to be a simple structure with standardized treatment of everyone. If they wish to achieve "equity" in benefits and financial contributions, policymakers must devote extra effort to defining these goals and enacting the legislation. In practice, every law—including statutory health insurance—is the outcome of legislative logrolling whereby influential interest groups try to limit their obligations and increase their benefits. Since every member is an independent political entrepreneur, Congress is vulnerable to such pressures; but as the closed rule in the initial House passage of the Medicare Catastrophic Coverage Act during 1987 showed, it is possible for a determined leadership to plan and pass simple legislation. The leadership must be forewarned and resolute, however, and the country must be sold on the unfamiliar (to Americans) ideas of equal benefits and social solidarity.

The self-employed are a nemesis in social security policy, and they are proving difficult in America as well as in Europe. But they fight over a different issue. European social security and health insurance expanded coverage by occupation; all employees of small business were covered; and the small urban employers could not block their obligations to pay normal payroll taxes for their workers. Their resistance came when policymakers wanted to cover the self-employed themselves at tax levels that would produce surpluses to cover the bad risks in other occupations.

In contrast, the Americans extended Social Security pension and related schemes to small business peacefully, with the self-employed eventually paying full payroll taxes for themselves as well as for their workers. An impasse arises now because most American proposals for statutory health insurance try to mandate employer-paid group insurance for all firms. The small businessmen do not wish to pay for their workers;[37] they use their considerable political leverage to block enactment of this form of universal coverage; the proponents try to salvage their bills by exempting all the very small firms. This sequence cannot occur in Europe, where entire occupations are covered by simply mandating that individuals join sickness funds, and their employers are required to do no more than pay normal payroll taxes.

Covering Pensioners and the Poor. Foreign experience shows—as Americans are discovering—that full health coverage of the elderly and the poor requires a highly redistributive financing system. If the United States enacts universal health insurance and folds Medicare and coverage of all the poor into it, it is impossible to collect more than nominal contributions from these groups. Automatic deductions from pension and unemployment checks are inevitable; the pension and unemployment benefit systems inevitably take this into account. Percentage deductions from pension checks tap ability to pay. But a considerable extra burden on the economically active is inevitable. (The United States actually has been practicing this for some time. By enacting a Social Security payroll tax for the Medicare Hospital Insurance Trust Fund without enacting comprehensive health insurance, the Americans in 1965 made Medicare redistributive from the start. Normal statutory health insurance would simply enact the rest of the payroll tax system, whereby the economically active pay for their own health protection.)

Adding the poor to a system financed by payroll taxes would increase these rates even more. This troublesome prospect will probably persuade the Americans—like the Europeans—to search for additional or substitute financing channels.

Notes

1. Commissie Structuur en Financiering Gezondheidszorg (W. Dekker and others), *Bereidheid tot verandering* (The Hague: Distributiecentrum Overheids-publikaties, 1987), especially pp. 11-12, 48-63; and *Derde Dekker-brief (Nota "Verandering verzekerd," 7 maart 1988)* (Rijswijk: Ministerie van Welzijn, Volksgezondheid en Cultuur, 1988), Tweede Kamer, zitting 1987-88, 19,945, nos. 27-28, Bijlage A-4.

2. I. M. Rubinow, *Standards of Health Insurance* (New York: Holt, Rinehart & Winston, 1916), pp. 90-93, 148.

3. The German regime is described in Horst Gerold, *Krankenversicherung der Landwirte*, 3rd ed. (Sankt Augustin: Asgard Verlag, 1982); and Kurt Noell, *Die Krankenversicherung der Landwirte*, 8th ed. (Kassel: Verlag Hans Meister, 1982). The French regime is described in Yves Saint-Jour, *La protection sociale agricole* (Paris: Librairie Générale de Droit et Jurisprudence, 1984); Cour des Comptes, *Rapport au Président de la République suivi des réponses des administrations, collectivités, organismes et entreprises* (Paris: Direction des Journaux Officiels, 1986), pp. 175-188; and *La Mutualité Sociale Agricole*, 2nd ed. (Paris: Union des Caisses Centrales de la Mutualité Agricole, 1984).

4. *Régime d'assurance maladie et maternité des non salariés* (Paris: Caisse National d'Assurance Maladie et Maternité des Travailleurs Non Salariés des Professions Non Agricoles, 1985); and Jean-Jacques Dupeyroux (ed.), "L'assurance maladie des travailleurs non salariés des professions non agricoles," special issue of *Droit Social*, vol. 33, no. 3 (March 1970).

5. The considerable understatement of incomes and underpayment of income taxes by the self-employed of France and Belgium are estimated in Philippe Madiner and others, *Les benefices déclarés par les entrepreneurs individuels non agricoles* (Paris: Documents du Centre d'Etude des Revenus et des Coûts, 1974), pp. 21-24, 107-112; Max Frank and others, "Problèmes methodologiques et statistiques relatifs à l'évaluation de la sous-estimation et de la fraude fiscale," in Max Frank (ed.), *L'exacte perception de l'impôt* (Brussels: Etablissements Emile Bruylant, 1973), pp. 147-200; and Max Frank, *Rapport à la Commission financière de la Chambre et du Sénat* (Brussels: Chambre de Réprésentants et Sénat, 1975). Besides underpaying their own social security taxes, the self-employed—particularly in construction—may understate their payrolls and not pay full social security taxes on all their workers: *Aperçu de la Sécurité sociale en Belgique* (Brussels: Ministère de la Prévoyance Sociale, 1981), pp. 41-42.

6. Alain Foulon and others, *Comparaison des régimes de Sécurité sociale* (Paris: Documents du Centre d'Etude des Revenus et des Coûts, 1982), vol. 1, passim.

7. The rules and administration for *aide médicale* (and all *aide sociale*) in

France during those years are summarized in Tony Lynes, *French Pensions* (London: G. Bell & Sons, 1967), chaps. 9–10.

8. For the case of Germany, see Hans Hungenberg and Jürgen Steffens, *Krankenversicherung der Rentner*, 3rd ed. (Sankt Augustin: Asgard Verlag, 1983).

9. The French medical welfare programs are described in Claude Fonroset, "L'aide médicale," *Revue française des affaires sociales*, vol. 34, no. 4 (Oct.–Dec. 1980), pp. 363–367; and Elie Alfandari, *Action et aide sociales*, 3rd ed. (Paris: Dalloz, 1987), pp. 363–367.

10. "Leefsituatie-onderzoek Nederlandse Bevolking 1983 Algemeen," Enquêtenummer 73, Question 112, Centraal Bureau voor de Statistiek.

11. Until recently such statistics were not calculated by social categories and therefore could not yield coverage rates. Statistical time series therefore have merely reordered total enrollments and have aggregated many carriers and policies. Few estimates antedate 1940. See Louis S. Reed, "Private Health Insurance: Coverage and Financial Experience, 1940–66," *Social Security Bulletin*, vol. 30, no. 11 (Nov. 1967), pp. 3–22; and Monroe Lerner and Odin W. Anderson, *Health Progress in the United States: 1900–1960* (Chicago: University of Chicago Press, 1963), chap. 29.

12. Herman Miles Somers and Anne Ramsay Somers, *Doctors, Patients, and Health Insurance* (Washington: Brookings Institution, 1961), pp. 364–365; and Ronald Andersen and others, *Two Decades of Health Services* (Cambridge, Mass.: Ballinger, 1976), chap. 4.

13. Tables 3.2 and 3.3 use the surveys especially designed for the study of coverage and utilization by the National Center for Health Services Research. The other reliable estimates—with similar results—arise from the Census Bureau's Survey of Income and Program Participation and are reported periodically in monographs such as Charles Nelson and Kathleen Short, *Health Insurance Coverage, 1986–88*, Current Population Reports, series P-70, no. 17 (Washington: Bureau of the Census, 1990).

14. The facts, policy options, and voluminous literature are summarized in two volumes prepared for congressional committees: *Health Insurance and the Uninsured: Background Data and Analysis* and *Insuring the Uninsured: Options and Analysis* (Washington: Congressional Research Service, Library of Congress, 1988). See also a series of reports to Congress by the General Accounting Office, particularly *Health Insurance: An Overview of the Working Uninsured* (Washington: General Accounting Office, 1989). A survey of employers—explaining why some do and some do not provide health insurance—is *Providing Employee Health Benefits: How Firms Differ* (Washington: Health Insurance Association of America, 1990).

15. Little research has been conducted to determine exactly how medical services have improved the health and longevity of populations: Barbara Starfield, *The Effectiveness of Medical Care* (Baltimore: Johns Hopkins University Press, 1985); Jack Hadley, *More Medical Care, Better Health?* (Washington: Urban Institute Press, 1982); Robert Blendon and David Rogers, "Cutting Medical

Care Costs," *Journal of the American Medical Association*, vol. 250, no. 14 (Oct. 14, 1983), pp. 1880-1885; and William Franklin Simpson, "Comparative Longevity in a College Cohort of Christian Scientists," *Journal of the American Medical Association*, vol. 262, no. 12 (Sept. 22-29, 1989), pp. 1657-1658. The deterioration of health services in the Soviet Union during the 1980s was accompanied by a deterioration in health indicators for the Soviet population, particularly in the acute conditions responsive to health care: Christopher M. Davis, "The Soviet Health System: A National Health Service in a Socialist Society," in Mark G. Field (ed.), *Success and Crisis in National Health Systems* (New York: Routledge, 1989), chap. 8. On the other hand, the two principal causal analyses of the history of improved health stress public health and preventive measures and minimize the effects of therapeutic interventions: Thomas McKeown, *The Role of Medicine: Dream, Mirage or Nemesis?*, 2nd ed. (Princeton: Princeton University Press, 1979); and Leonard A. Sagan, *The Health of Nations: True Causes of Sickness and Well-Being* (New York: Basic Books, 1987), especially chap. 4.

16. James DeLozier and others, *Ambulatory Care: Federal Republic of Germany and the United States 1981-83*, Vital and Health Statistics, series 5, no. 5 (Washington: National Center for Health Statistics, 1989).

17. Andrée Mizrahi, *Evolution à long terme des consommations médicales des populations agricoles* (Paris: CREDES, 1989).

18. Somers and Somers, *Doctors, Patients, and Health Insurance* (see note 12, above), passim, especially chap. 9, and the many sources cited.

19. Regina Loewenstein, "Early Effects of Medicare on the Health Care of the Aged," *Social Security Bulletin*, vol. 34, no. 4 (April 1971), pp. 3-20; Avedis Donabedian, "Effects of Medicare and Medicaid on Access to and Quality of Health Care," *Public Health Reports*, vol. 91, no. 4 (July–Aug. 1976), pp. 322–331; and Andersen and others, *Two Decades of Health Services* (see note 12, above), passim.

20. *Medicare and Medicaid: Problems, Issues, and Alternatives* (Washington: Committee on Finance, U.S. Senate, 91st Cong., 1st Sess., 1970), chap. 1.

21. Lu Ann Aday and others, *Access to Medical Care in the U.S.: Who Has It, Who Doesn't* (Chicago: Pluribus Press, 1984), passim and sources cited. For differential use of acute care, see Mark B. Wenneker, "The Association of Payer with Utilization of Cardiac Procedures in Massachusetts," *Journal of the American Medical Association*, vol. 264, no. 10 (Sept. 12, 1990), pp. 1255-1260.

22. Stephen M. Davidson, "Physician Participation in Medicaid: Background and Issues," *Journal of Health Politics, Policy and Law*, vol. 6, no. 4 (Winter 1982), pp. 707-717; and Janet B. Mitchell and Jerry Cromwell, "Medicaid Mills: Fact or Fiction," *Health Care Financing Review*, vol. 2, no. 1 (Summer 1980), pp. 37-49.

23. Rachel Benson Gold and others, *The Financing of Maternity Care in the United States* (New York: Alan Guttmacher Institute, 1987), chap. 6; Sara Rosenbaum, "Testimony of the Children's Defense Fund Before the Senate Finance Committee Regarding Child Health," May 1988; Paula Braveman and

others, "Adverse Outcomes and Lack of Health Insurance Among Newborns in an Eight-County Area of California, 1982 to 1986," *New England Journal of Medicine*, vol. 321, no. 8 (Aug. 24, 1989), pp. 508–531; Paul H. Wise and others, "Infant Mortality Increase Despite High Access to Tertiary Care," *Pediatrics*, vol. 81, no. 4 (April 1988), pp. 542–548; *Prenatal Care: Medicaid Recipients and Uninsured Women Obtain Insufficient Care* (Washington: General Accounting Office, 1987); and Michele C. Lynberg and Muin J. Khoury, "Contribution of Birth Defects to Infant Mortality Among Racial/Ethnic Minority Groups, United States, 1983," *Morbidity and Mortality Weekly Report* (Centers for Disease Control), vol. 39, no. SS-3 (July 1990), pp. 1–12. Compare the universal insured services described in *Having a Baby in Europe* (Copenhagen: World Health Organization Regional Office for Europe, 1985) and C. Arden Miller, *Maternal Health and Infant Survival* (Washington: National Center for Clinical Infant Programs, 1987). The superior clinical results are described in Embry Howell, "Socioeconomic Factors in Birth Outcomes: The United States and France" (Ph.D. dissertation, George Washington University, 1991).

    24. H. C. Chase, *International Comparison of Perinatal and Infant Mortality*, Vital and Health Statistics, series 3, no. 6 (Washington: National Center for Health Statistics, 1967). Since World War II, infant mortality diminished at a faster rate in Europe than in the United States, widening the differences. See Robert Maxwell, *Health Care: The Growing Dilemma*, 2nd ed. (New York: McKinsey and Company, 1975), pp. 8–9.

    25. All possible sociodemographic characteristics of mothers were examined during decades of inconclusive research. By the 1970s, some analysts hypothesized that prematurity, low birthweights, and infant mortality resulted from no or late access to prenatal care. But they did not take the next step and trace access to the absence of health insurance and the administration of Medicaid. See, for example, Joel C. Kleinman, "Trends and Variations in Birth Weight," in *Health: United States 1981* (Hyattsville, Md.: National Center for Health Statistics, 1981), pp. 7–13 and sources cited.

    26. Aday, *Access to Medical Care in the U.S.* (see note 21, above), passim; Steven A. Garfinkel and others, *Health Services Utilization in the U.S. Population by Health Insurance Coverage*, National Medical Center Utilization and Expenditure Survey, series B, descriptive report no. 13 (Washington: Health Care Financing Administration, Department of Health and Human Services, 1986), pp. 16, 23–24; Congressional Research Service, *Health Insurance and the Uninsured* (see note 13, above), pp. 229–242, 278–281; Fernando M. Trevino and Abigail J. Moss, "Health Insurance Coverage and Physician Visits Among Hispanic and Non-Hispanic People," in *Health: United States 1983* (Hyattsville, Md.: National Center for Health Statistics, 1983), pp. 45–48; Howard E. Freeman and others, "Uninsured Working-Age Adults: Characteristics and Consequences," *Health Services Research*, vol. 24, no. 6 (Feb. 1990), pp. 811–823; and Jack Hadley and others, "Comparison of Uninsured and Privately Insured Hospital Patients,"

Journal of the American Medical Association, vol. 265, no. 3 (Jan. 16, 1991), pp. 374-379.

27. Lower utilization of certain (not all) services by the lower classes in French statutory health insurance is reported in Andrée Mizrahi and others, *Medical Care, Morbidity and Costs* (Oxford: Pergamon Press, 1983), pp. 86-91, 159-161. Higher utilization of Britain's National Health Service by the lower classes is described in Martin Rein, "Social Class and the Utilization of Medical Care Services," *Hospitals*, vol. 43 (July 1, 1969), pp. 43-54. Since their morbidity is higher, the British lower classes may underutilize relative to need, according to Vivienne Walters, *Class Inequality and Health Care* (London: Croom Helm, 1980), chaps. 8-9.

28. Jean-Pierre Poullier, *Health OECD: Facts and Trends* (Paris: Organisation for Economic Co-operation and Development, 1991).

29. The limited importance of income and the role of other motives in location decisions by American doctors are summarized in Henry B. Steele and Gaston V. Rimlinger, "Income Opportunities and Physician Location Trends in the United States," *Western Economic Journal*, vol. 3, no. 2 (Spring 1965), pp. 182-194; James K. Cooper and others, "Rural or Urban Practice: Factors Influencing the Location Decision of Primary Care Physicians," *Inquiry*, vol. 12, no. 1 (March 1975), pp. 18-25; James K. Cooper and others, "The Decision for Rural Practice," *Journal of Medical Education*, vol. 47 (Dec. 1972), pp. 939-944; and Graduate Medical Education National Advisory Committee, *Report to the Secretary, Department of Health and Human Services: Geographic Distribution Technical Panel* (Washington: Department of Health and Human Services, 1980), vol. 3.

30. John C. Langenbrunner and others, "Physician Incomes and Work Patterns Across Specialties: 1975 and 1983-84," *Health Care Financing Review*, vol. 10, no. 2 (Winter 1988), p. 19.

31. Hermann Levy, *National Health Insurance: A Critical Study* (Cambridge: Cambridge University Press, 1944); John E. Pater, *The Making of the National Health Service* (London: King Edward's Hospital Fund for London, 1981); and Brian Abel-Smith, *The Hospitals 1800-1948* (London: Heinemann, 1964), chaps. 19-23.

32. Germany, the country that most closely resembles the American technocratic style of practice, also has the highest proportion of specialists, but nevertheless the proportion in general practice is 45 percent. See Bundesminister für Jugend, Familie, und Gesundheit, *Daten des Gesundheitswesens—Ausgabe 1989* (Stuttgart: Verlag W. Kohlhammer, 1989), p. 236. The proportion in general practice in France is nearly 47 percent. See Daniel Foulon and Jacqueline Gottely, "Quelques aspects de démographie médicale en France," *Solidarité santé— Etudes statistiques*, no. 1 (Jan.-Feb. 1987), p. 11. For the American distribution, see *Physician Characteristics and Distribution in the U.S.*, an annual volume of the American Medical Association.

33. See, for example, the studies of the Federal Employees Health Benefits

Program and other American insurance markets summarized in *Advances in Health Economics and Health Services Research,* vol. 6 (1985); and Steven M. Cassidy, "Alternative Benefit Choices by Employees with Dual Insurance Coverage," *Benefits Quarterly,* vol. 6 (First Quarter 1990), pp. 55–60.

34. Daniel C. Walden and others, *Consumer Knowledge of Health Insurance Coverage* (Washington: National Center for Health Services Research, 1982). So many people fail to understand whether they have any coverage at all that sample surveys of the population are unreliable. See Harris Meyer, "New Survey Suggests 31 Million Uninsured," *American Medical News,* July 7, 1989, pp. 1, 43–44.

35. Elisabeth Rosenthal, "Insurers Say Growing Fraud in Health Care Costs Billions," *New York Times,* July 5, 1990, pp. A1, B7.

36. See, for example, Pamela J. Farley, *Private Health Insurance in the United States* (Washington: National Center for Health Services Research, National Health Care Expenditures Study, 1986).

37. National Federation of Independent Business, "S.1265, 'Minimum Health Benefits for All Workers Act of 1987,' and Alternative Strategies for Extending Health Insurance Coverage to Employees of Small Firms," statement to the Labor and Human Resources Committee, U.S. Senate, Nov. 1987.

CHAPTER 4

The Structures
of Health Insurance

———————————— **Summary** ————————————

A variety of health insurance carriers now exist in every country with statutory or private coverage. Before laws were passed, each country had small carriers representing workers in particular industries, and some had nonprofit mutual insurance companies. At first, the occupationally based funds merely grew, and new ones were added. In a few countries, such as Germany, the occupational funds still exist, now supplemented by general-purpose funds for workers in less organized industries or for the retired. In some countries (such as Belgium and Holland), carriers were created by trade unions and ideological movements. Citizens could choose among them or join the occupational funds.

In order to protect the smaller carriers in less prosperous industries against decline, as well as to create large and efficient financial pools, some countries (such as Holland) have gradually merged the many small carriers. In other countries (such as France), the many small occupational funds are superseded by large public corporations that pool more money, manage more efficiently, and follow public policy.

Although each country's social insurance system has a different—and sometimes complicated—structure, they cover similar benefits and operate similarly. A few occupations have special political influence and obtain special regimes, so they can secure more generous benefits (such as miners and farmers) or can pay in less (such as the self-employed). In some countries, citizens may choose among carriers, resulting in competition by funds for the healthier risks. Elsewhere, the assignments are automatic, depending on one's occupation.

Once, social insurance funds were small and local. If they do not merge into larger entities, they join in associations that assume policy leadership, improve management, and represent all the carriers in negotiations with providers and government. Structures vary among countries. Since carriers began as democratic social movements, many funds and their national associations still have representative governments.

Where social insurance carriers cover mainstream benefits for the entire populations, private voluntary funds may survive. They cover supplementary benefits in general health insurance. Or they provide accident insurance. In a few countries (such as Germany today and Holland in the past), they still have a substantial market among those not required to join statutory health insurance.

Statutory health insurance is connected to the entire social security system, but the details vary among countries. The health insurance law may administer both, and government may contain the costs of both. The relations between the health insurance carriers and government also vary from country to country. Providers and the managers of the carriers usually try to preserve their autonomy.

Private health insurance is heterogeneous. The United States is the only country that has tried to cover all health care financing by an expanded private market, and the result is a complex and changing potpourri. The lack of standardization and the decentralization of decisions have advantages and disadvantages both for the public and for the carriers themselves.

Benefits

Every statutory health insurance system distinguishes between the basic and extra (optional) benefits:

- ☐ Basic benefits:
  - Ambulatory and inpatient care by doctors
  - Inpatient and outpatient hospital services (both acute and extended care)
  - Drugs
  - Several others (depending on the country's statute):
    - ★ Dentistry
    - ★ Ambulatory and inpatient care by certain other self-employed providers (midwives, community nurses, physiotherapists)
    - ★ Prostheses
    - ★ Thermal cures
  - Cash payments to the temporarily disabled worker if his wage is suspended
- ☐ Extra benefits:
  - Fee to the chief of service in the hospital
  - Private room in the hospital
  - Nursing homes

Social Insurance Carriers

The revenue and payments for the basic benefits in all European countries are administered by nonprofit carriers. They are called "sickness funds" in the various languages: *caisse maladie* in France and French-speaking Switzerland, *Krankenkasse* in Germany and German-speaking Switzerland, *ziekenfonds* in the Netherlands, and *mutualiteit* or *mutualité* in Belgium. These are always nonprofit entities. Usually they are private corporations, often centuries old and antedating the obligatory health insurance laws of the late nineteenth and twentieth centuries. Since 1945, the carriers in France have been autonomous government corporations.

In every country, health insurance today has a very complex structure. One might expect carriers within a country to be identical in organization and character, but they are not. All are obligated by law to pay for the same benefit package, but they differ in past history, in the political aims and power of their constituencies, in their methods of government, and in internal management. While the health insurance laws usually require all to submit annual financial reports to a government monitor, they have the political influence to block proposals to standardize their structures to an unacceptable degree. Militant social groups—such as farmers, miners, and railwaymen—can preserve their own sickness funds and social security programs as a tactic to avoid higher premiums and lower benefits.

This chapter surveys the structure of the carriers under statutory health insurance. Details about each country appear in Appendix A, which also outlines the history and explains why each country developed its current form.

Germany. The original guilds and mutual assistance societies united persons in the same occupation. Each urban craft had its own *Innungskrankenkasse*. During the nineteenth century, workers in each mine or factory created their own funds (*Knappschäfte* and *Betriebskrankenkassen*). The compulsory health insurance laws—first in the Kingdom of Prussia and later in the entire German Empire—required all workers in each workplace to join its sickness fund. The law required all the craftsmen in the city to join the appropriate municipal *Innungskrankenkasse*. Membership, budgets, and administrative work grew.

Since coverage of certain social strata was compulsory, the national health insurance law of the 1880s created special regional sickness funds (*Ortskrankenkassen*) to enroll persons whose workplaces lacked funds. Coverage was extended to other occupations, such as farmers and seamen, and special sickness funds were created for them. During the late nineteenth and early twentieth centuries, Germany had several thousand sickness funds. Most were small *Betriebskrankenkassen*. Most of the population was enrolled in the large catch-all *Ortskrankenkassen*.

Assignment to a particular sickness fund until recently was automatic for nearly everyone: one joined the fund for one's workplace or for one's occupation (if the fund enlisted persons from many small workplaces). Therefore, the German sickness funds did not compete for good risks and could not avoid accepting bad risks. Choice was confined to the elites in the following circumstances:

☐   Above a certain income level, periodically amended in the law, persons were
    exempt from obligatory health insurance. They were prosperous managers,
    professionals, civil servants, and the self-employed. Although they could join
    the sickness funds voluntarily, a large private health insurance market arose
    to cover them.

☐   If they were "salaried employees" rather than "wage workers," persons under
    obligatory insurance could opt out of the workplace sickness funds and
    enroll in a substitute. A few early mutual insurance companies specialized
    in this market rather than become sickness funds for the working class. They
    were called *Ersatzkassen* and enlisted managers, white-collar workers, and
    technicians who otherwise would have belonged to *Betriebskrankenkassen*
    and *Ortskrankenkassen*. For many years, the market was small.

The German health insurance structure became volatile during the 1970s
and 1980s. The system had little government regulation and little standardization, the sickness funds and *Ersatzkassen* insisted on autonomy and discretion
(*Selbstverwaltung*), and considerable change and competition resulted. The
number of *Betriebskrankenkassen* diminished for several reasons: many were too
small to be economically viable; many suffered declines in the number of workers
who paid contributions and increases in the elderly who incurred costs; their
more prosperous salaried members switched to the *Ersatzkassen;* and when business firms dissolved or merged, their *Betriebskrankenkassen* disappeared or were
reorganized. The *Ortskrankenkassen* grew in size, absorbing many workers from
dissolved *Betriebskrankenkassen* as well as many expensive pensioners.

Unexpectedly, the enrollment and economic strength of the *Ersatzkassen*
rose. The law increased the earnings ceiling for statutory health insurance, the
market for private commercial health insurance declined, and these persons selected the *Ersatzkassen* rather than the other sickness funds. Since the structure
of the German economy produced more salaried employees and fewer blue-collar
workers, more people could transfer from the *Betriebs-* and *Ortskrankenkassen*
to the *Ersatzkassen*. By the 1990s, only half the German population was covered
by *Betriebs-* and *Ortskrankenkassen,* and their share steadily diminished; more
than one-third belonged to the *Ersatzkassen,* and their share steadily grew.

The original occupational and workplace basis of social insurance survives in part in Germany. By now, however, most persons belong to more inclusive funds (the *Ortskrankenkassen* and *Ersatzkassen*) whose function is to create
large pools to cover all risks, not to promote the interests of single occupations.
Other countries have evolved even farther from the occupational and workplace
origins of social insurance.

Belgium. Belgium's long history of mutual protection funds has been
interrupted and restarted several times. When the *mutualités* were revived during
the nineteenth century, the organization around individual occupations was superseded by wider working-class movements. A number of local *mutualités* re-

gardless of occupation cooperated because they were united by socialist ideology. In order to counter the influence of Socialism among workers, the Catholic Church helped create rival *mutualités*. Therefore, Belgian social insurance was built on an ideological rather than occupational framework.

When an obligatory health insurance law was enacted during the 1890s, it could not (as in Germany) mandate that each person automatically join the one sickness fund in his workplace or in his craft. Belgians have always had free choice of sickness fund. The carriers compete for the more affluent and healthier risks. The law now requires universal coverage, and nearly everyone signs up voluntarily with a local fund affiliated with one of the five principal networks. Nearly half belong to the Catholic sickness funds, and slightly over one-quarter belong to the Socialist funds. If someone does not choose, he is assigned to a residual public fund, the *Caisse Auxiliaire d'Assurance Maladie-Invalidité*.

Each individual belongs to a local fund. The local funds of each faction— Catholic, Socialist, Liberal, and so forth—belong to regional federations. Each federation is part of a national union with its own headquarters.

France. Like Germany and Belgium, prewar France had a large number of mutual protection funds, most small and local. Many were created in one workplace and might have the employer's help; some were associations of workers in similar occupations; some had a religious or political character. Belgian *mutualités* were strengthened by fifty years of government subsidies before the enactment of statutory health insurance; since they acquired great political leverage through alliances with political parties and trade unions, the Belgian health insurance law made the *mutualités* the sole carrier.

The French *mutualités* had just enough political influence during the enactment of the first health insurance law in 1928 to prevent creation of official funds that would displace them. During the 1930s, these historic social protection funds received the payroll taxes and paid out the benefits, as in nearly all other countries with statutory health insurance. Members of certain occupations were required to accept cover and pay payroll taxes, but they could join any *mutualité*.

A comprehensive social security system was one of the war aims of the French Resistance—as in Britain and in several other countries—and it was enacted in 1945. Usually statutory health insurance is part of a country's social security laws, and the existing health insurance carriers have the political power to become the official carriers. Usually the pension system is administered by newly created official funds. Therefore, the structure of health insurance and that of the rest of social security differ. Examples are Germany and Belgium. However, the French *mutualités* in 1945 were obviously too small and impoverished to administer a massive new program. The Left was more interested in the success of social security than in the preservation of the *mutualités*.

By the 1990s, all the carriers for basic coverage of employees and farmers were autonomous public corporations monitored by the Ministries in the government. Nearly four-fifths of the population belong to the local agencies of the general regime (the *caisses primaires* of the *régime générale*). All managers, white-collar workers, and blue-collar workers belong, regardless of industry and specific occupation. A few industries—such as agriculture, the railroads, and mining—have their own regimes. The self-employed have a program of their own administered by a mixture of private health insurance carriers and *mutualités*.

The Netherlands. Despite its small size, Holland in the early twentieth century had more than six hundred sickness funds, each confined to a locality. Like those of neighboring countries, some were organized by workplace and some grouped all workers in a town with the same occupation. Much of Holland's nongovernmental organizational life was affiliated with churches, and the Catholics sponsored many sickness funds for workers. Many were prepayment arrangements created by doctors: if citizens in the community paid the doctor regular capitation fees, he would provide all necessary ambulatory and inpatient care.

During the 1940s, Holland adopted obligatory health insurance for about 70 percent of the population (under an earnings ceiling). The many small carriers could not administer efficiently the increased numbers of benefits and the new flow of money. The society secularized, so that the distinctions among Catholics, Protestants, and anticlericals were no longer relevant in the management of social protection. All sickness funds had to administer the same payroll taxes, benefits, and regulations under the national health insurance law. Individual small entities experienced financial imbalances and excessive administrative costs. At first, separate national associations were created for the physician-led, Christian, and occupational funds. Separate sickness funds within the same association merged in each locality, and by the 1970s only ninety distinct units existed throughout the country. During the 1980s, all the sickness funds within nearly every community merged, and all are united under the Union of Dutch Sickness Funds (the *Vereniging van Nederlandse Ziekenfondsen,* or VNZ). No one thinks of these new specially created entities as anything other than social insurance bureaucracies. It is the system as a whole that embodies social solidarity, not the local agencies.

Until the 1990s, Holland had two distinct health insurance markets with two different sets of carriers. Below a certain earnings threshold, everyone was covered by statutory health insurance and was required to join a sickness fund. Above the ceiling, one could self-insure or buy health insurance privately. During the 1980s, about seventy-five companies sold health insurance. The companies were either nonprofit mutual insurance firms or stock companies. A few had very large market shares; many had small numbers of subscribers. While each sickness fund after mergers had a local monopoly, any private insurance company could sell policies anywhere in the country and competition was vigorous. Six companies were affiliated with sickness funds (*bovenbouw*) and were less interested in expansion into a large market. They appealed to residents of their sickness funds' catchment areas, particularly those who rose above the earnings ceiling and were no longer obligatory members of the sickness funds.

The structure doubtless will change in the future, as the result of the reforms of the 1990s. Every Dutch citizen is now required to enroll under statutory health insurance, and all previously private carriers cover all benefits just like any sickness fund. Every social insurance carrier may offer all the supplementary policies that previously were the specialties of the private companies. Each carrier is free to sell policies everywhere in the country.

Switzerland. Like other European countries, Switzerland had many small mutual aid funds during the nineteenth century. The country was decentralized in political organization and local-minded in conceptions of social solidarity; most of the funds drew their members from small areas. The sponsors were varied: associations of workers and craftsmen, trade unions, religious associations, local governments, and so forth.

Switzerland has never had compulsory health insurance for the entire country. Several attempts to enact such a single national statute have been defeated, either within the national Parliament or—after passage there—in referenda of the country's electorate. A law was passed in 1911 and has been amended several times. Called the *Kranken- und Unfallversicherungsgesetz* (KUVG) or (in the country's other principal language) the *Loi sur l'assurance en cas de maladie et d'accidents* (LAMA), it allows each canton to make its own decision but authorizes the national government to subsidize those health insurance carriers that satisfy certain criteria. Accordingly, twenty-six systems exist—one for each of the country's twenty cantons and six half-cantons.

No canton had compulsory insurance for the entire population until Neuchâtel enacted it for 1981 and the years thereafter. A few cantons, such as the City of Basel, have come close to making coverage universal and compulsory. Nine cantons pass along the entire decision to their local governments, but in only a few have a majority of the communes made insurance compulsory. Nearly every canton in practice has a mosaic: some parts (or perhaps no part) of the population have compulsory coverage; the rest are encouraged to buy health insurance; besides certain basic coverage, a great variety of supplementary voluntary insurance policies are bought. At present, about 25 percent of the Swiss population has compulsory coverage, about 73 percent has voluntary coverage, and only 2 percent is not covered.

If they meet certain conditions in the law, sickness funds receive subsidies from the national government (the *Bund*). They must offer certain ambulatory and inpatient benefits, follow standard patient cost-sharing rules, not discriminate in acceptance of risks, and follow other rules. With the help of the national government subsidies and the increased number of subscribers, many sickness funds have grown substantially in scale. Several mutual insurance companies became nationwide; others became large entities within their home cantons. Despite their wide range in size and sponsorship, the sickness funds have become similar in work: all must satisfy the standard conditions for the *Bund* grants; all must fill out the same annual accounts questionnaires for the national government; all must cooperate within each cantonal association of carriers in negotiations with the medical association and the hospitals.

Hierarchies of Social Insurance Carriers

Since every country has a different history in the evolution of its social insurance funds, the horizontal structure of sickness funds across the population (that is, the mix of occupational, ideological, and other funds) differs among countries. Thus, there is no standard and simple structure of national health insurance.

Another dimension is the relation between center and periphery—that is, whether a country's health insurance structure is centralized or decentralized. If a country's sickness funds originated as workplace funds or local occupational associations, unification and centralization proceed very slowly. If the funds become involved in ideological rivalries within the working class, the funds in each camp cooperate under their own national and regional leaders, allied with the leaders of the movement's political party and trade union.

With the passage of national health insurance laws and the increasing intervention by national governments over health care costs, the small local sickness funds formed national and regional offices, and these offices became larger and more active. For example, every German sickness fund falls under one of several *Bundesverbände* (national associations). The public functions of the national offices are:

☐ Comment on legislative and regulatory proposals by the Ministry. In most countries, interest groups must have the right to recommend new laws and comment on the government's plans.

☐ Send representatives to standing public commissions that manage the health insurance system, plan the future in health finance, arbitrate disputes, and advise the Ministry.

☐ Receive subsidies from the national government, pass them on to the local sickness funds, and account for their use.

☐ Negotiate contracts and fee schedules with the medical association.

☐ Explain the national government's policies to the sickness fund managers throughout the country.

The national offices perform other management services for the sickness funds and their subscribers:

☐ Process data and issue statistical reports that help the local funds to monitor physicians and hospitals and improve their own efficiency.

☐ Advise the local funds about new methods of management and financial accounting.

☐ Issue publicity to persuade voluntary subscribers to join that association's carriers.

☐ Issue publicity to persuade all current subscribers to buy insurance policies to cover supplementary benefits.
☐ Send publications to subscribers in order to teach healthy lifestyles.
☐ Manage certain facilities used by all subscribers, such as sanatoria.
☐ Manage reinsurance funds to pay for unusually expensive cases.

If a network includes many sickness funds, the hierarchy includes regional offices that perform many of the foregoing tasks on behalf of the carriers in the region. Such a three-tier hierarchy exists in the French general regimes; since it is a system of governmentally owned and financed *caisses*, each higher level has considerable authority to regulate and audit the lower level. In the private hierarchies, the grass-roots sickness funds often have ultimate authority over the higher levels, since their delegates vote at their plenary assemblies and their subscription payments create the headquarters.

In federal systems of government—such as Germany—health is a provincial responsibility, and many decisions are made at that level about the payment of doctors and hospitals, facilities investment, planning, and so on. Therefore, the sickness funds have busy provincial offices (*Landesverbände*) to deal with provincial governments, medical associations, hospital associations, and the public. For example, each German hierarchy of sickness funds, such as the *Betriebs-krankenkassen*, has eleven *Landesverbände* as well as the one national *Bundesverband*.

In all countries—including the federal systems—health care financing steadily becomes more centralized. Health insurance increasingly depends on laws, regulations, subsidies, and taxing decisions by national governments. The executives in national headquarters of the sickness funds become important political figures. A large staff is necessary to monitor government proposals, participate in meetings of advisory committees, and lobby government for help. A large research staff is needed to provide these representatives with ammunition, to strengthen the headquarters' negotiators who face doctors and other providers, and to orient the member sickness funds to the overall situation.

The economics of social security and the requirements of modern financial management also force upward centralization. In Belgium, for example, each local mutual protection fund was once an active and self-sustaining association. To coordinate with the national trade unions and political parties and to negotiate with the national government over subsidies and regulations, they united in regional federations and national unions. The local *mutualités* could not survive for long as financially and managerially autonomous: some had adverse dependency ratios (too many heavy users and not enough payers), and equalization transfers were needed among sickness funds. Therefore, the federation office had to acquire financial control over the local *mutualités*. Moreover, modern accounting and computing can be installed efficiently at the region and not at the locality. Therefore, the local *mutualité* in Belgium is no longer a political club but has become the regional federation's local administrative office.

Private insurance companies are usually centralized: they sell the same policies throughout the country, often at the same premiums. Some sickness funds were originally nonprofit private companies and became carriers under the statutory scheme by conforming to certain laws and audits (as in Germany's *Ersatzkassen*) and, in addition, by accepting government subsidies (as in Switzerland). It is surprising to find such centralized sickness funds in countries with federal systems of government. In Germany and Switzerland, the same premiums are charged throughout the country and are included in a consolidated pool, despite the wide regional variations in fees to doctors and daily charges to hospitals. (All the other sickness funds in Germany belong to provincial and then to national associations.) The national sickness funds of Switzerland create unity in a health sector that otherwise is decentralized and heterogeneous.

Governing Sickness Funds

In countries where the carriers originated as small mutual protection societies of workers, they were ruled democratically. All the members met together, decided the premiums, approved expenditures, and hired the few employees. The first laws regulating mutual protection funds—such as those in France and Belgium during the 1890s—protected the members' sovereignty by guaranteeing regular meetings of members or subscribers' election of the governing board.

When government replaces these private carriers by public agencies, the democratic principle remains. Even though the public carriers' revenue, expenditures, and activities are fixed by the national health insurance law and its regulations, a large governing assembly or governing board is elected by the subscribers. The general public and the employers cannot vote; the sickness fund at first is still considered an association of workers. The electoral principle was a prominent issue when the new public *caisses* were created in France in 1946. A governing board (*conseil d'administration*) was created for every *caisse*. One possible procedure might have been appointment, with certain seats filled by each trade union. Instead, from 1947 to 1967, all the *caisses* were governed by "social elections." Three-quarters of the seats were to be filled by workers' representatives. Each trade union presented a slate for the workers' seats on the governing board, all campaigned, all *caisse* subscribers voted, and the seats on the board were distributed proportionate to the election results. All the local employers voted for their representatives in a similar fashion.[1]

This method had drawbacks. Unions competed for votes by promising better benefits, and costs rose excessively. The meetings of the governing boards and the affairs of the *caisses* were constantly embroiled in the rivalries among the unions. The governing boards were filled by union leaders and political militants inexperienced in health care finance. To manage the *caisses*, the winners of the elections selected union members rather than persons trained in insurance. The employers paid more than half the health insurance premiums, had no voice in management because of their few seats on the governing boards, and became critical of social security. The de Gaulle government reformed the structure and direction of the *caisses* in 1967 to strengthen governmental authority, improve management, and promote a social partnership between the workers and the employers. The governing boards in the general regime would be appointed and no longer elected. Workers and employers would have an equal number of seats selected by the principal trade unions and employers' associations. The system—with a recent revival of limited electoral methods—remains in place today for the general regime. (Other French regimes use a variety of electoral and appointive methods to select their governing bodies.)[2]

Private Insurance in Countries with Statutory Health Insurance

Nearly every country with national health insurance or a national health service has private health insurance in addition. Social groups are free to create mechanisms of social protection; private business firms are free to enter the market. But the problem for these organizations is to find a niche. If the population is forced to pay taxes and is fully entitled to benefits under the official scheme, why would anyone pay additional money for anything more? Since the possible niches vary among countries, the roles and structures of these supplementary schemes vary.

The Mutuelles *in France.* The *mutualités* in both France and Belgium at various times have been the carriers under statutory health insurance. In Belgium, they have steadily gained power and remain the carriers today: beginning in the 1890s, they have been subsidized by the national government; they became allied with all the political parties and trade unions; they could retain some of the insurance revenue for administrative costs; they were never regulated and audited strictly. In contrast, the French *mutualités* never became so powerful: having once been declared illegal by a liberal government (from 1791 to 1850), they have always sought maximum independence from government and from the political parties; they have never received subsidies from government; they have never formed alliances with the complete range of political parties and trade unions; most are very small and financially vulnerable, but they never united into strong associations. After World War II, the carrier function for the majority of subscribers under French statutory health insurance was taken from the *mutualités* and given to new governmental *caisses*.

Nevertheless, some niches exist in the French health insurance system—and the *mutuelles,* as they were recently renamed, fill them. These tasks and other details about the *mutuelles* are presented at greater length in Appendix A. The principal functions are:

☐ Insure the patient's cost sharing under statutory health insurance. The patient's bill is paid by two carriers: the largest share by his social insurance *caisse* and the rest by his *mutuelle.*

☐   Administer the patient's billing. Without a *mutuelle,* the patient must pay
    the doctor directly and then await reimbursement by his *caisse* (instead of
    turning the doctor's bill over to his *mutuelle,* which handles everything).
☐   Provide some services, such as pharmacies, dental care, and mental health.

An important role for *mutuelles* with large memberships of self-employed persons is to serve as the basic carriers for that regime (CANAM).

Instead of disappearing after losing their statutory health insurance role
in 1945, the *mutuelles* recently have been making a comeback. Nearly four-fifths
of the French population now subscribes. Usually one signs up with the *mutuelle*
at one's workplace.

Commercial Insurance Companies. Every country has insurance companies that insure for the nonhealth risks of their citizens and organizations.[3] Such
risks include destruction of buildings and property by fire and by natural disas-
ters; loss of ships, airplanes, and other vehicles and their cargoes during a voyage;
accidents to persons and property, such as automobile crashes; and so on. These
companies can be owned by:

☐   *Those who purchase the insurance policies.* In this case, the companies are
    consumer cooperatives. In American terminology, they are "mutual insur-
    ance companies." Extra earnings not absorbed by claims and administration
    result in dividends to policyholders or increases in the reserves. The board
    of directors is elected by the policyholders.
☐   *Private investors:*
    • Stockholders in that company. Extra earnings are distributed in divi-
      dends. The board of directors is elected by the stockholders.
    • Another company (or companies) that is itself owned by stockholders. If
      the board of directors exists as a separate entity, it is selected by the parent
      company (or companies). A family of legally separate but commonly held
      companies is common in countries—such as Germany—where insurance
      regulation requires that different lines be offered by separate companies
      with distinct financial accounts.
☐   *The government.* These are "nationalized companies." If they are organized
    and managed as autonomous public corporations (as in France during the
    1980s), they may relate to customers much like mutual insurance companies.
    The board of directors, if one exists, is selected by the responsible government
    Ministry with seats allocated to particular groups according to law.

Private insurance companies existed in every European country before the
development of statutory health insurance, accident, and disability laws. The first
workmen's compensation laws of the late nineteenth century required employers
to provide disability payments and medical care for workers injured on the job.
Employers insured against this risk by paying premiums to private insurance

companies, to workplace sickness funds, or to special new government work-accident funds. Different countries had different arrangements. Where the private carriers had the assignment, they acquired an important niche in health even before the national health insurance laws were enacted.[4]

Obligatory health insurance was enacted for the workers, and their sickness funds became the official carriers. Simultaneously, private insurance offered voluntary coverage to the self-employed, the managers, and the rich. These policies offered more generous benefits than did the statutory health insurance, since they covered private specialists' fees, private rooms in public and nonprofit hospitals, and the charges of private clinics. Gradually the upper classes have been added to statutory health insurance, but the private companies still have their niches:[5]

☐ Accidents:
- *Work.* In most countries, the principal statutory workmen's compensation coverage is now administered by special public funds or by the official sickness funds. But some countries still allow the private carriers to offer coverage. As competition between the sickness funds and the private insurers grew during the 1980s, some countries encouraged the private companies to enter the market more vigorously. For example, Switzerland in 1984 ended its policy of seventy-three years, eliminated the monopoly by the single national accident fund, and allowed the sickness funds and private companies to offer work accident coverage to employers.
- *Automobile accidents.* In every European country, drivers must buy private insurance covering both property and persons. The laws make the private policy primary: the patient must exhaust reimbursement from this source before billing the sickness fund. This is the most lucrative form of health insurance for the private companies, and the sickness funds have been eager to enter their markets.
- *Other losses.* Such cases include accidents or illnesses during vacations, while abroad, and under other unusual circumstances. The private policy is primary.
☐ Basic benefits for those still not required to join statutory health insurance. Examples are Holland (before 1990) and Germany—both described earlier. Nearly everyone buys coverage voluntarily, but most pick the private companies rather than the sickness funds since the premiums are lower and one can buy policies that cover the higher physician fees.
☐ Supplementary benefits for all persons covered by obligatory health insurance. The principal customers are the upper classes who have been added to the universal program. They can afford more generous services, like those they might have had under completely private voluntary health insurance. Their official social insurance carriers might or might not offer these benefits. If the ideology of social solidarity is strong, as in France and Belgium,

the sickness funds and *mutuelles* refuse to offer this coverage, so one must buy it privately.

☐ Insurance of the cost sharing under the statutory scheme, as in the market for the *mutuelles* in France. Usually the private companies do not offer such policies. Few countries have significant cost sharing. The administration is expensive.

☐ Carriers for basic benefits under obligatory health insurance:

• Nonprofit mutual insurance companies can accept the legislative conditions to administer the mainstream program. The German *Ersatzkassen* and many of the Swiss *Krankenkassen* began as private mutual insurance companies.

• Some regimes under the official schemes—usually the ones for the self-employed—allow subscribers to satisfy their obligation by insuring the specified risks with private companies. An example is the regime for the self-employed in France.

Because the private companies fill gaps in each country's statutory health insurance system, and because each structure varies, there is no standard pattern for private health insurance across Europe. The companies are important and visible in some countries (such as Holland and Germany) while hardly operating in others (such as Belgium). They have become integrated into statutory health insurance in some countries (such as Switzerland) while remaining distinct elsewhere. Their role fluctuates often; for example, the private companies recently began a competitive struggle with the sickness funds (or, in France, with the *mutuelles*) over supplementary policies.

Integration with Social Security

In every country, obligatory health insurance is part of the total social security system. But the precise connections are not the same everywhere. This helps explain why each country's health insurance structure is complicated and somewhat unique. Differences exist in the forms of legislation, methods of collecting money, and structures of the carriers:

☐ In several countries (for example, Germany, France, and Belgium), the health insurance law is part of the Social Security Code dealing with pensions, work disability, and other topics. When the United States enacted its single statutory health insurance program (Medicare), it became part of the Social Security Code. But in several other countries (such as Holland and Switzerland), the health insurance laws are separate.

☐ Payroll taxes can be set for statutory health insurance by the same principles as they are for other social security programs. The percentages are proposed by the Ministry responsible for the entire social security package, they are approved by the Ministry of Finance, and they are enacted together by the

Cabinet or the Parliament. All the revenue is collected from employers together and then distributed to the separate funds for sickness, pensions, and so on. This method is followed, for example, in France and Belgium. In contrast, the premiums and collections are administered separately in Germany and Switzerland.

☐ The same type of carrier may administer health insurance and other social security benefits. An example is France with its similar governmental funds in the general regime. But this arrangement is unusual, since the sickness funds have usually fought successfully to remain the carriers under the statutory scheme, while different types of agencies (such as centralized government pension institutes) administer pensions and other benefits.

☐ Equalization transfers can occur between the sickness funds and other social security units with surpluses. Such transfers occur in France but rarely elsewhere.

As later passages of this book will show, government finance officers may have jurisdiction over all the social security programs, but health is always the most troublesome:

☐ Spending on pensions can be predicted easily. Health constantly produces cost overruns and is the principal reason for deficits in social security.

☐ Pensions and some other programs can be administered easily. A massive computer system can send out pension checks automatically. But health involves a constant administrative effort to receive, investigate, and pay individual bills.

☐ In most social security programs, the funds deal only with the unsophisticated subscribers. But in health, the funds must deal with both the subscribers and the providers, who have quite different interests and styles.

☐ Payment of pensions and most other benefits follows formulas and procedural rules. But paying doctors and other health care providers involves frequent disputes.

Relations Between Health and Accident Funds. The structure of social security and health insurance is shaped by the political struggle among interest groups and among organizations. One might think that workmen's compensation and health insurance should be administered by the same funds, but this rarely happens. The ubiquity of self-interest in legislative politics was demonstrated in the first set of national social security laws enacted by the *Reichstag* of the new German Imperial Government during the 1880s. The first bill proposed administration by an Imperial Insurance Institute. Bismarck and his associates thought this strategy would induce the working class to favor the new national government. But the business and agricultural interests in the *Reichstag* opposed the financing provisions; and the provincial governments and conservatives opposed the expanded role of the national government. Work-accident legislation was repeatedly defeated over these issues and was finally enacted in 1885 when the proposal for an Imperial Insurance Institute was scrapped, oversight was given to agencies of the provincial governments, and special provincial local carriers were created for the financial management. The health insurance law was the first part of social security enacted in 1883, because the sickness funds already existed and were designated the carriers.

Work-accident insurance and health insurance remain separate to this day in Germany. The premiums are distinct and follow different formulas. The work-accident program is still administered by special carriers (*Gewerbliche Berufsgenossenschaften*) oriented toward employers. The health insurance program is still administered by *Krankenkassen* oriented toward subscribers and trade unions. An injured person must exhaust benefits from accident insurance before drawing health insurance coverage. The two networks, therefore, expend substantial effort in communications.[6] (The foregoing describes the industrial and commercial sectors. In the German agricultural regime, the accident funds and sickness funds are coordinated more closely.)

Relations Between Health and Pension Funds. In the past, the health insurance and pension carriers have had limited relationships. In many countries, the old-age pension funds pay the long-term disability pensions; in a few countries, they provide cash benefits for short-term disability. The person's eligibility is established by services received under statutory health insurance, and the sickness fund's control doctor may fill out the disability certificate for the pension fund. In some countries, the pension fund may pay for some health services, such as rehabilitation, while the sickness funds specialize in acute care.[7]

Long-term care is now producing new forms of collaboration between sickness funds and pension funds in many countries. The sickness funds have traditionally paid for acute care by doctors and hospitals—and, unlike the pension funds, they have had long experience with providers of services. Sickness funds have local field staffs, but pension systems often do not. In France, for example, the national pension fund in the general regime (CNAVTS) now makes large grants to the regional offices of the sickness funds (the CRAMs) so that the sickness funds can create home-care programs and other services that combine acute and social components. These new developments in long-term care financing are described in Chapter Fifteen.

Standardization

Sickness funds under social insurance become more alike. Commercial health insurers become more alike too. One reason is the list of benefits. The law and the oversight body (if the country has such a decision-making agency) list the same benefits for all the mainstream regimes. Therefore all the sickness funds do the same basic work. They deal with providers in the same way, usually forming common negotiating teams when settling fees and contracts with doctors and other providers. If the laws list slightly different benefits for some regimes—as for the self-employed in France—the differences are not great.

The supplementary benefits offered by sickness funds and private insurance companies eventually become standard too. If one company offers a new policy that attracts subscribers (such as dentistry), the others soon match it to keep their market shares. Aware of this regular experience, the private insurers often form a committee of their trade association to design an important new policy. For example, the long-term-care insurance policy offered by many German insurance firms during the mid-1980s was designed by a committee of the *Verband der privaten Krankenversicherung*.

The sickness funds become more alike because of laws and regulations. Their members are required to join, the law specifies their rights in participating in the management of the carriers, and the monitoring Ministry checks that their rights and health care benefits are respected. Since the sickness funds receive and use money from payroll taxes or compulsory premiums, an auditing agency of the government (such as Germany's *Bundesversicherungsamt* or France's *Ministère des Affaires Sociales*) requires everyone to submit an annual financial report. The law not only requires completion of the annual form but may require all sickness funds to keep their books according to the same chart of accounts. Schools and professional associations of social security accountants and insurance accountants teach standard methods.

All private insurance lines—including commercial health insurance—are monitored by an agency (such as Germany's *Bundesaufsichtsamt für das Versicherungswesen* and a division of France's *Ministère des Finances*). The agencies' regulations and financial audits protect the public from fraud and from the insolvency of the private companies. One result is to force some standardization in behavior and accounting upon the private carriers.

Even if local sickness funds remain independent, they become more alike under the leadership of regional and national associations. In Belgium, for example, the headquarters of each national union and those of the regional federations train the personnel of the local units, offer management advice, help install modern accounting and computing, and hold meetings for the exchange of experiences. The sickness fund officials of the past—steeped in the ideologies of the labor movement—are replaced by a new generation of financial managers. No longer responsive to the traditional ideologies and convinced that insurance can be administered efficiently only on a large scale, the managers press for unification of the carriers, as they did in Holland.

Relations to Government

Autonomy, responsibility, and accountability are constant issues between health insurance carriers and government. Whether nonprofit and private carriers have been created before or after enactment of the national health insurance laws, the managers guard their independence and claim they are responsible to their governing boards and thence to the boards' own constituencies. But the Ministry of Finance wants careful accounting of the tax money spent by the funds; the Ministries that regulate health services and social security want guarantees that the covered population receives its entitlements. Germany has generated many laws and court decisions defining the borderline between organizational autonomy (*Selbstverwaltung*) and statutory responsibility, and a considerable machinery of decision-making and oversight bodies is in place.[8] Other countries have a similar (although less voluminous) jurisprudence.

An Intermediary Council in Belgium. One method of relating government and the private carriers is to create a special autonomous public agency between them, an intermediary that is neither a simple government Ministry nor a completely private corporation. Belgium in 1963 created such agencies to govern all the social security programs. The one for health insurance is the *Institut National d'Assurance Maladie-Invalidité* (INAMI). The governing boards of all agencies are *paritaire*—that is, equal numbers of representatives are sent by the opposing private interest groups in the financing and implementation of each program. The INAMI board, for example, has equal numbers of representatives sent by the employers associations and trade unions and equal numbers of representatives sent by the *mutualités*, medical associations, and other associations of providers. A few leading citizens are appointed to each governing board in the name of the King; they act as chairmen and vice-chairmen, and they serve as liaisons between the government (particularly the Ministry of Social Affairs) and the agency. These leading citizens are not government officials assigned by the Cabinet or a Ministry; but they do serve at the pleasure of the government-of-the-day and transmit its policies, such as cost containment in health. Amidst the constant bickering among the rival interest groups, the neutral citizens hold the balance of power. Each agency has a staff of civil servants; since INAMI has many functions, its staff is large.

One task of INAMI is preparation of the detailed regulations for the *mutualités* and providers that implement the government's policies. The papers are prepared by the staff; they are debated by a standing committee (usually a *paritaire* body drawn from the *mutualités* and the providers); and often they are debated and approved by the governing council. One committee (supported by an office within INAMI) is the negotiating site between *mutualités* and the medical associations over the contracts, fee schedules, and pay rates of the doctors. Other INAMI committees and employees deal with the affairs of other providers. The INAMI staff also audits the annual financial and statistical reports of the *mutualités*.[9]

An Intermediary Council in the Netherlands. Holland has a similar Sickness Funds Council, the *Ziekenfondsraad*. As in Belgium, the governing board is *paritaire:* equal numbers of members come from the employers associations, the trade unions, the confederation of sickness funds, and the provider associations. As in Belgium, several independent citizens are appointed in the name of the Queen: they chair the full council and its special committees, they settle factional conflicts because they cast the swing votes, and they oversee implementation of the government's policies. A substantial staff of civil servants does research, prepares options papers for the committees, and drafts the contracts and regulations that will govern sectors of health insurance. Unlike Belgium's INAMI, the fees of Dutch doctors and hospitals are set elsewhere in another autonomous public commission. The *Ziekenfondsraad* staff performs the annual financial investigations leading to the payroll tax rates, but this task in Belgium is done by the government Ministries (as Chapter Five will explain).

A Private Market: The United States

Evolution of Private Carriers Under Statutory Health Insurance. After statutory health insurance is enacted in a country, the carriers survive but change. Survival and prosperity depend less on competition and marketing, more on management and reputation. Each carrier gains many more members and much more revenue. Basic benefits are fixed by law; although the carrier can try to attract young subscribers by offering a few extra benefits, it does not try to attract them by crafting a very different benefit package, and it cannot ward off deficits by reducing benefits. If faced with deficits from adverse selection, a carrier tries to add young subscribers, limit its expenditures, press government for subsidies, or merge with another carrier.

The number of carriers diminishes. Multiline insurance companies concentrate on their more remunerative and less troublesome business. Small carriers cannot cope with high administrative costs and the risk of a few expensive subscribers. Many mergers occur. Comparable sickness funds cooperate in associations.

Relations with providers change. Formerly many carriers paid fixed cash benefits and let the subscribers negotiate fees with doctors. Some private carriers tried to deliver services by employing doctors. Under statutory health insurance, providers separate from carriers; all doctors and hospitals can participate, patients and their referring physicians choose the hospitals, and carriers are obligated to pay the medical fees and hospital charges in full. A system of collective negotiation is created, and carriers develop a capacity to analyze health care utilization and costs, as well as a capacity to bargain with providers.

Carriers develop close relations with government. They must carry out the insurance laws and regulations, account for money from payroll taxes and government subsidies, and collaborate with government officials in setting and implementing expenditure targets.

The United States is the only comparison case, among developed countries, where none of this has happened. America's original private arrangements have been expanded and modernized, but there is a constant struggle to keep them afloat.

The American Evolution. The United States once resembled Europe. Until the 1930s, much health insurance was provided by mutual assistance funds, either as cash or as direct service through employed doctors. The funds were small local arrangements created by immigrants, trade unions, fraternal clubs, and others. Many employers in heavy industry employed doctors to care for victims of accidents; in return for extra pay from employers or subscriptions from the workers, some of these doctors provided general medical care to the workers and their families. Some commercial insurance companies—otherwise specializing in life and accident coverage—offered cash indemnity policies in case of hospitalization. But they were very cautious about medical care benefits, and this line of insurance periodically expanded and contracted.[10]

In Europe, the socialist and trade union movements steadily expanded the mutual assistance funds before enactment of statutory health insurance. But the United States lacked a strong socialist movement, it lacked a competing Christian labor movement, and its trade unions were too weak. While America's mutual assistance funds survived, they remained small and did not coalesce into larger associations or nationwide movements, as they did in Europe. They were vulnerable to economic depressions and to migration of their members to distant places.

A century ago, in all countries, financing of hospital and medical care benefits was separated. And the distinction continued during the early years of statutory health insurance: hospital costs were covered by their owners' charitable fund raising, by endowment income, and by governments; the mutual assistance funds covered the fees of doctors for office visits and home care. Gradually the sickness funds added hospital benefits. European statutory health insurance now covers both hospital and medical care benefits; every sickness fund now reimburses both hospitals and doctors from its unified budget. In contrast, the Anglo-Saxon countries have retained the distinction between hospital and physicians' financing—Great Britain and Canada by governmental payments, the United States through separate insurance accounts and even by separate insurance carriers.[11]

When the United States expanded its private health insurance, the priority was hospital finance rather than physicians' bills. During the 1930s, when the Depression had destroyed much of private insurance and patients' ability to pay cash, individual hospitals and state hospital associations created prepayment schemes. The subscribers could use the individual hospital or any of the participating hospitals. These "Blue Cross Plans" spread throughout the country. The American Hospital Association issued franchises to nonprofit organizations that used the logo, followed rules, collected premiums, negotiated rates with hospitals, and paid bills.[12] Some state and local medical societies created similar prepayment schemes for physicians, some even before the spread of Blue Cross Plans. Their benefits for a long time were adjuncts to hospital care: they paid for surgery and other expensive inpatient treatments. The physicians' schemes grew slowly and did not cover ambulatory care adequately until the 1950s and 1960s. For a while, these state and local "Blue Shield Plans" were franchised and guided by the American Medical Association.[13]

Blue Cross and Blue Shield received an unexpected stimulus during the 1940s: employers and unions could not negotiate for higher wages under wartime wage controls; they were allowed to add health care benefits, however, and employers retained the Blues to write the benefit packages in return for the premiums and other features settled in the labor/management contracts. To improve procedures and benefits and to be able to negotiate with employers, the Blue Cross and Blue Shield Plans in each state cooperated. Their two parent national associations cooperated. "Welfare bargaining" and employer group coverage spread in the United States during the 1950s and 1960s, thereby taking the steam out of any movement for statutory health insurance. The United States appeared to have developed a unique private alternative to a national health service. The labor movement preferred the American method, since the worker paid no payroll taxes and appeared to get health care "free" from the employer.[14]

This private solution, however, could not cover the entire population. In an effort to achieve universality, the national government in 1965 enacted two categorical programs to cover the retired and the unemployed. The elderly were to be covered by a unique type of statutory health insurance called Medicare: an act of Congress levied payroll taxes on all employees and employers, the money was administered by trust funds in the Social Security system, and the beneficiaries were the pensioners. In every other country, statutory health insurance taxed and covered the economically active, and the pensioners were added later by supplementary methods. Medicare was a copy of Blue Cross and Blue Shield: hospital and physician reimbursement were separated; the staffs of the Blues and those of the provider associations wrote the law, designed the benefit packages, and used their preferred reimbursement methods; Blue Cross and Blue Shield Plans administered Medicare under contracts from the national government in most parts of the country.[15]

The American unemployed and poor were to be covered by an expansion and improvement of the public welfare programs that every country maintains before enactment of universal statutory health insurance. Under the new Medicaid, state and local governments paid for the care of their poor in mainstream hospitals and medical practices; the national government reimbursed them for half or more of their costs. Medicaid's benefits and hospital reimbursement methods were copies of Medicare and therefore replicas of the Blues.[16]

During the 1960s, therefore, it looked as if American health care would be essentially Blue Cross and Blue Shield made universal by private employer contracts, by some individual and family policies, by Medicare, and by Medicaid. The Blue Cross and Blue Shield Plans cooperated and eventually merged within each state; their national associations cooperated and then merged.

This scenario foundered on the voluntary and competitive nature of a private market. Commercial insurance companies had been in and out of health for decades, selling policies directly to individuals: some offered fixed cash benefits in case of disability or hospitalization; a few offered an indemnity schedule for particular benefits. Some were mutual insurance companies, others were investor-owned. Some specialized in health, others were multiline. All sought a niche in the lucrative and apparently risk-free employer-group market.

At first, during the 1950s and 1960s, they sold "major medical" policies that supplemented the Blue Cross coverage: they paid for very high hospital and physician bills. Then, during the 1970s, the commercial companies competed directly with Blue Cross and Blue Shield for "comprehensive" major medical coverage, covering both hospital and medical benefits and paying both basic and catastrophic claims. The competition added physicians' ambulatory services to the traditional inpatient coverage. The competition then led to price wars: the commercial insurers offered to experience-rate every group strictly, and Blue Cross Plans were forced to do the same, losing the extra cash that enabled them to cover bad risks. The competition also led to thinner coverage for the beneficiaries and yet lower premiums for the employers: the commercial insurers reformulated their methods of indemnity insurance and offered lower premiums to groups that required every beneficiary to meet deductibles and coinsurance. To keep their group business, most Blue Cross/Blue Shield Plans were forced to abandon their goals of first-dollar coverage and restored patient cost sharing. In the market for individual and family policies, the commercial insurers expanded their benefits but tried to attract the better risks from the Blues by offering age-graded and medically underwritten premiums; to keep selling individual policies, many Blue Cross/Blue Shield Plans had to abandon community rates and open enrollment.[17]

In this flexible market, a few earlier forms endured. Some trade unions—such as those for miners, construction workers, and truck drivers—continued to maintain their own health benefits funds and (in the case of the miners) even ran their own services. Prepaid group practices—whereby insurers employed general practitioners or multispecialty groups—provided all necessary acute care to individuals, families, and employer-paid groups. Renamed "health maintenance organizations," they were eulogized by many American health policy analysts and were subsidized by the national government.[18]

The volatile health insurance system spawned new forms during the 1980s. Employers tried to control costs. They felt that the Blues and commercial plans were too permissive in paying hospitals and doctors, wanted to minimize the underwriting profits of the carriers, and wished to evade state regulations that required several generous benefits (such as mental health services) in all "insurance" policies. Within a few years during the 1980s, a substantial fraction of all employers "self-financed" instead of "insured" the health care benefits of their workers: instead of paying carriers large premiums that might exceed costs, some employers paid all claims from their operating budgets, hired insurance carriers on fixed fees only to administer claims, and bought insurance only for the risks of the large and few catastrophic bills; some employers dispensed with insurance companies completely and hired "third-party administrators" to administer all claims.[19]

   The Present Structure. In the late 1980s, a large number and bewildering variety of forms coexisted in American health insurance. Details appear in Appendix A. The principal private arrangements are:

☐ *Blue Cross and Blue Shield.* One or a few Plans operate in each state. All are guided by a national headquarters; all are nonprofit; almost all specialize in health insurance alone.

☐ *Commercial insurance companies.* Some are mutuals, others are stock companies. All are centrally managed and nationwide. Over one thousand exist.

☐ *Self-funded plans of individual employers.* The company pays for employees' health benefits as they are incurred. Many business firms now substitute these arrangements for traditional group health insurance. Many give the administrative work to Blue Cross/Blue Shield or a commercial carrier.

☐ *Prepaid multispecialty groups of physicians.* These groups include health maintenance organizations and independent practice associations.

The market is extremely competitive and volatile. The commercial carriers have steadily taken business from Blue Cross/Blue Shield. Individual companies enter and leave health insurance while retaining their other insurance products.

   All persons over the age of sixty-five are covered by Medicare, America's only form of statutory health insurance. Medicare claims are processed by the Blues or by commercial insurers, under contract with the Health Care Financing Administration (HCFA) of the national government.

Private Insurance in Countries with Full Public Financing

A system where the Treasury pays for all health care would seem to provide no opportunities for private health insurance. All or nearly all money comes from general taxation, none or nearly none from payroll taxes. All revenue goes into the government's general Treasury, none into special sickness funds selected by subscribers. All residents are covered by the public scheme, and none need purchase coverage from a private market. Government Ministries distribute money to providers and do not need private fiscal intermediaries. Examples are Great Britain, Canada, and Sweden. Spain and Italy are now in transition toward such arrangements after previous forms of statutory health insurance. Even so, limited opportunities for voluntary private health insurance do exist in such countries:

☐ Certain benefits may not be offered by the main public programs. For example, Canadian private insurance companies offer dental, pharmaceutical, and several other benefits not provided by the provincial plans.[20] Many policies are bought privately, but much Canadian coverage comes in groups. Employers buy it as part of the fringe benefits for their employees.

☐   Auto and work accident financing remains in the insurance industry after government assumes the financing of all other acute care.

☐   Some private medical practice and private hospitalization remain. They offer patients faster service and more personal attention than they can get in mainstream care. Private insurance companies offer policies to cover the costs. An example is Spain: a doctor's office is crowded during the hours he sees the general public under the official and universal reimbursement scheme (INSALUD); if the patient comes during the hours reserved for the privately insured, he is seen promptly and the doctor is less hurried. (Spanish private insurance is not bought in order to avoid the INSALUD hospitals and enter the private hospitals, however, for the INSALUD hospitals are considered superior.)

Private Health Insurance in Britain. British experience demonstrates how circumstances determine the magnitude, forms, and limitations of private health insurance. The National Health Service covers the entire population. It is fully funded through general taxes and through a special "social insurance" tax, provides many acute-care benefits without limit and almost without cost sharing by patients, and is implemented by providers that are numerous but of limited capacity.[21] Britain has one of the world's largest and most innovative insurance industries, enterprising in the development of new products and new niches. No law about health or insurance prevents an insurance company from devising and marketing a policy for any health benefit.[22]

The principal carriers are nonprofit mutual assistance associations that specialize in health insurance.[23] One, the British United Provident Association (BUPA), has always dominated the market and still enrolls over 60 percent of all subscribers. Commercial companies—some specializing in health and some multiline, some British and some multinational—have recently entered the market.

Subscribers are enrolled primarily through employed groups. Most groups are "franchised" arrangements: an employer negotiates a set of benefits and premiums with an insurance company, and the employer and carrier must then persuade each worker (and his family) to sign up and pay the premiums. In some group contracts, the employer pays the premium in full as fringe benefits for top managers; in a few companies, the managers are expected to pay part of their premiums. Almost all subscribers are members of the upper and middle classes. Britain has no noncontributory, contributory, or even franchise contracts for ordinary workers, and only a few contributory arrangements for skilled workers. Some individual policies also are bought. About 9 percent of the British population—subscribers and their dependents—was covered privately in the late 1980s.

Since everyone is fully entitled to use the National Health Service, the purchase of private health insurance—indeed, the mere existence of the carriers—depends on events that create a perceived need for a substitute or supplement. At various times since the creation of the NHS such conditions have occurred (leading to moderate or even rapid growth in private insurance sales) or have been absent (leading to stagnant sales). The demand for substitutes for NHS services has several sources:

☐ Both before and since the creation of the NHS, Britain has never had as many specialist physicians and hospital beds as Europe. Many British hospitals and specialists had waiting lists before the NHS, and they still do. As more serious cases are admitted, the delays in nonemergency care increase. The periodic strikes and slowdowns in NHS hospitals—particularly during the 1970s—lengthen waiting lists.[24] The principal appeal of private health insurance is coverage of nonemergency surgery and orthopedics in private hospitals.[25]

☐ NHS hospitals are busy high-tech sites. Once autonomous units run by the nursing staffs, today they are subordinate to the administrative agencies of the NHS. Private hospitals offer the smaller scale and the personal atmosphere of the pre-NHS voluntary hospital, and private insurance covers the costs.

☐ Until the mid-1970s, a patient could pay the NHS consultant privately and occupy a "pay-bed" in his NHS hospital for a small additional fee. But Labour Governments reduced the number of pay-beds, many hospital workers were hostile to such patients, and the consultants had to conduct their private practices completely outside. To cover the costs of private hospitalization, the market for private health insurance rapidly grew.

Similarly, the demand for NHS supplements has several sources:

☐ New treatments became common, were not offered by the NHS, but were covered by private health insurance. An example is discretionary abortions. (The NHS covers abortions meeting certain conditions and requires approvals.)

☐ The advertising of private health insurance appealed to the image and lifestyle aspirations of the new young professional class. Private medicine covered by private insurance was part of this lifestyle.

☐ The new managerial elite believes itself very busy at all times. Delay is expensive to the employer. Private medicine is said to be prompt and schedule-conscious, private doctors and private hospitals are solicitous of the split-second needs of management, and private insurance finances them.

A universal social or private insurance system can expand coverage, add benefits, cover higher costs, and raise premiums. But private health insurance in Britain must operate within limits: employers and individuals can choose not to buy it and can obtain care "free" from the NHS. During the late 1970s, British critics of the NHS (and all governmental services) predicted that the population would flock to private medicine and to private insurance. All private insurers promised to cover expensive benefits, and BUPA added blue-collar groups. The result was higher provider charges, higher utilization, and higher premiums. Expansion of coverage from the young managers and professionals to blue-collar groups and their families was expensive, since the workers and (especially) their dependents had more frequent and more serious morbidity. Expansion of benefits into high-tech procedures like heart surgery proved expensive. Promises to clear NHS waiting lists for nonemergency surgery proved expensive, as well, since a large hidden demand surfaced for benefits like hip replacements. As costs rose, adverse selection stabilized subscriptions and revenue during the 1980s: some employers and healthy individuals dropped their policies completely, others shopped for cheaper packages, and the principal carriers suffered underwriting losses.

Competition among private carriers prevented the larger ones (such as BUPA) from expanding their enrollments, benefits, and revenue. Smaller carriers took business away from the larger ones by offering lower premiums to employed groups (that is, experience rates minus discounts) and to individuals. Transfers became common. No carriers could build up reserves.

Since this imprudent venture into a vigorous free competition, the British private health insurance industry has become more cautious and more sensitive to the limitations and perils of its environment. Each company's benefits now highlight simpler surgery with predictable costs. Companies also avoid advanced surgery and long-term care with less predictable and less controllable costs, they avoid primary care (for which there is no private market outside the NHS), their lifetime total financial commitment per subscriber is limited, they avoid industries and age groups with bad risks, they negotiate maximum per diems with private hospitals, and they offer maximum fees to doctors. Whether private health insurance grows or contracts significantly depends entirely on the national government-of-the-day's provision of the National Health Service. The private health insurance industry cannot control its own future.

Relation to Full Public Financing. Tax-supported coverage of the entire population is supposed to make health care a right of citizenship and a public service. Clinical need, not cash, determines access and priorities. If private insurance supplies the patient with extra cash, he can "jump the queue" over the more needy, contrary to the intent of the public system. Two solutions are used:

☐ Privately insured care is delivered in sites separate from the workplaces for publicly provided care; these sites are created by private investment. For example, private practice within British NHS hospitals has diminished, and private insurance now is intended primarily to finance private hospitalization. But the law does not forbid duplication of NHS benefits.

☐ The law could forbid extra payments to hospitals and doctors, and it could forbid private insurance companies to supply such extra cash. Six of Canada's provinces and two territories forbid private carriers to offer any benefits already covered by the tax-supported and paid-in-full provincial health plans. Another motive for the Canadian regulation is consumer protection: the companies are not allowed to market policies for which they will never pay out. As a result, Canadian insurers concentrate on benefits not provided by the provinces.

Effects on Performance

What difference does it make? If a country's health insurance system uses one or another form of organization, does it enjoy greater or lesser benefits in its management, recruitment of subscribers, efficiency, relations with providers, and costs? Do any results follow for the health of the population?

Number of Carriers. The trend in statutory insurance systems is toward one or a few principal carriers in each community and in the country as a whole. If the original ideological distinctions become obsolete amidst preoccupations with merely administering a standard service, smaller carriers merge and even the larger ones merge. Many smaller carriers drop out of the troublesome health field and concentrate on other lines.

Concentration has several advantages. Economies of scale are achieved if more subscribers and claims are processed by the same number of employees, by the same high-capacity computers, in the same building. Expensive rivalries among independent managements are avoided. A large data file is created for utilization review of providers and subscribers. A single large fund has greater negotiating power when facing providers and the government. The government's oversight task is simplest with the smallest number of sickness funds.

On the other hand, the existence of a large number of funds has advantages for some people. If the funds differ in ideology and services, subscribers have wider choice. If the funds compete for subscribers, some may offer better service, greater benefits, and innovative methods. Medical associations and hospitals may be able to bargain more successfully with many independent carriers or with a joint negotiating committee than with a single powerful sickness fund.

While the number and concentration of sickness funds affect the administrative order and costs of a social insurance system, they probably make little difference in clinical outcomes. Likewise, other organizational variations have important administrative and financial outcomes but few (perhaps no) clinical effects. The features that determine the health of the population—access, the list of insured benefits, and the approved clinical techniques—are provided to everyone under all statutory health insurance arrangements, since all are designed to guarantee good medicine. Judgments about inclusion of benefits and payment for certain techniques are made by medical professionals and by government regulators, and the health insurance system (however structured) adopts them in all countries.

Centralized, Decentralized, and Local Structures. A sickness fund may cover a country from a single national office. It avoids disagreements with regional and local offices; the local offices are subordinate agencies and do not deviate in performance. The central office can administer large amounts of work with economies of scale in accounting, claims processing, and advertising. The entire business is a single risk pool: the headquarters can quote standard rates across the country and is not beset by adverse selection, insufficient enrollment, and deficits in individual regions. Benefits are not confined to the subscriber's home region; if he travels or moves, the carrier can pay for services anywhere in the country. An insurance structure consisting of many autonomous local funds cannot enjoy these advantages.

But regional and local carriers, the second option, can accomplish things beyond centralized national structures. Since the regional or local carrier's staff is part of the community, it can issue personalized appeals to the local market and discuss matters with the subscribers. Its staff can negotiate with, monitor, and mollify the local medical society and the hospitals. Its staff can observe the quality of medical care and can caution the providers directly on behalf of their subscribers; it can advise the more remotely situated government.

A third option is a decentralized national network: in Belgium, the national headquarters wields much delegated authority, the regional headquarters has much original authority, and the local offices are now subordinate; in the United States, the member Blue Cross/Blue Shield Plans have original authority but the national association is growing in functions and influence. Thus, a decentralized national network combines the advantages and avoids the separate disadvantages of the first two options. The national office unifies claims processing and certain other technical services for all its parts, coordinates the member offices' handling of traveling subscribers, administers interfund financial equalization, provides expert management help to the weak member funds, performs demonstration projects about new methods, conducts research, and represents all the member funds before the national government and the national association of providers. The regional offices do all the marketing, advise the subscribers, negotiate with doctors and hospitals, and monitor quality of care. The decentralized arrangements require consistent negotiations between the national and regional offices to ensure cooperation.

Governmental or Private Ownership and Management. A sickness fund may be a public corporation, as in France today or Sweden and Italy in the past. Or it can be a private nonprofit or for-profit corporation. (If a government Ministry pays providers from its general budget—as in Canada—I do not regard it as a governmentally based health insurance carrier.)

A governmental carrier has advantages and disadvantages, depending on one's point of view. It can command more professionally and technically trained staff and more advanced computers. It can be coordinated more closely with the social security system in both collection of payroll taxes and administration of benefits. It must conform to cost containment policies, including the implementation of fixed expenditure caps. It has greater bargaining power with medical associations, hospitals, and other providers. It is more likely than private carriers to receive public subsidies to cover deficits. Its policies and internal affairs are more open to public scrutiny.

A private carrier that has evolved from a political and labor movement may have executives less skilled in insurance, accounting, and health care. (However, the task is becoming so technical and so much less ideological nowadays that private carriers under statutory health insurance are becoming more professional.) A private carrier has greater freedom to pursue its own policies and methods and need conform less to standard government rules. Managing so much money, large private carriers can become important influences over government and not merely its instrument. Private carriers cooperate with cost containment policies unevenly. They insist on participating in the making of public policies in cost containment, provider reimbursement, and additional benefits. Since they compete against each other, private carriers—particularly the for-profits—are more secretive about their financial balance and internal affairs.

Ideological, Occupational, or Universal Character. Sickness funds were once parts of social movements, and some are still "socialist," "liberal," or "Catholic" in goals and certain management details, such as membership of the governing boards. These ideological heritages still have important advantages. Particularly the socialist, Marxist, and Catholic carriers remain bulwarks of the public policy of social solidarity; their healthier and better-paid subscribers are reminded of an obligation to pay beyond their actuarial costs. (In contrast, the "liberal" sickness funds attract small businessmen and professionals who resist social solidarity and redistributive financing. The literature and insurance policies of the "liberal" carriers are antiredistributive.) The ideological history helps a carrier to recruit many subscribers from those social circles, political parties, and trade unions; nowadays in every country, the carrier must also convey a second image of nonpartisan efficiency so that it can broaden its appeal as ideology and religion weaken. The ideological history recruits managers who think of the sickness fund as a lifelong cause, who are not on the lookout for better jobs in the insurance and health management sectors, who accept modest salaries, and who are honest.

Many sickness funds originated in certain industries and workplaces, and they still are identified with particular industries and occupations. When the industry grows, the sickness fund can expand membership with minimum marketing efforts, its benefits improve, and its public influence grows. Conversely, if the industry declines, the sickness fund's dependency ratio and finances deteriorate, and its occupational character is a barrier to recruitment of a new membership. An advantage of an occupational-based and employer-based sickness fund is help in management staffing and in financing from trade unions and employers; but such help becomes obsolete as modern health insurance requires professionally and technically trained managers and employees.

Compared to the other types, secular sickness funds have advantages and disadvantages. Each has a much wider potential membership base, none can start up from an assured base (thus making the market more competitive), and each may be unstable in financing, market share, and benefits. Secular carriers are quicker to hire professionally and technically trained staff, but they may lose them to competing offers. Secular carriers are quicker to adopt new management techniques. A drawback is the possible orientation of management to pecuniary gain—or whatever is the current fashion in schools of business—rather than to public service and social solidarity. Compared to the ideological and occupational carriers, the secular and universal carriers are less tied to a political party and less involved in politics; but, on the other hand, they may be politically active at times to promote their own organizational self-interest.

More or Less Competitive Market Structures. Where several sickness funds exist and subscribers have free choice, carriers compete for members. Health care economists depict competition that revolves around money: insurers compete for business by offering lower premiums; in order to operate within revenue and maximize profits, they cut their costs by avoiding bad health risks among subscribers, by discouraging utilization, and by paying providers lower prices. But this is a narrow conception of markets in health. Even when payroll taxes, provider fees, and utilization rules are standard among all carriers—and even when the law automatically assigns subscribers to certain insurers—the sickness funds still may compete. Their goals are greater size, superior reputation, public image, and financial solvency.

In statutory health insurance, the sickness funds compete by avoiding reputations for poor service to subscribers and (if possible) by improving services and benefits. They seek the healthier and more prosperous subscribers, so they can earn extra cash. Some offer extra benefits without extra premiums, such as dentistry, thermal cures, and (among the German *Ersatzkassen*) higher fees for physicians.

According to the American experience, a highly competitive, predominantly private, decentralized, and money-oriented market has the following advantages:

☐ Management methods are open to innovation. New forms of financial accounting and claims processing are quickly adopted. Lacking the methods of deciding reimbursement under social insurance—collective negotiation between carriers and medical associations, as well as public regulation of the rates of hospitals and pharmaceuticals—private carriers may invent their own versions. American commercial insurers and some Blue Cross/Blue Shield Plans attempt forms of "managed care," such as selective contracting with providers who accept lower fees. (But the competitive and decentralized structure of the American market limits the effectiveness of managed care: the country's antitrust laws and each carrier's desire to gain at competitors' expense mean that each carrier has its own distinct managed care methods without the strong market power necessary for results.) If an arrangement does not win enough subscribers, it is readily transformed or abandoned.[26]

☐ New benefit packages are quickly introduced. If they do not win enough subscribers, they are quickly withdrawn.

☐ Inefficient carriers are not protected by a guaranteed subscription list or public subsidies. They must reorganize or withdraw.

☐ Purchasers of insurance—employers and individuals—have a wide choice and can change easily. (In the American market, the employers are eager to switch to cheaper plans, since they do the paying and other persons are the patients. But the subscribers and prospective patients are more risk-averse and are reluctant to change, particularly if they must give up their customary doctors.)[27]

☐ Purchasers can decide to buy little or no health insurance and can use their money for other purposes.

Such a market has many disadvantages as well:

☐ Bad medical risks can be left uninsured. No carrier is obligated to take them, although many (not all) Blue Cross/Blue Shield Plans in America take some voluntarily. If a carrier takes a bad risk, it usually asks him for extra premiums.

☐ Competition for subscribers leads to cuts in premiums, and carriers lack the cash for the redistributive financing of social solidarity. Strong purchasers—such as large employers in the United States—force carriers to cut premiums and take great financial risks.[28]

☐ Benefits can be cut in order to reduce expenditures by strong purchasers and by carriers. For the same carrier, benefits can change from year to year, bewildering the subscriber.

☐ Considerable personnel and money go into marketing, while social insurance systems minimize them. If there are many carriers, each must have managers, employees, and office buildings, and total administrative costs exceed those in the social insurance system.[29]

☐ Salesmanship generates claims about remarkable benefit packages that are the best in the market. Since no carrier wants the buyer to make accurate comparisons, the benefit packages and their values are obscure to everyone except experts. Comparison shopping—the supposed essence of a competitive market—is difficult.

☐ Salesmanship plays on anxieties and sells people as much insurance as possible. Brokers often sell a person more health insurance than he needs—that is, more than he can collect on when the insured event occurs.[30]

☐ The health insurance market is less stable than other insurance markets,

because medical costs are difficult to predict and control and can easily
exceed revenue.

☐   The subscriber may find that his customary policy is no longer offered or that
his customary carrier has dropped out of the health line. In the American
system, employers change carriers every eight years (on the average), and the
individual subscribers within the group must adapt to new benefits and new
procedures.

☐   Carriers conceal facts and exaggerate their trends and solvency in order to
attract subscribers, investors, and loans. The truth is hard to learn. For example, the American health insurance market has at various times heard
exaggerated claims about the growth and success of HMOs and managed
care.

When evaluating a system and proposing fundamental reforms, one must
establish the facts and not merely recite the claims. While America's competitive
markets may generate many innovations and lower consumer prices in fields
other than health, innovations in its health services may not be as common as
Americans believe. This issue is examined further in Chapters Ten and Nineteen.
The offsetting disadvantages recur throughout this book.

Implications for the United States

Structure, Number, and Character of Funds. Since American health insurance is organized heterogeneously now, this condition will probably persist if the
country enacts statutory health insurance. The managers of carriers wish to keep
their jobs and autonomy; they resist becoming subordinates in a consolidated
organization. In some countries, the carrier has a tradition and special character,
and members may fight to preserve it. This loyalty is absent in America, but the
existing carriers will follow the usual organizational instinct to survive by pressing to retain that role under statutory insurance, as Blue Cross/Blue Shield did
in the design of Medicare. Foreign experience suggests that all carriers will press
for recognition in the same market—like the administration of the Federal Employees Health Benefits Program and unlike the single fiscal intermediary in
Medicare.

Dutch experience shows that carriers themselves can decide to streamline
the system by merging voluntarily. Mergers among business firms are common
in American economic sectors subject to antitrust laws. Mergers and all-payer
cooperation are even more possible in insurance today, since the sector is largely
exempt from the American antitrust laws. The exemption will doubtless be
strengthened under any American statutory health insurance.

The United States might enact statutory health insurance without requiring standard benefits. This step would be unusual, but America often differs from
other countries. If different packages of basic benefits can be offered, the carriers
might have a genuine basis for remaining distinct. At present, the only example

in the statutory markets abroad is the slightly different basic coverage of physicians' fees in Germany. The unstandardized private insurance market permits variations in supplementary benefit policies (offered by the sickness funds and by the private companies in many countries) and in basic policies in the voluntary market (still offered by private companies in Germany and formerly in Holland). New carriers cannot enter the statutory insurance market easily, but opportunities exist in the market for supplementary benefits. Americans can learn much about the design and fate of competing benefit packages from these European experiences. One lesson is the cycle of competition: new benefit packages may be distinctive for a while, some are financially unviable and wither, and the successful sellers are eventually emulated by everyone.

A decision to retain the existing health insurance companies as carriers under statutory health insurance raises the issue of profits. For-profit companies do not become carriers under obligatory health insurance abroad, since cash profits cannot be retained. If a carrier earns a surplus, it uses up the money by increasing its operating costs or (less often) by offering extra benefits. Or it is forced to transfer its surpluses to carriers with deficits. But profits are unusual abroad, because of the constant increase in health care costs. The United States has been pressed by the political influence of the private sector to guarantee profits to the for-profit and even to the supposedly nonprofit hospitals under Medicare's pre-DRG cost reimbursement. No doubt private commercial insurance companies will press for such opportunities—or even guarantees—under any national health insurance law.

The difficult debate over national health insurance in the United States therefore will be complicated by the issue—long settled in Europe—whether some carriers will have the right to collect extra revenue from the system or whether they will be exempt from suspicions of underservicing. (No problem arises for nonprofit plans or for mutual insurance companies, since they do not earn cash profits for owners.)

Clarity. A standardized health insurance system spelled out in a law would reduce the confusion and conflict that permeate American health care at present. The improvements will be:

☐ Patients will better understand their benefits, designated providers, and out-of-pocket obligations. Current uncertainties and denials by carriers are a leading cause of discontent. It will no longer be necessary for citizens to try to resolve their insecurities by buying additional and often unnecessarily duplicative policies.[31]

☐ The obligations of primary and secondary carriers will become clear. At present, coverage is a subject of tension among private carriers and (for elderly workers) between Medicare and the private insurance industry.

☐ Physicians who bill carriers directly will no longer have the infuriating experience of being rejected by one carrier on the grounds that another is primary. These events are important reasons why many American physicians refuse assignment of any claims and insist on full direct payment by patients (*tiers garant* rather than *tiers payant*).

Special Niches. The United States doubtless will retain its penchant for entrepreneurial innovation, even if a national law standardizes the definition and financing of basic benefits. Perhaps a free and competitive market will remain to cover statutory cost sharing by patients (as in France), extra acute-care benefits (as in Germany, Switzerland, and France), or cash benefits in case of illness (as in much of the private health insurance market in America today). An important opportunity for American carriers would be long-term care—if, as happens in nearly all countries today, America's statutory insurance focuses on acute care.

A Supervisory Commission. The United States would benefit greatly from a commission to govern statutory health insurance, a device used in the Netherlands and Belgium. It can be the standing site for managing adversarial matters, such as the negotiations over fees between sickness funds and medical associations. It can be the external auditor over the health insurance carriers, overseeing both finances and management, as in the Netherlands. With the help of an expert and nonpartisan staff, it can investigate and recommend proposed changes in benefits. It can be a focused channel of communication between government and private sickness funds. It can provide an important stage of responsible private self-government in a situation that might otherwise lead to the kind of extensive government intervention that Americans avoid.

When well led, a commission can settle conflicts, prevent trouble, and keep narrow issues out of the national legislature and out of the courts. The United States is prone to disputes because of the rarity of such intermediary commissions, but statutory health insurance should not overload Congress and the courts with disputes, and the adversarial style of litigation is inappropriate to health financing issues. A few precedents for such commissions exist in Medicare Part A and have demonstrated their value in the turbulent American scene: since the early 1970s, the small Provider Reimbursement Review Committee has settled disputes between fiscal intermediaries and providers; recently the Prospective Payment Assessment Commission (ProPAC), representing many interest groups, has become the screening panel for many financial and benefit issues in hospital reimbursement. (In Europe, the Ministry of Social Affairs and Parliament would let ProPAC settle these detailed issues and would give pro forma approval. But in the United States, Congress insists on the final say.)

Affiliation of Pensioners. The United States has an important coordination problem that Europe avoids. When Medicare was planned during the early 1960s, it was assumed that active workers received employer-paid group health insurance and the problem of coverage began only upon retirement at sixty-five. Therefore, persons started to receive both pensions and Medicare benefits at sixty-five; workers transferred neatly from their employer-paid group health insurance carriers to Medicare fiscal intermediaries on that date. Then the question of early retirement arose. Just before the enactment of Medicare in 1965, Congress allowed workers to draw actuarially reduced Social Security pensions as early as the age of sixty-two, but it underestimated the magnitude of early retirement and did not link the Medicare age. Many employers offered private pensions and lump-sum payments to persons retiring before sixty-two, and they dropped such workers from all group insurance membership.

The lapses in health insurance coverage have been an important reason for the increase in uninsured Americans, particularly spotlighted because of the widespread public sympathy for the deserving elderly.[32] Several stopgaps have been introduced in a typical American patchwork: some unions press employers to retain retirees in group health accounts, but many employers resist new agreements and weaken old ones; Congress mandated continued membership in such groups by all discharged and retired workers, but the workers must pay individual premiums.

In Europe, the affiliation problem does not arise, since separate sickness funds no longer exist for workers and pensioners: the worker and his family stay in his previous sickness fund or (if they move, as in Germany) transfer to a community fund with identical benefits. Transferring from employment to a pension fund has no effect on membership and benefits under health insurance. The problem—as later chapters will explain—is financing, since the pensioner no longer brings in an employer's payroll tax.

Notes

1. Henry C. Galant, *Histoire politique de la Sécurité sociale française 1945-1952* (Paris: Librairie Armand Colin, 1955); and *Dossier Doc.: Les élections des administrateurs de la Sécurité sociale* (Paris: Direction de l'Administration Générale, Caisse Nationale de l'Assurance Maladie des Travailleurs Salariés, 1982).

2. The effects of the electoral and other management reforms of 1967 are examined in Antoinette Catrice-Lorey, *Dynamique interne de la Sécurité sociale* (Paris: Centre de Recherches en Sciences Sociales du Travail, 1980).

3. Every country's private insurance industry is described in Robert M. Crowe (ed.), *Insurance in the World's Economies* (Philadelphia: Corporation for the Philadelphia World Insurance Congress, 1982); *Supervision of Private Insurance in Europe* (Paris: Organisation for Economic Co-operation and Development, 1963); and *Insurance Markets of the World* (Zurich: Swiss Reinsurance Company, 1964).

4. Workmen's compensation arrangements today in several countries are summarized in Robert H. Haveman and others, *Public Policy Toward Disabled Workers* (Ithaca: Cornell University Press, 1984), and in Marcus Rosenblum (ed.),

Compendium on Workmen's Compensation (Washington: National Commission on State Workmen's Compensation Laws, 1973), chap. 6.

5. For overviews of private health insurance in Europe, see G. W. de Wit, *Recueil technique maladie* and *Private Health Insurance Europe* (Paris: Comité Européen des Assurances, 1983 and 1985); and Hans Georg Timmer (ed.), *Technische Methoden der privaten Krankenversicherung in Europa* (Karlsruhe: Verlag Versicherungswirtschaft, 1990).

6. Past history and the current situation are summarized in Christa Altenstetter, *Implementation of National Health Insurance Seen from the Perspective of General Sickness Funds (AOKs) in the Federal Republic of Germany 1955-1975* (Berlin: Wissenschaftszentrum, 1982), pp. 129-150. The recent situation is described thoroughly in Hanns Podzun, *Die gesetzliche Unfallversicherung*, 7th ed. (Bonn: Asgard Verlag, 1975). For a summary of how accident insurance and health insurance fit into the total German health insurance system, see Dieter Schewe and others, *Übersicht über die Soziale Sicherung*, 10th ed. (Bonn: Bundesministerium für Arbeit und Sozialordnung, 1977).

7. Relations between German sickness funds and pension funds over these matters are summarized in Hans-Gunter Renk, *Die Beziehungen zwischen Krankenversicherung und Rentenversicherung* (Sankt Augustin: Asgard Verlag, 1984).

8. Dieter Leopold, *Die Selbstverwaltung in der Sozialversicherung*, 3rd ed. (Sankt Augustin: Asgard Verlag, 1980).

9. The public agencies governing all the sectors in social security are described in *Aperçu de la Sécurité Sociale en Belgique* (Brussels: Ministère de la Prévoyance Sociale, 1981), pp. 46-50. The organization and operations of INAMI are described in Tien Nguyen-Nam, *INAMI: Aperçu des processus de décisions* (Brussels: Groupe d'Etude pour une Réforme de la Médecine, 1979); and William A. Glaser, *Health Insurance Bargaining: Foreign Lessons for Americans* (New York: Gardner Press and John Wiley, 1978), chap. 4.

10. Paul Starr, *The Social Transformation of American Medicine* (New York: Basic Books, 1982), pp. 200-209, 240-243, and sources cited therein; and Pierce Williams, *The Purchase of Medical Care Through Fixed Periodic Payment* (New York: National Bureau of Economic Research, 1932).

11. The evolution in both Europe and North America is described in William A. Glaser, *Paying the Hospital* (San Francisco: Jossey-Bass, 1987), pp. 66-80.

12. For the history of Blue Cross, see Odin W. Anderson, *Blue Cross Since 1929: Accountability and the Public Trust* (Cambridge, Mass.: Ballinger, 1975).

13. Herman Miles Somers and Anne Ramsay Somers, *Doctors, Patients, and Health Insurance* (Washington: Brookings Institution, 1961), chap. 16.

14. Raymond Munts, *Bargaining for Health: Labor Unions, Health Insurance, and Medical Care* (Madison: University of Wisconsin Press, 1967).

15. Robert J. Myers, *Medicare* (Homewood, Ill.: Irwin, 1970); and Judith M. Feder, *Medicare: The Politics of Federal Hospital Insurance* (Lexington, Mass.: Lexington Books, 1977).

16. Robert Stevens and Rosemary Stevens, *Welfare Medicine in America* (New York: Free Press, 1974); and Stephen M. Davidson, *Medicaid Decisions* (Cambridge, Mass.: Ballinger, 1980).

17. For overviews of the turbulent private health insurance market of the 1970s and 1980s, see John R. Griffith, "The Role of Blue Cross and Blue Shield in the Future U.S. Health Care System," *Inquiry,* vol. 20 (Spring 1983), pp. 12-19; and Pamela Farley Short, "Trends in Employee Health Benefits," *Health Affairs,* vol. 7, no. 3 (Summer 1988), pp. 186-196.

18. Lawrence D. Brown, *Politics and Health Care Organization: HMO's as Federal Policy* (Washington: Brookings Institution, 1983).

19. The trend toward self-financing by employers can be traced in successive issues of *Employee Benefits in Medium and Large Firms* (Washington: Bureau of Labor Statistics, Department of Labor, annual). The trend is explained in Ross H. Arnett and Gordon R. Trapnell, "Private Health Insurance: New Measures of a Complex and Changing Industry," *Health Care Financing Review,* vol. 6, no. 2 (Winter 1984), pp. 31-42, and in Patricia McDonnell and others, "Self-Insured Health Plans," *Health Care Financing Review,* vol. 8, no. 2 (Winter 1986), pp. 1-15. The work of the third-party administrators is summarized in David Manley, "Tapping the Talents of a TPA," *Best's Review—Life/Health Insurance Edition,* vol. 88, no. 2 (June 1988), pp. 82-88.

20. *A Course in Group Life and Health Insurance,* rev. ed. (Washington: Health Insurance Association of America, 1985), pt. A, pp. 273-275.

21. Ruth Levitt and Andrew Wall, *The Reorganised National Health Service,* 3rd ed. (London: Croom Helm, 1984); and John Fry and others, *NHS Data Book* (Lancaster: MTP Press, 1984).

22. S. R. Diacon, *United Kingdom Insurance Industry: Structure, Development and Market Prospects to 1990* (London: Staniland Hall Associates, 1985).

23. Ben Griffith and others, *Banking on Sickness: Commercial Medicine in Britain and the USA* (London: Lawrence and Wishart, 1987), chap. 3; William Laing, *Private Health Care* (London: Office of Health Economics, 1985), chap. 3; and Nick Bosanquet, "Private Health Insurance in Britain and the National Health Service," *Geneva Papers on Risk and Insurance,* vol. 12, no. 45 (Oct. 1987), pp. 350-357.

24. Explained in Glaser, *Paying the Hospital* (see note 11 above), pp. 366-368.

25. Klim McPherson and others, "Increasing Use of Private Practice by Patients in Oxford Requiring Common Elective Surgical Operations," *British Medical Journal,* vol. 291, no. 6498 (Sept. 21, 1985), pp. 797-799.

26. Consider, for example, the recent attempts by some American HMOs to keep discontented subscribers by relaxing the "lock-in." In "open-ended HMOs," the patient may consult an out-of-plan doctor and receive partial reimbursement. See Judith A. Hale and Mary M. Hunter, *From HMO Movement to Managed Care Industry* (Excelsior, Minn.: InterStudy, 1988); and Robert Feldman and others, "Health Maintenance Organizations: The Beginning or the End?",

Health Services Research, vol. 24, no. 2 (June 1989), pp. 192–211. The open-ended option may increase the HMO's difficulties in fulfilling its commitments to its own provider panel and in staying within budget, according to early experience by the CIGNA Corporation, America's leading managed-care insurer. Disputes between the plan and its doctors over referrals and assumption of out-of-plan claims are described in Paul J. Kenkel, " 'Open-Ended' Plans Pose Risks to Providers," *Modern Healthcare,* vol. 19 (Aug. 25, 1989), pp. 68–69.

27. David Mechanic, "Consumer Choice Among Health Insurance Options," *Health Affairs,* vol. 8, no. 1 (Spring 1989), pp. 138–148; Fred J. Hellinger, "Selection Bias in Health Maintenance Organizations: Analysis of Recent Evidence," *Health Care Financing Review,* vol. 9, no. 2 (Winter 1987), pp. 55–63; and Michael D. Rosko and Robert W. Broyles, *The Economics of Health Care* (New York: Greenwood Press, 1988), pp. 332–336 and sources cited.

28. The chronic underwriting losses of the 1980s are reported in "Accident and Health Premiums," *Best's Review: Life/Health Insurance Edition,* annual in every December issue.

29. The less centralized a private market, the higher the administrative and marketing costs. See Roger D. Blair and Ronald Vogel, *The Cost of Health Insurance Administration: An Economic Analysis* (Lexington, Mass.: Heath, 1975). In the United States, Medicare has lower administrative costs and lower retention rates than private health insurance; the Social Security Administration and state Medicaid agencies have lower administrative costs than the private fiscal intermediaries, despite their higher wage rates: William Hsiao, "Public versus Private Administration of Health Insurance: A Study in Relative Economic Efficiency," *Inquiry,* vol. 15, no. 4 (Dec. 1978), pp. 379–387; Alice M. Rivlin and Joshua M. Wiener, *Caring for the Disabled Elderly* (Washington: Brookings Institution, 1988), p. 213. Within the United States, the more socially oriented Blue Cross Plans have lower administrative costs and lower retention ratios than the commercial carriers: Kuo-cheng Tseng, "Administrative Costs of Medicare Contractors: Blue Cross Plans versus Commercial Intermediaries," *Inquiry,* vol. 15, no. 4 (Dec. 1978), pp. 371–378. The American financing system has much higher administrative costs than the publicly administered National Health Service of Great Britain and the publicly financed Canadian arrangements: David U. Himmelstein and Steffie Woolhandler, "Cost Without Benefit: Administrative Waste in U.S. Health Care," *New England Journal of Medicine,* vol. 314 (Feb. 13, 1986), pp. 441–445.

30. Described in *Abuses in the Sale of Health Insurance to the Elderly in Supplementation of Medicare: A National Scandal,* Comm. Pub. 95-160 (Washington: Select Committee on Aging, U.S. House of Representatives, 1978); and in two public hearings that followed this report: *Abuses in the Sale of Health Insurance to the Elderly* and *Fraudulent Medical and Insurance Promotions: Cleveland, Ohio,* Comm. Pub. 95-165 and Comm. Pub. 97-369 (Washington: Select Committee on Aging, U.S. House of Representatives, 1978 and 1982).

31. M. Susan Marquis, "Consumers' Knowledge About Their Health In-

surance Coverage," *Health Care Financing Review*, vol. 5, no. 1 (Fall 1983), pp. 65–80; Nelda McCall and others, "Consumer Knowledge of Medicare and Supplemental Health Insurance Benefits," *Health Services Research*, vol. 20, no. 6 (Feb. 1986), pp. 633–657; and Thomas Rice and others, *Older Americans and Their Health Coverage* (Washington: Health Insurance Association of America, 1989), pp. 7–12.

32. Michael J. McNamara, "The OASDI Early Retirement-Medicare Gap," *Benefits Quarterly*, vol. 3, no. 2 (Second Quarter 1987), pp. 8–17; and Jonathan C. Dopkeen, "Postretirement Health Benefits," *Health Services Research*, vol. 21, no. 6 (Feb. 1987), pp. 795–848.

PART TWO

Financing
Health Insurance

The next five chapters describe the sources of money for health insurance under both statutory and private programs. Chapter Five summarizes the variations in payroll tax systems under social security among developed countries and discusses the place of the health insurance accounts in these programs. The equity and consequences of payroll taxes have been questioned in several countries, and Chapter Six presents the issues and summarizes the unsuccessful search for better methods.

Instead of percentage-of-earnings rates, private commercial insurance uses flat rates for classes of risks. These premium systems are described in Chapter Seven. (A few countries use age-of-entry lifetime premiums.) But payroll taxes are not adequate to cover all subscribers in systems dedicated to social solidarity and equal entitlement for all. Chapters Eight and Nine describe the government subsidies and interfund transfers that remedy shortfalls.

CHAPTER 5

Social Security
Payroll Taxes

───────────── **Summary** ─────────────

Social security in general and statutory health insurance in particular usually depend on payroll taxes. A proportion is levied on each employee's earnings, and the employer adds a matching or higher percentage. As health insurance costs have risen, the proportions rise—particularly on the employer—and the ceiling on taxable wages rises or is eliminated.

Payroll taxes are associated with statutory health insurance. The Parliament usually enacts specific rates on entire classes of the compulsorily insured. In Germany, an exceptional case, the principle of payroll taxes is obligatory, but each health insurance carrier may fix the rates it wishes in accord with its financial needs and design of benefits. Quoting lower rates may be an instrument of competition for subscribers, although usually carriers compete by offering more generous benefits and customer services.

Rates may vary by economic sector. Some politically influential occupations—such as farmers and the self-employed—may obtain slightly lower rates from Parliament without loss of benefits. In order to combat deficits, governments recently have begun to impose premiums on the elderly and unemployed. These persons' claims of financial deprivation conflict with the health insurance system's need to cover their costs.

Sickness funds used to be allowed considerable discretion in fixing their rates. Since the payroll taxes are really acts of government, however, finance officials now play a bigger role in examining the sickness funds' accounts and setting the rates. Governments now limit the annual increases in payroll taxes and impose cost containment upon the health insurance carriers and the providers.

Private insurance carriers do not become involved in these public decisions. Their premiums are related to the benefits purchased, not to the subscribers' incomes. Most of the essentially private American health financing market is governed by such independent decisions by insurance carriers. America's only form of statutory health insurance—Medicare—is part of Social Security, uses payroll taxes, and follows government decisions as in any other country.

Options

A health insurance carrier can obtain its revenues from any of the following sources:[1]

☐ *Capitation payments from each subscriber.* The same amount applies to each regardless of income, personal traits, or medical risk.
☐ *A flat rate to cover the subscriber's risk to the carrier:*
  • Individual rates may be calculated for each individual subscriber. Or rates may be calculated for different degrees of risk, and each subscriber is assigned to a class.
  • The entire group (such as all employees of one business firm or all members of a professional association) may be "experience-rated" by the group's past claims history. The employer or the association pays a lump sum to cover all members' probable costs for the next year.
☐ *A proportion of each subscriber's income.*

In theory, a carrier should be self-sustaining from its collection of premiums or statutory payroll taxes. In practice, however, sickness funds cannot cover their full costs and thus receive subsidies from government or equalization transfers from each other. These measures are discussed in Chapters Eight and Nine.

Under modern social insurance, there are several alternative methods of designing payroll taxes and premiums:

☐ Construction of rates:
  • Percentage of:
    ★ All income
    ★ Earnings from work
  • By class of risk, where risks are defined by:
    ★ Age (subscriber's current age or age of entry)
    ★ Sex
    ★ Occupation
    ★ Lifestyle
☐ Rates set by:
  • Law passed by Parliament
  • Rate regulator in government
  • Each sickness fund

☐   Uniformity:
  • Standard throughout the country
  • Varies among sickness funds according to:
    ★ Formula in the law
    ★ Each fund's costs and marketing strategy
☐   With or without an earnings ceiling
☐   Division between the subscriber and his employer
☐   Special rules for self-employed
☐   Reductions or exemptions for:
  • Pensioners
  • Disabled
  • Unemployed
  • Low-income earners
☐   Relation to other social security taxes
☐   Whether deductible from the income base of:
  • Subscriber
  • Employer
☐   Family coverage:
  • One premium for the entire family
  • Separate premiums for each family member

In the following discussion, I employ the American usage by calling stat-utory insurance deductions "payroll taxes." In other countries, the word "tax" is often reserved for levies on income or on business transactions that go into the Treasury. These countries refer to the health insurance and social security pay-ments as "contributions"—for example, *cotisations* in French and *Beiträge* in German.

Historical Development

For centuries, the guilds and mutual aid societies charged their members capi-tation rates—that is, a fixed amount of money per year. It was collected in one lump sum or in installments upon two or three feast days during the year. In addition, the guild collected an initiation fee when the person was admitted as a master or as a journeyman. These amounts did not vary by income or by family size.[2] Some guilds collected additional funds by charging the master a small amount of money for each product he sold to his customers. These total payments therefore were somewhat proportional to members' incomes.

But insurance companies had long charged risk-based premiums. If the owner of a ship bought insurance against its loss, he and the carrier negotiated a single premium for each voyage. If the owner of a building bought insurance against its destruction by fire, the carrier charged an annual premium that might remain the same or might vary as risks and costs changed. Commercial insurance companies entered health in the late nineteenth century, when governments passed laws defining accidents of workers as risks that employers should bear. Throughout Europe and North America, employers bought policies to cover their risks of liability for workers' medical care and invalidity payments, and they negotiated premiums with commercial insurance companies to cover the particular risks of their factories and work forces.

During the twentieth century, insurance companies began to offer individual policies providing cash benefits in case of illness. They used the customary actuarial reasoning of private insurance of individuals: premium classes were designed for the principal dimensions associated with differential risk (sex, age, occupation, and community). The morbidity and mortality experience of each class was calculated from demographic data. All persons falling into a class would share the rating of that class. The individual could buy more coverage by paying a premium calculated as a multiple of the class rate. This methodology has been followed in commercial health insurance ever since.

The mutual aid societies that became the carriers under statutory health insurance during the late nineteenth and early twentieth centuries could not adopt this method of charging premiums. The method would have led to much higher premiums for the elderly and the less healthy, much lower premiums for young men. Such actuarial discrimination fundamentally contradicted the philosophy of the mutual aid societies, which were often socialist or Catholic in origin. Since they practiced social solidarity—whereby everybody contributed to help the weaker—their capitation payments put all payers on the same footing. Instead of placing greater financial burdens on the weak, the changes in the capitation system went in the opposite direction: increasing the contributions from the better off. If rates varied by age, the older members were charged less, not more.

Even before governments began to enact compulsory health insurance laws in the late nineteenth century, some mutual aid societies tried to collect higher subscription fees from their members in the better-paid occupations. When governments enacted laws and specified the bases for contributions, the mutual aid societies could shed inhibitions about asking their members' earnings. The laws required disclosures of earnings, since they specified different ways of collecting more money from the better paid. Disclosure of each person's income for the entire social security package was necessary also because the new old-age and disability pension laws accompanying health insurance were based on earnings: the better paid would earn higher pensions by paying higher premiums.

At first, as in Germany, simple methods of graduated premiums were used by the sickness funds: all covered workers were placed in a few income classes, and each higher-income class made a slightly higher cash payment to the sickness fund. The income classes and premiums were discrete, not continuous, variables, but the actuaries who planned the policy options and monitored the funds thought in variable terms. Their papers reported that total revenue was a certain percentage of total wages, and it became easy to think of the average premium as this percentage of the average wage.

Another source of the shift toward percentage calculations was the upper limit in the first German health insurance law. The sickness funds were free to set any premiums, but the law forbade them to collect more than 1.5 percent of the daily wages of laborers in some funds and more than 2 to 3 percent of the daily wages of more skilled workers in certain other associations. Unexpectedly, these clauses became invitations to sickness funds to adopt those rates as standard for all.

For several decades, sickness funds and governmental social security laws adopted a great variety of capitation rates, progressive but discrete premiums, and percentage deductions.[3] Eventually all social security payroll taxes in nearly all countries became defined as percentages of each worker's earnings and percentages of each employer's payroll.

Percentage of Payroll for Basic Health Insurance

Basic Insurance Rates. In nearly every country today, social security pension funds are financed from payroll taxes. When statutory health insurance is an integral part of social security, it too is financed by payroll taxes. Here, for example, is an illustration from the Netherlands in 1987:

	Employer	*Employee*	*To be paid up to maximum earnings of*
Medical care	4.90%	4.90%	f. 161/day
Invalidity cash benefits	5.35%	1.00%	f. 262/day

The medical care accounts are distinguished from the invalidity payments accounts, governments can monitor their different trends in costs, and therefore the tax rates are often distinguished. But the sickness funds usually administer both.

Taxable earnings limits have existed in social security since the higher-paid managers, craftsmen, and self-employed were added. If any Dutch employee earned more than an average f. 161 per day, he paid no more than $(4.90) \times (f. 161)$ = f. 7.89 per day. (The exchange rate for the Dutch guilder in mid-1987 was f. 1 = $0.48 U.S.) The Dutch employer matches the worker's contribution to sickness insurance, using the same ceiling. In many countries, the employer's contribution is a higher percentage than the employee's, but both worker and employer are taxed up to the same ceiling.

Some groups are fully covered by the basic health insurance program, but they pay lower rates. Examples are the elderly and the unemployed. In some countries, these groups might be recorded in accounts separate from those of the economically active. An example was the pensioners in Holland until 1986, the *bejaardenverzekering.* The separate account was designed to identify the special category of sickness fund enrollees not covered by full payroll taxes who had unusual costs and needed special subsidies. But now the Dutch pensioners keep their previous social and private carriers, and their accounts are merged into each carrier's full membership.

Special Health Programs. Every country has several health-related programs under social security, each with its own funds and payroll taxes. Most countries cover medical and invalidity payments for work injuries as separate accounts financed by their own payroll taxes. In several countries, this was the first social security program enacted and settled a long dispute over employers' liability for work injuries. Because employers were usually considered fully liable for injuries in the absence of workers' negligence, they cover the payroll tax in full. Usually the rate varies among industries according to their risks (established by their history of accidents and occupational diseases). The rates apply to the employer's entire payroll, and there is no income ceiling.

The invalidity cash benefit rates in Holland quoted earlier are unusual—they are high and include a payroll tax on the workers—because they cover both work injury and temporary invalidity not caused by a work injury. Holland also has a special social security program for long-term care and other matters: the General Law for Exceptional Medical Expenses (the *Algemene Wet Bijzondere Ziektekosten,* or AWBZ). This too is financed by a payroll tax on earnings, according to its own formula, and is described in Chapter Fifteen.

Variations. A payroll tax is a law of the Parliament and is usually the same throughout the country for all carriers and regions. If the law leaves to the sickness fund the tasks of fixing and collecting the premiums, each fund might have a slightly different rate to cover its own risks. In Germany, for example, the law requires equal rates for worker and employer, but each sickness fund sets its own rates according to its financial needs. The German rates vary between 3.50 and 8.00 percent on the worker and the same on the employer. With younger membership and administrative support from employers, *Betriebskrankenkassen* have lower rates than *Ortskrankenkassen.*

If wages of health care employees cause medical costs to vary among regions, each sickness fund may keep its accounts by region and therefore charge different rates across the nation. Examples are countries (like Germany and Switzerland) with federal systems of government and federal systems of health care organization.

Division Between Worker and Employer. The guilds consisted of self-employed craftsmen and merchants, and each paid his own dues in full. The mutual aid societies at first were created entirely by workers and each member paid in full. Some mutual aid societies were created by the workers in a single plant, and employers in dangerous industries were interested in helping them. (If the sickness funds provided the workers satisfactory invalidity payments and medical care in case of accidents at work, the employer might not be held liable in a court case.) Before the enactment of statutory health insurance, therefore, owners of coal mines and dangerous factories in Germany, France, and Belgium encouraged creation of sickness funds with administrative support and cash grants.

When the imperial government of Germany adopted social security during the 1880s, each program was introduced to the Parliament and enacted separately. Political parties oriented toward employers held many seats, the government's leadership tilted toward business rather than toward workers, and business was expected to pay some but not most of the costs. Replacing employers' legal liability for accidents at the workplace, a separate accident insurance arrangement was financed entirely by employers. Therefore, health insurance covering non-work-connected illness and accidents was financed primarily but not entirely by the workers: the employer was required to pay to the sickness fund one-third of the worker's premium; in the many *Betriebskrankenkassen* located at the employer's factory and managed with his help, he might contribute more. Workers and employers equally divided the premiums for old-age and disability pensions.

Other countries followed in enacting a menu of social security programs, each with a different mix of employer/employee contributions. The trade unions and political parties of the Left were the principal forces urging governments to add new programs, expand benefits, and raise new money. They pressed to raise payroll taxes on the most promising source of new money: the employers. To demonstrate their social consciousness, governments of the Right sometimes expanded and improved the organization of social security. They preferred to distribute the tax burden between employers and employees, rather than burdening the employers excessively.

Eventually, after World War II, certain patterns evolved: the payroll taxes for pensions were divided nearly 50–50; accident insurance was paid for entirely by employers; unemployment insurance was paid for primarily by the employers. But there was no standard division, and employers paid higher proportions for pensions in some countries. Gradually employers were taxed at higher rates for health insurance, and their share is now half or (usually) more. By the 1980s, employers in developed countries paid in social security taxes between 20 and 30 percent of their payrolls. For health insurance alone and for the total social security package (pensions, work accidents, unemployment insurance, family allowances, and health), the rates as of July 1988 in percentage of wages were:[4]

| | Health insurance | | All social security | |
	Employer	Employee	Employer	Employee
France	12.60	5.90	37.77	15.41
West Germany	6.00	6.00	18.90	17.50
Belgium	6.00	3.70	34.83	12.07
Netherlands	14.80	5.90	26.08	34.58
United States	1.45	1.45	15.05	7.15

The German insurance rate in the table is an estimated average. The American rate is the one used for the only health component of Social Security (the hospital insurance part of Medicare).

Belgium seems to collect less money from employees than other European countries. But the percentage seems lower only because Belgium has no ceiling for health insurance: the full rate of 3.70 percent was collected from the higher-salaried as well as from the lower-paid. Belgium eliminated the ceiling for health insurance during the mid-1970s, one of the first countries to do so. Increasing the rate is more visible and more contentious politically.

Switzerland does not fit into the employer/employee format, since health insurance and work injuries are not financed by payroll taxes. The burden on German employers is higher than appears in the foregoing data, since they pay short-term invalidity payments by continuing to pay the workers' wages.

Earnings Ceilings. Every country's social security system has a limit. It might distinguish between the eligible and ineligible: persons above certain annual earnings are not required to join and are not taxed. Or the ceiling might define the limit of the taxable wage base. Higher earners may be compulsorily insured, but they pay contributions only on the specified earnings from work.

Usually countries increase the ceiling every year, since the revenue of social security must cover its costs, which constantly rise. The government rate setters may increase the ceiling every year in accordance with the rise in a national index of wages, as they do in the French Ministry of Social Affairs and the American Social Security Administration. This method, less contentious than consulting among interest groups every year, is more likely to yield increases in the ceiling that will bring in enough revenue to keep pace with mounting program costs.[5] On the other hand, increases determined automatically by the index without human judgment—as in the American Social Security system—are never practiced in Europe.

The taxable earnings ceiling may apply to some social security programs but not to others. In France, for example, it applies to the payroll taxes for pensions but not for health insurance. How France gradually lifted the ceiling for health insurance is described in Chapter Six.

Cash Flow. Collections are always administered by the employers, as one of their contributions to social security. They deduct all social taxes from the weekly or monthly paychecks of employees, add their own contributions, and send the total amounts to the collection agencies of the social security system.

Someone must make sure that every employer transmits the right amount for every worker. This immense task is always decentralized. There are two principal methods of decentralization:

☐   *By industrial sector.* The Dutch economy is divided into twenty-five sectors, each led by a trade association (a *bedrijfsvereniging*) governed by a council representing the workers and employers in that industry. The association performs several social security functions, including collecting the payroll taxes for all the employment-based social security programs, such as health insurance. Each trade association sends the money to the central funds of the different social security programs. For example, it sends the health insurance money to the central fund (the *Algemene Kas*) managed by the *Ziekenfondsraad*. The *Ziekenfondsraad* then distributes the money among the subscribers' sickness funds, who pay the subscribers' bills. Legally, all these agencies are nongovernmental.[6] Other Dutch health insurance programs, particularly AWBZ, have slightly different taxing systems and their own collection agencies.

☐ *By region.* The general regime of France has one collection agency (*union de recouvrement*) in each *département*, totaling 105 altogether. Each has a governing board representing trade unions and employers in the area. The *unions* collect all the payroll taxes for the health insurance, pensions, and family allowances in the general regime. Information in this highly automated system is processed at regional centers. The *unions* forward the cash to the central office in Paris, the *Agence Centrale des Organismes de Sécurité Sociale* (ACOSS), which also receives subsidies from the government. ACOSS then divides the money among the national *caisses* for health insurance, pensions, and family allowances. CNAMTS for health then passes the money down to the regional and grass-roots *caisses* to cover the costs of the subscribers. Legally, the *unions* are private entities in the public service whereas ACOSS is a government agency.[7] The other special regimes have their own collection agencies.

A large fraction of the country's money constantly passes through these channels. Nowadays the work is done electronically and through bank transfers, and it can be very efficient if organized and centralized properly. For example, the French system has handled steadily more money (1.5 trillion francs in 1986) and has absorbed a steadily smaller proportion in administration costs (0.47 percent in 1983).[8]

These agencies have the difficult task of pursuing employers who pay late or not at all. During business recessions, more employers fail to pay and—if they go out of business—never pay at all. In France in the mid-1980s, over 2 percent of the recorded obligations have been bad debts.[9] Despite their employers' default, the workers remain covered in full by the health insurance system. Apart from these shortfalls, a large and probably growing number of employers and workers evade social security taxes by operating in the "underground economy."

If a country still has many sickness funds and each employer's work force is spread among them, a method must channel the payroll taxes—varying among paychecks—to the right places. Belgium solves the problem by merely expecting the employer to send the money to the collection agency, not to keep track of his workers' affiliations. The employer deducts the premiums from the worker's paycheck and gives him a receipt. Each *mutualité* gathers the receipts from all its subscribers, sends them to the collection agency, and is paid its share of the payroll taxes and the government subsidy. The system is an incentive for competition among the *mutualités,* since the subsidy is based on the number of subscribers and receipts.

How Rates Are Decided

There are several methods for deciding the rates for a country's health insurance payroll taxes. The topics for decision are:

- ☐ Site of the decision:
  - Sickness funds
  - Ministry of the government (particularly Health or Finance)
- ☐ Whether the rate must be formally enacted by Parliament
- ☐ Use of indexes and other automatic formulas
- ☐ Criteria for an increase:
  - Prospective costs of health care
  - Fiscal capacity of the sickness funds
  - Effects on the economy (particularly on employment and manufacturers' sales prices)
  - Ability of the government to cover deficits by subsidies
- ☐ Relationship to the rest of social security:
  - Health insurance rates decided separately
  - Entire set of social security rates decided together

Following are the decision-making methods employed by the principal European countries.

The Netherlands. National governments were essential to the creation of modern health care financing: they enacted health insurance laws and required collection of the previously voluntary premiums. After these initial steps, governments were very permissive, allowing providers to increase their charges rapidly, permitting carriers to increase their premiums, and covering the premium increases in the tax laws. Recently all national governments have tried to control health care costs strictly. One method has been to limit the annual increases in the payroll taxes. In many cases, the procedure for deciding the rates has changed. A good example of this history is the Netherlands.

At one time, Dutch government was very limited. The sickness funds and health providers were private. Many sectors in the Dutch economy settled prices, wages, and other matters by negotiation, often through standing councils. Instead of allowing conflicts of interest to be settled by power bargaining and strikes, Holland tried to ensure social harmony by using generally accepted economic indexes. For example, wages in much of the economy might be tied to annual increases in the prices of a market basket of supplies.

From its creation in 1949, two of the most important functions of the *Ziekenfondsraad* were to evaluate the financial needs of the sickness funds and recommend the annual increases in payroll taxes. (The following discussion concentrates on statutory health insurance, but the *Ziekenfondsraad* performed the same tasks for AWBZ.) Its Statistical Department constantly monitored health care costs and utilization under insurance, noted trends in the reserves of the sickness funds, and predicted health insurance costs for the next year. The statisticians used the Central Planning Bureau's annual report about past and probable future trends in indexes of prices and wages as the most authoritative basis for predicting the future. Hospital wages, for example, were tied to these indexes. The *Ziekenfondsraad* administered the *Algemene Kas* of the health insurance system and sought payroll tax rates that would keep a reserve equal to 6 percent of annual expenditure. The Statistical Department recommended a rate—often several rates based on slightly different predictions about the economy.[10] The department sent a detailed report every year to the *Ziekenfondsraad* governing board, which adopted the rate recommendation with only rare and small changes (for example, 9.2 percent instead of 9.3 percent). The Ministry of Health nearly always accepted the advice, and the Parliament enacted the rate. Payroll taxes for health insurance and for each of the other social security programs were decided separately rather than in an integrated way. The economy grew and seemed able to support many rising payroll taxes; social security was expected to provide people with what they needed.

During the 1970s, the economies of Europe could no longer support such permissive rate setting. Health care costs were growing faster than the revenue of the sickness funds, even when the payroll tax rates rose every year. The Dutch national government was being pressed to cover deficits in the health insurance accounts by subsidies, but this measure simply transferred the deficits to the government's budget. The total payroll taxes for all social security programs had become very high, arousing complaints by employers and leading to high prices for manufactures and services.

The Dutch national government then intervened to control the costs of health insurance and social security generally, and its role has steadily grown. One method was direct control over the health provider costs that would be charged to health insurance. The leading example was creation of a strict agency that set hospital charges and managed the negotiation of physicians' fees.[11] The method of deciding the health insurance rates has been changed both in procedure and in sites. It is no longer merely a method of raising money to cover the costs of health care providers; it is now an integral part of the national government's financial decisions.

The Statistical Department of the *Ziekenfondsraad* still prepares an annual report about trends in health care costs, the revenue from payroll taxes, and the financial situations of the sickness funds. The *Ziekenfondsraad* governing board continues to examine the report, recommends health insurance premiums to achieve certain financial targets, and in midyear forwards the report and its recommendations to the Ministry of Health (at present called the *Ministerie van Welzijn, Volksgezondheid en Cultuur,* or WVC). At this point, the decisions about the payroll tax rate begin. The staff of the Finance and Control Division of WVC has developed its own research capability, studies the *Ziekenfondsraad* report, and consults with many officials in WVC and other Ministries concerning probable trends next year in health care costs and social security revenue. The WVC staff learns about new policies of the government that will reduce health costs, such as plans to reduce the number of hospital beds.

The payroll taxes for all social security programs are now decided together in accordance with the government's economic policies. During July and subsequent months, the Prime Minister and four other key economic Ministers (for Finance, Social Affairs, Economic Affairs, and Internal Affairs) set the goals for the budget, taxes, and policies next year. During the mid- and late 1980s—in order to eliminate the deficit and reduce taxes—they recommended overall cuts in three principal sectors: social insurance, the general budget, and government employment. The Ministries in each sector may be instructed to limit specific programs; more often, they have discretion to find and implement the cuts themselves.

At the end of August, civil servants from the Ministries of WVC, Social Affairs,[12] and Finance meet to discuss the payroll tax rates for all of social security, beginning next January. Their decisions depend on the policy goals set by the five key Ministers:

☐ If the goal is to put more cash into the hands of the population, the civil servants set the entire package of social security payroll taxes at a level lower than is actuarially required to maintain the current reserves in each fund.

☐ If the goal is to let the lower-income groups keep as much cash as possible, the payroll tax percentages are kept nearly the same.

☐ If the goal is to shift the tax burden more toward the higher earners, the earnings ceiling is increased while the percentages stay nearly the same.

Because of the constant pressure to cover mounting social costs, these policies have been implemented incompletely. During the 1980s, the income ceilings remained the same in Dutch basic health insurance but rose steadily according to a national wage index for pensions, AWBZ, and several other social security programs. Despite the aim of enabling the workers to keep more of their cash, the health insurance premiums have had to be increased slightly.

Formerly the burden was shifted from the worker to the employer in Holland and the rest of Europe by increasing the employer-paid share faster than the percentage on the worker's paycheck to meet the need for more revenue. The relative burden on the Dutch employer never reached the levels in other countries, such as France and Belgium, described earlier. It has long been customary in Holland that employers and workers pay the same proportions for basic health insurance (with the same earnings ceiling). During the period of economic over-confidence in the 1960s, the Dutch government placed upon the employers the entire payroll tax rate for the additional health insurance program (AWBZ). Dutch policymakers now share the widespread European fear—summarized in the next chapter—that the tax burden on employers makes exports too expensive and discourages employment. Therefore the Dutch continue to divide the payroll taxes equally between worker and employer.

Tradeoffs used to be made between raising payroll taxes and turning to the general Treasury. Originally health insurance was privately financed completely from premiums and the payroll taxes. During the 1970s, the ideology of social solidarity led to a change: leaders in the Dutch sickness funds and in the social insurance Ministries argued that it was more socially equitable to use revenue derived from progressive taxes (such as the income tax supporting government budgets) than from flat and regressive taxes (such as the social security payroll taxes on earnings from work). Normally opposed to this thinking, the Ministry of Finance went along, fearful that the payroll taxes were destroying exports and domestic employment.[13] Thus, the Ministry of Health budgets for several years in the late 1970s and 1980s contained steadily mounting subsidies for both basic health insurance and AWBZ. But these subsidies, described in Chapter Eight, merely transferred the deficit from the sickness funds to the national government's budget. During the 1980s, the Cabinet struggled to eliminate the government's budget deficit, to reduce the resulting inflation, and to lessen the public share in the economy. So, through the social security system, the government pressed either to limit expenditures to each program's payroll taxes or to substitute a special tax instead of the government subsidy (as in AWBZ). Basic health insurance was the only social security program still subsidized in the early 1990s—primarily to cover the costs of the elderly—but the trend even there was toward self-financing.

When setting the payroll tax rates and subsidies, the policymakers now deliberately try to force each social security program to impose economies upon its providers and beneficiaries so that the program can operate within its means. Often this requires changes in the statutes (written by the Ministry of Social Affairs and enacted by Parliament) and tighter administration. For example, the Dutch disability benefits program has long been thought too generous: many persons fit for some sort of work were receiving full benefits; a substantial payroll tax had to be paid by employers.[14] During the mid-1980s, the disability pension was reduced, eligibility was tightened, and its payroll tax could be reduced. The policymakers tried to force economies throughout health insurance by refusing to increase the payroll tax automatically to cover costs and maintain a reserve. The reserve in the *Algemene Kas* was reduced during the 1980s and turned into a deficit. The *Ziekenfondsraad* borrowed from banks to pay the sickness funds' claims. WVC used its regulatory powers over health care providers to limit their prices and curb the proliferation of facilities, but it expected the *Ziekenfondsraad* to make the sickness funds more cost conscious. The *Raad* tightened many guidelines about benefits and utilization. It instituted stricter reporting and accounting by sickness funds generally. It appointed caretaker managers for a few spendthrift sickness funds.

The national health insurance laws of Europe authorize the Minister of Health or Minister of Social Affairs to issue each year's specific payroll tax rates. Therefore, when the Dutch civil servants have agreed on details, the State Secretary for WVC announces the new rates and the income ceiling during the final months of the year, to take effect the following January 1. This procedure avoids the American experience—namely, a debilitating political fight in Parliament over each year's rates or, in order to avoid the struggle, fixing the rates automatically according to a multiyear economic index.

France. Holland illustrates the gradual evolution of government authority over the payroll tax in an originally private health insurance system. Even when the tax is fixed by law, government at first merely rubber-stamps private decisions. Eventually, the need to control taxes, spending, inflation, and employment places government in charge.

Where government itself is the carrier for health insurance, it decides from the start the health and other social security tax rates. An example is France. From 1945 to 1967, French social security for the general labor force had a single fund for both health insurance and pensions. It was financed throughout that time by a percentage of wages up to a ceiling, with the employer paying about two-thirds and the worker one-third. The employers' share approximately covered the current health care costs of the program; the workers' share approximately covered the current pension costs of the program. In 1960, for example, the employer had paid 12.50 percent and the worker 6.00 percent on every wage up to the annual ceiling of 7,080 F. As a result of the political disputes over the structure of the system, a separate *caisse* existed for the family allowances program, paid for entirely by the employer.[15] After 1967, health insurance and pensions were separated into distinct funds in the general regime and in the special regimes, and each had a distinct payroll tax, usually levied on employers and workers at different rates.

All these taxes are decided every year by the Prime Minister and the Cabinet on the basis of considerable research by several government agencies. Most work focuses on the payroll taxes of the general regimes. The principal analysts are in the Office for Administrative and Financial Affairs, Division of Social Security, Ministry of Social Affairs and Employment (*Ministère des Affaires Sociales*). For its calculations, the Office obtains information about recent trends and probable future scenarios from research offices in the Ministry of Social Affairs, the Bureau of the Census (INSEE), and the Ministry of Finance and Budget. The Office has the detailed annual reports of the authoritative nonpartisan *Commission des Comptes de la Sécurité Sociale*. From these sources the Office learns the recent trends and next year's prospects for numbers of workers (and, therefore, numbers of taxpayers), levels of salaries (and, therefore, revenue from the payroll taxes), retirement and births (and, therefore, the expected expenditures by the pension and family allowance funds), and prices (which will affect the expenditures for pensions, family allowances, and health care). Probable revenue and expenditures next year are simulated on the Ministry's computer. To estimate health care costs, the Office obtains data about recent utilization and spending from research offices within the Ministry of Social Affairs and CNAMTS.

The Office drafts its reports during the first half of the year (such as 1990) for payroll taxes that will go into effect next year (such as 1991). As the Office works, the data bearing on revenue and expenditure come in for the previous year (such as 1989). The Office monitors whether the current year's decisions have been successful—that is, whether ACOSS's collections are covering all health care bills under social security. While pensions and family allowances depend on easily predictable demography and rarely run unexpected deficits, health insurance has been chronically troublesome because of surprising increases in utilization, more expensive service intensity, and failure of cost containment policies. ACOSS could have obtained less revenue than expected because of a business recession or because the government's predictions of lower unemployment were disappointed. If deficits are being run currently, continuation or minor increases in current payroll tax rates will not be successful next year. (The goal is to maintain as a reserve in ACOSS at all times 10 to 12 percent of annual revenue.) If there is a current deficit in the current year's account, the Office of Administrative and Financial Affairs may recommend that the Cabinet increase the current payroll tax at once.

The Office must implement policy decisions by the Cabinet, since the majority party is committed to enacting the promises that got it elected. Some decisions have serious financial results—for example, the new Socialist government during 1981–1983 reduced the age for full pensions, increased family allowances, relaxed the eligibility for disability benefits, and altogether increased social security expenditures while reducing its revenue from payroll taxes. The Office must learn whether the Cabinet will continue its current level of subsidies to the social security accounts, whether more revenues must be sought from increasing the payroll taxes and raising the income ceiling, or whether—a perennial issue— the Cabinet will press for new forms of social security taxation. When preparing their final recommendations, the civil servants in the Office confer with their opposite numbers in the other Ministries (especially Finance and Budget). As well, they confer with their political superiors in the Cabinet: the Minister for Social Affairs and the Secretary of State for Social Security. If an important change is contemplated, the politicians might ask the leading interest groups (the trade unions and the employers association). A useful forum for discussion is the governing board of CNAMTS, where these interest groups are represented.

One option that the Office cannot recommend is saving money by reducing benefits. Whenever any government-of-the-day has proposed eliminating benefits or increasing patient cost sharing, it has been overwhelmed by protest demonstrations in the street of Paris and it has lost the next election. The Ministry tries to limit insurance costs by instructing its Division of Hospitals to regulate hospital rates more strictly and ration capital investment. But in the financing of statutory health insurance, the Office of Administration and Financial Affairs has only a limited choice among alternative taxes.

Late in the year, the Office sends its report and tax proposal for all social security programs in all regimes to its political superiors in the Ministry (that is, the Minister of Social Affairs, the Secretary of State for Social Security, and their personal staffs). Then the proposal about payroll taxes goes to the Prime Minister and the Cabinet. There it gets caught up in the annual struggle over the budget of the Ministry of Social Affairs. For some years, the budget has included subsidies enabling the general regime to cover the costs of its own subscribers who underpay (particularly the pensioners and the unemployed) and to cover transfers to other underfinanced regimes (particularly the farmers, miners, and railwaymen). The Ministry staff tries to avoid recommending higher payroll taxes by negotiating higher subsidies from the Ministry of Finance and Budget. The discussion over payroll taxes and subsidies occurs in midyear. Since Budget rarely gives Social Affairs as much as the latter wants, the issue is ultimately settled by the Prime Minister (and, often, by the President) during the autumn. During the 1970s and 1980s, the struggle over the accounts recurred every year and wore down its participants. Health care cost increases were the principal villain. But social security financing became more stable during the late 1980s, when health costs were controlled better.

The result in recent years has been a complex combination of several taxes with different formulas:

☐   Payroll taxes on employers and employees:
   •   Below and above the income ceiling. For many years, France—like other countries—levied the payroll tax on earnings up to a ceiling. From 1971 to 1984, in order to find more money, it levied two payroll taxes on both employer and worker: one rate on earnings up to the ceiling; a second one at a lower rate on the total earnings. Every few years, the proportion levied on total earnings rose. Finally, since 1984 the payroll taxes for both employer and worker have been collected from total earnings, resulting in very high collections from the highest earners. (The figures appear in Table 6.1.)
   •   Shares by employer and employee. To avoid burdening employment, the employer's rate has been kept the same since 1976. That rate was reduced slightly in 1984 to offset the elimination of the earnings ceiling on the employer's payroll tax. Increases in the payroll tax rates therefore have had to fall on the workers, but governments shrink from this step lest consumption be depressed and the voters be outraged. Nevertheless, the unavoidable emergency tax increase in mid-1987 had to fall on the workers. In late 1987, the rates were 12.6 percent on the employer and 5.9

percent on the worker. The once wide differential between employer and worker rates therefore narrowed.

- Other social security payroll taxes. Different rates with earnings ceilings were imposed at the same time for the retirement and family allowances programs.

☐ Special taxes levied from time to time and earmarked for the health insurance fund: for example, taxes on automobiles, tobacco, alcohol, and drug advertising.

☐ Special taxes on income that is not subject to payroll taxes. The money goes into the entire social security system; or it is earmarked at first for a politically appealing program and then can be used by the others under the equalization transfer system:

- A 1 percent tax on all personal income was imposed by the Socialist government from 1983 to 1986. This *impôt de solidarité* was officially earmarked for the family allowance fund, long a channel for transfers into others.

- A 1 percent tax on income from dividends and rents was imposed by the Conservative government as one of its emergency measures in 1987.

Belgium. Even if the sickness funds are strong private organizations with responsibility for administering benefits, government can decide the payroll taxes on the grounds that it is responsible for health insurance revenue and social security taxation. An example is Belgium.

Before Belgium enacted health insurance laws, the *mutualités* set and collected their own premiums. But government intervention in their revenue began early with annual subsidies from the 1890s. The premiums became a legal tax in 1963 when health insurance was added to the existing social security system, all programs to be financed by payroll taxes. The Ministry of Social Protection (*Ministère de la Prévoyance Sociale*) had long set policy for social security, including fixing the payroll taxes, and it simply added responsibility for health insurance revenue.

Belgium's INAMI—like Holland's *Ziekenfondsraad*—acts as an intermediary between the private health insurance carriers and the government. The governing boards and committees of both are drawn from the principal interest groups (the trade unions and employers) and from the adversaries in health care finance (the *mutualités*, the medical associations, and the other providers). While the research staff of the *Ziekenfondsraad* has long provided the initial input and (formerly) the predominant influence in setting the rates, the Ministry of Social Protection has never allowed INAMI to do this work. It is the Ministry of Social Protection and not INAMI that has the research staff and the data about the economy and labor force essential for insurance rate setting. INAMI collects utilization and expenditure information from the *mutualités* and passes it on to the Ministry's researchers. Their report about prospects for the social security system and the need for changes in the payroll taxes goes to the Minister for Social

Affairs, who is in charge of both the Ministry of Social Protection and the Ministry of Health.

All the decisions must be made inside the government, because they involve designing the payroll taxes and all other taxes together. Health insurance revenue comes from the payroll taxes and from subsidies from the general budgets of the Ministry of Social Protection and Ministry of Health. Every year, the taxes and subsidies are set by the Prime Minister and the leading members of the Cabinet. During the late 1970s and 1980s, Belgium was in constant financial crisis. The decisions—announced by the leading Cabinet members and then enacted by Parliament—have been designed not only to reduce the government's budgetary deficit but also to stimulate the economy. Increases in the payroll taxes—particularly the employers' shares—are avoided. Cuts are made in all government spending, and the subsidies to the sickness funds are reduced as well. The decisions include cuts in health insurance benefits. The Ministry of Health is pressed to tighten its regulations over hospital operating and capital costs, and it is instructed to order the closing of beds. INAMI is pressed to limit utilization of the ambulatory medical services.

Germany. When national health insurance is enacted, the premiums become part of the payroll taxes of social security, with percentages levied on workers and employers. As cost containment and tax restraint become more important, government exercises more authority over the rates.

One of the few exceptions is Germany, the first country that enacted national health insurance. The political tradeoffs in enacting the law produced a privatized rate-setting and collection method altogether different from the situation of the countries that followed. As often happens, the original political compromise acquired vested interests and is firmly implanted a century later.

As Chapter Three reported, Bismarck and Kaiser Wilhelm pushed statutory health insurance and other programs during the 1880s in large part to expand the functions of the new national government. An Imperial Insurance Institute would enroll members, collect payroll taxes, and pay benefits. Important blocs in the *Reichstag*—the businessmen, farmers, and trade unions—were willing to enact social security provided the national government did not administer it. The existing sickness funds were allowed to administer health insurance, and the *Ortskrankenkassen* were created as local units for those without workplace funds.[16] The statute merely required membership by certain classes of the population, authorized the sickness funds to collect premiums, set the division of the premium between employers and workers (now equal), authorized the national government to fix maximum premiums (a power long unused and now repealed), and listed the minimum benefits that the premiums must cover. Every sickness fund fiercely defends its autonomy from the government and sets whatever premiums it needs to cover its costs. The pension program under social security uses percentage-of-income payroll taxes, but it lacks special pension funds, so the sickness funds collect the pension premiums as well as their own. The employer deducts all the social security premiums from each worker's paycheck, adds his own contributions, and sends payments to the one or more sickness funds in his work force.

Every sickness fund has its own actuaries to calculate its own costs and set its own premiums.[17] Some uniformity in methods and results is due to regulations. Under the RVO statute, every sickness fund is supposed to be financially responsible with stable accounts and neither profits nor losses. An annual financial report with both recent costs and a prospective budget must be submitted to each sickness fund's own governing board (representing workers and employers). Then the report goes to a regulatory agency either of the provincial government (a *Landesversicherungsamt* for the sickness funds operating exclusively within the province) or of the national government (the *Bundesversicherungsamt* for the funds operating in more than one province, such as the *Ersatzkassen*). The regulatory agencies check that the interests of the subscribers are protected and the premiums are high enough to pay expected benefits. If the premiums seem too low or too high, the agency can order corrections. Considerable actuarial standardization results, because the reports and their accounting conventions apply to all sickness funds. (The national and provincial associations of sickness funds offer methodological guidance.) The national associations supply the individual funds with information about expected trends in the economy (affecting revenue) and trends in health care costs (affecting expenditures).

Because of decentralization, the demand for autonomy, and the variations in the funds' membership, the premiums differ more widely than under a fixed statutory payroll tax. Using community rating of their risks, the large *Ortskrankenkassen* do not vary so widely across Germany. Each must charge higher premiums if health care wages and costs are higher in its region, but these variations across Germany have been diminishing. *Betriebskrankenkassen* have low premiums if they are new, have many young workers, and have few retirees; but many have deteriorating dependency ratios, their premiums rise, and their young workers flee to the *Ersatzkassen*. The provincial association of *Betriebskrankenkassen* tries to limit the deterioration of viable funds by equalization transfers of money, but it guides others into mergers and dissolutions.[18]

United States. The Americans in 1934–1935 became the last developed country to enact social security. By then, payroll taxes on workers and employers were universal. If government injected money from general revenue, as in Belgium, these were limited subsidies intended to restrain increases in the payroll tax. The deductions from payrolls were thought part of a social compact between employers and workers.

The Americans were heirs of Anglo-Saxon self-interested individualism, and the European philosophy and methods of social solidarity were less influential. The Anglo-Saxons have defined social programs as charity, a fallback because of failures of private enterprise, to be paid for temporarily by government and phased out eventually. Britain, Canada, and other Anglo-Saxon countries have relied on full Treasury financing for certain programs that Europe supports by different methods. Therefore, the first American plans for a pension system during the early 1930s provided for a small payroll tax in the first years and predominantly Treasury financing thereafter. This design had a practical justi- fication as well: the Americans sometimes introduce major programs during severe crises when normal solutions are difficult. Old-age pensions, for example, were introduced at the depths of the Depression of the 1930s, when it was feared that workers and employers could not bear mounting payroll taxes and progres- sive taxation on the wealthy might provide a larger base.

The Roosevelt administration saw political dangers in general Treasury financing: when the conservatives and Big Business regained office, they would reduce Treasury funding and destroy the pension system. If the payroll tax be- came the primary financing method, however, the workers would feel they had personally paid for their pensions, they would protect Social Security against attack, and the program would be insulated from budgetary politics.[19]

Therefore, lacking a prior history of mutual assistance funds, the Amer- icans in 1935 created a European-type statutory pension program. A trust fund was created, governed by public trustees, managed generally by the Department of the Treasury, and monitored and planned in its financial details by actuaries in a special Social Security Administration. It has never received general revenue but has been financed fully by payroll taxes. The actuaries calculate whether payroll tax increases are needed to maintain "actuarial soundness" in the long run. Congress has the last word, often expanding benefits for political reasons and enacting increases in the payroll tax and the earnings base in order to pre- serve actuarial soundness.[20] Since the American Social Security system had been enacted late and would not mature for some time, it accumulated large surpluses in the trust funds. Thus, Congress optimistically expanded benefits during the 1950s and 1960s. When the actuaries recommended increases in the payroll taxes, Congress enacted them. The economy was prosperous, the initial rates had been set too low, and the increases seemed painless and reasonable.[21]

Medicare was enacted in 1965 as a hybrid: hospital finance would now become part of Social Security. Since physicians opposed integration into Social Security and preferred voluntary private insurance, an ambiguous (and ulti- mately unmanageable) method was devised. The hospital finance part mimicked the established pension and disability parts of Social Security: a Hospital Insur- ance Trust Fund joined the two other trust funds; it was financed by a payroll tax and would be managed by the Treasury and monitored by actuaries. Congress would have the final voice in deciding benefits and tax rates.[22] Medicare differs from every other country's statutory health insurance, since the payers of the payroll tax are entirely different from the beneficiaries. The payroll tax is small and unnoticed by nearly all payers; as previous pages in this chapter show, statutory health insurance for entire populations in Europe produces large and controversial payroll taxes.

By the late 1970s in the United States, both the Old Age and Survivors

Insurance and Hospital Insurance Trust Funds faced imminent deficits. Not only had Congress improved benefits for both, but spending was rising much faster than revenue from the payroll taxes. Congress had indexed pensions against inflation, and inflation increased rapidly while the economy—that is, the revenue base—stagnated. Hospital costs seemed uncontrollable. The aging of the population would have strained both programs even under the best of circumstances. The payroll taxes once had been kept stable for years at a time; now they were increased every few years and began to evoke protests.

Financial solutions in social security and statutory health insurance require consensus across political battle lines. Facing the same problems as the Americans during the 1970s and 1980s, the Europeans resolved them.[23] The Americans had previously maintained a consensus over the financial management of Social Security and Medicare despite the potential breakdowns arising from the separation of powers between Congress and the executive branch, as well as from the incessant rivalry between the Democratic and Republican parties. The consensus broke down after the election of 1980, when the White House was won by the faction of the Republican Party that had long opposed both Social Security pensions and Medicare—that is, the adversaries against whom the Roosevelt administration tried to ensure the permanent institutional protection of Social Security. This new administration threw the government into permanent fiscal chaos by reducing general taxes but increasing military spending. In 1982, it proposed short-term prevention of a Social Security pension deficit by cutting benefits; its eventual long-term proposals probably would have been drastic.[24] In 1982, the White House, the Senate, and the House of Representatives were controlled by different political parties and (within the Republican Party) by different factions, each ideological and militant. The House of Representatives was fragmented in response to interest groups pushing rival nostrums.

The United States then had to suspend the normal decision-making machinery and created a temporary coalition government for purposes of remedying the pension program. A National Commission for Social Security Reform was created, bringing together the leaders of the executive and legislative branches of government, the leaders of both political parties, all factions within both parties, and the principal interest groups. It was staffed by leading actuaries, who simulated everyone's favorite short-term and long-term policy options. The Commission conducted small and secret bargaining sessions as well as larger plenary deliberations. The American electorate contributed its all-important voice by reducing its Republican votes in the 1982 midterm election to Congress, in part because of the Reagan administration's suspected designs on Social Security. The Commission and its key participants worked out an elaborate compromise package combining moderate short-term payroll tax increases, moderate short-term benefit restraints, and other long-term changes. The essentials—the payroll tax method, the traditional benefits, and actuarial soundness without ad hoc public subsidies—were preserved. Congress quickly enacted the package, the President signed it, the Commission went out of existence, and the traditional decision-making sequence resumed. [25]

The same cycle might have been followed for Medicare's hospital insurance—namely, an impending deficit, resistance to payroll tax increases and to government subsidies, the Reagan administration's aspirations for fundamental restructuring of benefits and finances in the long term, [26] a public uproar, an impasse with Congress, and finally creation of a national commission to broker a politically realistic solution. But unexpected events made this sequence seem unnecessary: Medicare changed its method of paying hospitals, hospitals slowed their billings to Medicare, the Medicare payroll tax was increased slightly, and the Trust Fund was actuarially viable for a longer period.

Pandora's Box was finally opened in 1988 when Congress expanded the benefits under the Social Security part of Medicare—that is, reductions in cost sharing and in catastrophic liability of patients, drug prescriptions in ambulatory care, easier qualification for nursing home coverage, and more generous home care and hospice benefits. If any European country had so expanded benefits, it would have promptly increased either the payroll tax or government subsidies. But American politicians had painted themselves into a corner: a new article of faith was "no tax increases," and the Americans had long thought of the Social Security rates as "taxes"; government could not subsidize the Medicare account because it had never done so and because the general government budget now had enormous deficits; and all new benefits were supposed to be "budget neutral," thereby compelling cuts in other items in the program. Thus, Congress had to pay for its expanded benefits by sleight of hand—by revenue that was neither a payroll tax on workers nor a percentage deduction from the elderly beneficiaries' Social Security pensions.

Enacted under the Medicare Catastrophic Coverage Act of 1988, the result was ingenious, difficult to understand, and certain to outrage the payers: Medicare beneficiaries with higher incomes would pay an income tax surcharge earmarked for the Hospital Insurance Trust Fund. The surcharge was not a straightforward income tax on the elderly, since one of Washington's buzzwords was "no new taxes." But the benefits had to be financed. If a Medicare-eligible married couple filed an income tax return in 1989, and their joint income tax was $150 or less, they paid no surcharge. If their joint income tax ranged from $150 to $200, they paid an additional surcharge of $22. For every additional income tax of $50, they paid an additional surcharge of $7.50. For couples paying income taxes of $10,650 and over, they paid surcharges of $1,600 but no more. If only one member of the couple was Medicare-eligible, the surcharges were halved but could not exceed $800 per year. The rates automatically increased each year according to the rising costs of the additional Medicare benefits enacted by the law. The surcharge was proportional to the income tax but not progressive; but the underlying income tax was a progressive levy on the elderly person's income. This unique and troublesome financing method was adopted after the Congress had studied and rejected normal methods—increases in payroll taxes and Treasury subsidies—and had studied and rejected a clear-cut extra progressive income tax on the elderly.[27] The final handiwork was given a politically safe but misleading name: the "supplementary Medicare premium."

A formula method that had never been explained to politicians and the public and lacked political consensus could not survive. In a country without firm belief in social solidarity, the rich elderly did not want to subsidize the poor elderly. America's entrepreneurial political environment quickly produced political action committees that bombarded Congressmen and Senators with protests. Instead of leading, the two Presidents merely observed events during the enactment and backlash. Congress in 1989 quickly and overwhelmingly repealed the Medicare Catastrophic Coverage Act—the only time (except for some cutbacks in Australia) that a developed country has ever repealed a significant part of its social security.

Special Rates

When employees are added to social security—whether laborers or the highest managers—the familiar pattern of payroll taxes is extended to them. As a concession to the managers, so that they accept inclusion in social security, an earnings ceiling exempts the higher brackets. In order to raise more money for the increasingly expensive health insurance, the ceiling is steadily increased.

Completely new arrangements must be devised for those groups who do not fit the employment model. The political struggles that first shaped the social security and health insurance systems in each country now are repeated over the financial arrangements for the special groups. On the one hand, their political parties and pressure groups try to limit their financial contributions and protect their benefits. On the other hand, the government's finance officers try to make these accounts self-sustaining and limit the subsidies from the government's general budget.

Self-Employed. As Chapter Three explained, every country has added the self-employed to the statutory health insurance system in a different form. Since administrative arrangements and benefits vary, the rules about premium rates and income ceilings vary. The self-employed consistently resist paying rates exceeding their actuarial costs: social solidarity is the philosophy of the labor movement, not theirs. As more of the self-employed retire, however, their health insurance accounts must cover higher costs and the health insurance rates must rise. Unlike the low-income workers, they cannot openly extract special subsidies from the general government budget.

If the self-employed are obligatorily covered, they must all pay a tax resembling the employer/employee payroll tax. The self-employed resist the total rates collected from both employer and employee, but the government actuaries attempt to use the general regime's rate as an arithmetical starting point. The result is usually very complicated.

The goal in France, for example, is to bring enough money into the special regime (CANAM) that will cover the standard benefits of statutory health insurance. (The principal differences from the general regime for the workers are higher cost sharing for physicians' services for the self-employed and no cash benefits for occupational accidents or occupational diseases.) Before 1972, each self-employed occupation in France was assigned a flat premium category according to its field of work or the person's last declaration of annual income to the tax collection, but the rising costs of health care required more money. Since 1972, premiums are supposed to be a proportion of the self-employed person's actual income. But calculations have to be made on the basis of the person's last declaration of income—usually one year old and perhaps substantially understated. Unlike the United States, French social security and income tax collections are administered separately.

The earnings ceiling has disappeared from health insurance calculations in the French general regime but is still used in the self-employed's health insurance and in the general regime's pension tax rates. Two ceilings are used for the health insurance of the self-employed: one tax rate (3.10 percent in 1987) for all self-employed income between a certain floor and the standard social security annual ceiling (between 46,224 F and 115,560 F in 1987) and a second additional tax rate (8.45 percent in 1987) for all self-employed income between this ceiling and five times the ceiling (between 115,560 F and 577,800 F in 1987). A third figure is the minimum payment (5,338 F in 1987); every person must pay it even if he does not reach the lower ceiling; everyone else must pay it in addition to the results of the foregoing calculations. No one need pay more than an annual maximum (50,314 F in 1987).[28] Upper-income salaried people bring much more money into the sickness funds, because the rates are higher, no income ceiling exists in the calculations, no limit exists on the premium, and the *caisses primaires* collect the money more successfully.[29]

The self-employed's rates are examined every year by the Office of Administrative and Financial Affairs, Division of Social Security, Ministry of Social Affairs, at the same time it frames recommendations about the entire social security system, a process described earlier in this chapter. The Office uses the financial and statistical reports from each of the program headquarters—from the research staffs of CANAM as well as from CNAMTS and the others. The Office devotes most of its limited staff resources to making the general regime viable, since it is the principal part of social security and is used to earn surpluses and channel money into the underfunded regimes. The Office knows that the elected politicians will not change the premium rates, the ceilings, and the calculating methodology of CANAM unless the self-employed regime deteriorates substantially. The frequent small deficits in CANAM are papered over by means of annual equalization transfers from the general to the self-employed regime. Chapter Nine describes this method in France and other countries.

In countries where the self-employed are allowed to choose carriers and coverage, the transaction is freed of arguments and political pressures. The self-employed do not have to conceal income from a tax collector since the premiums are usually a flat rate, not related to income. Some self-employed may join sickness funds voluntarily, despite higher premiums, because these carriers make ideological appeals or guarantee coverage after retirement at the low pensioner's rates. More often, the self-employed pick commercial carriers with thinner benefits and lower premiums.

Retired in Belgium. Recent events in Belgium illustrate a common cycle. At first, the elderly were kept in the sickness funds without premiums until a financial crisis occurred in the accounts. Then, after much debate, the political parties in Parliament were forced to agree on premiums, since the alternative was massive subsidies by the Treasury. A mix of premiums and subsidies has prevailed ever since. Premiums have had to be increased, but the political parties deadlock over imposing very high rates.

Until the 1980s, a retired Belgian was fully covered by his *mutualité* without new premiums if he had been an employed subscriber for fifteen years. If he had been paying payroll taxes for less than fifteen years, he had to pay a small flat premium. During the general financial reforms of the troubled social security system in 1980, it was agreed that everyone should be expected to contribute something. Persons currently receiving social security, as well as private persons, were expected to make a "personal contribution" (*cotisation personnelle*). The rate was 2.18 percent of income in 1981 and 1.80 percent annually thereafter. The figure 1.80 was picked because it was the percentage levied on employees at that time. It is often argued that all pensioners are too poor to pay any health insurance premiums or to pay the normal patient cost sharing to providers. The Belgian compromise in 1980 was to exempt from premiums those receiving pensions below 21,615 FB per month (where 35 FB = $1 U.S. approximately at that time). The previous exemption from cost sharing by the very poor pensioners was continued.

While the government's problem was how to balance the social security accounts through payroll taxes and special premiums, the problem of the *mutualités* was how to cover the costs of elderly persons who paid no premiums but were heavy users. This was a particularly severe problem for the Socialist *mutualités* with their large numbers of widows and disabled from the smokestack industries. Invariably sickness funds press for government subsidies, but Belgian policymakers were trying to reduce the deficit in the government budget as well as in the social security accounts. The government had long subsidized the management costs of the *mutualités* and, more recently, had added lump-sum grants to help the sickness funds cover the costs of pensioners, widows, and disabled. These subsidies were continued during the 1980s, but under stricter rules. The Belgians have always avoided per capita grants lest more persons obtain the advantageous classifications and the totals exceed predictions.

Utilization and treatment costs for the elderly continued to rise, and government policymakers were pressed to increase both contribution rates and the subsidies to the *mutualités*. The payroll tax rates on the employees and self-employed had to be increased to 2.55 percent in late 1983, and the same increase was applied to all the elderly. But this was far enough for the precariously balanced coalition Cabinet. During the meetings to solve the crisis in the government budget during the spring of 1986, the Liberals (favoring a fiscally sound and less redistributive social security) recommended further increases in the premiums of the elderly; the Christians (more committed to social welfare policies) disagreed; and no premium increase was possible.

Retired in Germany. Traditionally, German health insurance was supposed to be completely self-financed through premiums without government subsidies. But the retired could not afford full actuarial premiums. For many years after the pensioners were added to health insurance in 1941, their coverage was a special project for the *Ortskrankenkassen*: the pension institute paid the sickness funds to cover the pensioners. At times, the elderly were charged small premiums, but the premiums were not kept for long. By the 1970s the elderly had become a substantial fraction of the beneficiaries of health insurance and accounted for much of the costs.

The question of how to finance their health insurance became caught up in the struggle among political parties over social security policy and the competition between the traditional sickness funds and the *Ersatzkassen* over market share. Germany during the 1970s was governed by a coalition Cabinet combining the Social Democrats (SPD) and the Free Democrats (FDP). The SPD favored traditional social insurance with compulsory universal membership, expansion of the official sickness funds (especially the *Ortskrankenkassen* and *Betriebskrankenkassen*), service benefits, price controls over providers, and no cost sharing by patients. The FDP favored free choice of carriers and providers, personal responsibility in paying premiums and provider bills, and more cost sharing by patients. The FDP wanted every pensioner to have enough cash to choose his own carrier, including the right to stay in the *Ersatzkasse* or private insurance carrier after retirement. The FDP pressed its coalition partners to change the method of paying for the pensioners' health insurance; since Germany traditionally used only payroll taxes and premiums, the SPD agreed during the late 1970s to a method whereby the pensioner pays premiums. The FDP, wishing to go much farther in reforming health insurance and health care finance, carried the disagreements with the SPD into the media. The Cabinet broke up, a new coalition between the Christian Democrats and the FDP took office, and the new government enacted what the FDP wanted.[30]

Every year, each pensioner is supposed to pay an average of 11.8 percent of his pension and of most of his extra earnings to a health insurance carrier. The figure 11.8 is the average premium percentage split between employer and employee for statutory health insurance. During the first year of a transitional period

(1982), the social security pension system paid this sum to the pensioner's preferred carrier. Thereafter, each year the pension institute paid a smaller percentage and the subscriber paid the balance, maintaining the 11.8 percent total—for
example, 10.8 percent and 1.0 percent in 1983; 8.8 percent and 3.0 percent in 1984;
6.8 percent and 5.0 percent in 1985. The social security pension fund increased its pension to the recipient every year to cover his payment. Therefore,
neither the pension fund nor the pensioner gained or lost cash. The premiums
were routed through the pensioner's personal accounts instead of being transferred directly by the pension fund to an *Ortskrankenkasse* or another official carrier.

One goal was the individual responsibility and flexibility much prized by
the FDP and other advocates of consumer choice in health insurance. Another
goal was greater market share by the *Ersatzkassen* and private insurers. The
pensioner would have more cash from his several public and private pensions and
would have the right to assign any social security deductions from outside earnings, so that he could pay *Ersatzkasse* and private premiums. Because of the
lifelong premium system (explained in Chapter Seven), a long-time subscriber to
a private company might wish to stay with it. *Ersatzkassen* can now keep their
long-time subscribers but—unlike the *Ortskrankenkassen*—are not obligated to
take the elderly as new enrollees.

One fact remaining the same is that the premiums paid to the carrier—
whether by the pension institute or by the pensioner himself—do not cover the
elderly person's full medical costs. The economically active have always paid
more than their actuarial costs in order to support the elderly and they still do.
In addition to the percentage of an economically active person's wage levied by
the sickness fund, 3.2 percent is a standard surcharge imposed by government (a
Zuschlag) to cover the costs of elderly and disabled members. Instead of each
carrier keeping its own surcharge, the money is pooled in an interfund equalization system (Chapter Nine).

Retired in France. A problem in every country is collecting enough premiums from the elderly to defray more of their costs. Faced by severe deficits
during the 1970s and 1980s, the French imposed several rates on different pensions. All retired persons must pay a 1 percent premium on the basic first-tier
pension from social security. A 2 percent premium is levied on the second-tier
pension paid by a private scheme. These are the more prosperous pensioners.[31]

A serious problem for social security in every country is the spread of early
retirement: the funds lose essential payroll tax revenue and pay out more in
pensions.[32] The French social security system imprudently encouraged early retirement in 1982 by reducing the age of full pensions to sixty. It does not encourage even earlier retirement: actuarially reduced pensions cannot be collected at
ages lower than sixty. In order to reduce unemployment of the young, the French
government created a special program whereby a worker between the ages of fifty-
five and sixty could get a stipend from the unemployment insurance fund, pro-

vided his job was given to a young unemployed worker. The social security system now tries to recapture some of the lost payroll tax revenue by imposing on these stipends the rate that the active workers pay on their wages (5.9 percent in late 1987).

Unemployed. Countries have long continued coverage after the worker has lost a fully covered job. But voluntary or obligatory premiums have seemed impossible, since the worker is receiving very low benefits and no longer can call upon contributions by an employer. One solution has been government subsidies to the sickness funds, rising along with the number of unemployed.

Germany has always tried to follow the premium model of revenue and to avoid government subsidies. The agency of the national government that administers unemployment benefits (the *Bundesanstalt für Arbeit*) has long paid the sickness fund premiums on behalf of the workers receiving these benefits. The *Bundesanstalt* once paid on behalf of every worker two-thirds of the average payroll tax; now it pays the full amount. The payment is the average payroll tax for all workers—both the employee's and the employer's shares—and not the premium customarily charged by each sickness fund. The program concerns the *Ortskrankenkasse*, since it has almost all the unemployed. If a worker has belonged to a *Betriebskrankenkasse*, the end of his employment automatically terminates his membership. By coincidence, each *Ortskrankenkasse* collects all the payroll taxes from local employers and workers for unemployment insurance as well as for all other social security programs. Before sending the money to the regional office of the *Bundesanstalt für Arbeit*, the *Ortskrankenkasse* deducts the premiums for its unemployed subscribers.

France in 1975 enacted a law protecting coverage of its growing number of unemployed. When a worker loses his job, he continues to be covered under the employer's and his last payroll tax payment for one month. He must then register with a labor exchange. This guarantees his continued protection by CNAMTS. For several years, the costs of the unemployed were paid for by the subsidies of government. These grants rapidly grew but still were not enough. A package of new social security taxes enacted by the Socialist government in 1982 and 1983 was designed to get contributions from groups that had not paid before. One measure was a deduction of 1 percent from every unemployment check, earmarked for the sickness fund. To relieve the very poor unemployed of hardship, their tax had a floor: only the amount exceeding the country's statutory minimum wage was taxable.

Effects on Utilization and Health

What difference does it make whether statutory health insurance is financed by payroll taxes or by some other method? What differences result from the detailed variations among types of payroll tax? Since these are financing instruments, they make a difference for the size of revenue, for the ease in quickly increasing and reducing it, and for fiscal administration. Payroll taxes and general revenue taxes have different consequences for the incidence within the population and possibly different consequences for the economy, as the next chapter explains. But effects on medical services and patient health are indirect and remote. Doctors, hospitals, and patients do not care how the money originated, so long as they get enough.

The payroll tax evolved out of the premiums of mutual assistance funds, which were associations of persons well aware that they were paying and benefiting. Government, its taxes, and its programs were more distant. For many years, payroll taxes were thought to symbolize grass-roots awareness of costs and services: they were bonds between subscribers and sickness funds. In practice, this symbolic distinction between payroll taxes and other taxes has weakened: both are deducted from paychecks; sickness funds are now becoming impersonal administrative agencies, increasingly like offices of local government. Payroll taxes are no longer thought to be a voluntary group action by the mutual assistance fund as part of its decisions about benefits and provider reimbursement; the benefits are fixed by law, and government in nearly every country decides the payroll taxes as well as other taxes.

Payroll taxes were once thought to be less generous sources of funding than general revenue. They could be raised only slowly whereas progressive general taxation could tap a larger base and could be increased suddenly. Therefore, when policymakers favored expansion of statutory health insurance benefits, they often called for large new public subsidies or for a change to full fiscalization. But when governments ran deficits during the economic downturn of the 1970s and 1980s, they had to control spending in general and medical care costs in particular. As a result, public subsidies and fully tax-financed health care systems were cut back.[33] Therefore, funding by general taxation can fluctuate more widely than funding by payroll taxes, which tend to grow steadily—faster or slower, depending on employment and wages—and are not drawn into budgetary politics so quickly.

Payroll taxes are associated with nonprofit private or autonomous public sickness funds, while general tax financing is associated with government agencies. Sickness funds are associated with negotiations with providers and flexible expenditure targets whereas government agencies are associated with greater governmental authority and expenditure caps. Providers—especially the medical associations—prefer the more flexible and less tempestuous environment associated with payroll taxes.

Implications for the United States

The Political Nature of Rate Setting. At first sight, fixing payroll taxes and premiums seems straightforward: actuaries should be able to make calculations and fix rates, as in any insurance company. However, the organization and financing of statutory health insurance vary from country to country. Each government must go through a series of never-ending decisions about the setting of rates, the division of revenue between payroll taxes and subsidies, and the response to cost increases.

A central lesson of this book is that the structure and financing of health insurance are not technical design tasks for actuaries and policy researchers alone. Rather, like all components of social protection, they are the outcome of struggles of self-interest among payers, beneficiaries, health care providers, and financial managers. Political will and political ingenuity are necessary to assimilate sound actuarial advice and produce a result that is satisfactory to the interest groups and administratively workable. The outcome is never simple, must be constantly monitored, and is sometimes amended.

Americans should be aware of the political nature of decisions in Social Security and statutory health insurance, in view of the political deadlock over Social Security pension reform in 1982-1983, described earlier in this chapter. However, many policy analysts in American health insurance are technically trained economists who believe that conflicts of interest can be settled by formulas. But this is not possible—and concentrating on formulas while neglecting political negotiation wastes resources and time.[34]

Creating Decision-Making Machinery. Of course, economists and actuarial research are indispensable. The problem is how to use them in the decision-making sequence—how to relate the technicians and framers of policy options to the leaders of government and interest groups. A harmonious permanent system of monitoring statutory health insurance, hearing the conflicting interest groups, evaluating possibilities, and making decisions is indispensable. Technical fields with conflicts of interest—such as rate setting in statutory health insurance and reimbursement of providers—cannot be thrown into a legislature without thorough preliminary investigation, without formulation of clear policy options, and without recommendations formulated either by the executive branch or by negotiations among the principal interest groups.

Other developed countries rely both on strong executive leadership (required under a parliamentary system of government) and on agreements negotiated among the private interest groups most affected by social security and statutory health insurance. America's impasse over Social Security reform in 1982-1983, as well as its intermittent difficulties in making Medicare policy, show that Congress cannot settle such matters without preliminary negotiations among interest groups and without leadership from the executive branch and from its own ranks.

Avoiding Fruitless Policies. Other democracies debate—and often seriously struggle over—major issues. Once they are settled, the country nowadays moves on to the new problems requiring solution. Europe learned after centuries of revolution and counterrevolution that reopening past settlements is not only expensive in emotions and resources but prevents solution of new matters. For example, hardly anyone in Europe now questions the existence and financing principles of social security and statutory health insurance. The problems in these fields now are managerial.

In contrast, the financing problems of American Social Security and Medicare in the 1970s and early 1980s provided the occasion for the free-market ideologists and the Reagan administration to question their existence. A passionate debate and complex political negotiations ensued. At the end, these programs were not altered at all, because they are fundamental institutions in the United States and in every other developed country. The only results were unnecessary trouble and delay in the necessary decisions.

Besides pretending to reverse a long-settled and essential social arrangement, another wasteful exercise is to abjure an indispensable instrument of public policy. American politicians did so by pledging "no new taxes" during the 1980s. But taxes are indispensable to the balancing of budgets, and no other developed country during the 1980s has hesitated to increase taxes—including the payroll tax for statutory health insurance. America's confusing financing of Medicare during the late 1980s, described earlier in this chapter, and its enormous budgetary deficits follow from its fruitless attitude toward taxes.

Notes

1. For valuable overview of current financing methods and recent trends, see Pierre Mouton, "Methods of Financing Social Security in Industrial Countries: An International Analysis," in *Financing Social Security: The Options* (Geneva: International Labour Office, 1984), pp. 3–32.

2. The revenue and financial management of French guilds and other brotherhoods (*confréries*) are described in Jean Bennet, *La Mutualité Française des origines à la Révolution de 1789* (Paris: Coopérative d'Information et d'Edition Mutaliste, 1981), pp. 291–363.

3. Full details about the development during the late nineteenth century appear throughout the encyclopedic "Workmen's Insurance and Compensation Systems in Europe," *Twenty-Fourth Annual Report of the Commissioner of Labor 1909* (Washington: Government Printing Office, 1911). Highlights are summarized in William Franklin Willoughby, *Workingmen's Insurance* (New York: Crowell, 1898).

4. The rates appear in several annual (or biennial) volumes: *Comparative Tables of the Social Security Schemes in the Member States of the European Communities* (Luxembourg: Commission of the European Communities); *Comparative Tables of the Social Security Systems of Council of Europe Member States Not Belonging to the European Communities* (Strasbourg: Council of Europe); and *Social Security Programs Throughout the World* (Washington: Social Security Administration, Department of Health and Human Services).

5. The managerial and financial reforms of social security in France in 1967 replaced political consultations among interest groups with decisions by

civil servants on the basis of an index. See Jacques Doublet, *Sécurité sociale,* 5th ed. (Paris: Presses Universitaires de France, 1972), p. 409.

6. The administrative organization of Holland's intricate social security system is described in Annemarie Kolkert and others, *Praktische informatie over sociale zekerheid,* 4th ed. (Deventer: Kluwer, 1987).

7. *L'A.C.O.S.S. et la Branche du Recouvrement* (Paris: Agence Centrale des Organismes de Sécurité Sociale, 1984); and Isabelle Courty and others, *Le service public du recouvrement et les relations avec les entreprises cotisantes* (Saint-Etienne: Centre National d'Etudes Supérieures de Sécurité Sociale, 1985).

8. *Régime Général: Le Recouvrement des Cotisations au Service de la Protection Sociale* (Paris: Agence Centrale des Organismes de Sécurité Sociale, 1985), pp. 9–10.

9. Jean-Pierre Dumont, *La Sécurité sociale: toujours en chantier* (Paris: Les Editions Ouvrières, 1981), p. 271, and the annual reports of the Commission des Comptes de la Sécurité Sociale. The proportion of uncollected payroll taxes may approach 3 percent in Belgium, according to the annual reports of the Office National de Sécurité Sociale in Brussels.

10. *Advies over de premie voor de verplichte ziekenfondsverzekering* (Amsterdam: Ziekenfondsraad, annual). The title of the annual report changed in subsequent years. The report with authoritative index numbers and projections is *Macro Economische Verkenning* (The Hague: Centraal Planbureau, annual).

11. William A. Glaser, *Paying the Hospital* (San Francisco: Jossey-Bass, 1987), pp. 96–103, 132–142.

12. The Ministry of Social Affairs has been studying a detailed financial report about all the other social security programs (like the report about health insurance sent by the *Ziekenfondsraad* to WVC). The authors are in the Social-Economic Department of the Social Insurance Council. See *De premiepercentages van de sociale verzekeringen* (Zoetermeer: Sociale Verzekeringsraad, annual).

13. Geert A. Tuinier, "The Relationship Between Social Security and Taxation in the Netherlands," in *Social Security and Taxation* (Geneva: International Social Security Association, 1979), pp. 109–112.

14. Han Emanuel and others, "Disability Policy in the Netherlands," in Robert Haveman and others, *Public Policy Toward Disabled Workers* (Ithaca: Cornell University Press, 1984), pp. 399–443.

15. Pierre Begault and others, "Le financement du régime général de Sécurité sociale," *Revue française des affaires sociales,* vol. 30, special number (July–Sept. 1976), pp. 59–60; and Alain Foulon and others, *Les revenues des français: La croissance et la crise (1960–1983)—Quatrième rapport de synthèse* (Paris: Documents du Centre d'Etude des Revenus et des Coûts, 1985), pp. 203–205.

16. Herbert Jacob, *German Administration Since Bismarck* (New Haven: Yale University Press, 1963), pp. 37–43.

17. Klaus-Kirk Henke and Hans Adam, *Die Finanzlage der sozialen Krankenversicherung 1960–1978* (Cologne: Deutsche Arzte-Verlag, 1983), pp. 77–86.

18. Paul-Helmut Huppertz and others, *Beitragssatzdifferenzen und adäquate Finanzausgleichsverfahren in der gesetzlichen Krankenversicherung* (Bonn: Bundesministerium für Arbeit und Sozialordnung, 1981); Reinhart Schmidt, *Materialen zu Kosten und Finanzierung des Gesundheitswesens* (Kiel: Institut für Gesundheits-System-Forschung, 1978); and Theo Giehler, "Unterschiedliche Beitragssätze in der gesetzlichen Krankenversicherung," *Betriebskrankenkasse*, vol. 69, no. 5 (May 1981), pp. 137–144.

19. The early financial decisions are summarized in Martha Derthick, *Policymaking for Social Security* (Washington: Brookings Institution, 1979), chap. 11.

20. The financial organization, actuarial methodology, and successive decisions in the pension system are described in Robert J. Myers, *Social Security*, 3rd ed. (Homewood, Ill.: Irwin, 1985), chaps. 3, 4, 10.

21. The full time series for benefits and payroll taxes are given in Alicia H. Munnell, *The Future of Social Security* (Washington: Brookings Institution, 1977), app.

22. Robert J. Myers, *Medicare* (Homewood, Ill.: Irwin, 1970), chaps. 8, 10.

23. Jean-Pierre Dumont, *L'impact de la crise économique sur les systèmes de protection sociale* (Geneva: International Labour Office, 1986).

24. See, for example, Peter Ferrara, *Social Security: The Inherent Contradiction* (San Francisco: Cato Institute, 1980), and Martin Feldstein, *The Optimal Financing of Social Security* (Cambridge: Harvard Institute of Economic Research, 1974).

25. Paul Light, *Artful Work: The Politics of Social Security Reform* (New York: Random House, 1985).

26. See, for example, proposals to convert Medicare to a voucher system in Rita Ricardo-Campbell, *The Economics and Politics of Health* (Chapel Hill: University of North Carolina Press, 1982), pp. 329–340, and President Reagan's message to Congress (Feb. 28, 1983) on behalf of a proposed Medicare Voucher Act of 1983. A voucher system is a form of indemnity benefits—a far cry from statutory health insurance and America's current Medicare. A subscriber receives a voucher representing a fixed amount of money. He selects providers, pays any prices, but receives only the value of the voucher from Medicare. The program would have no relations with providers. Design options, strengths, and weaknesses are examined at length in Randall R. Bovbjerg, "Vouchers for Medicare: The Impossible Dream?" in Mark V. Pauly and William L. Kissick (eds.), *Lessons from the First Twenty Years of Medicare* (Philadelphia: University of Pennsylvania Press, 1988), pp. 25–48.

27. "Statement of Rosemary D. Marcuss, Assistant Director for Tax Analysis, Congressional Budget Office Before the Committee on Finance, United States Senate, March 26, 1987."

28. The rate calculations and the accounts appear every year in

C.A.N.A.M.—Statistiques (Paris: Caisse Nationale d'Assurance Maladie et Maternité des Travailleurs Non Salariés des Professions Non Agricoles, annual).

29. Tax evasion by the French self-employed and lax collection by CANAM are described in Cour des Comptes, *Rapport au Président de la République* (Paris: Journaux Officiels, 1983), pp. 107–112.

30. For past history and recent changes, see Hans Hungenberg and Jürgen Steffens, *Krankenversicherung der Rentner*, 3rd ed. (Sankt Augustin: Asgard Verlag, 1983).

31. The rates vary among regimes: Commission des Comptes de la Sécurité Sociale, *Les comptes de la Sécurité sociale—Prévisions 1989 et 1990* (Paris: La Documentation Française, 1989), p. 133.

32. *Social Security, Unemployment and Premature Retirement* (Geneva: International Social Security Association, 1985), especially chap. 10.

33. Described in Glaser, *Paying the Hospital* (see note 11 above), chaps. 8, 13. Therefore, when post-Communist reformers in Eastern Europe sought to revitalize their health services and assure adequate financing, some recommended shifting from general revenue to earmarked payroll taxes. See, for example, Stanislawa Golinowska and others, *W Interesie Zdrowia Spoleczenstwa—Projekt Reformy Opieki Zdrowotnej*, Biuletyn Informacyjny no. 105 (Warsaw: Instytut Gospodarki Nadorowej, 1989).

34. An example is the policy making to reform reimbursement of physicians under Medicare during the late 1980s, described in William Glaser, "The Politics of Paying American Physicians," *Health Affairs*, vol. 8, no. 3 (Fall 1989), pp. 129–146, and William Glaser, "Designing Fee Schedules by Formulae, Politics, and Negotiations," *American Journal of Public Health*, vol. 80, no. 7 (July 1990), pp. 804–809.

CHAPTER 6

Altering or Replacing
Payroll Taxes

———————————————— Summary ————————————————

Payroll taxes have been the traditional source of money for social security and statutory health insurance. They are criticized on several counts, and countries grope for substitutes. But changes may lose more than they gain: some taxpayers would pay more and they resist; the substitutes might have adverse effects on the economy; changes always have unexpected effects and might yield less revenue, creating a crisis throughout social security.

Ideally, taxes should be "equitable." The earnings ceiling exempts very high income brackets and is said to make the payroll tax regressive, but the need to find more money for health insurance now leads to increases and even elimination of the ceiling. Even so, progressive payroll tax rates are not yet proposed.

Ideally, a tax should not have adverse effects on the economy. Some critics fear that high payroll taxes on employers discourage employment, overprice exports, motivate tax evasion, and lead to economic recession. As countries compete in world markets and integrate their economies, wide differences in payroll taxes on employers produce problems in coordination and handicap the high-tax nations. Some reforms are attempted, such as experiments with value-added taxes earmarked for social security. Some of these changes produce new complications, such as one-time general price inflation, and do not yield instant benefits in exports. It is very difficult to find a substitute that may not have even greater drawbacks.

Some countries have shifted in part or in whole to general revenue financing for several reasons: employers and trade unions resist increases in the visible payroll taxes and accept less visible burdens on the general public; general revenue is based on the progressive taxation and redistributive financing preferred

131

by the political Left; and government has stronger leverage over health care financing. A shift to full revenue financing is often resisted: the trade unions and health insurance carriers fear they will lose authority to government finance offices and Parliament; doctors and hospitals fear that government will impose expenditure caps. A few countries consider substituting flat rates on all income instead of the earnings-based payroll tax, but the new method may discourage reporting all income for all taxes.

Even when general revenue financing is introduced, the payroll tax is remarkably persistent. After many years of crisis in costs, social security and statutory health insurance have recently stabilized. Today any major change lacks a political consensus and is financially risky.

Policy Issues

The proportion-of-earnings payroll tax has been the standby of social security and statutory health insurance for a century. At times certain groups have been added, with flat-rate premiums equal for all new subscribers, like their arrangements under previous private insurance for pensions and health. But as in the case of the self-employed in France and elsewhere, percentage-of-income taxes eventually replace flat rates. From time to time the structure of payroll taxes is criticized and revised. In statutory health insurance, the chronic problem has been not enough money, and the usual reform has been to increase the rates and earnings ceilings.

The payroll tax system is being debated today on several grounds:

☐ Social justice is at issue:
  • Since the same rates apply to everyone, the poor are charged too much.
  • Since the same rates apply to everyone and collections stop at an earnings ceiling, the rich are not charged enough.
☐ The burden on the employer is excessive:
  • The payroll tax is so high that the industry's prices are too high and uncompetitive in international trade.
  • The payroll tax is so high that the employer is motivated not to hire workers.
  • Labor-intensive industries must support social security more than capital-intensive industries do.
  • Employers are forced to pay for costs—such as health care of the retired—that do not concern them.
☐ Earnings from employment and self-employment are an excessively narrow base. Other income should be taxed too.

Regressivity and Progressivity

When social security was introduced in the late nineteenth century, it covered a set of blue-collar occupations in a narrow band of income. It did not yet cover the poor or the rich. It had been customary to think of members of a mutual protection fund as a socially solidary group, all paying the same premiums. This practice continued during the early years of statutory social security.

At the same time, throughout the nineteenth century, both Europe and North America were involved in debates over the structure of taxes on personal income, real property, inheritance, and so on. Many persons—both tax theorists and socially oriented policymakers—argued that calculations should be based on equality of burden and not mere equality of the cash payments or equality of the rates. Instead of applying the same rates to all taxpayers, some laws were progressive, increasing the percentage rates as the taxable base rose.[1]

The ferment in tax policy did not affect payroll taxes for many years. The payroll tax until recently was not perceived as a "tax" but only as a regular obligatory contribution to social insurance funds, which previously had used voluntary methods to collect similar amounts of money from limited groups for the same purpose. A "tax" was perceived as an imposition on the general population to support the general Treasury of the government. Imposing progressive contributions upon the rich did not arise for many decades, since social security was designed for the less affluent and the less provident, and the rich did not belong. Persons in the more prosperous occupations or above a certain income ceiling were not required to join. The membership ceiling and the contributions ceiling at first were identical. If compulsory cover under a country's laws depended on a list of occupations and a richer person fell in, every social security system at first precluded any progressive contributions by mandating the opposite: he paid the payroll tax for his income only up to a ceiling, and the excess was exempt.

Upper-income managers, self-employed, and others then entered social security, either by mandatory coverage of entire industries or by use of an earnings ceiling for membership. Persons earning more were exempt. The membership ceiling was no longer identical with the contributions ceiling. One began to hear complaints that the payroll tax was "regressive" because of the ceiling on the taxable earnings base. Critics argued thus if they thought of the payroll taxes as revenue for just another government program. The ceiling for rates began for the pension part of social security and was automatically extended to health insurance. The defenders of the ceiling argued that old-age insurance was an income-related contributory benefit program in which payments yielded a commensurate pension; those paying more money each year under the fixed-percentage payroll tax received a higher pension. But pension systems under social security were moderately redistributive: unlike a private system that correlated contributions and pensions exactly, the replacement rate declined as incomes rose. If the earnings ceiling was eliminated, argued its defenders, upper-income participants would pay large amounts, would recover little in replacement rates under pensions, and would protest that they had been tricked by a change in the rules after they had joined. With their income not taxed under social security, upper-income persons were always expected to buy second-tier private annuities with whatever replacement rate they were willing to pay for.[2]

The ceiling could not be justified in statutory health insurance by the same logic. No country has earnings-related benefits within the official scheme. Everyone paying the standard payroll tax rate is fully covered for the identical benefits, regardless of whether his cash payments are low or high. Health insurance is completely redistributive in finance, while the pension program is only partly so.

During the 1960s, as statutory health insurance needed more money, government finance officers discovered that prosperity was raising workers' and managers' wages faster than the annual increase in the earnings ceiling.[3] Substantial fractions of every country's labor force had wages exceeding the ceiling, and these extra amounts were not taxed. Industries with small but well-paid labor forces—such as petrochemicals, data processing, and banking—were supporting the country's social security system less than industries with large numbers of manual workers.[4] During the late 1960s, governments raised the ceilings faster than they did before, and eventually some abandoned the ceilings in health insurance. Usually a major change in social security financing—such as elimination of the ceiling—is not done suddenly, since the taxpayer would experience a large immediate increase, the worker would protest that a historic social contract has been violated, and all employers would suddenly be liable to much higher costs. Thus, the change is phased. In France, the transition took more than a decade and is described in Table 6.1.

At the start of the transition in 1967, according to Table 6.1, both the French employee and employer paid taxes on the employee's earnings and up to the ceiling for that year. During the transition, every worker paid two payroll taxes—in 1976, for example, 2.50 percent on his earnings below 37,920 F and 1.50 percent in addition on his entire wages including anything over the ceiling. (The second percentage applied to the entire wage, not the difference between the ceiling and his total.) Likewise, during the transition every employer paid two payroll taxes for each worker: in 1976, for instance, 10.45 percent on the earnings below 37,920 F and 2.50 percent in addition on his entire wage.

If this graduated two-rate method had covered costs adequately, it would have been kept. But more money was needed. Several commissions and small work groups met during the 1970s and 1980s to examine options in expanding the financial base. Instead of a radical alteration of the principle of payroll taxes on earnings from work, a few early groups recommended eliminating the ceiling (déplafonnement). Besides raising more money, this also had the virtue of eliminating the regressive nature of the rates, thereby promoting greater equality among the French.[5] Within a few years—by 1984—the health insurance taxation was proportionate and no longer regressive. However, the employees' pension program and the entire self-employed regime retain earnings ceilings.

Eliminating the ceiling substantially increases collections. Suppose that someone earned a salary of 180,000 F in 1985. The health insurance payroll tax

Table 6.1. Gradual Elimination of the Earnings Ceiling in French Health Insurance.

Payroll tax rates on	1967	1968–1969	1970	1971–1975	1976	1977–1978	1979	1980	1981–1983	1984–1986
Employees										
Up to income ceiling	6	2.50	2.50	2.50	2.50	3.00	1.00	0	0	0
Total wage	0	1.00	1.00	1.00	1.50	1.50	3.50[a]	5.50	5.50	5.50
Employers										
Up to income ceiling	15	9.50	10.25	10.45	10.45	10.95	8.95	8.95	5.45	0
Total wage	0	2.00	2.00	2.00	2.50	2.50	4.50	4.50	8.00	12.60
Earnings ceiling[b]	13,680	14,400 16,320	18,000	19,800 21,900 24,480 27,840 33,000	37,920	43,320 48,000	53,640	60,120	68,760 79,080 88,920	97,320 104,760 113,760

[a]Later 4.50.

[b]Earnings ceilings for each year are given in current francs.

Note: Before 1968, the health insurance and pension *caisses* and their accounts were combined. The payroll taxes provided money for both. The rates for 1968 and later years shown here are for health insurance only.

Sources: Pierre Begault and others, "Le financement du Régime Général de Sécurité sociale," *Revue française des affaires sociales,* vol. 30, special number (July–Sept. 1976), pp. 59–60; and *Le Régime Général en 1984—Statistiques Diverses* (Paris: Caisse Nationale de l'Assurance Maladie des Travailleurs Salariés, 1986), pp. 21–24.

was 5.50 percent on the employee and 12.60 percent on the employer. If the ceiling was still in effect for health (104,760 F for the pension program in 1985), the total revenue for that person in health would be 18,962 F (5.50[104,760] +12.60[104,760] = 18,961.56). But the collection in 1987 actually was 32,580 F (5.50[180,000] + 12.60[180,000] = 32,580). (In mid-1987, 1 F = $0.16 U.S.)

While the French payroll taxes for employees' health insurance have ceased to be regressive, they are not progressive. The same percentages apply to everyone, and the poorest are not exempt. No one is supposed to work for less than the statutory minimum wage, and the payroll tax applies to it. Unlike the United States,[6] part-timers and low earners do not get refunds.

Adverse Effects on Employment

The rates on employers have risen faster than the rates on workers. By the 1970s and 1980s, employers in a few countries were paying five times the deduction from the employee. During the recession of the 1970s, the most extreme contrasts seemed linked to serious crises in employment.

The leading example was Italy. In 1973, the average payroll taxes as percentages of wages were:[7]

	Employer	Employee
Health and maternity	14.46	0.15
Old-age and disability pensions	13.75	6.90
Work-injury compensation	3.90	0
Unemployment insurance	2.50	0
Family allowances	12.50	0
	47.11	7.05

These high payroll taxes in Italy and elsewhere had two serious results. First, they were thought to discourage employment. Second, although they had reached a level where politicians shrank from increasing them further, they still were not high enough to pay program costs. Italy and other countries began large government subsidies to the social security funds. In Italy, the sickness funds still could not pay all the hospitals' bills, and the health insurance system became officially bankrupt.

Italy was the first developed country to detect that social security payroll taxes might reduce employment. Some of the reduction was real. Companies preferred laborsaving equipment and work organization over new hirings. They preferred overtime by current workers rather than hiring new full-time workers who might not be fully used. Once a worker reached the income ceiling, his overtime pay was exempt from payroll taxes, but the wages of a new employee were fully taxable. Even when European economies began to revive during the 1980s, unemployment rates—the highest since World War II—did not come down.

Another adverse consequence—widespread in Italy and ultimately else-where—was clandestine employment. Employers hired workers, did not list them in official records, and paid no social security taxes for them. If the worker had a primary job in the aboveground economy that was taxed and gave him full social security coverage, he was happy to accept an underground second job. Self-employed persons did much of their work for cash and did not report it for income and social security taxation. Even before the recession struck Europe during the mid-1970s, officially reported employment dropped below plausible levels.[8]

Alternative Financing. No one in Europe proposed repealing social secur-ity, making it voluntary, or reducing it to protection for the poor alone. Such changes are heard only in the United States.[9] In other developed countries, the complete menu of social security programs is an integral part of modern society and the notion of reducing it is inconceivable. Instead they try to make social security more cost-effective, less wasteful.[10]

Europeans searched for new methods of paying for social security that would permit reductions of the payroll taxes upon employers. A considerable literature accumulated,[11] without major contributions by the Americans, who had not yet reached such heavy burdens on employers.[12] According to the Euro-pean publications, the ideal financing of social security should satisfy several criteria:

☐ It should not motivate employers to reduce personnel. It should not discour-age employers from hiring the unemployed and should not encourage in-creasing overtime instead.

☐ There should be equity among industries. Financing the country's social security should not fall more heavily on labor-intensive industries than on capital-intensive industries, particularly if the latter are more profitable.

☐ There should be equity among countries. A country's commitment to gener-ous social benefits and a country's unfavorable dependency ratio should not result in higher labor costs and higher export prices, ultimately wiping out that country's exports.

☐ It should not aggravate inflation in labor costs and prices. If payroll taxes and insurance premiums are percentages of wages, they are inflationary.

☐ Financing of each social security program should be appropriate to its pur-pose, rather than using a payroll tax method for all. Payroll taxes are ap-propriate for insurance of active workers, as in invalidity, work accident, and unemployment insurance. But taxes on the employer's payroll are less ap-propriate for health, since the principal users are the retired.

☐ If the social security system is redistributive, progressive and not regressive taxes should be used. Payroll taxes on employees and the self-employed—particularly with earnings ceilings—are regressive.

Many specific proposals were offered during the 1970s and 1980s. As each was analyzed, a fundamental conflict of interest between the social security system and employers became obvious: some measures to reduce the burden on employment reduce social security revenue; some methods of raising revenue burden the employers even more than before. Serious remedies must be introduced by Prime Ministers, Ministers of Finance, and entire Cabinets, and they hesitate to solve one problem by creating new ones. Proposals included:

☐ Eliminating or reducing employers' payroll taxes on new hires of previously unemployed workers. This measure has not been adopted anywhere, since it aggravates the financial problems of the social security accounts: the worker is guaranteed full benefits without full funding.

☐ Making the payroll tax progressive. This measure has not been adopted in any country—except for Britain's National Insurance Contributions during the late 1980s—since it would increase the burden on employers.[13] It would infuriate the self-employed. It would result in concealment of higher incomes by the self-employed—already a problem—and by managers. It would discourage wage increases.

☐ Raising and even eliminating earnings ceilings. Faced by imminent deficits in the pension and health insurance accounts, all governments have done this. The measure has the political advantage of making it appear that the government has bravely "held the line" on tax rates. (But employers and the self-employed know that this method has been a principal reason for the great increase in their social security payments during the last decade.)

☐ Substituting general revenue grants for payroll taxes in part or in whole. This strategy has existed for many years in certain social security programs in some countries. There has never been any standard pattern: some countries have used general revenue in the pension program, others in health insurance, still others in several programs simultaneously. The reasons vary. Faced with serious deficits in health insurance and pensions during the late 1970s and 1980s—and reluctant to keep raising payroll taxes—most national governments increased their traditional subsidies or instituted new ones. However, this measure merely transferred the social security deficit to the Ministry of Social Affairs' accounts in the government's general expenditure budget. Faced with declining revenue during a recession, governments soon halted or reversed the growth of subsidies. (Subsidies are described in Chapter Eight.)

☐ Substituting value-added taxes for part of the employer's payroll taxes. This strategy once attracted attention in several countries, since it would finally obtain large contributions to social security by the profitable capital-intensive and laborsaving industries. (In the next section we will see how Belgium tested this remedy.)

☐ Containing the costs of social security. All governments have been seeking methods, particularly in health insurance and pensions, of curbing social security costs. Saving large amounts of money is difficult, though, because the populations age, service intensity in medicine rapidly increases, and governments shrink from reducing benefits to the population.

An Experiment in Belgium. Any modification of national health insurance and social security must apply to everyone in the entire country. Local and unrealistic experiments—like the demonstration projects much practiced in American health care—are not often attempted: their participants would win or lose compared to other beneficiaries, local results would be artificial, and results would not predict how the complete system would react. But officials are cautious about major reforms of the full system lest current problems be aggravated rather than reduced.

Belgium had such serious problems in the financing of social security and in its effects that the government tested a major change. In the 1970s, Belgium experienced serious stagflation and could not revive. Many workers remained unemployed. Export prices were high and uncompetitive. Heavy industries closed. Payroll taxes and government subsidies for the generous social security programs were already very high. For all social security programs in the mid-1970s, employers paid 30 percent of payroll in taxes.

Policymakers decided that the payroll taxes on all employers should be reduced and an equivalent amount of money should be raised and earmarked for social security by taxing all added value.[14] The value-added tax (VAT) used throughout Europe would simply have a higher rate in Belgium. Export prices would drop and would not rise so fast every future year. The value-added tax would increase prices throughout the country during the first year but would not cause subsequent annual increases. The government's planning office simulated many schemes with its massive data files about the economy.[15]

The experiment—called *Opération Maribel*—was then implemented. Social security taxes on employers of manual workers were reduced 6.17 percent in 1981. An equivalent amount of money was raised by increasing the value-added tax and several excise taxes. The increased revenue went to the social security funds, particularly pensions. Rebates were payable on the VAT as usual. The government was nervous about unexpected outcomes and would not allow the planners to implement their full proposals. These plans had called for a large reduction of the payroll tax, reliance exclusively on the VAT and not on excise taxes, a larger increase in the VAT, inclusion of all employers and all payrolls, permanent adoption of the changes, and avoidance of other major changes in economic policy.[16]

The secular rise in Belgian labor costs reversed, and Belgian prices became more competitive. A one-time inflationary increase occurred, but secular trends in inflation were stopped. Intentions were fulfilled despite the limited scope of the experiment and despite other contradictory economic policies. Long-term effects petered out because of the weakness of the original stimulus and changing social security policies by government.

Cautious Conclusions. Payroll tax rates and public expenditures happened to peak at the time of a recession in Europe and elsewhere. After the Belgian experiment and after cross-national statistical comparisons, the relation between specific revenue instruments and employment did not seem so clear-cut. Payroll tax rates do not correlate highly with unemployment rates. Business decline results from many problems, and the cost of labor is only one. The cost of labor is determined by many causes, and the social security financing system is only one. Business firms' choices between hiring workers and substituting capital are determined by many causes, and earnings-related payroll taxes are only one.[17]

Short-term manipulation of a country's social security taxes will not stimulate the country's economy. A payroll tax is a crude device designed for particular purposes. To achieve different purposes—such as persuading employers to hire young unemployed workers—direct methods (such as subsidies) are more efficient and cheaper for government. The direct methods can be targeted at certain industries, regions, and time periods, but manipulating social security taxes cannot. Trying to fine-tune social security taxes will make social security even more complicated and may underfund the system.[18]

The much discussed substitution of a value-added tax for the employer's payroll tax may be very difficult to implement on a large scale. Greatly increasing the tax burden on capital-intensive industries may dampen a country's economic growth. Capital-intensive industries might flee offshore. The concept of value-added in each firm's production process may be too inexact for a national tax base. Value-added taxes may be underestimated in their tax bases and underpaid in their collections even more seriously than social security payroll and self-employment taxes are.[19]

A great variety of business and household taxes may be proposed as substitutes for the reductions in the employers' payroll taxes. Each new tax has advantages and disadvantages from the standpoint of particular business firms, their customers, and the economy.[20] Since the outcome is uncertain, changing taxes is a gamble.

Expanding the Revenue Base

The yield from payroll taxes cannot keep pace with the mounting costs of health insurance. Moreover, very high payroll taxes are suspected of having adverse effects on the strength of certain industries and on a country's prices in world markets. Thus, the 1980s witnessed a widespread search for new revenue sources.

Complete Fiscalization. The problem has been to assign specific taxes to the sickness funds instead of merely increasing their historic payroll taxes. A few developed countries have avoided the issue by changing financing from private premiums to full Treasury financing through the government. Instead of perpetuating the sickness funds, imposing payroll taxes on their behalf, and covering shortfalls with annual special subsidies from the Ministry of Health budget, the sickness funds are abolished and the Ministry of Health budget becomes the conduit for all operating and capital costs of providers. A complete change in financing health care is justified on functional grounds.[21] Traditional payroll taxes on earnings are said to be appropriate for work-related benefits, such as deferred wages for retirement income, insurance against unemployment, and income in case of disability due to work accidents. But health care not attributable to work is a different matter. It is provided by society to preserve human capital and to fulfill humanitarian values. The principal users of health care benefits—the elderly—are no longer employed and should not be supported by active workers and by employers in a current pay-as-you-go financing system.

But attempting a complete change in financing is easier than actually accomplishing it. The payroll taxes on workers and employers are so intimately connected with the idea of social protection that they are levied even by countries that have supposedly governmentalized all their health care financing and even by countries that have never had statutory health insurance. In the USSR and other Eastern European countries, for example, a payroll tax on employers is earmarked for health care in the government accounts. The employers are nationalized industries. The workers pay no payroll taxes. The complete operating and capital costs of the governmentally owned health services are paid by the Ministry of Health budget, derived primarily from general revenue but also using the payroll taxes. Canadian provinces use various devices. Quebec levies a 3 percent payroll tax on employers for the health care account of the Ministry of Social Affairs. Ontario, Alberta, and British Columbia levy flat health premiums on all citizens.

The Soviet Union and Canada have never had statutory health insurance financed by payroll taxes. A few others, such as Great Britain and Italy, enacted national health services that were supposed to be financed completely from general revenue, but payroll taxes have been kept as financially inescapable.

Great Britain had statutory National Health Insurance from 1911 to the advent of the National Health Service in 1948. The Friendly Societies were financed by payroll taxes on employers and employees.[22] When the NHS and other new social security programs began after World War II, the prewar payroll taxes were retained to finance pensions, disability benefits, and other programs. The NHS was supposed to be financed entirely from the Ministry of Health budget, and so it was during 1949 and 1950. But the Cabinet capped the funding from general revenue, requiring the Ministry to seek its additional money by charging patients and sharing in the National Insurance Fund derived from the National Insurance Contributions levied on employers and employees. The NHS has depended on the latter ever since—from 6 to 16 percent of its total budget each year. To cover the costs of all social security and to permit increases in the transfers from the fund to the NHS, Parliament raises the contributions from time to time.[23]

Italy replaced its national health insurance by a national health service in

1978 for financial as well as organizational reasons. By abandoning exclusive reliance on payroll taxes, more money would be available from a wider range of sources, employers would not be burdened disproportionately, and collections would improve. As in Britain, payroll taxes would continue to be levied for the rest of social security but would be replaced by general revenue financing in health. A National Health Fund was created to handle the mixture of money from payroll taxes and the government budget during the transition.

During the 1980s, the payroll taxes for health were reduced slightly and streamlined. The Italian financing system had been very complicated, with variations in rates among sickness funds and occupations. But health care costs rose too much (cost containment methods were not yet installed), and the government budget could not afford large transfers. Thus, the payroll taxes could not be phased out, new amendments added new complications, the burden on employers from the complete social security tax system remained high, and payroll taxes remained the principal source of health care funding.[24]

Payroll-like Taxes on Total Income. A solution that would preserve the payroll tax is a change in the taxable base. The tax no longer would be levied on earnings from work but would apply to all income. As countries seem to have reached the limit of yield from the present payroll tax on work, this change is seriously proposed for social security as a whole or for health insurance alone. For example, it was recommended during the 1980s by the French national commission that screened all proposed reforms.[25] The proportionate principle would remain the same, but the base would change. The idea has several advantages:

☐   The addition of many high earners—who make no contribution to social security now because the bulk of their income does not come from work— would help. Some of them now have small incomes from work, pay payroll taxes on this base, and get full health insurance coverage. But lower-income workers pay higher contributions.

☐   The system would no longer encourage unearned income and discourage earnings. It would no longer encourage tax dodges to avoid the social security payroll taxes.

☐   If the payroll taxes on employers were reduced or eliminated, employment and export sales might improve. Tax evasion might become more difficult, since the Treasury may be more effective than the social security collection agencies.

☐   If the population is taxed according to the same principles, the separate regimes for different occupations may no longer be necessary. They may merge and simplify administration.

One might think that everyone would welcome the additional revenue and other advantages from expanding the tax base. However, the idea evokes politically important resistance:

☐ The trade unions oppose any fundamental change in traditional structures in social security, including financing by the payroll taxes on earnings from work. At present, the trade unions and the employers associations fill the seats in the governing boards of the sickness funds, the other social security funds, the monitoring bodies, and the agencies that collect the payroll taxes from the employers. These boards have equal numbers of labor and employer representatives (*paritaire*) with no voting members from government Ministries. The trade unions for decades have tried to protect their predominance in the social security machinery in the face of increasing governmental monitoring intended to control costs and prevent increases in the payroll taxes. The trade unions fear that any shift from taxing workers' wages to taxing the general public's entire incomes will greatly increase the power of the Ministry of Finance and the government generally in the social security system. In the past, seats on the governing board have been redistributed when one side (usually the employers) has paid more of the payroll taxes. Thus, a shift of the revenue source would be the opportunity for government to take control. The general taxpayer would need to be represented, and government would be his representative.

☐ The self-employed, farmers, and others in special regimes oppose any form of general taxation tapping their presently underreported and undertaxed income. Part of their income attributable to their capital investment in their businesses is now exempt from the self-employed and farmers' social security taxes. Attempts by government finance officers to expand the definition of taxable self-employment has already created recurrent disputes in France.

☐ Expanding the definition of income taxable under social security—particularly if there is no ceiling—may aggravate flights of capital from one's own economy to nearby countries.

☐ Each of the principal policy antagonists predicts that its fears will be vindicated:

  • The Right predicts that the shift to open-ended taxing powers of government will result in excessive expansion of social security. Since general taxes going into the Treasury are not specifically tied to individual programs, the public will not realize that irresponsible improvements in benefits greatly increase the tax burden.

  • The Left suspects that the shift of social security taxes from business firms' payrolls to the population's full personal income will enable the upper classes to reduce its tax burden, underfund social security, and shift the burden to the general public.

☐ European governments would have to create new tax collection capabilities. At present, the payroll taxes on wages and self-employment and, on the other hand, the general income tax are collected by separate agencies. In most countries, the collection units for payroll taxes are legally private entities. The United States is one of the few countries where the same government agency collects both the income tax and the social security tax and where the final accounting for the year is spelled out on the income tax return. European Ministries of Finance are operated by people who oppose new taxes and more work.

☐ In several countries, such as Germany and Switzerland, health insurance is still so close to its original private arrangements that it cannot question subscribers about their total incomes and cannot compel payments from nonwork income. To broaden the funding base, these health insurance systems would have to become transformed. The Swiss health insurance system would have to become connected with the rest of social security, because it still uses flat premiums while the rest of social security uses proportional payroll taxes.

Hybrid Arrangements. A perennial problem with good ideas is how to reach them from the present situation. Scandinavian experience suggests that once payroll taxes are the principal source for collecting revenue, they are very difficult to give up on the employer side; thus, fiscalization takes the form of replacing the payroll tax on workers with a general earmarked income tax on all citizens. Replacing the payroll tax on the worker with a special tax on all his income is hardly noticeable and produces no political resistance: the final paychecks are nearly the same. More revenue is collected from the recipients of unearned income who previously were untouched by payroll taxes, but they can mobilize little resistance in countries (like Scandinavia) where social solidarity is a leading principle. Health insurance coverage is universal there, and the tax is accepted as properly universal too.

Fiscalizing the entire financing of health insurance requires eliminating the payroll tax on employers and creating an earmarked income tax on the entire population. The great increase in the income tax on persons would produce a political explosion and complaints about windfall business profits. Instead, the search elsewhere in Europe is not for a form of general revenue substitution for the employer's payroll tax, but rather substitution of another and broader tax on business firms—that is, the recent proposals for substituting a higher value-added tax. Scandinavians have not yet proposed such schemes.

The Scandinavian result has been a mixture.[26] Each country has a different pattern. Changes are frequent—usually in the direction of including more health care costs under the general government budget. A further complication is that the structure of taxes for health is not the same as the one for other social security programs. The substantial payroll taxes on employers and the self-employed are kept in most (not all) Scandinavian countries. Workers pay very low or no payroll taxes. If they pay none, the entire population pays low flat-rate earmarked income taxes. The national government subsidizes the sickness funds from its general revenue. The sickness funds are relieved of major costs, since the hospitals and ambulatory health centers are paid for from the budgets of the national or regional governments. Ultimately the money comes from general revenue.

Both Norway and Finland, for example, retain the payroll taxes on employers. Both levy flat taxes on all taxpayers to support pensions and health insurance: 4.7 percent in Norway for each program in 1983; 1.8 percent for the pension fund and 1.7 percent for the health insurance fund in Finland in 1983. The amounts are reported on the taxpayer's annual income tax form and are paid at that time. The calculations are kept separate, however, since the income tax is progressive.

After a long evolution from a typical European payroll tax system, Sweden still levies a substantial amount on the employer but now collects neither a payroll tax from the worker nor a flat earmarked income tax from the citizen. Rather, the balance of health care costs beyond the employers' contributions is covered from general tax revenue, depending on the steeply progressive income taxes on the population. The sickness funds (which primarily pay doctors' ambulatory charges and drugs) are subsidized by the national government. The county councils operate and pay for the hospitals.

These hybrid arrangements—mixing both payroll taxes and special flat-rate earmarked income taxes—are possible only in countries where government dominates the decisions and collection machinery in health care. They are not proposed in countries like Germany and Switzerland, where the sickness funds guard their independence from government and collect their own premiums by methods long accepted by their subscribers. If they tried to increase collections from their subscribers according to ability to pay and unearned income, the subscribers would refuse to cooperate.

Special Taxes. In the search for more revenue, some governments levy flat-rate excise taxes and the yield is earmarked for the sickness funds. The taxes are completely independent of earnings from employment and from payroll taxes. They are levied on activities and objects that create higher costs for the sickness funds and therefore are a tax on moral hazard. Persons pay for their risky behavior. They can avoid payment by not engaging in the activity, thereby reducing the costs to the sickness funds.

The taxes are levied on the producer and collected from him. They are included in the prices of the goods and services, and the ultimate consumer pays. The special agency that collects the payroll taxes and manages their distribution to the sickness funds—such as ACOSS in France—collects these special taxes. The agency then implements the formula for distribution among the sickness funds as spelled out in the Parliament's law enacting the tax. The method is used in countries—like France and Belgium—where the national government is prominent in overseeing the sickness funds' finance, administering their flow of payroll tax revenue, and granting them subsidies.

Once these excise taxes are enacted, the sickness funds cannot do without them. Thus, they become permanent. At times, the rates may be increased, particularly when deficits must be reduced. Examples are taxes on:

☐ *Automobile insurance premiums.* They were the first targets of special taxes, beginning in France in 1967. The justification was (and still is) that auto traffic greatly increases health care costs for drivers, passengers, and pedestrians. Although auto accident policies are the primary insurers in paying medical care expenses, additional health care costs and disability benefits must be borne by the sickness funds. The excise taxes have risen substantially: in France, they began in 1967 at 3 percent of the insurance premium and by 1982 reached 12 percent. The rates vary among countries: Belgium levies 5 percent.

☐ *Alcohol.* Usually the tax is a flat amount per unit. In France, for example, it is 10 F per liter on all sales of drinks containing more than 25 percent alcohol.

☐ *Tobacco.* Usually the tax is a percentage of the sales price. In France, for example, the rate was 25 percent when the tax went to CNAMTS. (At times the tax went entirely to the French Treasury; at other times it was divided between the Treasury and CNAMTS.)

So far, these three obvious health care risks have been the objects of special taxes. One might think of others, such as taxes on entire industries or on individual plants that pollute the environment, increasing the burden on the sickness funds.[27] But at a time when European governments worry that social security taxes are overburdening their industries, no special pollution tax has been seriously considered. Rather, governments prefer direct regulation, informal persuasion, and fines for specific violations. (The premium imposed on an industry for its work-accident insurance under social security reflects its safety performance for its workers, but that is different from the environmental pollutants that affect utilization of national health insurance by the general population.)

Occasionally a government may try to tax an industry that profits excessively from health care, but such a target is not as vulnerable as another industry that clearly increases morbidity, and the taxpayers' political friends may be able to reverse the decision. For example, the French Socialist government in 1983 levied a 5 percent tax on all advertising by drug companies for drugs reimbursed under national health insurance. The revenue went to CNAMTS. The government thought such special action long overdue: the pharmaceutical industry was highly profitable; advertising, cultural habits, and permissive third-party reimbursement had made the French nearly the highest per capita consumers of drugs in the world. When the conservatives won the 1986 parliamentary election, they quickly repealed the tax. But this measure reduced CNAMTS' revenue and worsened its deficit. So the government reduced CNAMTS' expenditures (and made the drug companies even happier) by reducing the value-added tax on all pharmaceuticals.

Despite their occasional prominence in political debates, these special taxes are only minor sources of revenue. In 1984—when all the foregoing taxes were being levied and earmarked for CNAMTS—they yielded only 2.6 percent of the agency's total income of 320 F billion. The payroll tax on employers yielded 65.6 percent.[28]

Implications for the United States

A generous social security system for an elderly population is expensive. The United States has not yet fully faced the problems because its social security system is limited, it lacks national health insurance, and its population is younger.

A serious issue is the method of raising revenue, as well as the level. Each form of taxation involves conflicts of interest and difficulties in economic policy, particularly in periods of recession and unemployment. General social security based on payroll taxes presumes prosperity and full employment. The United States during the early 1980s experienced some of these difficulties and conflicts on a small scale in OASI, but it avoided such wrangles in statutory health insurance by the simple expedient of not having it.

The United States has adopted typical social security payroll taxes for its pension and Medicare programs. The last debate over national health insurance during the 1970s inspired a Grand Bazaar of financing schemes rather than a consensus: the bills proposed complete financing by employers, payroll taxes paid primarily by employers, 50-50 payroll taxes, premiums paid entirely by beneficiaries, complete national public financing, and numerous variations and combinations of the foregoing. Other schemes envisioned a mélange of state programs, each financed by a public fund in each state. Some bills specified very low payroll taxes and premiums; they foresaw separate funding for the expensive elderly patients, counted on extensive cost sharing by patients, and assumed that costs would be low.[29]

In the light of foreign experience and American politics, many of these explicit proposals and implicit assumptions will be hard to implement in the United States for several reasons:

☐ *Complete or predominant financing by employers:*
  • Such levels may harm exports.
  • Such levels may discourage employment in certain industries. They may encourage underreporting of income and employment by some business firms. This hurts income tax collections as well as the social security system. America is trying to reduce, not increase, its ominous levels of tax evasion and fraud.[30]
  • American business would block enactment of any health insurance laws that it would have to finance completely or predominantly. On the other hand, American trade unions might turn against laws requiring the rates of payroll taxes on employees that are normal abroad.
  • This option is fast becoming unrealistic during the 1990s, as employers require contributory premiums from workers and full premiums for their dependents.
☐ *Public financing in whole.* This is not "insurance," even if the word is used in the program's title. Therefore, I have not described it in this survey. An

example is Canada, whose experiences are well known to American medical and hospital associations. Because government will eventually impose strict controls over costs, enactment of any such system will be blocked by American providers. And because government administers the financing and uses existing insurance carriers only as subordinate fiscal intermediaries, enactment of any such system will be blocked by the American insurance industry.

☐ *Public financing in part:*
- The specific drawbacks of subsidies are summarized in Chapter Eight.
- Public subsidies make for unstable financial management in health insurance. At first, the immediate burdens of the payroll taxes on the employer, worker, and subscriber are frozen. The burdens from subsidies on the Treasury rise and cause deficits in the government budget. Eventually the subsidies are capped or even reduced, and the payroll tax rates and premiums are again raised. The United States has already experienced such a cycle in Medicare Part B.
- Insurance carriers would encounter drawbacks, such as strict audits of public money and restrictions on profits.
- Special taxes other than payroll taxes might be used. Capital-intensive industries therefore would contribute in accordance with their fiscal capacity. Designing and collecting such taxes is difficult. The American proposals for national health insurance have not yet suggested any.

☐ *Premiums from subscribers alone:*
- Such premiums require supplementation by subsidies, since individual premiums underfund the system.
- This option would be welcomed by employers, who now pay most of America's health insurance premiums. It would be welcomed as well by small businessmen who now fight the limited current proposals to mandate benefits.
- But this option is unrealistic. If individuals who can pay only low premiums or none at all are not fully covered, then this proposal does not create genuine modern obligatory health insurance. The difficult financing problems are evaded, and the present jumble of categorical programs is preserved.

☐ *Diverse design and financing.* Every carrier can design and charge its own premiums and methods of paying providers. Perhaps the benefit package would be variable. Only coverage and payment of some sort of premium would be obligatory.
- This approach would enact the flexibility and scope for innovation so dear to Americans. It would enable Congress to "pass a bill," avoid all difficult decisions, and "let the market decide."
- No country at present administers anything so amorphous and potentially so heterogeneous. At first, national health insurance laws allowed considerable diversity in financial practices and in benefits—partly to

allow carriers to preserve their previous methods and partly to appease troublesome new groups (such as the self-employed). But eventually financial methods become standardized in order to raise enough money from more prosperous subscribers, avoid preferred-risk selection by carriers, avoid adverse selection by subscribers, and manage the total system efficiently.

- Enacting an amorphous law and postponing specific financial decisions invite constant deadlocks, disputes, cost overruns, and crises in the financial accounts. Examples are America's Medicare (both Part A and Part B at various times), the French social security accounts for the self-employed, and Italy's statutory health insurance.

Unable to make difficult financial design decisions—because of political deadlocks, the complex nature of the subject, or a utopian search for a method that is equitable and pleasing to all—Americans may settle for yet more research. America sponsors more research on health care financing than the rest of the world combined, but it has no health care financing system. It has no system because it has no policy, and no more research is needed in order to create a policy. That requires political will to create statutory health insurance, to opt for certain designs, to build political support, and to face down opponents. The knowledge needed for policy making already exists.

Notes

1. Edwin R. Seligman, *Progressive Taxation in Theory and Practice,* 2nd ed. (Princeton: American Economic Association and Princeton University Press, 1908).

2. For an American and a European critique of the payroll tax system and its earnings ceiling, see John A. Brittain, *The Payroll Tax for Social Security* (Washington: Brookings Institution, 1972); and Alain Euzéby and Chantal Euzéby, "The Significance of Ceilings on Social Security Contributions in Europe," *Benefits International,* vol. 12, no. 3 (Sept. 1982), pp. 20–24. An American rebuttal is Robert J. Myers, *Social Security,* 3rd ed. (Homewood, Ill.: Irwin, 1985), pp. 455–458.

3. During the late 1950s, more than one-sixth of all employees insured under the French general regime had earnings exceeding the ceiling. See Jacques Doublet, *Sécurité Sociale,* 5th ed. (Paris: Presses Universitaires de France, 1972), p. 409. Even after the substantial increases in the ceiling during the 1960s and 1970s, one-fifth of all the wages exceeded it. See V. Maillet, *Eléments de réflexion sur la réforme de l'assiette des cotisations sociales* (Paris: Direction de la Sécurité Sociale, Ministère de la Solidarité Nationale, 1981), app. 3, table 1.

4. Léon Boutbien, "Les problèmes posés par la Sécurité sociale," *Droit Social,* vol. 38, no. 3 (March 1975), pp. 198–206.

5. The *Rapport Granger* was issued at a time of mounting deficits and

precipitated the end of the ceilings. It is summarized in Christian Rollet, "Pourquoi modifier l'assiette des cotisations sociales?," *Droit Social*, vol. 4, nos. 9–10 (Sept.–Oct. 1978), pp. 128–133.

6. Myers, *Social Security* (see note 3, above), p. 458.

7. Martin B. Tracy, "Payroll Taxes Under Social Security Programs: Cross-National Survey," *Social Security Bulletin*, vol. 38, no. 12 (Dec. 1975), p. 6. (The total shares of employers and employees in every developed country in 1973 are given on p. 5.)

8. Onorato Castellino, "Italy," in Jean-Jacques Rosa (ed.), *The World Crisis in Social Security* (Paris: Fondation Nationale d'Economie Politique, 1982), chap. 4. The development of the underground economy—largely to evade social security and other taxes—is described in Raffaele de Grazia, *Clandestine Employment* (Geneva: International Labour Office, 1984), and Rosine Klatzmann, *Le travail noir* (Paris: Presses Universitaires de France, 1982). The adverse effect on Italian social security tax collections is estimated in *Osservazioni e proposte sul finanziamento del Servizio Sanitario Nazionale* (Rome: Consiglio Nazionale dell'Economia e del Lavoro, 1985), pp. 101–112.

9. As in Peter J. Ferrara, *Social Security* (San Francisco: Cato Institute, 1980).

10. See the essays from several countries in Else Oyen (ed.), *Comparing Welfare States and Their Futures* (Aldershot: Gower, 1986). See also the overview in Jean-Pierre Dumont, *L'impact de la crise économique sur les systèmes de protection sociale* (Geneva: International Labour Office, 1986), especially pp. 189–194.

11. *Financing Social Security: The Options* (Geneva: International Labour Office, 1984); *Social Security Financing: A Study by a Group of Independent Experts* (Brussels: Commission of the European Communities, 1986); Bernhard Weissmann, "Sozialversicherungsbeiträge und Lohnsteuer als Jobkiller?," *Zeitschrift für Sozialreform*, vol. 31, nos. 9–10 (Sept.–Oct. 1985), pp. 513–532, 590–603; Jan Peeters, "Modes alternatifs de financement de la Sécurité sociale et leurs incidences sur l'emploi," *Revue belge de Sécurité sociale*, vol. 26, nos. 11–12 (Nov.–Dec. 1984), pp. 795–831; and Alain Euzéby and Chantal Euzéby, "Sécurité sociale, coût de la main-d'oeuvre et compétivité des entreprises," *Revue d'économie politique*, vol. 91, no. 5 (Sept.–Oct. 1981), pp. 579–591.

12. The American critics of social security do not stress Europeans' fears that payroll taxes may discourage hiring by employers but argue principally that social security reduces savings and ambition. See the many sources evaluated in Henry J. Aaron, *Economic Effects of Social Security* (Washington: Brookings Institution, 1982). But, of course, adverse effects on employment are not completely unexamined in the American literature. They are considered in John Brittain's exhaustive *The Payroll Tax for Social Security* (see note 2, above).

13. For Britain's case see Nicholas Barr, *The Economics of the Welfare State* (London: Weidenfeld & Nicolson, 1987), p. 171.

14. Herman Deleeck, "Les cotisations à la Sécurité sociale et leurs

conséquences sur la distribution des charges sociales et sur l'emploi," *Revue belge de Sécurité sociale*, vol. 25, no. 2 (Feb. 1983), pp. 302–316.

15. A government's tax decisions do not follow automatically from such eonomic research, of course, but result from its own strategy in its somewhat unique situation. The French government performed similar simulations and decided to apply remedies other than reducing the payroll tax and increasing the VAT. See Maillet, *Eléments de réflexion* (see note 3, above).

16. *Rapport général sur la Sécurité sociale 1981* (Brussels: Ministère de la Prévoyance Sociale, 1982), pp. iii–xxviii; and Richard de Falleur, *L'opération Maribel et les calculs nationaux sur lesquels elle répose* (Brussels: Bureau du Plan, 1985).

17. Alain Euzéby and Alan Maynard, *Social Security Financing and Effects on Employment* (Brussels: Commission of the European Communities, 1983), especially pt. 1, pp. 28–32, 41, 45–52.

18. Ibid., pp. 67–74.

19. Ibid., pp. 60–63, 74–82, 95; and *Social Security Financing: A Study by a Group of Independent Experts* (Brussels: Commission of the European Communities, 1986), pp. 35–39.

20. Spelled out for the French situation in Denis Kessler and Dominique Strauss-Kahn, "Les modes alternatifs de financement de la Sécurité sociale," *Politiques et management public*, vol. 4, no. 2 (June 1986), pp. 1–33.

21. For functional justification of different modes of social security financing, see Guy Perrin, "Rationalisation of Social Security Financing," in *Financing Social Security: The Options* (Geneva: International Labour Office, 1984), pp. 124–126 and 130; and *Methods of Financing Social Security: Their Economic and Social Effects* (Geneva: International Social Security Association, 1979), pp. 3–7, 83–85.

22. R. W. Harris, *National Health Insurance in Great Britain 1911–1946* (London: Allen & Unwin, 1946).

23. *Compendium of Health Statistics*, 5th ed. (London: Office of Health Economics, 1984), table 2.8; and Almont Lindsey, *Socialized Medicine in England and Wales* (Chapel Hill: University of North Carolina Press, 1962), pp. 105–106, 116–118.

24. *Osservazioni e proposte sul finanziamento del Servizio Sanitario Nazionale* (see note 9, above), pp. 34–35, 82–94.

25. *Rapport du Comité des Sages* (Paris: Etats Généraux de la Sécurité Sociale, 1987), pp. 62–63, 90–92, 138–148 passim.

26. For the history of organization and financing in Swedish health insurance, see *Den svenska sjukkasserorelsen historia* (Stockholm: Svenska Sjukkasseforbundet, 1949); Rolf Broberg, *Sa formades tryggheten: Socialforsakringens historia 1946–1972* (Stockholm: Forsakringskasseforbundet, 1973); and Hirobumi Ito, *The Development of the Health Care System and Modernization in Denmark and Sweden 1850–1950* (Copenhagen: Institute of Social Medicine, 1982), pp. 37–62. Denmark evolved from payroll tax financing of health to general budget

financing earlier than other Scandinavian countries, as can be seen in Ito's monograph. Social security financing was subsequently fiscalized in Denmark, resulting in complications and still unsettled debates on tax policy, summarized by Jorn Henrik Petersen, "Financing Social Security by Means of Taxation," in *Methods of Financing Social Security: Their Economic and Social Effects* (Geneva: International Social Security Association, 1979), pp. 50–60.

27. *The Polluter Pays Principle* (Paris: Organisation for Economic Cooperation and Development, 1975); and William J. Baumol and Alan S. Blinder, *Economics,* 2nd ed. (New York: Harcourt Brace Jovanovich, 1982), pp. 580–583. In the many OECD reports, the Europeans do not propose earmarking charges for the country's entire system for sickness funds but only for depositing them in superfunds for cleanups and prevention. Without any system of health insurance, the Americans too can think only of using the charges for cleanup superfunds.

28. Commission des Comptes de la Sécurité Sociale, *Rapport* (Paris: Ministère des Affaires Sociales et de l'Emploi, 1986), vol. 2, p. 9.

29. Saul Waldman, *National Health Insurance Proposals: Provisions of Bills Introduced in the 94th Congress* (Washington: Office of Research and Statistics, Social Security Administration, Department of Health, Education and Welfare, 1976).

30. "Income Tax Compliance Research: Estimates for 1973–1981" (Washington: Research Division, Office of Assistant Commissioner for Planning, Finance and Research, Internal Revenue Service, 1983). In most years, the shortfalls in collection exceed the deficits in the general budget.

CHAPTER 7

Flat-Rate Premium Systems

─────────────────────── **Summary** ───────────────────────

If health insurance is not financed by payroll taxes, some sort of premium system is used. Payroll taxes are imposed by government as part of the entire social security system, while premiums are usually associated with voluntary health insurance. Payroll taxes are usually enacted by Parliament for large classes of the population, while premiums are set by each carrier in order to cover its unique costs.

Nonprofit carriers devoted to a social policy would like to collect average-risk premiums, whereby the healthier risks pay more than their actuarial costs and subsidize the poorer and less healthy subscribers. But this policy cannot survive in free competitive markets. The young and healthy resist such over-charging and refuse to participate. New insurance companies offer them low premiums and thinner benefits, and the established carriers are left with the more expensive risks. In order to survive, the established carriers match the competition by quoting age-graded premiums and underwriting more of their applicants.

Graduated premiums have the disadvantage of charging the elderly a great deal, thereby inviting government intervention. Switzerland is the only country where private carriers using premiums cover the entire population under statutory health insurance. It uses age-of-entry level premiums to guarantee adequate financing, to avoid high but actuarially necessary rates at older ages, and to prevent cutthroat competition among the carriers.

The United States organizes its private market through group contracts between employers and insurance carriers. Group premiums are experience-rated if insurance calculations are used; or the employer simply pays for all claims for the employees' care. No other country covers the population in this manner.

Uniform Contribution Systems for Individuals

Almost every country uses payroll taxes for statutory health insurance, including the United States for its one obligatory program, Medicare. The alternative methods for individual policies are not related to income. Flat-rate premiums based on class of risk are charged by classifying the person according to sex, age, state of health, occupation, and community. These are "uniform contribution systems," because everyone falling into the same class pays identical monthly or quarterly premiums. People in different classes pay different premiums. A payroll tax system is not "uniform" in the same sense: while the same rate applies to everyone, individuals vary in financial contributions as their incomes vary.

Three types of premium systems exist for individual (that is, nongroup) policies:

☐ *Average risk.* None or few of the foregoing classifications are used. Large classes result. The same premium is charged all subscribers.
☐ *Graduated.* As the subscriber ages, his premium increases.
☐ *Level.* The subscriber's premium depends on his age of initial enrollment. All subscribers with the same age of entry pay the same premium. If the subscriber stays with that carrier, he pays the same premium for life. Rate increases apply to all subscribers in order to cover the costs of the entire enrollment.

An important issue is the base used by the carrier for its calculation of costs and prices:

☐ *Entire community.* One carrier may have a very large share of the market—a large and representative "portfolio" in insurance terminology—and can use the demographic and economic data regularly and publicly reported by government. Or several competing companies may use the same aggregate data.
☐ *Carrier's own subscribers (its own "portfolio").* The data and the calculations become trade secrets concealed from competitors and itinerant researchers.

Premium calculations depend on the costs incurred by the subscribers. Therefore, each carrier must consistently monitor the characteristics of its membership, particularly the "age of the portfolio" in comparison to the entire community and competitors.

Premiums are used in national health insurance instead of payroll taxes for any of the following reasons:

☐ Typical statutory health insurance was defeated politically, usually because the employers opposed paying payroll taxes. Therefore, health financing was left to the private insurance industry and to the voluntary purchase of policies. One example is Switzerland. For all health insurance except the coverage of accidents at work, citizens buy policies from private companies, they pay premiums, and employers contribute nothing. (Accident insurance is compulsory under law, however, and employers support it by paying a percentage of payroll.) Another example is the United States. Except for Medicare, business interests and medical associations have blocked enactment of statutory health insurance, and the private sector handles the finance.

☐ Statutory health insurance was never extended to the wealthy—for either obligatory or voluntary enrollment—and they must buy policies from private companies. The last important remaining example was the Netherlands, where between 30 and 38 percent of the population had to insure privately. (The exact percentage varied from year to year according to the numbers of persons who earned more than the income ceiling for membership.)

☐ Voluntary insurance exists for extra benefits, such as private hospital rooms and fees for hospital doctors. These policies may be sold by sickness funds that collect payroll taxes for basic benefits. Supplementary benefit policies are found in every country, with varying premium structures.

Since the premium is calculated according to the insured person's characteristics, often each member of the family must have an individual policy. An example is Switzerland. Many Swiss companies put all family members' separate premiums on the same bill, but each member is priced separately.

Usually individuals pay for their own insurance out-of-pocket. Unlike the statutory payroll-tax system described in the last two chapters, the employers are not obligated to contribute. If employers do participate in the private health insurance of their workers, it is through group contracts between the employers and the private insurance companies. These are the principal forms of health insurance coverage in the United States, but they are unusual abroad, where protection is established by national health insurance or by national health services. The Netherlands has had group contracts, since it once had the largest market share not covered by statutory insurance. Group contracts are described at the end of this chapter.

Uniform contribution systems are used almost entirely in private health insurance. Usually the policies are bought by the upper-income groups who can afford them. If someone lacks the money, he does not buy private insurance but can fall back on the statutory health insurance system. The only country where premiums—community rates, graduated, or lifelong level—are used in the population's basic insurance is Switzerland. A law patterned on the German precedent was enacted by the Swiss Parliament in 1900 but was defeated in a public referendum. The Left prefers payroll taxes and more generous financing, but employers oppose them for health, since they already pay payroll taxes for other social security programs. The Swiss population has voted down several subsequent attempts to substitute payroll taxes, most recently in 1980.

Once a few Swiss cantons (such as Bern) allowed sickness funds to collect higher premiums from upper-income subscribers. This method led to concealment and protests, however, and the variations by income have been abandoned. Therefore, all Swiss members of a sickness fund now pay the same rates regardless of income.

Under standard premium methods—whether in Switzerland or elsewhere—everyone can join or not join a carrier and pay the premiums, regardless of income and occupation. Thus, the health insurance system is not wracked by controversies—inspired by the self-employed or by certain occupations—over creating special regimes or conceding special terms in the general regime.

Payroll taxes are associated with government programs, are levied on a large scale, and change only occasionally (after the laborious public decisions described in Chapter Five). Premiums are associated with private insurance carriers, who are autonomous in their financing decisions and compete for business. Therefore, premiums are more volatile than payroll taxes. The companies may cut premiums during competitive struggles for market share. At times, premiums may be too low to cover costs.

Average Premiums, Community Rates

Private mutual insurance companies often start off trying to do for the middle and upper classes what the sickness funds do for the workers. Large numbers of people are to be covered by a simple rate structure. Everyone is charged the same, covering the probable average costs of care and administration for those social classes and that list of benefits. Benefits are more generous than those under statutory health insurance and include services desired by the middle and upper classes, such as payment for personal care by doctors and private rooms in hospitals.

For most of their history, Blue Cross/Blue Shield Plans throughout the United States tried to enroll as many people as possible and charged average rates. Blue Cross/Blue Shield often practiced open enrollment of individuals, accepting bad risks who might be rejected by private commercial insurance companies. The Blues could cover these expensive persons—provided that most citizens joined and believed that the rates were reasonable. Blue Cross/Blue Shield also enjoyed special advantages: governments exempted them from premium taxes on the grounds they performed a public service and were not business firms; several state governments required that hospitals grant the Blues discounts from their normal charges; the Blues had many profitable group contracts that might cross-subsidize the individual contracts.[1]

Blue Cross/Blue Shield still advertises community rates. Each of the seventy-six Blue Cross Plans covers a region. A rate is calculated for each region or for an area. The rates per quarter for the principal policies sold in one Plan during 1987 were:

Type of coverage	Individual	Family
Extensive hospital and physician benefits ("Million Dollar Major Medical")	$318.75	$866.55
Hospitalization up to 120 days	$139.95	$326.70
Inpatient hospital bills		
Payment in full (less patient cost sharing)	$81.60	$216.45
Indemnity reimbursement	$55.05	$145.50

Several policies are offered at slight discounts if the applicant joins as a member of a group with three or more persons. Thus, subscribers have an incentive to bring in their friends. Such small groupings are economical in marketing, collections, and administration of benefits. (Most Blue Cross/Blue Shield business comes from employer-based groups, described at the end of this chapter.)

Some nonprofit mutual insurance companies in Europe also charged average community rates rather than graduated premiums differentiated by age, sex, and other characteristics. For example, several major insurance companies (Nationale Nederlanden, Delta-Lloyd, and others) for decades dominated the large Dutch market for persons not obligated to join and to pay payroll taxes to the sickness funds. Each had a large market share, the philosophy of public service was widespread, the companies tried only to break even, and community rates were the standard method.[2]

Unless mandated by law for the entire health insurance industry, community rates cannot survive. In a free market, new companies try to capture business by offering lower premiums to the better risks, particularly the younger. The community rates of the established companies average premiums over everybody, overcharging the young and healthy and undercharging the older and less healthy. As early as the 1950s, Blue Cross in America was threatened by commercial health insurers and searched for modifications of community rates.[3] In the early 1970s the established Dutch companies were forced to match their new competitors by substituting graduated for average premiums.[4] The changes in the Dutch method are described in the following section.

Most Blue Cross/Blue Shield Plans still try to use community rating for individual policies. But the few detailed comparisons of rate making by the Blues and commercials in the United States reveal fewer differences than is generally supposed.[5] In many states where the Blues and commercials compete for young subscribers, the Blues have been forced to adopt age-graduated premiums. The U.S. Congress in 1986 repealed the Blues' exemption from the federal corporation income tax on the grounds they were no longer nonprofit social welfare entities and were really little different from the commercial carriers.

When the United States government offered to place HMOs on a preferred "qualified" list during the 1970s, community rates were a statutory condition. These HMOs would be the vanguard of public policy. But such rates were too high for healthy individual subscribers who could buy policies from commercial insurers, and they were too high for employers who could obtain experience rates from the Blues and commercial carriers. During the 1980s, Congress ended the rating requirements and HMOs moved toward graduated individual premiums and experience group rates.[6]

Graduated Premiums

Graduated premium systems always calculate rates that will actuarially cover the costs for that class of insured persons. The costs, in turn, depend on the benefits covered for that class. Premium tables include several dimensions:

☐ *Age.* These systems always include "step rates"—that is, each subscriber is charged a higher rate as he grows older. The increases cover the higher medical costs as subscribers age. Each age may be charged a unique premium. Or, more often, subscribers are grouped: for example, persons aged thirty to thirty-nine are charged less than those aged forty to forty-nine. The interval usually occurs after five or ten years.

☐ *Sex.* Women were once charged higher rates than men because of their higher costs. The trend in many countries is to eliminate the difference in favor of unisex rates because of new government regulations or unfavorable publicity in the market—both inspired by women's movements.[7]

☐ *Benefits.* The European subscriber can choose between ordinary, semiprivate, and private hospital room coverage in return for higher rates. The basic policy may vary in coverage of certain other benefits, such as dentistry, but usually these are sold as separate policies with their own premium tables.

☐ *Cost sharing.* In much of Europe, the private carriers offer subscribers a lower premium in each class if they are willing to pay more of the costs out-of-pocket. The structure of the premium table otherwise remains the same.

The methods of calculating rates by age and sex are similar in all countries. First, estimate the carrier's own utilization of the insured benefits by age and sex (if the carrier has enough experience), or the average utilization in the country by age and sex (if the insurance industry or government issues data), or the carrier's expected future experience. Then estimate the cost per benefit and the aggregate cost per age-sex class. The categories with higher utilization and higher costs (such as older women) will have higher premiums than others (such as younger men). To this "pure premium" for each category, add a "loading"—usually a standard markup—to cover administration, marketing, and any profit. These premiums might be reduced for some classes with offsetting increases for others, according to the marketing strategy of the carrier.[8]

Other variations in the premiums result from negotiations between the agent and the subscriber pursuant to an underwriter's manual written by the carrier's headquarters:

☐ *Occupation.* The manual may list hundreds of occupations and rate their safety for purposes of health insurance. For persons in the more dangerous occupations, the underwriter may refuse to sell a policy or may charge an extra premium according to the carrier's guidelines and the individual circumstances. Although basic premium tables are advertised, the manuals are not widely known by the public.[9]

☐ *State of health.* After seeing the results of a medical examination, the underwriter may deny the applicant any coverage or may offer it only for an extra premium, according to the home office's guidelines and the individual circumstances.[10]

Each carrier in a competitive private market tries to develop policies that it can advertise as unique and superior to anyone else's. Therefore, premium tables vary within each country along with more or less variation in the basic package of benefits. The shopper can never compare different companies' premiums exactly to identify the best buy.[11]

The Netherlands. Holland's experience demonstrates how a competitive private market can destroy community rates and then produce flux in graduated rates. During the 1970s, new insurance companies tried to enter the market for persons above the statutory income ceiling. The newcomers tried to win the younger subscribers by offering premiums lower than the established companies' community rates. The latter then had to adopt step rates in defense. They also needed to keep their older subscribers who had been with them for some years. Different companies offered different premium tables in order to appeal to the young, avoid antagonizing the older, and break even across all their business.

One method was a separate premium for each age.[12] Every subscriber's premium rose every year. (In addition, the entire premium table might have to be increased every few years to keep pace with cost inflation in health.) Table 7.1 shows a company's table so designed. From the ages of twenty-one through fifty, the premium increases every year; then it stays the same, thereby protecting the older subscribers. The premium for the couple does not cover children; for each child, an additional premium is collected. The carrier starts paying after the subscriber satisfies a deductible of f. 1,000. (In 1986, f. 1 = $0.40 U.S.)

The Dutch private insurance system is pay-as-you-go. This year's revenue from premiums must cover this year's costs. In a highly differentiated step-rate system like the one in Table 7.1 each rate should be enough to cover each age group's costs. A true actuarial premium for persons in their sixties, however, would be very high—so much higher than the previous community rate as to arouse embarrassing protests. The rates for everyone are slightly higher than actuarial costs in Table 7.1 in order to cover the elderly. The company hoped that its reputation would attract young subscribers and that the young would not go to competing firms with lower premiums. If a person joins for the first time after the age of fifty in order to enjoy a bargain, he is charged a permanent monthly supplement. Until 1986, the private companies could refuse to keep a subscriber

Table 7.1. Premiums Appealing to Both Young and Old in Holland.

Age of subscriber	General room in hospital		Semiprivate room		Private room	
	Individual	*Married couple*	*Individual*	*Married couple*	*Individual*	*Married couple*
21	52.84	123.89	83.58	191.34	100.29	229.61
22	54.87	128.66	86.79	198.70	104.15	238.44
23	56.90	133.42	90.01	206.05	108.01	247.27
.						
.						
35	81.29	190.60	128.58	294.36	154.30	353.24
36	83.32	195.37	131.80	301.72	158.16	362.07
.						
.						
49	109.72	257.31	173.59	397.39	208.30	476.88
50	111.77	262.08	176.80	404.75	212.16	485.71

Note: Premiums are given in 1986 Dutch guilders per month.

after the age of sixty-five, and he joined the special program for the elderly in statutory health insurance (the now defunct *bejaardenverzekering*).

Other Dutch companies developed different premium tables in accordance with other strategies. One aiming particularly at the young market, for example, designed a set of rates for different age levels such as the one shown in Table 7.2. The young were charged little until they entered age groups when they had higher incomes and higher medical costs. Then they were charged steadily more until their private coverage ceased at age sixty-five. In order to offer lower premiums, insurance companies designed sliding scales whereby lower premiums were charged in return for higher cost sharing by patients. Such sliding scales became very common in Dutch private health insurance design; greater cost sharing meant that the patient was ready to pay for most of his visits to the general practitioner.

Competitors offered even lower premiums to attract young subscribers. In response, several established companies joined to offer a policy with a premium table like the one shown in Table 7.3. The companies were expected to break even on these rates, instead of earning extra revenue to cover the costs of older subscribers. The goal was to prevent losses to the smaller price-cutting firms. Subscribers were promised a stable premium after the age of forty at a rate individually negotiated but higher than the one at age thirty-nine. The smaller competitors oriented toward the young market might not be able to cover the over-40s, but the established companies hoped to attract the young with a longer view.

Actuaries in the established companies worried that although the strategy in Table 7.3 would protect their large market shares, it would lose money. The higher premiums after the age of forty would cover costs, but not for long. New enrollees after the age of forty might be asked for permanent extra premiums ("solidarity payments"). Those enrolled under the arrangement before the age of forty would not be expected to pay them, since the rates at each upward step—at ages twenty-one, twenty-five, thirty, and thirty-five—had produced small solidarity payments exceeding actuarial costs. But competition for the young wiped out the large extra revenue that was once earned from them in general in order to cover the extra costs of the older. A further difficulty in every step-rate system is loss of the more desirable subscribers in the years when the individual crosses an age threshold and must suddenly pay a higher rate (that is, adverse selection).

Since women are more expensive users of care than men at all ages under seventy,[13] the health insurance companies might construct premium tables by sex. The Dutch companies avoided doing this overtly, since the social insurance system did not vary payroll taxes by sex and the companies avoided antagonizing any possible customers. Meetings of Common Market committees sometimes discuss the reduction of economic inequalities burdensome to women, their higher insurance premiums are occasionally mentioned, and the Dutch private companies believed that unisex premiums eventually would be mandated. Thus, the extra charges for women were hidden: the premium for the couple in Tables 7.1

Table 7.2. Premiums Appealing to the Young in Holland.

Age of subscriber	General room			Semiprivate room			Private room		
	f. 1,000 deduct.	f. 1,500 deduct.	f. 2,000 deduct.	f. 1,000 deduct.	f. 1,500 deduct.	f. 2,000 deduct.	f. 1,000 deduct.	f. 1,500 deduct.	f. 2,000 deduct.
To 44									
Individual	733	598	553	1,028	893	848	1,204	1,069	1,024
Married couple	1,541	1,296	1,191	2,206	1,961	1,856	2,588	2,343	2,238
45–49									
Individual	826	691	646	1,154	1,019	974	1,329	1,194	1,149
Married couple	1,761	1,516	1,411	2,488	2,243	2,138	2,877	2,632	2,527
50–54									
Individual	984	849	804	1,374	1,239	1,194	1,587	1,452	1,407
Married couple	2,118	1,873	1,768	2,992	2,747	2,642	3,471	3,226	3,121
55–59									
Individual	1,118	983	938	1,559	1,424	1,379	1,799	1,664	1,619
Married couple	2,399	2,154	2,049	3,378	3,183	3,028	3,911	3,666	3,561
60–64									
Individual	1,299	1,164	1,119	1,956	1,821	1,776	2,277	2,142	2,097
Married couple	2,794	2,594	2,444	4,088	3,843	3,738	4,690	4,445	4,340

Note: Premiums are given in 1979 guilders per year. Premiums vary by benefits (that is, type of room in the hospital) and by the size of the annual deductible.

Table 7.3. Premiums Strongly Appealing to the Young in Holland But Risking Losses.

Age of subscriber	General room			Semiprivate room			Private room		
	f. 500 deduct.	f. 750 deduct.	f. 1,000 deduct.	f. 500 deduct.	f. 750 deduct.	f. 1,000 deduct.	f. 500 deduct.	f. 750 deduct.	f. 1,000 deduct.
21–24									
Individual	59.96	53.83	48.63	84.23	76.63	69.98	95.95	87.75	80.50
Married couple	128.32	116.47	105.90	179.31	165.36	152.41	203.58	188.76	174.86
25–29									
Individual	68.53	61.53	55.58	96.27	87.57	79.98	109.66	100.28	92.00
Married couple	146.65	133.11	121.03	204.93	188.98	174.19	232.66	215.73	199.84
30–34									
Individual	77.09	69.22	62.53	108.30	98.52	89.98	123.37	112.82	103.50
Married couple	164.98	149.75	136.16	230.55	212.60	195.96	261.75	242.69	224.82
35–39									
Individual	85.66	76.91	69.47	120.33	109.47	99.97	137.08	125.36	115.00
Married couple	183.31	166.39	151.29	256.16	236.22	217.73	290.83	269.66	249.80

Note: Premiums are given in 1986 guilders per month.

through 7.3 is more than twice the premium for the (usually male) individual subscriber. Some additional money comes from the individual premiums, as well, which are set higher than the actuarial costs of that class.

Graduated premium systems exist in highly competitive markets with unpredictable turnover of subscribers. At the time when the actuaries fix the rates—always using past data about costs—one cannot be sure of the number and prices of sales during the next year. Therefore, the company must try to cover the costs of each class of subscribers by a rate calculated for it. An unexpected loss in one class then will not produce a great financial loss in the complete accounts. If affiliations are more stable, the carrier can adopt level premiums set at the subscriber's age of entry. This method has become common in the German private market and in all of Swiss health insurance.

Level Premiums

As health insurance became an integral part of social security throughout Europe, graduated premiums became an embarrassment to the insurance industry. Charging the young very little, charging the elderly a great deal, and driving the retired onto social welfare violated social solidarity. Campaigns to extend statutory health insurance to entire populations pointed to the fate of the older workers and the pensioners under private insurance. If everyone belonged to social sickness funds supported by standard payroll taxes from all workers and employers, solidarity would be achieved among generations: the older would not pay higher rates than the younger, regardless of utilization. Expensive age groups would no longer be dumped onto government welfare.

In order to safeguard their images and head off moves to enact universal statutory insurance, insurance companies searched for actuarially sound methods that would protect individual subscribers from steady and steep increases in payment. A model was the life insurance policies sold by the health insurance carriers or their affiliated companies. They charged level premiums: a subscriber paid upon entry a premium based on his age and expected life span. The premiums and investment yield over his lifetime fully capitalized the face value upon death.

A solution was first sought in Germany. Private insurance companies previously used graduated premiums, but the costs rose for the elderly when their incomes were dropping. The privately insured elderly could not flee and join the low-priced sickness funds where they had never been subscribers. The insurance companies needed to demonstrate they could provide the same lifetime protection as the sickness funds, making unnecessary the enactment of universal obligatory health insurance.

During the 1930s, several German actuaries devised level premium systems in health insurance, using the methodology of life insurance.[14] The lifelong premium would be calculated to provide benefits to the average subscriber between the age of enrollment and the expected age of death. In order to cover the excessive costs of the young subscribers later in life, the health insurance company would have to maintain a substantial reserve from their payments in excess of their costs.

After World War II, German private health insurance companies competed among themselves for the many managers, self-employed people, and upper-income persons who still were not required to enroll in the statutory sickness funds. They also competed with the sickness funds for a new market: the persons who earned higher salaries, passed over the membership ceiling for obligatory coverage, and could choose between continued membership in the sickness funds and buying private coverage. Deutsche Krankenversicherung A.G. (DKV) and a few others offered the option of level premiums rather than graduated premiums. The attraction to subscribers was a guarantee of affordable premiums during old age and retirement, when they could no longer rejoin the sickness funds.

In a population with a great penchant for saving and great worries about security in the future, the lifelong premium system was very persuasive. DKV quickly became the most successful health insurance company in Germany. The usual cycle in a competitive market then followed: in order to survive, every other company offered level premiums. The government regulatory agency that monitors private insurance policies—the *Bundesaufsichtsamt für das Versicherungswesen* (BAV), which checked that current premiums and reserves were sufficient to cover contractual benefits for current subscribers—clearly preferred capitalized methods to arrangements with greater lapse rates and more financial uncertainties. By 1990, graduated premiums had nearly disappeared from basic health insurance. All companies calculate their premiums and reserves by nearly the same methods.[15] (Switzerland quickly emulated Germany but on a larger scale: since statutory health insurance with payroll taxes does not exist in Switzerland, and since private companies service the entire market, level premiums are paid by everyone.)

Table 7.4 is a typical example of a level premium table like ones used by a company in Germany for basic health insurance coverage. This company—like most others—does not accept new members after the age of sixty. The example represents one of many company policies, each with a different monetary scale but all with the same structure by sex and age. One can buy coverage for ambulatory care, hospital care, dentistry, nursing home care, and others in any combination. For each coverage, one can elect higher cost sharing and lower premiums. Different scales are offered civil servants and certain other occupations. Each member of the family has his or her own policy; its premiums depend on the age of entry.

If one changes carriers, he must pay premiums at the new age of entry, although the pressure of competition may persuade the company not to charge the full increase. (Swiss law guarantees continuation of the original age of entry if the subscriber was forced to leave the insurer involuntarily because of its bankruptcy or his job-related change of community.) The change of entry age when the subscriber switches carriers voluntarily has unexpectedly reduced competition. If the subscriber has stayed with a company for several years, he is usually

Table 7.4. Ambulatory and Hospital Care Without Cost Sharing in 1986.

Age of entry	Men (DM/month)[a]	Women (DM/month)[a]
0–14	145.10	145.10
15–19	145.10	167.60
20–24	250.20	394.40
25–29	280.00	417.40
30–34	313.60	434.90
35–39	354.60	455.30
40–44	399.60	488.50
45–49	448.00	525.90
50–54	496.60	563.20
55–59	547.80	598.10

[a]In 1986, 1 DM = $0.47 U.S.

locked in forever, since a voluntary change results in a permanent increase in premiums. This is one of the many barriers facing new insurance experiments such as HMOs. The age-of-entry method strengthens the position of large nationwide insurance companies and contributes to the demise of small local ones: if the subscriber moves, he can continue coverage by the same carrier at the same entry age elsewhere in the country.

Sliding Scales. Statutory health insurance has standard payroll tax rates and standard cost-sharing rules for everyone. But private companies are very competitive and tempt customers by offering a great range of policies. In particular, the young and healthy are offered lower premiums by means of policies with higher deductibles. The subscriber keeps his age of entry throughout his affiliation with that company but can alter his cost-sharing rate from time to time in return for lower or higher premiums. Therefore, each company in Holland and many in Germany and Switzerland offer a variety of policies for the same benefits and the same age groups. For example, another German company offers several combinations of coverage for ambulatory health service, such as the following:

Sample ages of entry	None	Premium in DM per month for the following annual maximum deductibles			
		360 DM	720 DM	1,320 DM	2,400 DM
Men					
25–29	99.37	80.41	48.94	23.95	5.32
45–49	210.95	176.60	121.64	65.82	14.62
Women					
25–29	155.99	123.18	81.19	44.17	3.69
45–49	238.10	194.52	140.70	89.39	6.84

The premium tables are calculated by each company's actuaries based on past claims experience. Each company has been in business for some time and has accumulated considerable data files for such decisions. New products are priced cautiously and are corrected after a few years experience. BAV monitors the premium tables in order to prevent either underpricing or overpricing. In private insurance, each premium class should pay for its own costs; therefore, the company should not lose from adverse selection of the coverage with lower cost sharing.

The supplementary policies for extra benefits can also have a sliding scale of premiums related to a scale of cost sharing by the subscriber. Swiss insurance companies are prevented by law from varying the cost sharing and premiums for basic coverage, but they may do so for the supplementary policies that are free of government regulation. The premiums for the extra policies are based on the same age-of-entry classifications as the basic insurance.

Reserves. Community-rated and graduated premiums can be used in pay-as-you-go systems. If enough cash can be raised from all current subscribers, all current costs and obligations are covered. If few new contracts replace lapsed and deceased subscribers, revenue drops; but costs drop as well, and the carrier is no longer obligated to former subscribers.

Under lifelong premiums, however, the older subscriber's current actuarial costs exceed his current premium. Since he paid more than his actuarial costs during the early years, his lifetime payments plus accumulated interest should be enough to cover his expected lifetime costs without counting on revenue from the company's new subscribers.[16] The company has a lifetime obligation to the subscriber, even if it cannot enlist new subscribers.

Countries using pay-as-you-go methods maintain small reserves in their sickness funds, sufficient to pay bills promptly despite short-term dips in collection of premiums. Countries using lifelong premium methods must maintain large reserves sufficient to guarantee fulfillment of all current contracts until the end of subscribers' lives. One task of the government regulatory agency for the insurance industry is making sure that the reserves are sufficient.

Problems. Level premium systems are difficult to manage. Premiums in life insurance are predictable and stable, since they guarantee payment of a fixed amount. If inflation causes deterioration in the value of the contractual amount, it is the subscriber who has taken the risk. If he wants to preserve his original protection, he must buy more coverage. Inflation is a windfall for the company, since its investment yield from the reserve rises.

But in health insurance it is the carrier who bears the risk—and it is serious. The policy obligates the carrier to pay the bills of providers over the subscriber's lifetime. The original premiums invested at an interest rate—in normal times around 4 percent—should cover lifetime increases in utilization and medical prices. But the explosion in health care costs during the 1970s and 1980s outran the capacity of the original premiums and reserves even in Germany and Switzerland, the countries with the lowest rate of inflation. The entire table of health insurance premiums has had to be increased regularly.[17] The lifelong premium system therefore required a regular injection of pay-as-you-go financing not originally anticipated. Formerly the companies had advertised that their claims experience and administrative efficiency kept their premiums below the payroll taxes of statutory health insurance and below the graduated premiums of traditional private insurance, but such differences diminished.

Other European countries cannot escape problems with their current systems by substituting lifelong premium methods with capitalized reserves. When community rating in the private health insurance market crumbled during the 1970s in Holland, it was tempting for carriers to appeal to new young subscribers but also to build stable attachments by offering low age-of-entry premiums for life. But health care cost inflation was exploding in Holland at the same time—annual increases ultimately approached 20 percent—and a capitalized method could not be adopted.

Countries with universal coverage and pay-as-you-go cannot switch financing methods. Everyone would have to pay two premiums in order to pay current bills of the population and start building up the reserves. Too much money would be tied up, and the burden of social security on the economy would be doubled. (The debate in France was cited in Chapter Two.)

How Rates Are Decided in Switzerland. Swiss sickness funds and the private insurance companies elsewhere compete for subscribers and reputation, and they keep secret their actuarial methods and complete financial position. There is no standard methodology calculated by a Ministry for all or imposed on them by regulation.[18] Therefore, the carriers calculate their level premiums a bit differently. Some limits exist on discretion in Switzerland, since there are statutory conditions for receiving subsidies from the national government.

A leading Swiss company uses the following method. As in all the sickness funds, all calculations are performed by the head office. Claims data are kept there, and the structure of premiums is calculated every five years. Tabulations of the last three years' utilization and expenditures by the company are run by age—by five-year bands, such as 21–25 and 41–45—and by sex. Average lifetime costs are then calculated for persons entering in each age bracket. A man entering at age twenty-eight, for example, will incur the lifetime costs of three times the annual average in the 26–30 bracket, five times the annual average in the 31–35 bracket, and so on to the postulated average final year of enrollment. The same calculation is then made for the average person at each age of entry. A young entrant will accumulate more total lifetime costs than an older entrant, but his average annual costs will be lower, since they will spread over more years. For example, someone entering at age twenty-six will accumulate 63,000 SFr. lifetime treatment costs while someone entering at fifty-one will accumulate 33,000 SFr. The former will be enrolled on the average for forty-five years while the latter will be enrolled for twenty; but the former's annual costs will be only 1,400 SFr. (63,000 ÷ 45 = 1,400) while the latter's will be 1,650 SFr. (33,000 ÷ 20 = 1,650).

Average annual costs must then be compared between the various dates of enrollment and expected termination in order to calculate premiums. The average annual cost in the age bracket 26–30 is taken as the baseline (that is, 100), and each of the other age groups is lower or higher. For example:

Age	Weight in premium calculations
0–15	33
16–20	50
21–25	75
26–30	100
31–35	110
.	
.	
.	
51–55	170
.	
.	
.	
66+	300

As a result, someone who enrolled at the age of twenty-two will always pay 75 percent of the rate charged the person who enrolled at twenty-eight. Someone who enrolled at fifty-four will always pay 170 percent of the rate of the person who enrolled at twenty-eight. The methodology permits corrections for future enrollees. As the costs of caring for the elderly have risen, for example, the foregoing weights for the elderly have risen. As a result, expected lifetime costs for all age groups have risen; but the age-of-entry premiums for the elderly have risen relative to the others.

The structure of the premiums also varies by region. Persons living in areas with more expensive health care must pay correspondingly higher premiums. If everyone was charged an average national rate, the residents of cheaper areas would protest and competing sickness funds would attract them by offering lower rates covering local costs. But charging a unique rate in each locality is too difficult to administer. The actuaries in the head office of this sickness fund compare the age-adjusted per capita health care costs in all localities throughout the country. Adjustments are made for cantons with notoriously permissive cost-containment practices. Lower premiums can be quoted if the canton or commune subsidizes poor subscribers. Premiums must be lower if competition with other sickness funds is vigorous. The actuaries assign localities throughout Switzerland with similar costs to the same category and set the same premiums for all subscribers living there. Premiums are about 6 percent higher for each successive regional category.

Premiums also vary by sex. In Switzerland, as in other countries, women incur higher health care costs than men between the ages of twenty and seventy. Both annual and lifetime costs are higher.[19] Formerly the companies were allowed by law to charge the actuarial difference—up to 25 percent higher for women. In 1964, the national law reduced the differential to 10 percent, and the national government's subsidy is designed primarily to compensate the sickness funds for the balance. Four cantons (Geneva, Neuchâtel, Fribourg, and Ticino) now require unisex premium tables.

The structure of the premium tables remains the same for five years. However, the home office's computers have become so efficient that it may soon recalculate annually. While the structures of the tables remain the same for several years, the financial charges increase every year so that the sickness fund can keep pace with rising health care costs and pay all claims. Everyone keeps the same age-of-entry premium; all premiums rise a few percentage points every year, equally throughout the country.[20]

By raising the entire premium table to pay all current costs, the sickness funds do not need to maintain huge reserves. They must simply maintain reserves to guard against sudden losses of younger members whose payments exceed their current costs and to cover catastrophic cases. Reserves of the larger carriers equal about 30 or 40 percent of annual claims. The smaller carriers must maintain greater reserves.

If a subscriber moves from one area to another and retains the same carrier, he keeps the same age-of-entry premium but must pay a higher or lower amount than before, depending on the regional differences. If he changes carriers, he starts at the new one with a higher age-of-entry premium. Whether he actually pays more cash depends on the comparative levels of charges in the two cantons and the differences in regions if (as usually happens) his move has carried him across the country.

Normally it is payroll taxes rather than premiums that yield redistributive financing. As Chapters Five and Six showed, payroll taxes collect extra cash from the healthier and more affluent people, while the poor and pensioners incur health care costs exceeding their payments. Premiums are usually associated with private insurance, whose competitive market motivates companies to reduce premiums for the good risks and for the rich—leaving no extra cash for the poor risks and leading to preferred risk selection. However, public policy might intervene. In Switzerland, the carriers administer basic benefits for the entire population, receive subsidies from the national government, and are therefore expected to serve the public interest. Thus they set premiums higher than those of a highly competitive market and can cover their more expensive subscribers, such as the elderly.[21]

The design of level premium systems depends on the character and size of the market. The Swiss sickness fund designs a premium table for its basic health insurance coverage for a large and stable enrollment. The principal company, Helvetia, covers nearly one-fifth of the entire Swiss population. For the basic coverage, the benefit package is prescribed by law. In their calculations, the actuaries must take into account wide variations in individual subscribers' expected lifetime costs, regional variations in costs, government subsidies, and regulations about allowable differentials in premiums among classes of subscribers (particularly men and women). The Swiss company can offer sliding scales (that is, lower premiums for higher cost sharing) for its supplementary health insurance but not for its basic coverage.

How Rates Are Decided in Germany. The German situation differs. The level premium system is used by Germany's private insurance carriers for their basic and supplementary coverage of subscribers who are neither obligatory nor voluntary subscribers to the *Krankenkassen* and *Ersatzkassen.* The actuarial logic of calculating lifetime costs covered by age-of-entry premiums is the same in Germany as in Switzerland.[22] However, the methods are used differently:

☐ *Many apparently unique policies.* The German companies are very competitive, and each tries to market policies that seem to differ from the others' in benefits, premiums, and labels. New policies are frequently offered, and old subscribers may switch. Old policies may be phased out, and their subscribers may be transferred to equivalent ones.

☐ *Sliding scales.* For many policies in each German company, the subscriber can elect a lower premium for a higher deductible. The subscriber is usually free to change the option at least once a year.

The entire German insurance industry, as noted earlier, is overseen by an agency of the national government: the *Bundesaufsichtsamt für das Versicherungswesen* (BAV). Its aim is to prevent a common malady of private insurance markets: competition for market share may tempt a company to cut premiums so low that it cannot cover its contractual obligations. German health insurance must be offered by independent specialized companies; it cannot be cross-subsidized by other lines. The individual policies cannot cross-subsidize each other: each policy must provide a premium table and reserves to cover its benefits, including the obligations to holders of lifelong contracts. Every new policy must be approved by BAV on the basis of a detailed actuarial plan (a *Geschäftsplan*). Revisions of the premiums must be approved by BAV on the basis of an amended *Geschäftsplan,* describing the claims experience and explaining the revenue shortfall.

Within each company, new policies are designed by committees representing the departments for marketing, legal contracts, actuary, and finance. Ultimately the decisions must settle on a *Geschäftsplan* that BAV will approve. A proposal will be shelved if it cannot be widely sold or cannot be financed under a viable *Geschäftsplan.* No company reveals these documents to competitors or to researchers, lest another competitor discover that it can offer a comparable product at a lower premium. BAV keeps all the papers confidential.[23]

Since the German companies are private business firms, they can reject bad risks. Usually the underwriter evaluates the case and recommends a supplement to the basic age-of-entry premium. The supplement may be temporary or permanent. This has become the general practice among all companies, lest each company lose customers to the other private firms or to the sickness funds. Because of the complexities in all the companies' papers and rates, the subscriber may never realize that he is being charged a supplement.

Under the rules of the European Economic Community, business firms can sell goods and services across national boundaries. Insurance companies can therefore offer policies in other countries provided only that they conform to local regulations. The principal German carrier, Deutsche Krankenversicherung A.G. (DKV), has tried to enter nearby markets, offering the lifelong security of level premiums and noncancellable policies. So far, its sales in France and Belgium—its first two targets—have been limited. Both countries have universal statutory insurance without the voluntary sector that constitutes the private market in Germany. The private companies in France and Belgium concentrate on supplementary health insurance, use graduated premiums, and do not carry the elderly. Therefore, the young are not yet willing to pay DKV's higher lifelong premiums. However, DKV hopes to find a niche as carriers under the obligatory schemes for the self-employed in France and Belgium. It will need to educate these markets in the advantages of level premiums. Anticipating stronger German competition and the appeal of guaranteed lifelong protection, a few French companies have begun to offer age-of-entry premiums in addition to traditional policies.

Group Contracts

United States. Employment-related private contracts are the principal basis for health insurance coverage in the United States. During the late 1980s, approximately 65 percent of the population depended on private insurance from Blue Cross and Blue Shield, insurance companies, and special plans. Of this number, approximately 84 percent were in groups, either as the breadwinner or as dependents.[24] (Other estimates of the large market share by group contracts are offered in Appendix A.) During the 1980s and early 1990s the only serious proposals in Congress to expand American health insurance coverage substantially have been to require all employers to cover workers and dependents.[25]

The United States is the only country that has widely spread health insurance coverage as a private arrangement negotiated between trade unions and employers or granted by employers voluntarily as a form of employee benefits. As noted in Chapter Four, the method developed unexpectedly during the 1940s, when collective bargaining included fringe benefits as well as wages. The method is an important reason why the labor movement has not pressed for statutory health insurance in the United States as urgently as it has in Europe.[26]

The first step in traditional group coverage was the annual (or periodic) collective bargaining between union and employer over wages, working conditions, fringe benefits, and other matters. The contract might govern several plants by a national employer or one plant by a local employer. Usually the contract specified the health care benefits, beneficiaries (employees alone, retirees, dependents), worker contributions to the premium, patient sharing of provider charges, and certain other matters. Usually contracts did not specify the financial value of the employer's commitment.[27]

The employer then bought the benefit package from a health insurance carrier. He might shop by looking for the lowest premium—he could not cut the benefit list—and the best management of claims. American health insurance carriers developed skills in estimating the probable utilization and costs of various work forces (in cases of completely new accounts), in studying past experience of a transfer (in case of an employer seeking a possible change), and in studying past experience of a current account being renewed. The carrier needed to charge the employer enough to cover claims costs, marketing and administration ("retention"), profit, and (among many Blue Cross Plans during the early years) extra cash to cover bad risks in their community portfolio. The carrier was usually at risk for deficits, unless it obtained a guarantee during the first year of a new account. The carrier could keep profits; but since the group premium used an experience rate, the employer would insist on paying less upon the annual renewal. One could not generalize about the size of group premiums across the country: not only did each group pay a different amount according to its expected or actual experience, but the amount changed every year for every group and the carriers concealed this information.[28]

During the 1980s, competition led to a deterioration of the workers' benefits. Where unions existed, they could still insist on the traditional benefits, minimum patient cost sharing, and minimum contribution to the premiums. In the traditional industries that had set the pattern in welfare bargaining, employment and union membership declined. Other employers had customarily granted health insurance to show workers that unionization was unnecessary, and workers in these industries never had protectors. Competing to keep foreign and domestic markets, employers made cuts in their labor costs and their increasingly expensive health care premiums were singled out. During the 1980s, employers routinely expected dependents to contribute substantially to the group premiums, initiated and then increased contributions by the workers, and increased point-of-service cost sharing by patients.[29]

Employers forced insurance carriers to compete for group contracts. Blue Cross/Blue Shield had much of the group business before 1970, but employers increasingly solicited competitive bids for new accounts and renewals, and the pressure lowered group premiums. Blue Cross/Blue Shield lost market share, no longer earned extra cash from its contracts, and therefore could not cross-subsidize its community business. Some employers forced carriers to sign "experience refund" clauses rebating windfall profits; the carriers might still be at risk for deficits.

To eliminate payment for carrier loadings, prevent payment of windfall profits, control health care costs more strictly, and retain any interest earned from the health care accounts, many employers abandoned traditional insurance and self-financed in the forms described in Chapter Four and Appendix A. Insurance companies were hired merely to administer claims; or they might even be dispensed with altogether. Within a decade, the group health insurance market had been transformed completely: by the late 1980s, most large groups that still used insurance carriers had "administrative services only" or "minimum premium plans" (described in Appendix A); few still had conventional insurance. This trend was one reason the private health insurance industry was often in deficit.[30]

Americans once imagined they could cover the population through group contracts. This was never possible, however, since many persons worked for small business, which did not fit the group model at all. Noticing the financial squeeze and reduced market in their traditional large group business during the 1970s and 1980s, many commercial insurers and some Blue Cross/Blue Shield Plans tried to compensate by entering the small business market. But this venture worsened rather than improved their balance sheets, since they competed for sales in a voluntary market among resistant purchasers. Government played no role in setting minimum premiums or mandating coverage. The carriers were competitors and could not create large and efficient marketing efforts and underwriting pools.

Small groups in a voluntary market are expensive and risky even under the best of circumstances. Marketing and administration are expensive. The carrier cannot investigate and medically underwrite individuals in any groups: while the workers may be healthy, bad risks may lurk among the dependents. Adverse selection is a consistent threat: the small firm may choose to buy group insurance for the first time because the owner needs to cover a dependent's costs, and he chooses a group rather than a family policy in order to avoid medical underwriting. Since every worker must contribute to the premium, each must sign up voluntarily; the healthier ones may not. Thus, the carrier cannot calculate its full revenue until the enrollment period has ended—and this occurs long after it has set the first year's premium.

When setting premiums for previously uninsured small groups, the Blue Cross/Blue Shield Plans had benchmarks in their community rates for local individual and family policies. They hoped to offer these rates (less discounts) for local individual and family policies. But the commercial insurers had no such starting point; they aimed at rates that would attract purchasers (that is, the small businessmen) who were accustomed to buying insurance for themselves but had never seen the need to buy it for their workers. In order to win business, all the carriers (including the Blues) offered premiums that were too low to cover subsequent years lest the employers cancel altogether. They hoped to practice the "underwriting cycle" once accepted by large employer group purchasers and by state insurance rate regulators—namely, make up for intervening losses and replenish reserves by raising rates substantially every few years. But the participating small groups would have canceled and no new business could be found.[31] Therefore, among small groups even more than large ones, customary actuarial premium setting was not possible in a real-life competitive free market.

The Netherlands. Employer-paid groups exist in only a few European countries where statutory health insurance leaves a substantial private niche. The principal market was in the Netherlands, where one-third of the population insured privately. About 37 percent of the nearly 5 million privately insured belonged to employer-based or other groups.[32] Creating a privately insured group was more complicated in Holland than in the United States, because the entire labor force of a firm was not automatically covered. The participants could be only those persons earning more than the annual membership ceiling for obligatory coverage in the *ziekenfonds* (f. 49,150.00 in 1987). Therefore, a carrier could find group business only in those firms with large numbers of employees earning more, such as banks, universities, and government agencies.

The Dutch insurance company and the employer negotiated a package of benefits much like that available in the carrier's private individual insurance. The subscriber could choose higher deductibles for lower premiums. The actuaries estimated the cost of the first year, and the employer agreed. The employer usually planned to recover half or one-quarter of the cost by deducting premiums from employees' paychecks. The attraction for the employees was lower premiums than those in the private individual market. Another attraction for individuals was that the worse risks who might be rejected or charged a supplement for a private individual policy could not be singled out and rejected by the carrier; if they were members of the group, they received standard coverage. The employees (led by their trade unions) were then polled: if about three-quarters agreed to subscribe, the plan was implemented; if fewer approved, the carrier withdrew the offer.

Rate setting pitted two business firms against each other: the employer and the carrier. During the first years under the originally agreed lump sum, the carrier might suffer losses or might earn very high profits. Perhaps the original contract allowed the carrier—in case of a serious financial emergency—to increase cost sharing by patients. After the end of the initial one-year or two-year contract, the lump sum was adjusted in the light of claims experience. The negotiations were based on power bargaining rather than agreed financial facts, since the carrier concealed the full truth (especially windfall profits) from the employer. If the terms seemed very advantageous to them, the employer and the trade union sought long contracts—up to five years. Since health care costs and utilization rose unpredictably, the carrier usually preferred shorter contracts.

The carrier collected no premiums from the employee. The division of the costs was a private arrangement between company and worker. The carrier administered all the employee's claims according to the policy. The employee could not opt out of the contract, collect cash, and use it as he liked. In some firms without groups, the employer might give employees extra cash earmarked for purchase of private policies.

Before World War II, a few large Dutch employers maintained their own free medical services for their employees and their families. A few, such as Phillips, still do. This was the forerunner of modern group insurance. Until statutory health insurance became universal during the 1990s, nearly all employers split their coverage between statutory health insurance (for workers below the membership ceiling) and private group insurance (for workers above). The employers covered these benefits by paying payroll taxes to the *ziekenfonds* and lump sums to the private carriers. No Dutch company self-insured and hired a private carrier for an "administrative services only" role, as in the United States.

France. Several countries have private employer-assisted health insurance that supplements the basic statutory health insurance financed by payroll taxes. Usually these fringe benefits provide a second tier of pensions over the basic social security coverage. Health and accident coverage is an appendage.

The leading example is France.[33] According to a national labor/management agreement (signed in 1961), every employer is expected to contribute to a second tier of pensions for all workers. In addition, many private firms and government agencies have *mutuelles*, governed and financed by the workers, covering extra health benefits. Although some employers contribute to the *mutuelles*, most believe they already contribute enough in social security payroll taxes.

Some employers—either unilaterally or in response to demands by the local trade union—contract with a private insurance company to cover the managers alone or all ranks. The benefits can include life insurance, off-the-job accident insurance, and certain health care benefits. The carrier usually covers the employer's obligations in work accidents and second-tier pensions. In practice, the benefits and financing of the health insurance component are much like those of a *mutuelle*. The employer may contribute to the other parts of the group insurance, but rarely for the health coverage.[34]

Great Britain. The private insurance sector in Britain—described in Chapter Four—depends heavily on group contracts. Since everyone can use the National Health Service, all private practice and private insurance depend on voluntary extra payments. If the patient has private insurance, he is helped in paying for inpatient care in a private nonprofit or private for-profit hospital; he can pay the specialist a private fee.

In 1984, some 4,367,000 people (almost 8 percent of the United Kingdom) were covered by private health insurance. Of these people, 51 percent belonged to groups completely paid for by employers; 21 percent belonged to groups organized at the workplace but paid for by workers' premiums; and 28 percent bought individual policies.[35] (In some employer-paid groups, dependents are fully covered; in others, they must pay premiums.)

The private health care market is very unpredictable and unstable. Unlike countries with national health insurance, Britain lacks data about utilization and provider prices that can be guidelines for the carriers. The private hospitals and pay-beds inside the NHS hospitals are a small market of their own. Private insurance has considerable turnover of subscribers and changes in claims experience. Thus, the private carriers have learned to be cautious.

Only a few carriers exist, and one of them (the British United Provident Association, or BUPA) controls two-thirds of the private insurance market. About half its groups are large enough and have stayed with BUPA long enough so that BUPA and the employer negotiate an experience rate. For the other groups—particularly those where the employees will pay the premiums—BUPA offers the same benefits as in the individual policies and charges the same premiums (less a discount). These premiums are moderately age-graduated; by overcharging the young and undercharging the old, they approach community rating. The group contracts are reexamined and renewed annually, so the carrier can correct the lump sum negotiated with the employer and so the carrier can correct the benefit schedule.

Germany. At first sight, Germany's many *Betriebskrankenkassen* might seem to resemble American group insurance, but the differences are fundamental. A *Betriebskrankenkasse* must cover a list of benefits and follow many other statutory requirements; the American arrangement is completely private and almost unregulated. The German sickness fund must cover all dependents; the American group contracts need not and have significantly reduced dependent coverage during the 1980s. If a *Betriebskrankenkasse* terminates, its subscribers continue coverage automatically elsewhere with employer contributions; American groups can be terminated or revised, eliminating all coverage of their members.

Effects on Utilization and Health

What difference does it make whether health insurance is financed by premiums or by some other method? As in the case of payroll taxes, these are financing instruments, they affect the volume of revenue and fiscal administration, but they are remote from the work of providers and from the clinical experience of patients.

In practice, premiums are usually associated with private competitive markets. In order to attract individual and group business, carriers are pressed to quote lower premiums barely sufficient to cover the costs of each category of subscribers. No extra money is generated so that the carrier can cover the bad risks and the uninsured. But government or a consensus in the insurance industry can intervene to limit the price cutting by carriers and therefore preserve some redistributive financing, as in Switzerland.

Premiums are often associated with arrangements wherein either the subscriber or the employer pays, but not both. In these cases, revenue is low, providers might be paid little, subscribers may be pressed to pay providers out-of-pocket, and no extra money is generated for the bad risks and uninsured. In such arrangements, utilization might be inhibited, the population's illnesses are untreated, and the providers are underfinanced. Public policy steps in with subsidies, as in Switzerland. Or, as in the American case of employer-paid premiums, the workers are pressed to contribute to the premiums.

Since premiums rise with age and medical risk, the elderly and bad risks are priced out of the market. Government must then step in with special subsidized programs for the elderly and the unhealthy, as in Holland and the United States. The health insurance industry may try to protect the elderly and bad risks by adopting community rates or lifelong level rates, but government regulation or a consensus in the insurance industry is needed to protect these rates from price-cutting appeals to the younger and healthier subscribers.

Implications for the United States

The problems in designing a premium system have not been faced by American public policy, since most employed persons receive health insurance as a fringe benefit of employment, the retired are covered by Social Security payroll taxes on the employed, and many others are not covered. The Americans who buy individual insurance—including the aged who buy Medigap—are confused by the complicated market, are frequently overcharged for their coverage, and often buy duplicating coverage.

If America enacts national health insurance and bases it on individual premiums, this arrangement may not mesh easily with Medicare (assuming the latter is retained as part of Social Security). America has a propensity for enacting a range of categorical programs, however, so perhaps they will indeed coexist.

Americans are accustomed to graduated premiums in health insurance, but such a premium system is troublesome on a large scale because of the overpricing or dumping of the elderly. The United States already experienced that problem once, and it was remedied by Medicare.

Americans are accustomed to level premiums in life insurance, but the method would be a novelty in their health insurance. It is a trend in other developed countries that used premium financing of statutory and voluntary health insurance. A few American carriers are offering lifelong level premiums for their new long-term-care insurance policies. The method has several advantages: it gives subscribers an incentive to begin insuring long before need and reduces adverse selection; it discourages lapses; it enables the carrier to accumulate reserves.

If America enacts national health insurance, advocates of competition and flexibility would prefer a premium system to the standardized and highly redistributive payroll taxes. Premiums differ among insurance companies according to their costs and membership. A variety of policies can be offered with different cost-sharing rates and benefits. However, competition produces constant innovation and instability in premiums and policies. In particular, companies try to capture market share by appealing to the young with lower premiums. This tactic produces serious financial problems for the established companies (who must raise the money to cover the older subscribers), and it creates public policy responsibilities for government—which Americans do not yet foresee and debate. All this demonstrates the common outcome in competitive insurance markets offering alternative packages: adverse selection and premium spirals feed on each other, and there is no inevitable equilibrium that stabilizes the market.[36]

Any premium system shows up the contradictions between a public policy of free-market economic competition and a public policy of universal social protection and predictability. Uninhibited economic competition directed at payers' self-interest reduces revenue to the actuarial costs of each group—or even less. The population can be protected only by creation of a parallel set of public programs and subsidies, perhaps overshadowing the competitive premium-paid market in size and in public discussion. Under statutory health insurance—whether financed by premiums or by payroll taxes—Americans will have to focus "competition" on socially constructive efforts, such as the quality of service, rather than on unstabilizing activities.

Or Americans could preserve a competitive economic market in second-tier health insurance. Several European countries distinguish between basic services financed through social insurance and extra services financed through voluntary insurance. Payroll taxes or community-rated premiums could cover the basic and universal set of services. Subscribers could then buy the extra services through voluntary insurance. The carriers could design many packages, quote various premium tables, and compete for business. The American health care economists would still have a market to study.

No country bases health care finance on employer-paid groups, and it is not likely that the Americans can do so. Nearly all legislative bills for national health insurance since the early 1970s have mandated coverage through employer groups, and the subject is debated at length in the 1990s, but none of these proposals can be enacted or administered. Large American employers are trying to reduce their role in health care, not increase it. They want to spend less, not more. They do not want a bigger responsibility in interpreting acts of Congress, shopping among carriers for the most attractive contract, and monitoring the performance of carriers and providers. Small business can block enactment of any law requiring it to carry and administer standard levels of health insurance. Legislative mandates of universal employer coverage will leave many loopholes and variations in benefits. They will leave in place the separate categorical programs for the aged and unemployed. They will aggravate, not alleviate, the American problems of administrative complexity and administrative cost.

Notes

1. Duncan M. MacIntyre, *Voluntary Health Insurance and Rate Making* (Ithaca: Cornell University Press, 1962), pp. 54–64, 70, 136–137, 162–165, 173–175, 188–190, 248–269, 286–292.

2. The techniques were summarized in G. W. de Wit, "Ziektekostenverzek-

ering: Technische grondslagen van de Nederlandse ziektekostenverzekering," *Verzekerings-Archief,* vol. 45, no. 3 (Oct. 1969), pp. 141–154.

3. Herman Somers and Anne Somers, *Doctors, Patients, and Health Insurance* (Washington: Brookings Institution, 1961), pp. 310–313.

4. G. W. de Wit, *De financiering van ziektekostenverzekering* (Rotterdam: Nationale-Nederlanden, 1986), pp. 37–38.

5. MacIntyre, *Voluntary Health Insurance and Rate Making* (see note 1, above); and *Health Insurance: Comparing Blue Cross and Blue Shield Plans with Commercial Insurers,* (Washington: General Accounting Office, 1986), especially pp. 16–18, 28–30.

6. "Cooperative HMO Stays Strong by Keeping Enrollees Involved," *Modern Healthcare,* vol. 19, no. 31 (Aug. 4, 1989), pp. 22–23; and Paul J. Kenkel, "Kaiser Breaks with Tradition with New Rate Change That Reflects Expected Use," *Modern Healthcare,* vol. 19, no. 43 (Oct. 27, 1989), p. 76.

7. Deborah Benjamin and others, "Two Sexes—One Rate," *Best's Review—Life/Health Insurance Edition,* vol. 89, no. 2 (June 1988), pp. 52–56, 138.

8. *A Course in Individual Health Insurance,* rev. ed. (Washington: Health Insurance Association of America, 1983), pt. A, chap. 4.

9. They may have to be filed with the government agency that regulates the private insurance industry of that country. Parts of the manuals of the leading private American carriers were published in *Commercial Health and Accident Insurance Industry: Hearings Before the Subcommittee on Antitrust and Monopoly of the Committee on the Judiciary, United States Senate, Ninety-Second Congress, Second Session* (Washington: Government Printing Office, 1972), pp. 124–170 passim, 306–307, 537–554, 948–963, 1260–1276, 1389–1406. American home office underwriting methods for individual medical expense and disability insurance are described in *A Course in Individual Health Insurance* (see note 8, above), pt. A, chap. 6; and O. D. Dickerson, *Health Insurance,* 3rd ed. (Homewood, Ill.: Irwin, 1968), chap. 17.

10. *Medical Testing and Health Insurance* (Washington: Office of Technology Assessment, Congress of the United States, 1988).

11. For examples of the difficulties in making comparisons, see *Commercial Health and Accident Insurance Industry* (see note 9, above), pp. 567–568. Even the American Medigap policies—designed to cover only the Medicare cost sharing—are unclear and noncomparable to the average purchaser. See *Catastrophic Health Insurance: The "Medigap" Crisis,* Comm. Pub. 99-576 (Washington: Select Committee on Aging, U.S. House of Representatives, 1986), pp. 55–106; and Nelda McCall and others, "Consumer Knowledge of Medicare and Supplemental Health Insurance Benefits," *Health Services Research,* vol. 20, no. 6, pt. 1 (Feb. 1986), pp. 648–655.

12. The technical methodology used by all the Dutch firms—before the variations reflecting their marketing strategies—is summarized in Wim de Wit, "Technische Methoden der privaten Krankenversicherung in den Nederlanden," in Hans Georg Timmer (ed.), *Technische Methoden der privaten Krankenversi-*

cherung in Europa (Karlsruhe: Verlag Versicherungswirtschaft, 1990), pp. 161–177.

13. *KISG85: Jaarboek 1985* (Houten: Stichting KLOZ Informatiesysteem Gezondheidszorg, 1986), pp. 77–82.

14. A. Tosberg, "Rechnungsgrundlagen und Schadentafeln der Krankheitskostenversicherung," *Veröffentlichungen des Deutschen Vereins für Versicherungswissenschaft*, vol. 66 (1940); F. Rusam, "Grundzuge der Mathematik der privaten Krankheitskostenversicherung," *Zwölfter Internationale Kongress der Versicherungsmathematik*, vol. 4 (1940), pp. 147–167; and many other papers by Tosberg and Rusam during the late 1930s.

15. Described in the widely used manual by Klaus Bohn, *Die Mathematik der deutschen privaten Krankenversicherung* (Karlsruhe: Verlag Versicherungswirtschaft, 1980); summarized in Christian Brünjes, "Technische Methoden der privaten Krankenversicherung in Deutschland," in Timmer, *Technische Methoden* (see note 12, above), pp. 44–62. For an overview of German practices when level premiums were spreading, see G. Jäger, *Die versicherungstechnischen Grundlagen der deutschen privaten Krankheitskostenversicherung* (Berlin: Duncker und Humblot, 1958).

16. Dickerson, *Health Insurance* (see note 9, above), pp. 588, 606–609; and *A Course in Individual Health Insurance* (see note 8, above), pt. A, pp. 122–127.

17. Hans Georg Timmer, "Die Prämienanpassungsautomatik in der Krankenversicherung," *Blätter der Deutschen Gesellschaft für Versicherungsmathematik*, vol. 11 (1973), pp. 123–130.

18. Some general principles appear in Rudolf Haberthür, "Technische Methoden der privaten Krankenversicherung in der Schweiz," in Timmer, *Technische Methoden* (see note 12, above), pp. 199–215.

19. Heinz Schmid and others, *Datenanalyse in der Krankenversicherung* (Aarau: Schweizerisches Institut für Gesundheits- und Krankenhauswesen, 1985), vol. 1, sec. 377.

20. Because of rising health care costs and the national government's limits on its subsidies, the leading Swiss sickness fund in 1984 was charging seven times its 1966 rates. See *Jahresbericht* (Zurich: Schweizerische Krankenkasse Helvetia, 1985), pp. 1–4.

21. René L. Frey and Robert E. Leu, *Der Sozialstaat unter der Lupe: Wohlstandsverteilung und Wohlstandsumverteilung in der Schweiz* (Basel: Verlag Helbing und Lichtenhahn, 1988), pp. 249–276.

22. Apparently all the German actuaries depend on Bohn, *Die Mathematik der deutschen privaten Krankenversicherung* (see note 10, above), especially chap. 6.

23. How to write a *Geschäftsplan* is explained by Hartmut Herde, "Erstellung technischer Geschäftspläne in der privaten Krankenversicherung," *Versicherungswirtschaft*, vol. 31, no. 17 (Sept. 1, 1976), pp. 967–982. The work of BAV is described in *Die Versicherungsaufsicht in der Bundesrepublik Deutschland* (Berlin: Bundesaufsichtsamt für das Versicherungswesen, 1984). The work of

BAV and all other European monitoring agencies is summarized in OECD Insurance Committee, *Supervision of Private Insurance in Europe* (Paris: Organisation for European Co-Operation and Development, 1963).

24. The precise figures are unknown because the United States has many programs, overlapping coverage, no systematic national surveys on the subject, and much uncertainty in the population. The proportions are my best estimate pieced together from the following sources: *1988 Update: Source Book of Health Insurance Data* (Washington: Health Insurance Association of America, 1988); *Fact Book 1981* (Chicago: Blue Cross and Blue Shield Associations, 1981); and Gail Lee Cafferata, *Private Health Insurance: Premium Expenditures and Sources of Payment*, National Health Care Expenditures Study Data Preview, no. 17 (Rockville, Md.: National Center for Health Services Research, 1984).

25. *Government Mandating of Employee Benefits* (Washington: Employee Benefit Research Institute, 1987), pt. 2.

26. The origins and early evolution are described in Raymond Munts, *Bargaining for Health: Labor Unions, Health Insurance, and Medical Care* (Madison: University of Wisconsin Press, 1962), pt. 1; and Beth Stevens, *Complementing the Welfare State: The Development of Private Pension, Health Insurance and Other Employee Benefits in the United States* (Geneva: International Labour Office, 1986).

27. Munts, *Bargaining for Health*, pt. 2 (see note 26, above); and Joseph W. Garbarino, *Health Plans and Collective Bargaining* (Berkeley: University of California Press, 1960).

28. The American health insurance industry had to develop a considerable methodology about negotiating, pricing, and administering group accounts. See, for example, the methods in Robert D. Eilers and Robert M. Crowe, *Group Insurance Handbook* (Homewood, Ill.: Irwin, 1965); and *A Course in Group Life and Health Insurance*, rev. ed. (Washington: Health Insurance Association of America, 1985), 3 vol.

29. The increase in contributions by worker and dependents, as well as the increase in cost sharing by patients, are described in successive issues of *Employee Benefits in Medium and Large Firms* (Washington: Bureau of Labor Statistics, Department of Labor, annual). The changes were sugar-coated by an apparent improvement in benefits: plans covered all patient costs over a limit ("stop-loss"). But few cases were catastrophic, and the rare savings by a few patients did not offset the increased out-of-pockets by all.

30. Steven DiCarlo and Jon Gabel, "Conventional Health Insurance: A Decade Later," *Health Care Financing Review*, vol. 10, no. 3 (Spring 1989), pp. 77–89; and the sources cited in Chapter Four, note 19. Carriers could still use their languishing underwriting skills in calculating the catastrophic-cost premiums they charged employers under "minimum premium plans."

31. Howard J. Bolnick, "It's Time to Pay the Piper," *Best's Review—Life/ Health Insurance Edition*, vol. 88, no. 8 (Dec. 1987), pp. 18, 21, 134. Bolnick's earlier warnings about the life cycle of small-group accounts are in his "Why

Small Group Programs Fail," *Best's Review—Life/Health Insurance Edition,* vol. 84, no. 6 (Oct. 1983), pp. 16, 18, 104, 106.

32. *KISG85* (see note 13, above), pp. 18, 21-22.

33. Thomas Coutrot and Philippe Madinier, *Les compléments du salaire* (Paris: Documents du Centre d'Etude des Revenus et des Coûts, 1987), especially pp. 55-64.

34. The only manual of methods is *Guide de l'assurance de groupe* (Paris: Bureau Commun d'Assurance Collective), a looseleaf volume that is periodically updated. Part 5 of the manual deals with health insurance.

35. See the sources cited in Chapter Four, note 23.

36. Michael Rothschild and Joseph Stiglitz, "Equilibrium in Competitive Insurance Markets: An Essay on the Economics of Imperfect Information," *Quarterly Journal of Economics,* vol. 90, no. 4 (Nov. 1976), pp. 629-650. Even if people persist with their policies in a confusing multiple-choice market, the escalating premiums of high-option plans during premium spirals cause the better risks to flee. See Joachim Neipp and Richard Zeckhauser, "Persistence in the Choice of Health Plans," *Advances in Health Economics and Health Services Research,* vol. 6 (1985), pp. 63-64.

CHAPTER 8

Government Subsidies

──────────────────────────── **Summary** ────────────────────────────

Statutory health insurance in most countries was designed to be financially self-supporting and independent of government budgets. But the increase in health care costs and the extension of health insurance to the poor, the unemployed, and pensioners induce government to fill shortfalls with grants to the sickness funds. As payroll taxes reach their limits, pressures build for government help.

Subsidy policy takes different forms. Government has long granted money to Belgian nonprofit carriers in order to support their administration and make public corporations unnecessary. In lieu of normal social security payroll taxes on employers, the Swiss national government has long made direct grants to all sickness funds. Grants to carriers make up for the excess of health costs over premiums by the aged and unemployed in France, in Holland, and in American Medicare.

Some governments grant money to providers in order to reduce the claims charged to health insurance carriers. Examples are capital grants to hospitals in several countries and Swiss cantonal sharing of hospital operating budgets.

Starting subsidies in periods of prosperity is politically popular; but controlling them during recessions touches off great political controversies. The need to limit increases in payroll taxes and public subsidies leads national governments to intervene in the once independent health care market by controlling provider costs.

The Role of Government

Under a completely private health insurance system, premiums, benefits, and other matters are private transactions between subscriber and carrier. Payments to health care providers are private transactions between carriers and providers. Disputes involve government as administrator of the courts. Government's principal role is to regulate the premium and the carrier's accounts to make sure that the carriers can pay all claims. Insurance regulation is one of the earliest and most common forms of government regulation. It is encountered in every developed country.

Under national health insurance, by way of contrast, the government enacts a law requiring certain occupations to join carriers, specifying the methods of financing, setting minimum benefits, and fixing other rules. Government may create public corporations and carriers, as in France and American Medicare. Government may collect the health insurance funding as part of the package of social security payroll taxes and then distribute the cash to the sickness funds. Government may also provide subsidies from general revenue—the subject of this chapter.

Government may take over financing completely.[1] Providers are paid from the Ministry of Health budget, which is part of the government's total budget based on general revenue. This is not health insurance, and this book does not describe such systems. (Examples are Great Britain, Italy, Canada, and Eastern Europe.) A few countries had national health insurance before switching to full government ownership of hospitals, full government financing of all services, and full entitlement of the entire population. Great Britain's National Health Insurance was incomplete—it covered only workers and not dependents, only general practice and not specialty care or hospital service—and the complete system had to be reorganized completely in the 1940s. Italy's statutory health insurance was underfunded, hospital costs were inadequately controlled, and the system went bankrupt.

Types of Government Subsidy

General revenue may be injected into the health insurance stream in several ways for different reasons:[2]

☐   Grants to the sickness funds (usually by the national government):
  - To cover the costs of subscribers who pay very low or no premiums, such as pensioners, the unemployed, and farm workers. Examples: France and the Netherlands.
  - To make up for the absence of payroll taxes from employers. Several governments once encouraged voluntary health insurance by offering subsidies to the sickness funds, matching the premiums of subscribers.[3] When laws made membership compulsory, payroll taxes were levied on employers and replaced the subsidies. The only country that retains the older system is Switzerland.
  - To cover the administrative costs of the sickness funds and to defray costs

of certain public welfare programs they carry out, thereby relieving government of the task. Example: Belgium.
- To cover the costs of certain public health services that government otherwise would have to provide or finance. Example: Switzerland.
☐ Grants to hospitals enabling them to charge lower rates to the sickness funds, thereby reducing the funds' expenditures and premiums. Usually from provincial governments.[4]
- Capital investment. Example: Germany.
- A share of operating costs. Examples: Switzerland and Belgium.
☐ Payments to sickness funds on behalf of impoverished subscribers unable to pay their premiums. Usually from provincial or local governments. Example: Switzerland.

Some subsidies have existed for many decades, and statutory health insurance was originally designed to include them. Examples are Switzerland and Belgium. In the other cases, government came to the financial rescue of the sickness funds after making them responsible for beneficiaries or for tasks that could not be covered by conventional payroll taxes and premiums.

Grants to Sickness Funds

Since the sickness funds receive tax money and must account for it, only the nonprofit carriers are eligible. In such countries—Switzerland, Belgium, and Holland, for instance—only nonprofit funds can afford to participate in statutory health insurance and the for-profit companies are confined to extra benefits and accident insurance.

Purposes. In subsidy policy as in many other respects, health insurance must be viewed as part of the complete social security system. Every country—even the United States in Medicare Part B—provides subsidies to some sectors of social security. The patterns vary among countries: Germany subsidizes the pension but not the health insurance funds; Switzerland subsidizes the sickness funds more than the pension funds; Belgium unifies the finances for the entire system at the collection stage and adds general revenue to the total. France tries to limit general revenue grants to the deficit-ridden programs by unifying all the regimes and by transferring money from programs with surpluses (such as family allowances) to those with deficits (such as health insurance).

Usually a subsidy policy has specific rather than general aims; instead of helping health insurance on general principles, the government compensates for specific shortfalls. For example, the Swiss national government has subsidized all sickness funds since 1911 to make up for the absence of contributions by employers, to keep women's and children's premiums lower than their actuarial costs, and to make high cost sharing by patients unnecessary. The method has been per capita payments to each sickness fund: the ones with more women and children get more money. Per capita annual payments at various times in Swiss francs have been:[5]

	Men	*Women*	*Children*
1950	5.00	8.00	6.50
1970	18.30	99.50	30.50
1985	41.23	220.69	55.48

A subsidy policy may become obsolete in design as new problems arise. For example, the Swiss classification originated when subscribers were young workers, and it uses the women and children who were the high-cost problems. But after the 1950s, life expectancy greatly lengthened—and the elderly are much more expensive than the young. Sickness funds with an older membership have severe financial problems, but they are not helped by traditional methods of calculation. Each carrier must cover the excess costs of the pensioners from the excess premiums of the employed, a substantial effort of social solidarity that subsidies were supposed to make unnecessary. After a prolonged national debate,[6] the Swiss government in 1989 revised the subsidy formulas, adding a per capita annual payment for each pensioner and reducing the extra payment for each woman. The changes reduced the need for the sickness funds to cover the costs of the elderly by overcharging the young.

Deciding the Amounts. The size of subsidies can be determined by any of the following approaches:

☐ *Billing by sickness funds.* In this case, the sickness funds incur costs and bill the government. While the private carriers in all countries have considerable discretion in increasing their premiums—the laws regulating insurance require them to cover their costs—no government abdicates control over its own budget in this way.

☐ *Law of Parliament.* Democratic legislatures insist on enacting the annual budget, and subsidies to sickness funds are an item in the sections for the Ministries of Social Affairs and Health. Likewise, Parliaments insist on setting the social security payroll taxes.

☐ *The Cabinet.* In this case, the Cabinet is exercising discretion on behalf of Parliament. This is possible only in countries with very powerful all-party coalition cabinets. For many years, Swiss national subsidies were set annually by the Cabinet (the *Bundesrat*).

☐ *Formula.* This approach represents a compromise between sickness funds' constant requests for more money and the financing Ministries' preferences for freezes. Formulas are apparently objective and automatic solutions, relieving the Cabinet and the Parliament of the political pressures for distribution of money. Formulas fix annual increases in subsidies according to rises in the country's consumer prices, wages, medical care costs, or some other variable. Many governments during the 1960s adopted formulas as guidelines in deciding annual increases in pensions, the prices paid by sickness funds to doctors and hospitals, and other components of social security.

Usually governments do not allow such an important part of the annual budget to be predetermined by formula; Parliament and the Cabinet decide the amount every year, along with the payroll tax rates. However, if a government wishes to avoid annual legislative wrangles, it enacts a formula. For example, the Swiss national health insurance law after 1964 specified that the annual per capita subsidy should be calculated from the average cost incurred the previous year in the country as a whole: 10 percent of each man's cost, 35 percent of each woman's cost, and 30 percent of each child's cost.

Grants have followed a definite cycle. At first, they are small in scale and earmarked for particular purposes. During the 1960s and 1970s, they grew substantially in every country as coverage was extended to pensioners and the poor and medical costs kept rising. Since industrial countries prospered during the 1960s and 1970s, few worried and the grumbling from Ministries of Finance was ignored. But since the mid-1970s, all developed countries have experienced recession, unemployment, and difficulty in financing all public services. Social security generally and statutory health insurance in particular produced serious government crises. Their costs went up substantially, since they were entitlement programs resulting from the population's age and since they were linked to inflation. Payroll taxes had been going up rapidly and now were considered high enough, but they yielded less money because of reduced employment. The subsidies had been increasing rapidly during the 1970s, but governments now needed to reduce the deficits in their general budgets.

Government finance officers everywhere became hostile toward health care and toward the managers of the statutory health insurance system. Previously, when subsidies were low and the economy was prosperous, the tax-writers were the only officials of the central control Ministries concerned with the health care accounts, since they had to agree to increases in the payroll taxes. As subsidies increased and as governments needed to control their deficits, the budget-writers—often housed in a new Ministry of Budget—became more powerful generally and more involved in health insurance. In their view, the pension part of social security seems easy to predict since its costs are determined by the age of the population and the rate of inflation; but health care costs always seem out of control because of irresponsible demands by doctors, hospitals, and patients. During the 1970s and 1980s, the Ministries of Finance and Budget tried to limit further payroll tax increases, tried to cut back subsidies, and insisted that the Ministry of Social Affairs and the sickness funds control health care costs.[7] Since they are ideological conservatives, most government finance officers would like to cut health insurance benefits by imposing deductibles or by privatizing the program. But such drastic action would require legislation, and no elected politician dares make even small cutbacks.

When the payroll taxes are set by the national government, both the tax rates and the subsidies are decided by the same people in the same sessions. The methods in France and the Netherlands were described in Chapter Five. The financial specialists in health insurance in the French Ministry of Health and in the Dutch *Ziekenfondsraad* produce reports about the current situation and future prospects of the health insurance accounts; they recommend payroll tax rates in accordance with recent government policy; and they recommend higher subsidies. The Cabinet, led by the Ministries of Finance and Budget, then sets next year's payroll tax rate and the health insurance subsidy in next year's government budget.[8]

If the government does not set the carrier's payroll taxes and premiums, it decides the subsidies completely according to its own budget policies. Then it lets the carriers find the rest of the money. If government must reduce its own spending by cutting its own subsidies—as in Switzerland during the 1980s—it assumes that the carriers must raise their rates. The government officials feel this is the sickness funds' responsibility, not theirs.

Switzerland. Swiss experience illustrates the stages in the interaction between the demands of the health sector and the often contradictory fiscal capacity of government. For many years—before the 1930s—the health sector was stable in prices, utilization, and service intensity; the country generally was stable in prices and in government revenue; and the national government every year paid the same per capita subsidies. The sickness funds could always improve their benefits and raise their own premiums. Government revenue dropped during the Depression, Parliament had to reduce the national budget, the subsidies were reduced, and the sickness funds were allowed to impose higher cost sharing on patients. After World War II, the national government could restore subsidies to pre-Depression levels, cost sharing by patients was reduced, and the Cabinet thereafter raised subsidies only occasionally.

In its general revision of the national health insurance law of 1964, the Swiss government shared the worldwide economic optimism and generosity in health financing. The amendments included an automatic annual formula, and subsidies multiplied five times between 1964 and 1978. When the economic recession of the 1970s left the national government with the most un-Swiss problems of a budget deficit and inflation, the Cabinet abandoned the formula. The Cabinet proposed a 10 percent cut in 1974 (which was not implemented), froze all the per capita payments in 1979, imposed a 5 percent cut in 1981, and has frozen the reduced amounts ever since. The annual proportion of all sickness fund revenue coming from the *Bund* subsidy dropped from 17 percent during the 1960s and 1970s to 10 percent in 1985.[9] The law was amended to allow higher cost sharing by patients in 1986. The sickness funds remain free to raise their own premiums, but competition inhibits large increases. The national government invited the cantonal governments to fill the void by increasing the subsidies that some provide the local offices of the sickness funds. But few did so, since they already pay other subsidies and they too have budgetary difficulties.

In unitary systems of government, major public subsidies of health care usually come from the national government, while help for the poor and specialized grants come from local governments. In federal systems of government, the provincial governments always have constitutional responsibility for health and are the source of major public subsidies. But a trend after World War II was expansion of health financing by cost sharing between national and provincial governments. The large grants by the Swiss national government directly to the sickness funds without cantonal mediation is unusual. It results from the national government's need to preserve a healthy insurance program without payroll taxes on employers. Meanwhile, all cantonal governments subsidize the hospitals, and some subsidize the sickness funds and the individual subscribers.

The national government's finance officers and some reformers have recently proposed a more typical federal system: all subsidies of sickness funds would be divided 50-50 between the national and cantonal governments.[10] Since the cantonal and not the national government has constitutional authority over health care providers, the cantons would then be motivated to impose stricter cost containment over providers. This transfer of funding is opposed by the cantons and therefore cannot be enacted. It does not take into account the varying fiscal capacities, the current cantonal subsidy practices, and the political priorities of the cantons. And it contradicts the worldwide trend of recent years: shared-cost programs in many fields have been abandoned in other federal systems, either by delegating full responsibility to the provinces or by substituting national block grants to the provinces.[11]

Belgium. If a country has a long history of subsidizing the sickness funds, the criteria may be adjusted in response to unexpected difficulties but are never overtly reformed. If a country has several goals in its subsidy policies, the result is complex and sometimes internally inconsistent. An example is Belgium.

Keeping down payroll taxes has always been a goal. If its sickness funds had used graduated premiums, Belgium might have used for its subsidy formula a per capita payment for each member, increasing it for those with higher actuarial premiums (as in Switzerland). But Belgium had percentage-of-wage payroll taxes. So, for nearly a century, the Belgian national government has supplemented each sickness fund's revenue from its payroll taxes by a standard percentage. This policy seemed plausible for many years, when all subscribers' incomes were similar. But recently more affluent persons have been added, income is inverse to health care costs, and the carriers with more affluent members (such as the Christians) get higher per capita subsidies than those with members who earn lower incomes and incur higher costs (such as the Socialists). The result is yet a new controversy between the two rival confederations and their political factions: the Socialists are demanding a completely new approach to public subsidies.

Covering the costs of expensive patients who pay low premiums (or none at all) has become a reason for government subsidies everywhere. It is one of the purposes in Belgium, as well, although its administration seems to merge it into the principal subsidy allocation method described above. The special subsidy is supposed to cover the costs of certain widows, disabled, and orphans (VIPOs). Instituted recently, it eventually became larger than the subsidy designed to supplement the payroll taxes of all subscribers. The distribution of the two subsidies is administered by the public commission that monitors the entire health insurance system (INAMI). The agency cannot estimate the exact extra costs of VIPOs, and in practice it seems to distribute all the subsidies as a percentage of payroll tax revenue. The Socialist sickness funds regularly complain, and the INAMI financial officers may give them extra money in order to buy peace. But the result is imprecise and somewhat clandestine calculations. Neither officially nor unofficially does Belgium have a system to distribute subsidies according to the extra costs of its members. The result would be more money to the carriers with many pensioners, a group much larger than the VIPOs. The Socialist sickness funds would welcome such a policy. But the government's finance officers oppose it, fearing that carriers would increase costs rather than control them.

Covering the costs of administration is yet another goal. Belgium has subsidized the managements of mutual aid societies since the late nineteenth century. Because the larger funds served more people and provided more services than the small ones, the national government sought a formula based on size: at first, a per capita payment for each member; then a percentage of revenue from payroll taxes (with a slightly lower percentage for the largest carriers). Since administrative burdens varied with activity rather than income, the formula was changed to percentage of costs in 1963. When the health care cost explosion began during the 1970s, government finance officers feared that the formula provided a perverse incentive for the sickness funds to increase costs. So the formula during the late 1970s again became a percentage of receipts. But the national government was encountering large budget deficits and needed to control the growth in all its payments. After 1982, therefore, the subsidy for each sickness fund became last year's subsidy plus a percentage increment that is standard for every carrier. The result gives the budget officers more predictability and gives the sickness funds an incentive to stabilize total operations. None of these decisions were made by the civil servants alone; all had to be made by the elected politicians who voted the budget, either by act of Parliament or by regulation in the Cabinet.

United States. American Social Security has always followed the principle of self-financing through payroll taxes. This rule was long easy to obey, since the pension funds faced no deficit until the 1980s. Congress in 1944 authorized the use of general revenue to avoid increases in the payroll tax, but subsidies were never paid and the clause was repealed in 1950. During the general reforms of

1983, Congress enacted its only subsidy: a single grant to cover pension benefits to veterans that accumulated during wars but had not been matched by payroll taxes.[12]

The hospital financing part of Medicare was incorporated into the Social Security machinery and therefore shared the general presumption of financing entirely by payroll taxes. When the Hospital Insurance Trust Fund teetered toward deficit during the late 1970s and early 1980s, government subsidies or complete fiscalization were seriously proposed. But the payroll taxes were increased, hospital costs were controlled, and no subsidies were necessary.

The payment of doctors under Medicare has been entirely different. The principle of self-financing fell victim to political confusion. When Medicare was created, the medical associations, the Republican Party, and business interests opposed the idea of including physicians' services under Social Security, since this introduced the power of the national government over doctors and might foreshadow statutory health insurance. (In contrast, American hospitals welcomed the secure financing of Social Security's universal and obligatory payroll taxes.) In great haste, a politically logrolled method was enacted by Congress: physicians' services were not part of Social Security but were covered by voluntary insurance bought by the elderly and administered by the national government ("Supplementary Medical Insurance"); the pensioner was charged a flat premium, but the figure was unrealistically low ($3/month at the start in 1966); since no payroll taxes were levied on employers and since the elderly should not be burdened, the Treasury would contribute the same amount to the SMI Trust Fund.[13]

But fees and utilization were not constrained, the program lacked structures to monitor trends and control expenditures, and the utopian hopes failed. For the next fifteen years, costs paid by the SMI Trust Fund rose constantly, the premiums charged the elderly had to be raised frequently, the Treasury subsidies no longer merely matched the premiums but had to be raised to whatever physicians' charges required, and the elderly had to pay more to the doctors out-of-pocket.[14] Permissive politics therefore forced the United States government to deliver unlimited cash subsidies to satisfy providers' demands—an outcome avoided in all other countries. When the Treasury subsidies reached three-fourths of the Trust Fund's annual expenditures during the late 1980s, Congress enacted thereafter a permanent division: one-quarter from subscriber premiums and three-quarters from the Treasury. But this measure only required automatic increases in the elderly's premiums; it did not fix a lid on total expenditures or on the Treasury subsidies. By 1987, the subsidy had exceeded $20 billion—14 percent of the national government's entire budget deficit.[15] Congress then belatedly struggled to learn and possibly even enact forms of "expenditure target" or "expenditure cap."

America is supposed to rely on private enterprise and the competitive free market to insure the population under sixty-five. Therefore, ideology and political rivalry exclude all thoughts of subsidizing all private carriers (in the manner of Switzerland and Belgium). But there is one class of private health insurance carrier that was long thought to be a benchmark for reforming the entire system and that has infatuated both Republicans and Democrats: health maintenance organizations. Since these are private nonprofit and for-profit entities in a supposedly competitive market, an overt and systematic subsidy was never created for them. Instead, the national government has supported many with a stream of "demonstration grants" throughout the 1970s and 1980s.

Grants to Providers

Governments regularly subsidize health care providers for several motives:

☐ *Ideology.* General revenue draws upon progressive taxes on income and taxes from business. Payroll taxes are constantly proportionate in arithmetic, are often limited to an earnings ceiling, and are often regressive in incidence. Governments of the Left prefer public grants to increases in payroll taxes. Grants to providers reduce demands on the social security system and reduce the need to raise payroll taxes.

☐ *Adequate funding of particular services.* Health insurance carriers have limited revenues and may squeeze certain providers. Competition may prevent them from raising premiums or may lead them to spend on things that will strengthen their own marketing. Government grants target programs that the carriers underfund.

☐ *Cost containment.* If money goes through many uncoordinated channels, the result is uncontrollable. Providers can bargain advantageously with small and disunited sickness funds. Much duplication can result. If government provides much of the money, it can bring all other payers into a joint arrangement that sets and implements prospective budgets for a health sector. Such is the trend in hospital operating costs outside the United States.[16]

☐ *Facilities planning.* Health care providers have long been individualistic and fiercely resist system-wide planning. Results include duplication and inappropriate location of facilities. Individual insurance carriers usually lack any conception of a total health system, since their role is passively helping citizens pay established providers. Government plans are futile without incentives and sanctions. Thus, governments often provide investment funds to induce hospitals and other organizations to develop according to plans.

Public subsidies are welcomed by hospitals, since the establishments cover operating deficits and can modernize their facilities. (For the same reason, the hospitals are a principal political support for the enactment of statutory health insurance.) When government later tightens grant conditions and audits use of the money more carefully, hospital administrators are less enthusiastic.

If government pays money to practicing doctors, the form is direct employment in municipal or provincial hospitals and health centers. Office doctors initially oppose both statutory health insurance and public grants programs, fearing government controls over professional autonomy and over their incomes. Therefore, direct public grants to office doctors are never made. But subsidies are made regularly in a few countries to private institutional providers of ambulatory services.

Grants for Capital Investment. Many developed countries provide most or all of the money for hospital buildings and heavy equipment through direct public subsidies or through special public revolving funds. In these cases, the sickness funds had been paying low daily rates, amortization of capital costs was not included in hospitals' operating costs, investment had always come from owners and charitable donors, and only government had the resources to modernize hospitals when the need arose after World War I. In these countries today (such as France), health insurance covers operating costs and tax money pays for new buildings, major renovations, and heavy equipment.

In a few countries, hospital operating cost accounting has included interest, depreciation, and the repayment of debt. Self-financing under statutory health insurance grew and survives today in the Netherlands. But self-financing has been replaced by government subsidies in West Germany, providing the best example of coordination between public grants and the insurance system. For decades before 1972, hospitals paid for capital from the daily charges negotiated with sickness funds, but the carriers agreed only to low payments. Compared to other countries, German hospitals were underfunded, understaffed, and underequipped. The new Social Democratic government of the late 1960s and early 1970s wanted the insurance system to channel more money into a modernized hospital industry: short-term invalidity payments were shifted to employers, and capital costs were shifted to government. Provincial governments had constitutional responsibility in health services—as in all federal systems—but provinces varied in fiscal capacity and in willingness to subsidize hospitals. Germany's constitution was amended to allow shared-cost programs in health and in other fields: the national government would pay a large proportion of the provincial governments' capital grants to the hospitals.

The new law (the *Krankenhausfinanzierungsgesetz*, or KHG) was enacted in 1972. At first, it accomplished all its goals: sickness funds agreed to higher daily rates; hospitals could afford to employ more workers and give them normal wages and hours; hospitals obtained generous capital funds from the provinces and rapidly modernized. But the general economy soon experienced a recession. The shock to the health sector was greater in Germany than in other developed countries, because its economy had steadily grown after World War II and the KHG had produced a sudden boom in health. The national government's tax revenue dropped, its budget went into deficit, and it cut capital grants to the provincial governments. For the next decade, the provinces and hospitals were outraged and accused Bonn of reneging on the carefully designed agreement of 1972.

During these years, the interest groups, political parties, and provincial governments struggled over a new allocation of financing responsibilities. The governments and the hospitals wanted the sickness funds to resume financing the capital costs of the hospitals as part of total operating costs—this time under guidelines following provincial plans and requiring the carriers to be generous. But the sickness funds resisted on the grounds the recession had cut their revenue too. The compromise enacted in 1985 ended the automatic federal/provincial shared-cost formulas, assigned capital financing to the provinces, and obligated the national government to give a series of diminishing block grants to the provinces. Doubtless budget constraints and total political priorities will determine the subsidies the provincial governments can afford to grant the hospitals.[17]

Germany has never provided direct government subsidies to its principal sickness funds. The original attempt to make health insurance a government program was defeated in the 1880s, as Chapters Four and Five explained, and the health insurance system has tried to maintain its private character and autonomy (*Selbstverwaltung*) ever since. Direct government subsidies have been feared by the sickness funds as a lever for government control.[18] If there had been large subsidies, they would have been reduced in the national government's budgetary cutbacks of the 1970s and 1980s and the carriers would have experienced serious problems. The pension system had been the subsidized part of social security, and it had to adjust to cuts in the national government's grants.[19] In order to make clear that the health insurance system depended completely on payroll taxes and premiums and not on subsidies from any source, the pension funds' payment of the elderly's health insurance coverage was replaced during the 1980s by premiums personally paid by each pensioner (as Chapter Five explained).

The U.S. government's one program to subsidize hospital construction had a convoluted relation to its insurance program—or, more accurately, to the absence of insurance. In other countries, construction grants are designed to reinforce statutory health insurance by creating the capacity to satisfy the demand or relieve the sickness funds of the costs of amortizing the construction. But America had no statutory insurance. Instead, hospitals long had to bear bad debts. The Hill-Burton Hospital Construction Act (1948-1973) made such charity care official and obligatory. The law required the hospital to repay its grant by providing "a reasonable volume of service to persons unable to pay therefor"—an ambiguous standard that led to disputes and regulations until each hospital was deemed to have satisfied its obligations and the entire program was finally terminated.[20] Since Hill-Burton was never coordinated with actual insurance coverage, it ultimately produced overcapacity in many regions.

Grants for Operating Costs. The reason for enacting statutory health insurance is to pay doctors and hospitals in full without bad debts. Doctors and hospitals in all developed countries with statutory insurance expect high revenue, thereby driving up payroll taxes on all workers and employers. Because the usual financing method was blocked during the creation of the original law in 1911,

Switzerland's sickness funds have been able to collect premiums only from the subscribers and not from the employers. To make up the difference, governments subsidize the health sector from tax revenue in several ways: the national government and several cantons subsidize the operating costs of all the sickness funds; all the cantonal governments pay part of the operating costs and most of the capital costs of their private nonprofit and public hospitals.

Every cantonal government's Ministry of Health decides the precise shares of hospital operating costs to be charged to the sickness funds and to the cantonal budget. The higher the amount paid by the government, the lower the premiums the carriers need charge the population in that canton. Usually the cantonal government screens every hospital budget and then sets as its share a standard percentage of all the hospital budgets in the canton. Among the twenty-six cantons and half-cantons, the percentage varies widely between 18 and 72 percent. The government's share is higher if the canton's population has higher incomes and therefore higher fiscal capacity; if its leaders' ideology prefers progressive taxation to regressive methods of revenue; and if there are several very expensive teaching hospitals.[21]

Subsidies to Help the Poor

Before the advent of statutory health insurance, private charitable associations (such as churches) and municipal welfare services provided direct care to the poor or helped pay their bills. So long as health insurance applied only to the employed covered by payroll taxes or premiums, charity and public welfare continued for others. When its coverage was extended to the lower-income workers, to the widows of the formerly insured, and to the unemployed, the health insurance system had to accept members capable of only low premiums or none at all. One solution in several countries has been a law fixing as a special premium a low percentage of the unemployed person's benefits check or the elderly person's pension. The sickness fund then tries to cover all the members' costs redistributively: the employed persons' payroll taxes must be enough to cover their own costs and the deficits from the underpayers. Another solution is a government subsidy either to the sickness fund or to needy individuals.

A country gives subsidies to the sickness funds if it is strongly committed to social solidarity and grants entitlements to large classes of people. A country gives subsidies to specific individuals (upon a means test) if its ideology is more individualistic—if it presumes that every person normally buys health insurance and other services with his own money, if it wishes to target the taxpayers' money only upon those few persons in true need.

Subsidies to the Carriers. All social security funds are pay-as-you-go: current revenue pays for current benefits for the same or (more often) for different persons. An individual carrier can run a deficit—even if the entire nationwide system is balanced or in surplus—for several reasons:

☐ Unfavorable dependency ratio—that is, too many pensioners relative to workers. Example: sickness funds and pension funds in industries with a declining work force, such as railroads and mining.

☐ Wide variations in wealth within the fund. Example: carriers for farmers and the self-employed. (Some members underreport incomes.)

☐ Lower payroll taxes despite sharing the same benefits as the rest of social security. Example: political concessions to farmers in some countries.

☐ High medical costs and early invalidity payments. Example: carriers for miners.

☐ More generous benefits than in the rest of social security. Example: lower cost sharing for miners and railroad workers.

For a century, the national government of France has subsidized social security funds when their payroll taxes and other forms of revenue could not cover the full costs of benefits required or authorized by law. The subsidies began with grants to the mutual aid societies enabling them to add old-age pensions to their other health and welfare benefits.[22] The solution for such deficits in health care financing could be postponed until the passage of obligatory health insurance after World War I and until the rise in health costs. If the thousands of mutual aid societies had continued to be the carriers under statutory health insurance, a bewildering mosaic of deficits and surpluses would have resulted, but a few major official sickness funds displaced them as the principal insurers after World War II. The principal fund (the *Caisse Nationale de l'Assurance Maladie des Travailleurs Salariés*, or CNAMTS) mixed the pensioners into the bulk of the French labor force. A few special occupations insisted on keeping their own mutual aid societies—the miners, railwaymen, farmers, and a few others—and these were destined to run deficits.

Due to the increase in health costs and the aging of the population, a definite cycle developed in France after 1960. All sickness funds provided the same generous benefits. When the general regime (CNAMTS) was in deficit, the national Treasury loaned it money. Whenever the payroll taxes for health were increased, the general regime was in surplus, repaid the Treasury, and might even improve its benefits. The special funds might achieve a precarious balance if they adopted the same tax rise, but sometimes they did not. In general, their members were paid less than the rest of the labor force and therefore the same taxes yielded lower per capita revenue. The special funds had unfavorable dependency ratios, often higher per capita medical costs, and sometimes more generous benefits because of lower cost sharing.

Every year the financial monitors of the social security system (the Ministries of Social Affairs, Health, Finance, and Budget) adopted "temporary" measures to cover the deficits. Money was given to those funds by transfer from other funds or by grants from the annual budget enacted by Parliament. Along with "temporary" subsidies, the French government during the 1970s enacted permanent measures intended to reestablish equilibrium—measures such as higher payroll taxes, elimination of the earnings ceiling, and premiums automatically deducted from old-age pensions and unemployment compensation. By the 1980s, both the old-age pension funds and CNAMTS had joined the special regimes in chronic deficit, and the government had to acknowledge that subsidies were a permanent policy. In view of adverse effects on employment, increasing the heavy payroll taxes was no longer possible. But subsidies from general revenue merely transferred the deficit to the government's budget. The rapid increase in social security deficits and subsidies has become one of the principal problems of French government. It regularly dominates newspaper headlines and must be managed at the highest levels of government.[23]

Subsidies to the Poor. The spread of the ideology of social solidarity along with the enactment of social security usually eliminates the scrutiny of individual needs and the calibration of specific benefits by degrees of need. Means tests have been discredited. However, Switzerland, despite the enactment of several social security programs, retains its philosophy of individual self-reliance and family responsibility for the needy.

Switzerland's national government has been influenced by the idea of a negative income tax: people should buy services (including insurance coverage) with cash from earnings or pensions. If a means test shows they do not have enough, they are given the difference. The money passes through the national social security pension funds for old age and disability. Since the money is additional to the pensions paid for by social security payroll taxes, it originates as a subsidy by the national government to the pension funds. The national government enacts a definition of the poverty line. Beneficiaries are evaluated and the cash is distributed not by government but by three networks of voluntary associations who are active in all communities (*Pro Senectute, Pro Infirmis,* and *Pro Juventute*). The social workers at the grass roots help the beneficiaries pay their insurance premiums, rent, home-care services, and other bills with the combined income from their basic pensions and the extra cash. Some cantonal governments with expensive hospitals and expensive health insurance, such as Vaud, add their supplements to the national government's subsidies.[24]

Effects on Utilization and Health

Payroll taxes and premiums are financial instruments and do not produce subtle differences in utilization and the population's health. Public subsidies do make a difference because they expand provider revenue and citizen access. Without subsidies, the insurance system may have considerably less money and may not be able to guarantee lavish and technically advanced care. The health care system may have to economize for all or for particular groups that pay in less.

Subsidies often are introduced to guarantee equal services regardless of ability to pay taxes and premiums. Social solidarity is thereby financed, since the taxpayers who contribute to the general budget cannot trace the course of their money and hence cannot compare their payments and benefits with those of other taxpayers. The elderly and the poor are the ones who create the initial deficits leading to the subsidies, and it is they who benefit from the resulting guarantees of equal treatment.

Government subsidies can be increased faster than the yield from payroll taxes and premiums. In theory, subsidies may also be reduced quickly. In some countries where all health care financing is run through the general budgets of government—such as Great Britain and Canada—the need to control the general budget restrains provider revenue, modernization of capital, and speedy access. However, where public subsidies are only a supplement to insurance revenue, abrupt reductions do not occur in a manner that affects subscribers and providers. The sickness funds have their normal revenue and can rearrange their funding if government restrains the annual growth in subsidies, as Switzerland demonstrates. The sickness funds are articulate interest groups and can persuade government finance officers to compromise over their cuts and turn to less protected parts of the budgets.

Implications for the United States

The long-term trend has been to approach the limits of yield from payroll taxes and to add subsidies from government. Adding pensioners, the poor, and the unemployed to mainstream statutory health insurance produces a mounting imbalance in the accounts. Statutory health insurance was designed so that workers and their employers pay for the needs of those same workers, restoring them to the job. Payroll taxes on work seemed relevant to that mission, a large redistributive role seemed irrelevant, and it seemed during the 1970s that statutory health insurance depended so much on mounting subsidies that it would have to be fiscalized outright.

However, statutory health insurance has become stabilized in Europe: most revenue comes from payroll taxes or premiums; some of the surplus revenue from these sources is redistributed to pay for the extra costs of the elderly, the unemployed, and the bad risks; subsidies make up for those who pay low contributions; costs have been controlled; and the shares covered by subsidies have stabilized. Thus, the current financing system will survive longer.

The decline of the crisis provides a breathing space to think through the rationale for relying on payroll taxes and on subsidies. In Europe they were mixed to balance budgets in the face of an unexpected increase in subscribers who incurred high costs and paid little. Instead of merely protecting the working class—its original mission—health insurance has become a mechanism of social redistribution whereby the economically active pay for heavy consumption by the inactive. Some argue that this part of health care financing is a societal policy problem and not a problem for employers and workers. Therefore, they conclude, the costs of the pensioners and unemployed should be covered completely by public funding—in no part from the payroll taxes levied on the economically active. Then the full costs of the pensioners and unemployed would be manifest and employment would be burdened less.[25]

Whether this idea is meritorious or not, at least it is a considered policy. American health care financing should be based on a policy. But it is not: subsidies are adopted or not by political accident; if subsidies grow, often the reason is the error in omitting any method of containing costs. American results can be bizarre: one part of Medicare (Part A for hospitals) uses no subsidies and depends entirely on payroll taxes; the other part of the same program (Part B for physicians) depends overwhelmingly on subsidies and uses no payroll taxes. One would expect the opposite: if American doctors are so hostile to government interference, why does every one draw a substantial fraction of his income from the Treasury?

Notes

1. When government takes over ownership and management as well as financing, the result is a "national health service" (an NHS). The arrangements in Great Britain, Sweden, the Soviet Union, and China are described in Victor W. Sidel and Ruth Sidel, *A Healthy State*, 2nd ed. (New York: Pantheon Press, 1983).

2. For an overview see Aviva Ron, "Government Participation in Social Security Health Insurance Budgets," *International Social Security Review*, vol. 39, no. 1 (1986), pp. 52–63.

3. Barbara Armstrong, *Insuring the Essentials* (New York: Macmillan, 1932), pp. 316–321, 330–334.

4. Described in William Glaser, *Paying the Hospital* (San Francisco: Jossey-Bass, 1987), chaps. 7–9 passim.

5. *Statistik über die Krankenversicherung vom Bunde anerkannte Versicherungsträger 1985* (Bern: Bundesamt für Sozialversicherung, 1987), pp. 84–85. For the history and current practices in Swiss government subsidies in all sectors of social security see *Rapport sur les aspects actuariels, financiers et économiques de la sécurité sociale* (Bern: Bundesamt für Sozialversicherung, 1982), pp. 149–163; and *Message sur la révision partielle de l'assurance-maladie du 19 août 1981* (Bern: Bundesamt für Sozialversicherung, 1981).

6. *Message . . .* (see note 5, above), pp. 70–71.

7. See, for example, "Netherlands, 1975–82: Containing the Public Sector," in *Why Economic Policies Change Course: Eleven Case Studies* (Paris: Organization for Economic Co-Operation and Development, 1988), pp. 90–98.

8. For a description of how the budget of the Ministry of Social Affairs is written see Pierre Lequéret, *Le Budget de l'État* (Paris: La Documentation Française, 1982), p. 2.

9. *Statistik über die Krankenversicherung* (see note 5, above), p. 35.

10. *Message . . .* (see note 5, above), pp. 75–77.

11. I described shared-cost programs in health and the early stages in their

abandonment in Glaser, *Federalism in Canada and West Germany: Lessons for the United States* (New York: Center for the Social Sciences, Columbia University, 1979), a report to the National Center for Health Services Research.

12. James H. Schulz, *The Economics of Aging*, 4th ed. (Dover, Mass.: Auburn House, 1988), pp. 181–183. Proposals for regular inclusion of general revenue in pension financing are summarized in Robert J. Myers, *Social Security*, 3rd ed. (Homewood, Ill.: Richard D. Irwin, 1985), pp. 447–449.

13. Sheri I. David, *With Dignity: The Search for Medicare and Medicaid* (Westport, Conn.: Greenwood, 1985); and Frank D. Campion, *The AMA and U.S. Health Policy Since 1940* (Chicago: Chicago Review Press, 1984), chap. 15.

14. The first warnings about the trend were in *Medicare and Medicaid: Problems, Issues, and Alternatives* (Washington: Committee on Finance, U.S. Senate, 91st Congress, 1st Session, 1970), especially chaps. 1, 5, 7.

15. *The Federal Supplementary Medical Insurance Trust Fund: Communication from the Board of Trustees Transmitting the 1988 Annual Report* (Washington: Government Printing Office, 100th Congress, 2nd Session, House Document 100-194, 1988), p. 18. The total deficit in fiscal year 1987 was slightly over $148 billion.

16. Described in Glaser, *Paying the Hospital* (see note 4, above), chaps. 8 and 13.

17. Capital grants to hospitals in Germany and other countries are described in Glaser, *Paying the Hospital*, chap. 9, and *Federalism in Canada and West Germany* (see note 11, above), chap. 14, pp. 54–61, and chap. 15, pp. 20–24.

18. The only exceptions have been the two special regimes with dependency ratios so adverse that they could not self-finance completely: the farmers and the miners. The exceptions in Germany demonstrate that a completely self-financed system is impossible without public subsidies or interfund transfers (or both).

19. W. Adamy and S. Koeppinghoff, "Zur Krisenanfälligkeit der Rentenversicherung," *Konjunkturpolitik*, vol. 29 (1983), pp. 285–313; and Klaus Mackscheidt and others, "Der Finanzausgleich zwischen dem Bund und der Rentenversicherung," *Finanzarchiv*, vol. 39, no. 3 (1981), pp. 383–407.

20. Everett A. Veldman, "Hill-Burton Charity Care," in William O. Cleverley (ed.), *Handbook of Health Care Accounting and Finance* (Rockville, Md.: Aspen Systems, 1982), chap. 52.

21. William Glaser, *Paying the Hospital in Switzerland* (New York: Center for the Social Sciences, Columbia University, 1979), chap. 7.

22. Early workmen's insurance and compensation systems in Europe are described in *Twenty-Fourth Annual Report of the Commissioner of Labor 1909* (Washington: Government Printing Office, 1911), pp. 810, 868–869.

23. Current subsidies are summarized in Commission des Comptes de la Sécurité Sociale, *Les comptes de la Sécurité sociale—Prévisions 1989 et 1990* (Paris: La Documentation Française, 1989), pp. 37, 106. The annual struggle to

remedy the deficit is chronicled in Jean-Pierre Dumont, *La Sécurité sociale toujours en chantier* (Paris: Les Editions Ouvrières, 1981), chap. 9.

24. *Rapport annuel—AVS, AI, APG* (Bern: Bundesamt für Sozialversicherung, annual); *EL-Statistik: Statistik der Ergänzungsleistungen zu den AHV/IV-Renten in den Kanton Bern und St. Gallen 1983* (Bern: Bundesamt für Sozialversicherung, 1985); and Guy Métrailler, "L'assurance maladie des personnes âgées dans le canton de Vaud," *Âinés*, vol. 10, no. 6 (June 1980), pp. 26–27.

25. Guy Perrin, "L'avenir de la protection sociale dans les pays industriels," *Futuribles*, nos. 92–93 (Oct.–Nov. 1985), pp. 49–52; and Perrin, "Rationalisation of Social Security Financing," in *Financing Social Security: The Options* (Geneva: International Labour Office, 1984), pp. 121–145. This viewpoint was summarized earlier in Chapter Six.

CHAPTER 9

Transfers
Among Insurance Funds

———————————— Summary ————————————

If a health insurance scheme is universal and unified in one sickness fund, the overpayers cover the costs of the overusers. Social solidarity is fulfilled. But if the carriers are separate, different social classes and different medical risks often gravitate to different funds. The carriers may then select risks and vary coverage in order to improve profits and image. As a result, some sickness funds are stronger financially than others. And without intervention by government or the health insurance industry, the imbalance may worsen.

Instead of reducing the imbalance through subsidies, government may insist that the carriers redistribute their revenue according to need. In other words, the industry is pressed to practice social solidarity rather than competitive preferred-risk selection. How can balance be maintained without destroying incentives for efficiency? How much competition and flexibility can be allowed in the social insurance market? Critics of interfund transfers say that some arrangements contradict social solidarity. For example, in France, the more affluent regime for the self-employed receives rather than sends transfers, thereby easing the tax burden on its members.

Private health insurance companies create their own autonomous accounts and resist losing money to their competitors. They participate in transfers only to head off the threat of universal statutory health insurance, as in Holland during the 1980s. Or, as in the United States, they are forced to pay out extra money as the result of government reversal of the effects of free markets. Some state governments in the United States tax the health insurance companies or add surcharges to their hospital bills in order to generate money for the uninsured citizens or for the hospitals with operating deficits due to the uninsured. These private transfers are only temporary stopgaps until the government adopts a new comprehensive policy.

Different Financial Balances

Health insurance carriers experience surpluses, exact balances, or deficits in each year's accounts because their revenue is higher or lower than costs. A social insurance carrier can increase revenue temporarily by increasing premiums or by government subsidies, but it may face chronically high costs because it has many elderly and disabled members. A commercial insurance carrier may increase its general premiums slightly, but more often it tries to avoid deficits by not enrolling poor risks or by charging them higher individual premiums.

Some argue that each fund should live with its own finances, enjoying its own profits and suffering its own deficits. The balance sheet would reflect good performance in managing finances, selecting members, and offering benefits. Only then will the less efficient have an incentive to improve performance. If a fund is guaranteed against losses, it will become wasteful in management, permissive in the payment of providers, and lax in allowing overutilization. If a carrier loses its savings, it will try to use up all its extra cash in frills for managers.

Others, however, advocate temporary or permanent machinery whereby the carriers with surpluses help those with deficits. In many cases, they say, the deficits are due to the differential performance of social obligations: the carriers with surpluses minimize their costs by conducting preferred-risk selection—by dumping the elderly and disabled on the sickness funds who cannot refuse. If a country's insurance structure is based on occupation, sickness funds in declining industries experience inevitable deterioration in their dependency ratios. Financial transfers are a reasonable alternative to the bankruptcy and mergers that will disrupt the subscribers and cause the carrier managers to lose their jobs. Social solidarity implies that all sickness funds should unite, and equalization transfers achieve the same result while preserving the traditional structure of many independent carriers. If any carriers have surpluses, it is better to use them in the insurance system than burden government with subsidies for the deficit-ridden. In practice, many countries have interfund transfers. As in many other features of health insurance, the purposes and forms vary.

Transfers Among Social Security Funds

A policy of social solidarity assumes that everyone receives the same benefits. It can best be implemented when everyone belongs to the same fund. Members pay according to financial ability, and the reimbursement of cash benefits and medical services works redistributively.

When a health insurance system is decentralized—even if all persons must join and are assigned automatically to particular carriers—the results are not random and equal. Social insurance funds differ in the ratios between revenue and costs. This is particularly true when the funds represent different occupations, as in France and Germany. The carriers vary in:

☐ *Age distribution of members.* The older the members then:
  • The fewer the number of active workers and employers who pay full premiums
  • The larger the number of pensioners and disabled who pay little and incur large costs
☐ *Income level.* The lower the income, the lower the revenue, even if payroll tax rates are the same throughout statutory health insurance.
☐ *Tax rates.* Because of political influence, some occupations pay lower rates than others.
☐ *Benefits.* Because of political influence, some occupations may receive more generous benefits than others—for example, their cost-sharing rates may be lower.

France. Parliament has repeatedly enunciated the policy of a unified social security system with standard benefits. But several occupations have refused to join the general regime and have preserved their own sickness funds and other social security funds. Because many are in declining industries—special protection was a goal of their independence—their accounts are seriously strained and steadily deteriorate. For example, the ratios of number of active workers to number of pensioners in several regimes in France were:[1]

Regime	1960	1970	1979
General	4.6	4.4	3.1
Miners	1.7	0.7	0.4
Railwaymen	1.3	1.1	1.0
Self-employed businessmen	3.5	1.9	1.3
Self-employed farmers	3.7	1.7	1.1

Note: If the ratio exceeds 1.0, the employed outnumber the pensioners. If the ratio is below 1.0, the pensioners outnumber the employed.

Even though the same or even more generous benefits were guaranteed in the special regimes, their revenue per taxpayer was often lower for two reasons. First, their average wages were often lower than the bulk of the country's wages in the general regime—for example, the farm workers. (But not always: the miners and railwaymen were well paid.) Second, nearly all paid lower tax rates than the general regime. Even when the rate on the worker is the same, the rate on the employer is lower.[2]

Before 1974, special laws regulated equalization transfers between the general regime and the seriously underfunded sickness funds for farm workers, miners, railwaymen, and sailors. Each was a separate "bilateral" arrangement with different goals and different formulas.[3] A "general" system of transfers was substituted in late 1974—supposedly to prepare for a complete consolidation of all social security regimes, but still in effect today. To avoid annual disputes governed by political pressures and lacking long-term predictability, the calculations are based on formulas. All social security regimes are involved in the calculations and the financial transfers, either as payers or as recipients.

The calculations postulate a benefit package in health, pensions, family allowances, and other social security benefits that all regimes should be equally able to pay for. The formulas distribute the total of social security money among carriers according to their numbers of subscribers weighted by dependency ratios. Those with fewer economically active persons and more pensioners receive extra money from total revenue. The original plan was to base all transfers on the dependency ratios: the general regime would lose money and those with unfavorable dependency ratios (such as miners and small businessmen) would gain. But this simple method would provide financial windfalls for those regimes with low payroll taxes and earnings ceilings (particularly the self-employed) and for those with early retirement (such as miners and railwaymen). To limit these effects, the formulas were supplemented by additional weights. Besides the general arrangement, bilateral transfers are still made among regimes for pensions and certain other benefits.[4]

Pursuant to the original law and the regulations, the calculations are made by a special commission. They are based on each year's actual financial collections and dependency ratios when the numbers are available a year later. The agency that administers all social security revenue (ACOSS) then makes the retroactive transfers from the current year's cash. For example, the commission approved the calculations for 1985 in January 1987, and ACOSS then distributed its 1987 collections with retroactive revisions.

The French transfer system has often been criticized:[5]

☐ Regimes with low tax burdens and permissive collections—particularly those for the self-employed and farmers—get transfers when they should be contributing. The political influence in Parliament that created special regimes has also protected their windfalls under the transfer system. The formulas do not distinguish between low revenue due to low fiscal effort and low revenue due to low base incomes.

☐ Likewise, regimes with excessively generous benefits are not penalized.

☐ The transfers do not pave the way to a unification of all the regimes. They provide incentives for the special regimes to remain independent.

☐ The formulas cannot be understood easily. The complete system is incoherent.

☐ The system obscures the true financial state of each regime.

☐ In actual practice, the formulas do not produce stable and predictable results from year to year.

Some suggest that the obscurity of the system and the lack of clear accounts in each regime are deliberately cultivated. These characteristics conceal the political concessions to several occupations in fiscal effort and in benefits.[6]

German Statutory Pension Insurance. Everyone in the German social security pension system benefits from the same rules and from administration by public agencies. Pensions are based on the individual's past earnings and are not supposed to vary among provinces. The payroll tax rates for pensions are the same throughout the country. No interregional equalization problems would have arisen if the law had created a single national pension fund, as in the United States. But the German political compromise of the 1880s created a separate Insurance Institute in each provincial government and a national coordinating office.

The provincial Insurance Institutes obtain widely different revenue from the same payroll taxes, since some provinces have higher earnings than others. For example, Hamburg is much richer than the Saar. Some occupations have special pension rules and separate accounts—such as railwaymen and miners—but cannot cover the costs from their own wage-earners because of adverse dependency ratios. So that all the Insurance Institutes and special regimes can pay pensions according to standard nationwide formulas, money from the payroll taxes has long been transferred among them and is now supplemented by subsidies from the national government. The calculations are performed every year by the national government's social security Insurance Institute (the *Bundesversicherungsamt*).[7]

German Statutory Health Insurance. The sickness funds were never supposed to be mere fiscal administrators for a standardized program. Each sickness fund is supposed to be autonomous and responsible for its own economic survival. Unlike the pension system, with nationally standardized payroll taxes enacted by Parliament, each sickness fund is free to set its own rates.

As Chapter Four explained, most workers and their families are assigned automatically to certain sickness funds. (See also Appendix A.) However, a substantial and increasing number can choose between the *Ersatzkassen* and the other sickness funds. The *Ersatzkassen* attract the healthier and more profitable risks, while the other carriers are left with the less desirable portfolios. During the 1970s and 1980s, two rival policies were pushed:[8]

☐ Advocates of social solidarity argued that all statutory health insurance should be considered one pool. All carriers—including the *Ersatzkassen*—should participate in financial equalization among funds. The *Ersatzkassen* should be denied their incentives for preferred-risk selection. The *Ortskrankenkassen* in particular pressed for interfund equalization that would alleviate their own financial strains. In Parliament, they were supported by the

Social Democrats (SPD). Some research projects demonstrated interfund equalization methods.[9]

☐ Advocates of free markets argued for the continued right of all sickness funds to select their own subscribers and set premiums and benefits accordingly. Competition will maximize citizen choice and carrier efficiency. The *Ersatzkassen* defended the current situation. In Parliament, they were supported by the Free Democrats (FDP).

Equalization to cover some risks has always been inevitable. A sickness fund has always had an incentive to dump the poorest risks—particularly the elderly—on the *Ortskrankenkassen*. To compensate the *Ortskrankenkassen* and eliminate preferred-risk selection of pensioners by the other sickness funds, the special financing system for the elderly (the *Krankenversicherung der Rentner*) since 1977 transfers money among the carriers.

Each carrier collects premiums to cover some of the costs of its own pensioners. The sickness funds lack discretion in setting premiums for their pensioners. Once—as Chapters Five and Seven explained—the pension funds paid a standard per capita subsidy to the sickness fund. Now the pensioner pays proportions of his social security pension and other income. These rates are standard throughout the country. In addition, every statutory health insurance subscriber—including every member of the *Ersatzkassen*—pays a surcharge in his premiums to help cover the costs of that carrier's own pensioners. This too is standard throughout the country. For example, in 1986, the surcharge was 3.2 percent of earnings divided equally between workers and employers. Interfund transfers are still required, since every carrier still loses money from these premiums and benefits from sending the pensioners elsewhere. Unlike the French transfer system, the German transfers are not merely per capita subsidies to equalize differences in the collection of premiums. Rather, the German aim is to equalize the burden from costs of medical care. Each sickness fund calculates the medical care costs attributed to members on pensions. It calculates its revenue from these pensioners and from the extra premium it charges its employed subscribers in order to cover the elderly. Each sickness fund—for example, every *Ortskrankenkasse*—reports these figures and its entire accounts to the *Bundesversicherungsamt* every month. This office makes the calculations, deducting money from sickness funds with surpluses and transferring it to those sickness funds with strains attributable to the costs of their numerous, less affluent, and less healthy pensioners. The agency for the health insurance system that administers the monthly flow of premiums from the pension programs to the sickness funds (the *Bundesversicherungsanstalt für Angestellte*) makes the deductions and adds the supplements.[10]

The arrangement is required by amendments to the RVO enacted in 1977. Key decisions are made by the *Bundesversicherungsamt* after meeting representatives of the national associations of sickness funds, including the *Ersatzkassen*. Just before the start of each year, the conferees estimate the expected medical costs of all pensioners, the revenue from the pensioner's premiums, and the surcharge on all the employed that will be needed to cover the deficit. Since the medical costs for the elderly rise faster than the fiscal capacity of the insured labor force (the *Grundlohnsumme*), the surcharge usually is increased slightly every year. At the start of the year, the conferees agree on the general pattern of transfers to be followed during subsequent months. At periodic meetings during the year, they may adjust the transfers. They agree on a final settlement when the year's total costs and revenue for the pensioners are known.

This equalization system has been criticized on several grounds:

☐ It violates the principle that every sickness fund is completely autonomous and completely responsible for its own finances.

☐ Claims for transfers are based on costs and not on automatic criteria such as the numbers and ages of pensioners. Sickness funds may include in their estimates of the pensioners' costs amounts that really were due to the other economically active subscribers.

☐ Since a sickness fund loses its revenue if it underspends and gains transfers if it overspends, it has an incentive to be wasteful rather than efficient. It might grant frills that please subscribers but lack medical value—such as trips to spas and (in the case of *Ersatzkassen*) extra fees to doctors.[11] Subsequent amendments to the law have attempted to limit abuses by restricting costs to medically necessary treatments and auditing carriers' cost reports.

Preferred-risk selection by the *Ersatzkassen* and adverse selection by the public seemed to accelerate during the 1980s. Parliament finally abandoned tradition and enacted general interfund transfers to begin in 1989 and be in full operation during the 1990s. Since Germany was governed by a Center-Right coalition (CDU, CSU, and FDP) and not by the Left, transfers would be limited in scope to clinical costs due to difficulty of cases. Moreover, they would be implemented by negotiations among the associations of sickness funds. The transfers would not be imposed by government and would not achieve full-scale equalization. Transfers would occur among carriers within each province experiencing financial problems, not across the entire country. There are two types of transfers:

☐ *Payments by Ersatzkassen.* The medical costs per member would be calculated for all the social sickness funds together (*RVO-Kassen*) and for all the *Ersatzkassen*. If the former exceeds the latter—because of more difficult medical cases—the *Ersatzkassen* within the province will pay a lump-sum assessment to a joint committee of the province's sickness funds.

☐ *Payments among the sickness funds.* Calculations and transfers take place within each province. If one sickness fund has per capita clinical costs more than 10 percent above the average in the province, the others are obligated to help it. If one sickness fund faces a financial crisis because its clinical costs have risen 12.5 percent over the national average annual increase in costs for its type of carrier, the others are obligated to help it. The methods are designed to save a carrier from bankruptcy and prevent a prohibitive increase in premiums. These methods make universal and official what a few associations of sickness funds had already been doing voluntarily.

Belgium. An equalization system redistributes premium revenue from sickness funds with surpluses to those with deficits. In several countries, such as Belgium, this is precluded by the wording of the original law fixing each carrier's own financial responsibility: if one has a deficit, it must solve the problem alone—by temporarily tapping reserves, by eventually reestablishing balance through increase in premiums, and by controlling costs.

These financial rules were enacted in Belgium at a time before so many elderly patients incurred such high medical costs. Policymakers did not yet realize that the occupational and demographic characteristics of sickness funds would produce chronic deficits in some and surpluses in others. They did not foresee that some social insurance carriers could send many elderly subscribers to others. How can the principles of social solidarity and equity among carriers be preserved in the face of the original statutory language? This issue has led to controversies and deadlocks in Belgium and elsewhere. The Belgian sickness funds with many pensioners and deficits (such as the Socialists) press for a general equalization system while the sickness funds in balance (particularly the Christians) successfully block such a fundamental revision of the law.[12]

An alternative would be government subsidies for those sickness funds with many pensioners and high costs. It is difficult to target grants only at those with deficits: every sickness fund wants a share; critics of public subsidies argue that the deficits are due primarily to inefficiency. The subsidies covering the costs of the VIPOs—described in Chapter Eight—help the Socialist sickness funds, but their many other pensioners are not so covered. INAMI distributes its administrative subsidies to provide some extra relief to the Socialist sickness funds, but the help is less than the effects of a full-scale equalization formula. The leadership of the Christian *mutualités* allows this informal distribution in order to avoid open disputes and make the system work.

United States. Four trust funds are part of the Social Security system: Old Age and Survivors Insurance (OASI), Disability Insurance (DI), Hospital Insurance (HI for Medicare Part A), and Supplementary Medical Insurance (SMI for Medicare Part B). They were always supposed to be completely self-financing: the OASI, DI, and HI payroll taxes were regularly monitored and occasionally fine-tuned by Congress to ensure balances within each fund. But the OASI Trust Fund encountered cash-flow problems during the early 1980s, and Congress enacted authority for interfund loans among the OASI, DI, and HI Trust Funds according to precise formulas. OASI borrowed from DI and HI, repaid the money in the mid-1980s, and no other loans or outright transfers have ever occurred.[13]

The two parts of Medicare—the HI and SMI Trust Funds—have been kept rigorously separate even though both deal with health and both were created in the same law. No serious proposal has ever been made to relieve the Treasury of its uncontrollable SMI subsidies by tapping the payroll tax money that sometimes produces considerable surpluses in the other trust funds.[14]

Transfers Within Associations of Sickness Funds

If the financing of the health insurance system depends on standard payroll taxes, government must compensate for their differences in yield and in their adequacy to cover the costs of the several carriers. Therefore, an equalization system exists for German pension funds. But if the management of health insurance is private and each sickness fund can set its own premiums, government is expected to let the carriers settle their own financial problems.

Germany. While autonomous in many respects, German sickness funds cannot balance their budgets by rejecting the bad risks. Assignment of many subscribers is set by law—as outlined in Chapter Four and Appendix A—and the carriers cannot impose their own surcharges on the premiums of less healthy individual risks. The carriers with expensive underpayers cannot greatly increase their standard premiums, since the most desirable subscribers can transfer to the *Ersatzkassen* or to private insurance. Helping deficit-ridden sickness funds has been one of the tasks of the provincial association of carriers in that category (for example, the *Landesverband der Betriebskrankenkassen*). The German interfund transfer law of December 1988, described earlier, made this function universal and official. It gave provincial association officials authority to compel contributions from member sickness funds that did not want to help their brethren.

During the years of voluntary transactions, the principal equalization funding was performed among the workplace carriers—that is, the *Betriebskrankenkassen*. Under law, the employer is supposed to pay deficits. But if the underlying problem is the decline of the industry, the employer is less able to help. The employer would prefer to dissolve the sickness fund and let its members transfer to the *Ortskrankenkassen* and *Ersatzkassen*. The troubled fund must then turn to its *Landesverband*. Two provincial associations during the 1980s created equalization funds financed by a surcharge on every subscriber in the province. The trigger for help was the need of a workplace fund to raise its premium higher than the rate for the local *Ortskrankenkasse*.[15]

United States. Every American health insurance company is a self-centered competitor. It tries to gain over its rivals, not save them from decline. Extra cash goes into new benefits, more marketing, higher executive salaries, more lavish headquarters, and (in the case of stock companies) dividends to owners. But, as noted in Chapters Four and Seven, competition at times reduces profits for everyone and then there is no extra cash to share.

If competing American carriers prefer to impose deficits on their rivals rather than rescue them, one might expect collaborators to create their own equalization system. The model should be the Blue Cross and Blue Shield Association. Its headquarters controls the logos and franchises member Plans that meet several standards. The headquarters staff provides information and advice about financial management to all members. A telecommunication system and interfund bank have been created to permit a Plan to administer the payment of its local providers on behalf of subscribers belonging to other member Plans. Each Plan regularly pays dues to the association to cover headquarters' regular functions and special projects.

But Blue Cross/Blue Shield—unlike European associations of sickness funds—has no standing equalization system or even a permanent interfund rescue method. Because of the privatized and decentralized character of American health insurance, past proposals by the association's leadership have never progressed far. Each member Plan wishes to run its own affairs and limit the power of the association. Occasionally an impecunious Plan negotiates a loan or permanent transfer from an affluent Plan in another part of the country without involving the Chicago headquarters. The recipient therefore remains independent both of the headquarters and of the other Plans in its region. Each member Plan with a surplus wishes to earn interest on the surplus, rather than let the association earn it.

The vagaries of American insurance regulation—decentralized among the states and not uniform under the national government—give the association a reason not to maintain a rescue fund. In many state governments, the insurance department sets the rates for the Blues' nongroup policies. The Blues' rate-increase applications always arouse political controversy, but insolvency would embarrass the state government-of-the-day even more. If the Blue Cross/Blue Shield Association had an equalization fund, the state regulators would deny rate increases and force the local Plan to collect the money from the Chicago headquarters. By not maintaining a fund, the association can force all the state regulators to grant minimum rate increases pursuant to the various state financing laws.

If a Plan has a serious problem, it is handled according to the American preference for ad hoc solutions instead of standing machinery. The association headquarters requires submission of regular management and financial reports by member Plans and monitors them. If a Plan seems to have deteriorated, it is investigated and counseled by a committee of managers and actuaries from other member Plans, supported by the headquarters staff. If necessary, a special assessment might be levied on all member Plans by vote of the association at its annual conference or by its Board of Directors (in case of a sudden emergency). But the preferred solution is improvement of management, improvement of the benefit packages, and rate adjustments.

Transfers from the Private to the Social Sector

Private insurance companies can reject bad risks or quietly charge extra premiums as a condition for coverage. The sickness funds under statutory health insurance cannot. Mandatory assignment rules in some countries ensure that the most vulnerable patients and poorest subscribers go to the social insurance carriers. Meanwhile, in the name of competition, the private insurance companies may attract the healthier and more affluent persons with offers of lower premiums, better benefits, or both. The sickness funds and the political Left denounce the private insurance companies for cream-skimming, profiteering, and undermining social solidarity. They demand universal statutory health insurance that would either drive the private companies out of the market or make them function like sickness funds.

Before 1986, all Dutch citizens below a certain income ceiling were obligatory members of the sickness funds. Payroll taxes were standard, and the healthy had to contribute to the costs of the higher users. Persons over the income ceiling could remain voluntary subscribers of the sickness funds—with the same payroll taxes for the same benefits—or they could buy private insurance. The private companies could attract the young and better risks by offering the same benefits for premiums lower than the sickness fund rates, since their subscribers had lower utilization. As the private market became more competitive, the companies attracted subscribers from the sickness funds and from each other by offering a menu of policies with lower premiums made possible by greater cost sharing and fewer benefits (for example, by omitting general practice).

The problem is how to finance coverage of subscribers after retirement. As noted in Chapter Seven, the Dutch market once was dominated by a few large companies who charged everyone community rates and could afford to keep their older subscribers. Pensioners could stay with these private companies or switch back to sickness funds. As competition grew in the private market, new companies sought better risks by offering lower premiums and the established companies had to match them by adopting age-graduated premiums—and the pensioners became financially undesirable. Some companies refused to keep the pensioners on the grounds that they could return to the sickness funds for the full coverage they needed. Other companies charged high extra premiums. Special accounts for pensioners were set up in the statutory health insurance system (the *bejaardenverzekering*) and were subsidized by the national government. Refused outright by some private carriers or charged high and unsubsidized premiums by others, many pensioners switched back to the sickness funds. In 1982, the private companies enrolled over 35 percent of the Dutch population under age sixty-five but only 17 percent of those over that age.[16]

The social insurance carriers and many political factions denounced the private health insurance industry for profiteering and for violating social solidarity. The national government struggled to limit its budget deficit, caused in part by the need to subsidize the sickness funds' accounts for the aged. Universal statutory health insurance had been discussed but dropped during the 1970s, as the private companies argued that their role in a voluntary market served the public interest. The proposals for universal insurance administered entirely by the sickness funds revived, and the private companies needed to head them off.

The association of private health insurance companies (the *Kontaktorgaan Landelijke Organisaties van Ziektekostenverzekeraars*, or KLOZ) with the help of a management consulting firm estimated the numbers of pensioners in the social insurance sector and among its own members. Then it estimated the extra costs to the sickness funds due to their larger share: f.180 million in 1985. KLOZ met with the association of sickness funds (the *Vereniging van Nederlandse Zieken-fondsen*, or VNZ), and they agreed on such a transfer during the 1984–85 fiscal year. KLOZ collected it from its member companies in proportion to their total premium income. Estimates were that more pensioners would be kept by the private companies in 1986, and the transfer was reduced to f. 160 million during the 1985–86 fiscal year.

Parliament then enacted a redefinition of health insurance membership, eliminating voluntary assignments and the possibility of preferred-risk selection by the private sector. Above the membership earnings ceiling, no one could stay in the sickness funds and everyone must depend on the private market. Every private company must continue to insure its members after retirement, must offer its pensioners full coverage comparable to social insurance, and must charge no more than an actuarial rate set by the Minister of WVC. An equalization system was required in case the elderly were still overrepresented in the sickness funds. The *Ziekenfondsraad* calculated the distribution of the elderly, and a new special agency (the *Stichting uitvoering MOOZ*) administered the financial transfers. When a transfer was necessary, the money was raised by a surcharge on every private health insurance premium; every subscriber knew he was making this contribution. During the first fiscal year of the program (1986–87), the Minister recommended f. 135 a month as the private companies' premium for the full coverage of each elderly person. Every carrier adopted it. None took the option of charging a lower basic premium for its own revenue. All complained that true actuarial costs for the elderly were higher and they must now overcharge their young subscribers, in contrast to the competitive price cutting of the past.[17] They charged each younger subscriber at least f. 170 a month for the standard policy.

To eliminate the possibility of preferred-risk selection and avoid the need for a transfer system, Holland during the 1990s adopted universal obligatory insurance using both the private companies and sickness funds as carriers. A central agency collects all revenue and distributes it among carriers according to their numbers of subscribers weighted by risk, including age.[18] MOOZ was no longer necessary in its original form. In order to cover the elderly whose costs exceeded their premiums, all subscribers had to pay surcharges on their payroll taxes. The extra money was pooled, and the pool was shared among all carriers according to their numbers of pensioners.

Transfers Among Private Insurance Carriers

Private commercial insurance companies in all countries—whether nonprofit cooperatives or stockholder-owned—are considered self-interested profit maxi-mizers. The greater the net revenue, the higher the dividends to policyholders or to the stockholders. They conceal their financial affairs as much as possible and pay only taxes to outsiders. They are expected to outperform their competitors, not help them out. Governments require them to compensate the social insurance carriers in case of preferred-risk selection, but not to compensate each other.

The Netherlands. If the private companies seem on the brink of conversion into social insurance carriers, the industry's leadership may create an equalization system and government will endorse it. That happened in Holland during the 1980s after a decade of unhappy experience with a highly competitive private market.

When KLOZ devised the transfers between the private industry and the sickness funds, it also designed an equalization system among the private carriers to offset the competition that left some companies with older portfolios. The companies with younger portfolios must pay to those with older portfolios. The farther the company from the industry average in age, the greater the payments or receipts. The method did not equalize all costs, since that result would reward the wasteful and penalize the efficient. (Differentials in profitability were rewards and penalties in a market that was still supposed to be competitive.) Rather, the method was designed to narrow the wide range in premiums and prevent widespread desertion by subscribers of high-premium carriers when such differentials resulted from extreme variations in the ages of portfolios accumulated in past years. The system was administered by KLOZ and an affiliated financial agency. The government's role was to require participation of all private carriers, possible only by enacting a law.[19]

The arrangement lapsed during the 1900s. Statutory health insurance became universal, and all sickness funds and insurance companies could participate. A single equalization fund, described in previous paragraphs, was created.

Reinsurance. The only consistent financial pooling in private health insurance in Europe and North America is the universal practice of reinsurance. Every direct insurer ("ceding company") can purchase a commitment from and pay premiums to a reinsuring company. If the original direct insurer has a catastrophically expensive case listed in the contract, it can collect some of the costs from the reinsurance company. But this is part of the risk-sharing practice of the insurance industry, not a method whereby the more profitable companies regularly transfer money to those with frequent losses. All direct insurers—regardless of profitability—buy reinsurance and pay the premiums that are standard under a treaty or specially negotiated for the case at hand.

Reinsurance is more common in lines other than health, where an unexpected disaster may cause many large losses of property and lives concentrated in a few carriers in a few localities. The methods of reinsurance are flexible and varied.[20] Among the reforms of 1986 in Holland, KLOZ recommended and Parliament enacted a special fund that helped private insurance companies pay for catastrophic cases. With such a backup, a small Dutch insurance company was more likely to accept a bad health risk that it would have rejected earlier. It was one of the measures supporting the spread of social solidarity into the private Dutch health insurance sector before the complete adoption of universal social insurance.

Other European sickness funds have long had reinsurance treaties to protect local carriers from epidemics of serious diseases or from very expensive catastrophic cases. When the situation arises, the signatories share the costs. Associations of sickness funds—for example, provincial associations of *Betriebskrankenkassen* in Germany—sponsor such arrangements.

Some reinsurance pools are funds with administrative staffs and large reserves. For example, many Swiss sickness funds throughout the country participate in such a pool. Originally organized to cover the costs of poliomyelitis, it has been expanded to cover heart surgery, renal dialysis, and treatment of other catastrophic diseases. During the year, each participating sickness fund sends premiums. The sickness fund pays all provider bills and then asks the pool for full reimbursement of the eligible bills at the end of the year. As in all reinsurance programs in health, cost control is often questioned: the carriers who pay more than they recover complain that other sickness funds have paid providers too much. The pool's managers do not confront the providers but can only appeal to members for tighter practices.

Effects on Utilization and Health

Since interfund transfers are intended to substitute for public subsidies, some results are the same. They enable financially strained sickness funds to survive longer, to accept more bad risks, to maintain their full benefit packages, and to preserve their administrative service. Providers are still willing to accept those subscribers, since they will continue to be paid promptly and in full.

Unlike public subsidies, interfund transfers are redistributive. They level downward as well as upward. The carriers with a younger and healthier portfolio lose their financial advantages, since they become only a cog in a social insurance system. They no longer have so much extra cash to offer subscribers extra benefits and to offer doctors extra payments. They have less cash to market, glamorize their image, and recruit new members. Human service may replace preferred-risk selection in the organization's goals: the elderly and less healthy are no longer so undesirable, and the carrier is more willing to keep subscribers for life.

Implications for the United States

America has never had to develop a system of equalization transfers in health insurance, because it has never had a comprehensive official program with many carriers. Since it has never had public subsidies of insurance carriers, government budget officers have always assumed that the insurance industry rather than the Treasury should cover shortfalls. America has always encouraged competition among health insurance companies, and preferred-risk selection by each carrier has been a legitimate tactic.

State Pools. Even if the American private system lacks interfund equalization, the cause of the European problem (and the European solution) exists in the United States too. A significant number of persons with high costs can afford only low premiums or none at all. Government has finally had to create the American analog: pools to cover the health costs of the persons not covered by employer groups and unable to afford nongroup premiums (the "uninsured") and the bad risks rejected by carriers ("the uninsurables").

The state governments with such pools finance them by a rudimentary interfund transfer method. Part of the customary state taxes on group and nongroup premiums are earmarked for the pools. Because costs far exceed this revenue, the subscribers are charged (often high) premiums and the state government usually adds a subsidy from general revenue.[21]

The method demonstrates that no insurance system—no matter how privatized or how dedicated to competitive principles—can avoid a showdown over social equity. However, the American method has serious limitations: only a small number of states have them; subscriber premiums are unavoidable and deter many potential enrollees. The vagaries of employee benefits law create a serious loophole: increasing numbers of employees and insurance companies evade contributions and all premium taxes by signing administrative-services-only contracts rather than insurance contracts.

Interfund Mechanisms. In any design of NHI, Americans will have to think through the problem of interfund relations in advance. In a system with standard payroll taxes (or premiums), standard benefits, and many nonprofit and for-profit carriers, every fund will avoid bad risks and seek the better risks. Government will soon need to provide coverage for the bad risks, requiring either public subsidies or strict assignment rules for coverage of subscribers. If the system has voluntary coverage, public subsidies, and profits, voices will soon call for redistribution of the profits before burdening the taxpayer.

Financial equilibrium without interfund transfers is possible if only one sickness fund exists for all subscribers. Social Security uses unified funds: nearly everyone is in the OASI and DI Trust Funds with identical payroll taxes and identical benefits; everyone is covered by the HI Trust Fund. If the United States enacts NHI, it will decide whether to create such an unusual unified fund for all acute-care coverage throughout the country or adopt the usual European practice of using the many established carriers. In either case, America will need to stabilize its basic health insurance market with many rules. It can pursue its penchant for minimally regulated markets only in second-tier voluntary health insurance.

America's favorite alternative to European-type statutory health insurance is a proposed requirement that all employers buy private health insurance for their workers and dependents. This would merely expand the present arrangement. Any national law would be incomplete: political concessions would leave out many employees of small business, part-time workers, and the unemployed. If this becomes the American version of statutory health insurance, pools for the uninsured and uninsurable would have to be created throughout the country. They might be financed by taxes on small business without insurance, by taxes on all health insurance premiums, and by government subsidies. The short-lived Massachusetts Health Security Act of 1988 attempted to mandate universal employer-based health insurance. But it had to create several special pools to cover employees of small business firms that opted out, the unemployed, and other uncovered individuals.

Notes

1. Jean-Pierre Dumont, *La Sécurité sociale: Toujours en chantier* (Paris: Les Editions Ouvrières, 1981), p. 185.

2. Commission des Comptes de la Sécurité Sociale, *Les comptes de la Sécurité sociale—Prévisions 1989 et 1990* (Paris: La Documentation Française, 1989), p. 132.

3. The formulas are in Jean-François Chadelat, "La compensation," *Droit social,* vol. 41, nos. 9-10 (Sept.-Oct. 1978), pp. 87-94.

4. Ibid., pp. 95-115; *La compensation* (Paris: Direction de l'Administration Générale, Caisse Nationale de l'Assurance Maladie, 1983); and François Durin, "Les transferts sociaux," *Solidarité santé—études statistiques,* no. 2 (March-April 1988), pp. 21-28.

5. See M. Bougon and others, *Rapport sur l'évaluation des mécanismes de la compensation entre régimes de la Sécurité sociale* (Paris: La Documentation Française, 1987).

6. Pierre Begault and others, "Le financement du régime général de Sécurité sociale," *Revue française des affaires sociales,* vol. 30, special number (July-Sept. 1976), pp. 15-21, 61-62; and Alain Foulon, *Comparaison des régimes de Sécurité sociale: cotisations et prestations* (Paris: Documents du Centre d'Etude des Revenus et des Coûts, 1982), pp. 40-62.

7. For an analysis of all the interfund transfers in social security and the *Bund* subsidies for pensions see Klaus Mackscheidt, "Finanzausgleichsbeziehungen innerhalb und ausserhalb der gesetzlichen Rentenversicherung," in Sozialbeirat, *Langfristige Probleme der Alterssicherung in der Bundesrepublik Deutschland* (Bonn: Bundesminister für Arbeit und Sozialordnung, 1981), pp. 143-204. Mackscheidt compares the intentions and consequences of the transfer methods.

8. They were part of a larger and prolonged debate over the reorganization (*Strukturreform*) of German health insurance. See *Strukturfragen im Gesundheitswesen in der Bundesrepublik Deutschland* (Bonn: Wissenschaftliches Institut der Ortskrankenkassen, 1983), especially pp. 45-108. Evidence of the unequal distribution of the less healthy subscribers among carriers appears in Guntram Bauer and Peter Pick, "Besondere Risikogruppen in der GKV," *Die Ortskranken-*

kasse, vol. 70, no. 5 (March 7, 1988), pp. 145–148; and Guntram Bauer and Franz Schönhofen, "Risikostrukturen und Beitragssatzunterschiede in der GKV," *Die Ortskrankenkasse,* vol. 70, no. 22 (November 15, 1988), pp. 649–655.

9. See, for example, Heinz Jaschke and Manfred Kops, *Die Ursachen der Überdurchschnittlich der gesetzlichen Krankenkassen in Münsterland und die Möglichkeiten einer Beitragssätzverringerung mit Hilfe von Finanzausgleichsverfahren* (Cologne: Finanzwissenschaftliches Forschungsinstitut an der Universität zu Koln, 1981).

10. *Belastungsausgleich in der Krankenversicherung der Rentner (KVdR)* (Essen: Bundesverband der Betriebskrankenkassen, 1984); and Hans Hungenberg and Jürgen Steffens, *Krankenversicherung der Rentner,* 3rd ed. (Sankt Augustin: Asgard Verlag, 1983), pp. 120–131.

11. Günter Kübler, "KVdR-Finanzausgleich ist Korrekturbedurftig," *Die Krankenversicherung,* March 1986, pp. 77–80.

12. The greater concentration of pensioners in the socialist than in the Christian *mutualités* is evident in *Rapport général: Rapport statistique* (Brussels: INAMI, 1984), p. 3, pp. 19–22, 61.

13. Robert J. Myers, *Social Security,* 3rd ed. (Homewood, Ill.: Richard D. Irwin, 1985), pp. 131–132.

14. Alicia H. Munnell and Lynn E. Blais, "Do We Want Large Social Security Surpluses?" *Generation Journal,* vol. 1, no. 1 (April 1988), pp. 21–36. A typical discussion of the unexpected enormous increase in OASI reserves, the article mentions possible transfers to the HI Trust Fund if it encounters strains in the future. But the article does not mention using the OASI surplus to rescue the SMI Trust Fund from its current and chronic problems.

15. Kurt Friede, *Die Betriebskrankenkassen in der Bundesrepublik Deutschland,* 2nd ed. (Essen: Fachverlag C. W. Haarfeld, 1979), p. 62.

16. My calculations from data in *KISG83: Jaarboek 1983* (Houten: Stichting KLOZ Informatiesysteem Gezondheidszorg, 1984), pp. 8, 69–70.

17. A. Lugtenberg (ed.), *Nieuwe wetgeving ziektekostenverzekeringen* (The Hague: VUGA Uitgeverij, 1986), especially pp. 216–224; and G. W. de Wit, *De financiering van ziektekostenverzekering* (Rotterdam: Nationale-Nederlanden, 1986), pp. 43–47.

18. Commissie Structuur en Financiering Gezondheidszorg (W. Dekker and others), *Bereidheid tot verandering* (The Hague: Distributiecentrum Overheidspublikaties, 1987), pp. 14–15, 54–57.

19. Lugtenberg, *Nieuwe wetgeving ziektekostenverzekeringen* (see note 17, above), especially pp. 225–230; and de Wit, *De financiering* (see note 17, above), pp. 39–43.

20. Some sort of reinsurance is needed within each country and in international coverage. The basic ideas and technical methodology are universal. Some leading textbooks are Robert L. Carter, *Reinsurance* (Brentford, England: Kluwer, 1979); Klaus Gerathewohl, *Rückversicherung Grundlagen und Praxis* (Karlsruhe: Verlag Versicherungswirtschaft, 1976); and Robert W. Strain (ed.), *Reinsurance* (New York: College of Insurance, 1980).

21. Randall R. Bovbjerg and Christopher F. Koller, "State Health Insurance Pools: Current Performance, Future Prospects," *Inquiry,* vol. 23, no. 2 (Summer 1986), pp. 111–121; and *Health Insurance: Risk Pools for the Medically Uninsurable* (Washington: General Accounting Office, 1988).

PART THREE

Health Insurance Benefits

The next five chapters describe the benefits covered by statutory health insurance and private health insurance in all countries: physicians' services, hospital care, pharmaceuticals, dentistry, and mental health. Details vary among countries. Chapters Ten to Fourteen describe the methods of reimbursing providers and deciding reimbursement rates.

Long-term care for the increasing numbers of aged is needed in every country, and Chapter Fifteen describes the diverse methods of delivering and financing it. The relationship to statutory health insurance and the addition of other financing streams vary among countries.

Medical care is always evolving. New methods are being developed at an accelerating rate, their clinical value is often uncertain, and their costs are high. Chapter Sixteen describes the methods of deciding the addition of new benefits in health insurance.

CHAPTER 10

Physician Services

———————————————— **Summary** ————————————————

Once the large majority of physicians were insecure and earned little, and they welcomed contracts with mutual aid funds. The trend has been to create strong professional organizations and to become independent of the health insurance carriers. Now the doctors insist on negotiating the rules of practice and pay rates with the carriers. The medical associations have become powerful political interest groups. Direct employment of doctors for patient care by health insurance carriers has become unusual.

Mutual aid funds once contracted with closed panels of physicians, particularly general practitioners. The remaining doctors opposed exclusion from insurance practice, and every medical association has fought against limited panels. Every statutory health insurance law now guarantees participation by all office doctors and free choice of doctors by insured patients. Therefore, the doctor and patient make all the choices in a free market. The health insurance funds merely pay for practice; they no longer organize it. Selective contracting with particular doctors and locking patients into closed panels are possible only in the United States, where no health insurance statute exists.

In nearly all ambulatory and specialty care paid for directly by social insurance carriers, the unit of payment is fee-for-service. The fee schedule and rates are decided for the entire medical profession by collective negotiations be-

Note: This chapter gives highlights of the relationship between the medical profession and the health insurance system. Full details appear in my books *Paying the Doctor* (Baltimore: Johns Hopkins Press, 1970) and *Health Insurance Bargaining* (New York: Gardner Press and John Wiley, 1978).

tween medical associations and sickness funds. (Salaries are earned for patient care only by doctors employed by hospitals and health centers, where the insurance carriers pay the operating costs of the organizations and do not pay the doctors.) Capitation fees have declined in use. In most countries, carriers pay doctors directly; in some, they reimburse the patient.

In some countries, the official fee is payment in full under statutory health insurance, particularly if the carrier pays the doctor directly. In a few, the doctor has the right to extra-bill patients, but nowadays the frequency and financial amounts are limited. At times, extra-billing becomes very contentious. Specialists rely on extra-billing private patients for a substantial part of their income, since they are now treating increasing proportions of the socially insured at fixed fees.

Health insurance carriers and governments would like to review physicians' work in order to limit costs and prevent dangerous work. This is difficult to do, because of the fierce independence of the medical profession and because of doctors' claims to expertise. Health insurance carriers have installed computers to compare individual doctors with their peers. And they employ control doctors who investigate and counsel those who seem to violate the norm. Medical associations now insist that utilization review is one of the activities administered jointly with the sickness funds. The methodology and the criteria for judgment are still being developed. Statistical profiles merely identify deviation from the average—excessive rapidity or fraudulent billing, for example—but the method does not control excessive treatment by the entire profession. Guidelines for good practice are being defined and computerized only now, but they have not yet gained strong professional consensus. Some unorthodox practices may still be legitimate. Even under disciplined medical organization and standardized statutory health insurance systems, practice styles may vary widely among localities within a country.

Relations Between Sickness Funds and Doctors

Enabling people to pay doctors is what health insurance is all about. Different paths can be designed between the step where subscribers pay sickness funds and the step where the doctor collects money for his work.

Employment of Doctors by Sickness Funds. The early mutual assistance funds provided cash to compensate families for loss of income as well as heightened living costs during illnesses. They did not pay doctors. Physicians scrambled to make a living in unregulated private practice: they charged patients fees. Members of mutual assistance funds might use their cash payments to pay doctors, but the transaction was not organized by the carrier.

Mutual assistance funds added medical benefits to income replacement and death benefits during the nineteenth century. They did so in a simple fashion: each carrier retained one or a few doctors to be responsible for its members. In the style of that time, the doctor treated most of his patients in their homes; the sickness fund did not maintain a health center or buy advanced equipment. Since the doctor had an enduring contract with a definite number of subscribers, he could be paid accordingly—by a retainer, salary, or capitation fees—rather than by the itemized fees he charged in the free market. The subscribers joined such a fund in order to be guaranteed care by those doctors rather than paying fees out-of-pocket in the private market. The participating doctors welcomed the guaranteed income and competed for appointments.[1]

The first laws about compulsory membership and compulsory financing of health insurance—by German provinces during the mid-nineteenth century and by the German national government in 1883—assumed the existing method of organizing medical care. Providing care was thought the responsibility of the sickness funds—to be organized in the manner they judged best. The laws said nothing about the funds' relationship to their doctors and set no minimum standards for medical practice. The German sickness funds continued to employ closed panels of doctors and continued to pay many of them flat rates according to the number of subscribers. Since coverage and financing expanded under the law, more doctors were employed and paid in this manner.

Decades of dispute resulted. The doctors in the German panels complained they were underpaid and overworked. The sickness funds could always force the numerous doctors to compete for appointments, no matter how low the pay, and they were free to hire physicians who were not yet fully credentialed. The sickness funds added new members without appointing more doctors and without increasing doctors' pay at the same rate as their rise in revenue. Doctors not in the panels demanded access to these patients. Both groups of doctors organized trade unions: the panel doctors, to obtain better terms from individual sickness funds or to obtain amendments to the law; the nonpanel doctors, to lobby the government for statutory change. Strikes by the panel doctors were common and destabilized health care.[2]

Doctors in all other countries heeded the German uproar and organized medical associations to protect themselves against sickness funds and obtain favorable clauses in health insurance laws. No new laws conferred exclusive clinical responsibility on the sickness funds; all laws explicitly guaranteed that every licensed physician could treat any patient under statutory health insurance and that any beneficiary could choose any doctor. (The only exception was the unsuccessful and short-lived British National Health Insurance Act of 1911, to be described in this chapter.) In a few countries, such as France after the political compromise of 1960, either the law or the contracts negotiated between the medical associations and carriers forbade the sickness funds to operate health centers and deliver care by employing doctors.

If sickness funds had previously employed closed panels of doctors and operated health centers, they could keep these arrangements. But they could no longer lock their subscribers into using only those providers. Fully covered by statutory health insurance, the patient was free to consult any out-of-plan physician, who could bill the sickness fund for normal reimbursement. If the sickness fund had paid an annual capitation rate to the patient's prepaid panel, the carrier could deduct the itemized out-of-plan bills from the monthly capitation payments so that it would not be paying twice.

In order to persuade subscribers to use the panel doctors and therefore to cover their costs, the sickness funds must use incentives rather than contractual obligations or sanctions. France is one of the few countries where the law provides the opportunity for such incentives. Several *mutuelles* have employed doctors—usually part-timers on salary—for a century. The contracts forbidding health centers apply to the official *caisses maladie* and not to the *mutuelles.* If a patient subscribes to a *mutuelle,* his subscription fee entitles him to use the *mutuelle's* doctors without the usual cost sharing; the *mutuelle* bills the *caisse* on the patient's behalf without requiring his initial outlay of cash; and the patient can use the other health center services (dentistry, drugs, eyeglasses, medical supplies) at less-than-market prices. Loyal members of the *mutualist* movement still patronize their health centers, but most French patients use the office doctors and private practice has become the professional norm.[3]

The *mutualist* health centers vary widely in management, budget, and internal harmony. In some, managers and doctors quarrel. In some, patients complain about underservicing.[4] Doctors and patients would rebel if the arrangements became universal. But they are only an option for a few; discontented doctors and patients can elect conventional office practice. The *mutualist* groups no longer set the norms for office practice, but the office doctors set the standards for judging the groups.

The German panel physicians chipped away at the sickness funds' powers, ultimately achieving nearly the same degrees of free access as in other European countries. First, all the separate unions representing doctors in each panel coalesced into provincial associations (*Kassenärtzliche Vereinigungen,* or KVs). Instead of each sickness fund dictating pay to each individual doctor, all the provincial carriers transfer all their money to each KV, which pays all the doctors according to a fee schedule. At first the entire province was treated as a large closed panel: any member of a KV could treat and bill for any insured person, but the KV only admitted a fixed number of doctors in ratio to the number of subscribers. Protests by the unadmitted physicians led to increases in the ratios after World War II. Their lawsuit finally led to a decision by the constitutional court of Germany that invalidated any *numerus clausus* as an infringement on every doctor's right to earn a living.[5] Therefore, every licensed doctor in office practice may treat any insured patient, as in other countries. (A vestige of the earlier restrictions is a ban on insurance practice by full-time salaried hospital specialists.) Because of the present state of health insurance case law, Germany— once a system built around closed panels—no longer can have them.[6]

If closed panels survive under statutory health insurance, the law must explicitly preserve them, require a lock-in for their subscribers, and refuse to pay for out-of-plan care initiated by the subscribers. Such a law can be enacted only if carriers with closed panels are numerous and politically powerful, only if the medical association is politically weak, and only if the remaining doctors can survive in a large private market. British experience suggests that—in the unlikely case of legislative enactment—such a system cannot be implemented successfully thereafter. Despite the early rumblings of trouble in Germany, Great Britain enacted such a National Health Insurance Act for the working class in 1911. Defeated in Parliament by a determined Prime Minister and a large coalition of trade unionists and sickness funds, the British Medical Association denounced the arrangements for decades thereafter.

The sickness funds proved inept administrators.[7] When the Labour Government in 1946 moved to cover the entire population for all medical services, the mosaic of sickness funds and closed medical panels proved administratively and financially unworkable—as well as politically unacceptable to both the medical profession and the population. In its publicly financed and governmentally administered system, Britain then followed the experience of other countries with statutory health insurance: all licensed physicians may be admitted to practice; any patient may choose any primary physician.[8] (The only restriction is to limit the opening of new practices in overdoctored communities, a control that can be implemented more easily in a government-operated national health service than under national health insurance.)

Since health insurance carriers with their own closed panels can survive only in countries lacking universal health insurance laws, today they exist only in the United States. Typical European sickness funds connected with trade unions, isolated employers, and immigrant communities were common in America during the nineteenth and early twentieth centuries. A sickness fund collected subscription fees, hired one or a few doctors, paid the doctors salaries or capitation fees, and covered subscribers and their families only for within-plan services. Some carriers maintained offices as workplaces for the doctors. Since doctors wish to be independent professionals and not employees of the laymen who manage insurance carriers, compromise arrangements were developed: some closed panels were medical groups who directed their own affairs and contracted with the carriers.[9]

Among the few laws about health insurance ever enacted by the United States Congress are attempts to encourage the growth of these arrangements: the Health Maintenance Organization Act of 1973 subsidized prepaid groups that met conditions for enrollment, rates, and benefits; employers who offered group insurance to their workers also must give them an option to join an HMO; the health insurance programs for the national government's civil servants gives the option to enroll in many HMOs as well as in conventional insurance; Medicare offers annual capitation rates for any HMO that enrolls its beneficiaries.[10] The United States government has filed lawsuits under the antitrust laws against associations of office doctors who try to drive HMOs out of their communities.[11]

Left to the free market, carrier-sponsored closed panels have had uneven experiences in the United States. Some groups of physicians have been willing to practice in health centers for salaries or—more often—for fees divided according to work. Some employer groups and individuals have been willing to enroll with these carriers, primarily in the Western part of the country. But after many years of energetic marketing and optimistic forecasting, only 5.3 percent of the entire population in 1989 was enrolled in such "staff-model" and "group-model" HMOs.

More flexible arrangements have been created by insurance companies and lists of office doctors—called variously "network-model HMOs," "independent practice associations" (IPAs), and "preferred provider organizations" (PPOs). The insurer signs up the doctor by promising to steer its subscribers to that doctor. The doctor agrees to charge according to the carrier's fee schedules (less than the payments by his out-of-plan patients). What the doctor loses in unit prices he hopes to regain from higher volume. The incentive for the subscriber—as in a French *mutuelle*—is lower cost sharing (or none at all) for use of a within-plan doctor and higher cost sharing for use of any other physician.[12] While many patients and doctors participate in insurance that provides a PPO option, very few claims actually use this route. In 1987, for example, 43.3 percent of American doctors had contracts with PPOs but only 12 percent of their revenue came through this arrangement. A quarter of these doctors had no PPO patients and no PPO revenue at all.[13]

HMOs have long been the Holy Grail in American health service reform, and drafts of national health insurance laws try to guarantee their survival and growth. The authors hope for a voluntary preference for HMOs over conventional health insurance—motivated by potentially lower premiums and lower cost sharing. Since these differentials are unlikely to be large enough to wean the population from the traditional office practice, doctors are unlikely to be under great pressure to sign up.[14] If HMOs lose money whenever subscribers use their legal rights to see out-of-plan doctors, they cannot survive. American-style closed-panel HMOs collapsed in Ontario when universal public financing authorized every patient to consult any doctor outside the panels—at the expense of each HMO's capitation rate.[15]

In contrast, the American PPO is the germ of what every country has enacted in statutory health insurance: abroad every citizen and every doctor participate, and all bills are paid according to a controlled fee schedule. But unlike an American PPO, the payers under statutory health insurance cannot contract selectively among all the doctors admitted to practice and the payers cannot steer patients to preferred doctors.

Contractual Relations Between Sickness Funds and the Medical Profession. Direct employment of general practitioners and specialists by insurance carriers has become unusual, particularly under statutory systems. The usual method is a collective and general relationship between all the insurance carriers and the entire medical profession to set the ground rules, rather than specific employment relations between individual carriers and, on the other hand, subordinate individual doctors and small medical groups. For each service provided subscribers, the carrier pays the physician according to the collective agreements.

Since neither government nor the sickness funds can dictate to the medical profession, a bilateral negotiating system is set up:[16]

☐ *Sickness funds.* If all have been merged into one, its national headquarters meets with the medical association. If there are several carriers, their leaderships form a joint negotiating committee, usually with the largest carrier as chairman. In federal systems, the provincial headquarters and provincial joint negotiating committees meet with the provincial leaderships of the medical association.

☐ *Medical association.* The specialties are usually rivals for money. The association commonly becomes an elaborate system of government for the medical profession, prioritizing the demands of the specialties and working out a consensus to present to the sickness funds. If the concerns of a particular specialty are being negotiated—such as the redesign of its part of the fee schedule—its leaders join the negotiating team from the medical association. If there are several medical associations, they merge in a single federation or form a joint negotiating committee to face the carriers. If there are several medical associations and they are rivals—as in France and Belgium—the negotiations become complicated.

☐ *Government.* It enacts the law that constitutes the framework for the negotiations. But both the sickness funds and the medical associations try to keep health insurance a private transaction. Government usually does not participate in the negotiations except to arbitrate deadlocks. However, as costs and payroll taxes rise, governments now try to influence the bargaining by transmitting guidelines with limits on the annual increases in fees, as Chapter Seventeen will explain.

The sickness funds and the medical association negotiate a contract, a fee schedule (a "relative-values scale"), and the financial prices for the fee schedule (the "conversion factors"). Later pages of this chapter will describe the content of these documents and the negotiating process.

Direct Payment of the Doctor by the Sickness Fund. The foregoing negotiating arrangements are used both in the countries where the sickness funds pay the doctor directly (*tiers payant* in French) and in the countries where the sickness fund reimburses the patient after he has paid the doctor (*tiers garant*). In several (such as Holland and Switzerland), the doctors have become accustomed to billing the sickness funds directly and receiving full payment directly. But in several countries with histories of conflict between the doctors and sickness funds, other methods have been designed to symbolize the doctors' professional independence from the lowly insurance clerks: in Germany, for example, a special agency representing all the doctors in each province (the *Kassenärztliche Vereinigung,* mentioned earlier) is paid monthly installments by the sickness funds. The KV receives the bills from the doctors and pays them.

Reimbursement of the Patient. Under this method, the doctor can preserve the fiction that his clinical and financial transactions with the patient are completely private and discretionary—that both statutory and private commercial health insurance are the concern only of the patient and the laymen in the carriers. The patient pays the doctor and is reimbursed by the sickness fund (*tiers garant*).

The medical profession favors such arrangements because they symbolize professional independence: they enable each doctor to bill according to his own evaluation of his own eminence and the patient's financial capacity. However, the patients complain they are already paying payroll taxes and are not getting their money's worth. And government and the sickness funds argue that all doctors must conform to the law, contracts, and fee schedules that underlie the system. The medical association replies that it has negotiated a patient indemnity schedule, not a binding fee schedule without rights of extra-billing. The indignant doctors may strike. Strong governments (as in France in 1960) may force the doctors to bill according to the fee schedule, even though *tiers garant* remains. Weak governments (as in Belgium and the United States) cannot force the entire medical profession to conform, but the medical associations now induce doctors to minimize extra-billing in order to defuse the controversy.

American Medicare is one of the few statutory health insurance programs with an option. A "participating physician" who accepts assignment in all cases is rewarded—with listing in a brochure sent to patients, with prompt payment of his claims, and with annual increases in the controlled fees. His patients are relieved of having to pay high fees out-of-pocket. Nevertheless, the incentives have not fully overcome the desire for professional freedom and the collection of extra charges. By 1990, fewer than half the doctors were fully "participating physicians," although the proportion has slowly increased.[17] They experience little market pressure to join: most patients do not understand the rules and can see no advantage in switching from nonparticipating to participating physicians.[18]

The Belgian government and sickness funds discovered that a shift from reimbursement to direct third-party payment may complicate utilization control and unexpectedly raise costs. Under the contracts, Belgian doctors had the right to elect *tiers payant* and by 1986 half had done so. Offering a *tiers payant* arrangement that relieved the patient of a large cash outlay was a principal tactic in doctors' competition for patients. But if the patient no longer received a bill and if he no longer calculated a cash outlay, a doctor could add bogus treatment to the claim he sent to the patient's sickness fund. He might even submit completely false bills for patients that he did not see. In the competition for patients, the doctor might waive the coinsurance, which the Belgian system had preserved as a market disincentive against overutilization. The doctor could offset his loss of the coinsurance by multiplying services. Therefore, the direct third-party payment route, long favored by the world's sickness funds as the best control over medical practice and over costs, might be manipulated to increase costs. The Belgian government and sickness funds in 1986, as one of their cost containment reforms, banned direct third-party payment of physicians' bills.[19]

Units of Payment

The actual cash for work can be transferred in several ways:[20]

☐ *Fee-for-service*. A specific amount is provided for each treatment. The doctor itemizes his services on a bill after the completion of care, and the sickness fund pays him or reimburses the patient. This is the usual form of billing by self-employed doctors, both for ambulatory and hospital inpatient services.

☐ *Capitation fee*. Every subscriber to a sickness fund is on the list of a general practitioner. The sickness fund pays the GP a fixed amount per year for each subscriber, regardless of the work required. For ordinary care, the GP sends no bills and collects no itemized fees. Once common, capitation fees have often been replaced in whole or in part by fee-for-service systems. The medical profession usually prefers fee-for-service, since rewards are related to work. Sickness funds may prefer fee-for-service because the claims forms yield knowledge about work performed whereas the capitation system does not. Capitation fees fit primary care but are not used for specialists, who lack a continuing relationship with a group of subscribers.

☐ *Salary*. A fixed amount is paid for time at work, either full-time or part-time. Salary is associated with an employment relation or contractual relation with an organization.

☐ *Case payment*. A fixed amount is paid for providing all necessary care to each type of patient, classified by diagnosis. Occasionally it has been used by patients and sickness funds to pay for certain predictable care, such as normal deliveries in obstetrics. Used by some payers for inpatient hospital care in the United States, the method has been suggested for the payment of American doctors. It is rarely used in practice.

For the arms-length transactions that usually characterize sickness funds and doctors, the payments are fee-for-service. If a doctor is employed by a sickness fund, he usually receives a salary or capitation fees. Some closed panels caring for sickness funds' subscribers receive lump sums but may distribute them among the doctors by fee-for-service, prorated to keep within the total budget. A recent trend is payment of hospital-based specialists by full-time or part-time salary. In these cases, the doctors' salaries are included in the total inpatient costs; the sickness fund pays the hospital per diems, case payments, or a share of global budget; the carrier pays the hospital, not the salaried hospital doctor.

Ground Rules

In the medical profession's utopia, society would provide all necessary resources for optimum care. The doctor would deal only with the patient, would be paid only by the patient, and would be governed only by the principles of medical ethics and other rules formulated by the medical association. Complete professional autonomy is restricted by private health insurance and clearly cannot survive when statutory health insurance is enacted for the general population: government guarantees the money by enacting payroll taxes and contributing subsidies; the carriers must control their budgets; government and the carriers claim the responsibility to protect the dependent and ill-informed patient from overcharging and mistreatment.

The Law. One set of ground rules affecting the physician is in the statute enacted by Parliament and in the implementing regulations issued by the President, Prime Minister, and Minister of Social Affairs. Most of the law deals not with doctors but with the identity and responsibilities of taxpayers, the rights of insured persons, and the organization and functions of sickness funds. Nevertheless, the law deals with benefits and reimbursement in ways that affect the medical profession:

- [ ] It lists every benefit that insured persons can claim. This implies the need to define appropriate work sites and to decide a payment method for each benefit.
- [ ] It grants the right to bill the sickness funds by any other practitioners—such as midwives—who are recognized by the country's medical practice laws.
- [ ] It decides whether the sickness fund pays the doctor or reimburses the patient. If the doctor refuses to accept assignment—that is, if he "opts out"— the law decides whether the patient can be reimbursed by the sickness fund and (if so) whether he is reimbursed in full.
- [ ] It determines whether the official payment rates are payment in full. If the subject is not mentioned in the law or regulations, the doctor can extra-bill at his discretion.
- [ ] It includes some provisions about the containment of costs. If the medical association is foresighted, it can visualize future disputes with government and the sickness funds over fees and utilization.
- [ ] It stipulates how disputes are resolved.

The medical profession welcomes increases in public expenditure that will improve patients' access, resources for medical practice, and their own incomes. But it always opposes restrictions on its own autonomy. It is always wary of statutory health insurance proposals because eventually insurance will become restrictive. Often the first legislative drafts include the following clauses:

☐ Direct payment of doctors by the sickness funds (*tiers payant*) is opposed (unless this was the custom under voluntary health insurance).
☐ The fee schedule is payment in full without rights of extra-billing.
☐ If the doctor refuses to accept assignment, the sickness fund will reimburse the patient little or nothing (that is, *tiers garant* is not allowed).
☐ Government and the sickness funds may contain costs by unilateral action.

Objecting to such clauses, the medical association then opposes the entire scheme.

If the original law does not contain such restrictions but they are proposed later, the political battle between the medical association and the payers breaks out at this later time. But usually the divisive issues appear at the time of the original proposal of the law, and a protracted struggle ensues.[21] Several clauses desired by the doctors are usually inserted into the final law to mollify the medical association, prove to conservative legislators and pressure groups that medical care is not being politicized, and gain the cooperation of doctors during implementation. The clauses include:

☐ The government shall not interfere in the clinical practice of medicine.
☐ Every insured patient shall have free choice of doctor.
☐ Every licensed physician may practice under NHI and shall have free choice of patient.
☐ Licensed doctors shall not be compelled to practice under NHI but may practice privately.

After the law is enacted, the disputes fade. The medical association becomes a system of self-government so that the profession can formulate its demands, fix priorities, settle its internal rivalries, and negotiate with government and the sickness funds. The medical association develops an extensive system of committees, hires a large staff of administrators and researchers, moves into a larger headquarters, and acquires a politically sophisticated leadership. After a generation, the new medical practitioners take for granted the framework for practice and reimbursement.

The law and the regulations usually are left alone for many years. Everyone can learn them and the arrangements eventually stabilize. Developed countries avoid making changes until it is clear that serious problems need to be remedied, and they fear that frequent changes create confusion. They adjust details through the standing negotiations described below. An exception to this practice is the United States. The Congress left Medicare alone for several years after the initial passage in 1965. However, during the 1980s and 1990s, the Congress—particularly the House of Representatives—has revised both Parts A and B of Medicare annually in a futile effort to satisfy all interest groups and resolve a growing list of problems. The constant tinkering becomes a principal source of difficulty and dispute.

In other developed countries, the law remains simple and stable because the details are left to standing negotiations between the medical associations and sickness funds. But American Medicare lacks any such negotiating mechanisms, and Congress does not trust the discretion of the Department of Health and Human Services. Thus it is Congress that resolves all the details in the payment of doctors and hospitals, thereby seriously overloading itself.

Contract. Every country with either national health insurance or a national health service has some form of standing negotiating machinery to settle administrative and financial details. Under NHI, the medical association and the sickness funds negotiate and the government provides guidelines to limit costs. Under NHS, the medical association faces the Ministry of Health and a special arbitration body resolves deadlocks.[22]

Usually the two sides sign a contract that runs for about five years. The contract spells out the details of doctor/carrier relations—the procedures admitting doctors to insurance practice, how to submit bills, payment procedures, acts that may or may not be billed separately, rules governing the exceptional cases of extra-billing, utilization control, the composition of negotiating committees, and so on.

Many clauses are not controversial. They may merely implement parts of the law. Or perhaps they were negotiated in earlier contracts and are retained. But some new proposals by the sickness funds may elicit resistance from the medical association on the grounds they impinge on the financial and clinical prerogatives of the doctors—any revision of rights of extra-billing, for example, or any tightening of utilization control. Deadlocks may postpone a new agreement until the old one has expired. During the interim, health insurance continues under the procedures spelled out in the previous contract. Usually there is no arbitration machinery to resolve deadlocks over the contract, and government does not intervene since the outstanding issues are few. Without a change, the status quo persists.

Fee Schedule. A standing committee from the medical association and the sickness funds oversees the fee schedule. While bargaining over contracts and money is adversarial, the fee schedule is discussed in a more technical and collegial spirit. The numbers of representatives from the medical association and sickness funds need not be equal. All members are doctors. Each side may be accompanied by statisticians with data about costs of practice and utilization of the various procedures.

When national health insurance is first enacted, the sickness funds accept one of the crude fee schedules that the medical societies or health insurers wrote to guide private transactions. Therefore, modern fee schedules have a long and continuous lineage. The medical association still has a special interest in the fee schedule's revision, and proposed changes usually originate in the specialty societies within the association. But the country's fee schedule no longer can be promulgated by the medical association alone. Legally, it is an appendix to the contract between the medical association and sickness funds. In some countries, government issues it as a regulation that is binding on doctors, patients, and carriers in case of dispute.

The negotiating committee is busy with changes, adding new procedures, eliminating obsolete procedures, and reducing the relative value of acts that have become simpler. The medical association often is asked by doctors to clarify certain lines in the fee schedule and the committee issues explanations. For the routine work, the committee meets every few months throughout the year.

Occasionally an entire fee schedule is revised. Technological progress may have changed a specialty. Or the medical specialties and the sickness funds may complain that the fee schedule is biased on behalf of the technical and surgical specialties and call for higher weights for primary care and for social supports. Rewriting part or all of a fee schedule requires frequent meetings over at least a year by the tariff committee within the medical association and by the joint committee of the association and the carriers. When the schedule for a specialty is considered by the joint committee, the association is represented by leaders of the specialty society, supported by the association's statisticians.

Cash Values. A fee schedule is a relative-value scale giving each procedure a weight: 10, 15, 18, 21, and so forth. A basic financial unit (a "conversion factor"), such as 18 F or 9.12 DM, must be multiplied by the weight of each procedure to establish the cash payment by the sickness fund to the doctor for that procedure. The doctor fills out his bill by consulting the fee schedule; he enters on the bill either the procedure code alone, the weight alone (as in France), or (as in most countries) both. In the few countries where the entire fee schedule is reprinted every year in its current financial values (as in Holland), the doctor may enter both the procedure code and the financial price.

The fee schedule stays essentially the same for many years, but the conversion factor usually is increased every year. The top leadership of the medical association, with statistical ammunition from its research staff, initiates the request for more money. The association argues that the costs of practice have risen substantially during the last year and that doctors' incomes have not risen as fast as the incomes of other elite occupations. At the bargaining sessions, the leaders of the sickness funds (supported by their statisticians) rebut these claims and argue that the rise of all health care costs leaves them with little new money for the doctors. The negotiations are adversarial and often acrimonious. The sickness funds prefer a deadlock to a large award, since they continue to pay at the old conversion factor. The medical association may threaten an administrative strike: the doctors will bill patients according to their proposed conversion factor, and the patients will recover what they can from the sickness funds. To avoid turmoil, the two sides usually agree on a figure.

Agreement once was easy. The sickness funds conceded higher fees to the doctors and obtained higher payroll taxes from government. But hospital costs rose rapidly during the 1960s and 1970s, straining sickness funds and governments everywhere. As statutory health insurance (and all of social security) became too expensive and as governments were pressed to subsidize the sickness funds, the Ministries of Finance and Health urged the sickness funds—either informally or in written guidelines—to limit the annual awards to the doctors.

In Germany—which stresses that decisions are made by negotiations among private groups—the sickness funds, the association of insurance doctors, and other providers and payers meet once or twice a year in a forum staffed by the Ministry of Labor: the *Konzertierte Aktion im Gesundheitswesens,* or KA. Data are presented about the fiscal capacity of the sickness funds and about trends in utilization of physicians' services. The KA formulates recommendations about economically feasible increases in spending for physicians' services, and the negotiators in each province follow the guidelines in settling on either the total amount available for all physicians' services (the *Kopfpauschale*) or on the conversion factor. The provincial association of insurance doctors cannot press for more, because the dispute would then go to an arbitrator who would follow the KA guidelines. (Additional details and citations about the KA appear in Chapter Seventeen.)

Throughout Europe during the 1980s, sickness funds granted only small increases in the conversion factor. Medical associations became remarkably cooperative on this point, since the new research data showed unexpectedly that many doctors increased their total incomes substantially even with small increases in unit prices. Earnings rose because aging populations visited doctors more often and because technological progress led to more use of expensive items in the fee schedule. In other words, utilization and service intensity—which were not bargained during the negotiating sessions over conversion factors—rose steadily.

Rivals when seeking members and prestige, sickness funds unite when bargaining with doctors and hospitals. None wish to waste their money by paying more than the others for the same services. The only exception is the *Ersatzkassen* of Germany. They use the same fee schedule as the other sickness funds, but they pay by a conversion factor that is about 10 percent higher. (The differential varies by province: the *Ersatzkassen* have uniform national rates, whereas the sickness funds' rates vary among provinces.) The *Ersatzkassen* claim they need to obtain favorable attention for their members by paying the doctors higher fees, since they compete for subscribers with the private insurance companies. They use this image also to compete with the sickness funds for members. The *Ersatzkassen* have more extra cash than the sickness funds, since their members are healthier.

Utilization Control

The review of doctors' performance by health insurance carriers (or on their behalf) is designed to detect, punish, and prevent venality, waste, and poor quality in the following forms:

☐ Bills may be submitted in order to earn without giving the specified care to the subscribers. Or the bills might be false. Or the doctor might have seen the patient, given rapid and perfunctory care, and the examinations and treatments were too hasty to be effective.

☐ Care may have been given, but with a proliferation of remunerative services that were inappropriate or too repetitious for that diagnosis.

☐ Care may have been given, but it was ineffectively delivered. Or the wrong treatments were given for that diagnosis.

Utilization controls of some sort exist in all organized payment arrangements. How they work depends on the organization of the country's providers and that of the sickness funds. The number of doctors reviewed and the severity of the procedures depend on the structure of the hospitals:

☐ *Closed medical staffs on salary.* If most of the senior doctors and all the juniors are full-time salaried, they do not bill the sickness funds for fees, but the salaries are covered in the hospitals' operating costs. The chief of service is responsible for the efficiency and quality of work in his service. Any lapses are problems of hospital management and of government—until recently, the sickness funds were not involved. The carriers' control doctors hesitated to challenge the chiefs' performance.

☐ *Hospital staffs paid by fee-for-service.* They may be closed staffs in the sense that limited numbers of doctors belong and most physicians remain in office practice. (Examples are certain nonprofit hospital systems—as in Holland—and the many private clinics in Europe.) Or they may be open-staff hospitals that allow office doctors to hospitalize and treat their patients without referral to a permanent staff. (Examples are the United States and Canada.) In all these arrangements, the sickness funds have a considerable monitoring task, since they receive and pay for bills submitted both by these hospital doctors and by the many office doctors. The specialists' bills include many technically advanced, potentially dangerous, and remunerative acts. The hospitals' weak medical staff structures lack the internal controls to review efficiency and quality.

☐ *Office doctors.* They generate most of the bills processed by sickness funds. Almost always, the bills are itemized and the doctors are paid fees. Under an all-payer system covering the entire population, the volume of bills can be enormous. The more technically advanced work was once done only in hospitals. But now office doctors everywhere are buying and amortizing new equipment, and the sickness funds must monitor large bills and risky procedures.

Prerogatives of the Sickness Funds. Governments and sickness funds have always been aware that a doctor might bill excessively—either by submitting false bills or by multiplying services for more than clinical needs. The utilization review problem exists because sickness funds under NHI can no longer contract selectively with those doctors who are most restrained and most efficient. The sickness funds must pay all doctors regardless of practice style.

But the sickness funds cannot impose whatever utilization review arrangements they like. Medical associations have always challenged investigations by insurance carriers on principle: associations think that clinical work is the responsibility of the medical profession; any complaints about performance can legitimately be filed only by patients or other doctors and can be investigated only by disciplinary bodies of the medical profession; sickness funds must presume that every bill signed by the attending doctor is both legally and clinically legitimate. As a professional body, the medical association fosters efficiency and quality in giving care. But as the doctors' trade union in facing the payers, the association defends the individual physician from the sickness funds and government.

The sickness funds that had once employed their own doctors were accustomed to monitoring both their doctors and subscribers. When they tried to extend such scrutiny to the other doctors in office practice, the medical association reacted explosively. Such was the experience of the French *mutuelles* during the 1930s: some office doctors submitted bills that were suspected of being false, and the *mutuelles'* salaried control doctors examined the patients to verify the claims.[23]

The German sickness funds solved the problem by turning both the payment and monitoring of doctors over to a special medical association. Utilization control became an essential part of the payment method. From the early 1930s through the 1950s, the sickness funds negotiated a lump sum (*Kopfpauschale*) for all ambulatory and private clinic fees with an association representing all the insurance doctors (the *Kassenärztliche Vereinigung*, or KV). The KV used a relative-values scale to pay fees to members for their claims. Fees were prorated to keep total payments within the *Kopfpauschale*. If a doctor submitted too many bills or suspiciously high bills, he gained at the expense of the other doctors who practiced and billed honestly. The KVs created the first comparative statistical files to detect the doctors (the *Kassenlöwen* or "sickness fund lions") who submitted exceptionally many bills. They were not paid in full.[24]

Statistical Profiles. The KV's methods were very simple but foreshadowed later developments. The German sickness fund issued to each patient a form (a *Krankenschein*) that the patient gave to one doctor, who provided all ambulatory care for one calendar quarter. The doctor recorded all treatments on the form and then sent it to the KV. The clerks at the KV classified all forms by doctor, compared doctors, and notified the KV managers that some doctors were submitting forms that were implausible in the complexity and number of the listed procedures. Because the work was manual, the analysis was limited to comparing the doctors' aggregate totals. The clerks could not classify data by patient and procedure. They could not calculate annual totals. And they could not compare different stages in a physician's time series.

In all other countries, the claims forms are received, analyzed, and reimbursed by the sickness funds themselves and not (as in Germany) by an agency of the medical profession. But the medical association will not tolerate unilateral judgments by sickness funds that any doctors are billing fraudulently and wastefully or practicing inefficiently and dangerously. The issues then become:

☐ Roles of the medical association, the sickness funds, and government in the design and implementation of the complete control system
☐ Methodology
☐ Criteria for identifying physicians with suspicious billing practices
☐ Communicating with the deviant physicians
☐ Goals of control: exclude deviants from practice under statutory insurance or teach them to practice better medicine
☐ Sanctions
☐ Appeals

Roles. Unable to block the development of statistical profiles and judgments about individual doctors, the medical associations everywhere have agreed to incorporate utilization review into the standing negotiating machinery with sickness funds. As in France, the national contract discusses the subject and creates joint committees to supervise and to authorize contacts with individual doctors. In France, a national joint committee oversees the entire methodology, local joint committees supervise the control doctors' contacts with individual office doctors, and the national joint committee deals with disputes and appeals.[25] In Belgium, the standing joint committee within INAMI oversees utilization review, as well as all other relations between health insurance and doctors.

As in many other respects, the United States is different. It has no general law on health insurance for the entire population. It has no standing negotiating arrangements between payers and medical associations. Utilization review of individual doctors is performed unilaterally and separately by each payer—as by Blue Shield, the private fiscal intermediaries under contract to Medicare, and the government agencies that administer Medicaid. Since the medical profession does not collaborate in any stable arrangement in utilization review and cost containment, the doctors often wrangle with the payers, who then buy peace by backing away.

Methodology. The basic concepts of utilization control are similar everywhere and the methods, now computerized, have become common: all claims forms are read into the computer, statistical profiles are calculated for each procedure for all doctors in the same specialty, and the identical profile is generated for each doctor. Usually separate profiles can be calculated for every procedure in the fee schedule. (The only exception is France, where the claims form bears not the code number for an individual procedure but a key letter for class of procedures (such as K or Z) and a number giving the relative weight for that procedure in the conversion to payment in francs. Therefore, a French reviewer can only identify a doctor who submitted bills for many more weights in general than his peers.)

The strategic job of calculating and initially examining the statistical profiles is in the hands of the recipient of the claims form. In every country except Germany, the computer center and the employees are in the sickness fund— thereby causing great discomfort in the medical association. In Germany, the work is done by the KV—arousing the sickness funds' misgivings about cover-ups.

All data from all payers might be merged if the sickness funds cooperate, as in the Netherlands. The result is a very large data base. However, often the sickness funds are competitors for market share, they conceal their utilization and financial accounts from each other, and they process their claims forms separately. They cooperate in setting rates for doctors and hospitals, but not yet in utilization review.

Particularly troublesome procedures are given special attention. During the early years of utilization review, the prescribing of drugs by general practitioners accelerated and the profiling staffs in many countries were instructed to identify the high prescribers. When radiodiagnostic tests and laboratory tests exploded during the 1970s, profiling staffs identified the doctors who prescribed and performed them, as well as the laboratories that performed them.

Since conclusions are drawn from very large numbers of individual claims forms, the bills must be filled out accurately, collected completely, and read into the system accurately. Medical associations fight off implementation of utilization review for years—as in France and Belgium—by arguing that the data are incomplete and contain too many errors. The sickness funds respond that it is the medical profession's own fault, since it is the doctors who fill out the forms. Special studies of the accuracy of the data and the quality of the sickness funds' data management are often conducted before utilization review is fully implemented.

Criteria for Identifying Deviance. The object is to identify billing that takes money from the sickness funds without clinical justification. The offense could be either:

☐ *Fraud.* The doctor did not give the care but sent a bill to the sickness fund.
☐ *Upcoding.* The doctor gave care but billed for a procedure that is more expensive than his actual treatment.
☐ *Overproduction.* The doctor gave far more tests and treatments than are clinically justified.

The statistical profile system is designed to detect overproduction. If the doctor has given far more tests and treatments than his peers, the computer flags him. The next step requires personal communication to learn whether he is unusually busy or the director of a group.

The profile system cannot detect fraud or upcoding unless the doctor has also submitted a suspiciously large number of claims. Fraud and upcoding occur in a payment system where the provider bills the sickness fund without notifying the patient (*tiers payant*). They are unlikely under a reimbursement system where the doctor first bills the patient (*tiers garant*): here the patient is the sentinel for utilization control. During the 1980s, when utilization review was being phased into Belgian health insurance, INAMI's investigators discovered that some pharmacists, physiotherapists, and home health nurses (who bill under *tiers payant*) were submitting false claims.[26] Lest these practices spread into medicine, the Belgian government in 1986 amended the law to require *tiers garant* and forbid *tiers payant* in medical practice. The medical association agreed, since it preferred that the doctors be monitored by the patients and not by INAMI's auditors.

Communicating with the Deviant Physician. In countries where the sickness funds cooperate among themselves in utilization review, the joint committee (composed of the carriers' control doctors and the medical association) scrutinizes the statistical profiles of office doctors who submit very many or suspiciously expensive bills. It then authorizes one of the control doctors to approach the practitioner. If each sickness fund performs its own utilization review, its control doctor makes the preliminary judgment and the visit himself. This delicate task is presented at first as a request for information and an explanation. The control doctor shows the practitioner how his profile differs from that of his peers generally. (The work of the control doctors is described further in Chapter Seventeen.)

Goals and Sanctions. The control doctor presumes that the practitioner who performs an unusual number of services is inefficient or has an excessively interventionist style of practice, not that he is venal. If the style is not professionally unacceptable, the control doctor's role must be educational rather than punitive. He explains how other doctors practice, agrees to pay all the practitioner's pending claims, and hopes that the physician will become more restrained in the future. The doctor is now aware that he is being monitored and that the rest of the medical profession practices differently.

The control doctor and the sickness funds may privately judge some doctors to be venal overproducers, but they are cautious about saying so openly. Not only are the sickness funds and government powerless to exclude the doctor from insurance practice, but the medical association defends the doctor in the absence of strong evidence, and the atmosphere would be poisoned. To deal with such borderline cases, the sickness funds in many countries now favor expenditure caps over medical practice, like a German *Kopfpauschale*. If an excessive number of bills will create a deficit, then the sickness funds can reduce their unit payments below the levels of the fee schedule. These doctors will then have a financial incentive to reduce their overproduction without punitive intervention. The weakness of a profession-wide cap is that it affects all doctors equally and is not targeted upon the individual overproducers. To protect the majority, the medical association must then identify and caution the deviant members. (Application of expenditures targets and caps to doctors is discussed further in Chapter Seventeen.)

Fraud is a crime under statutory health insurance, since the provider has sworn falsely on the claim form and has taken tax money. Usually the provider must be prosecuted in a court case if the money is to be recovered or his license to practice is jeopardized. More often, the doctor and the sickness funds settle quietly by dropping him from insurance practice permanently or temporarily.

Upcoding is a crime too. But it is difficult to detect—since some care was given—and it is not as blatant as submitting fraudulent bills. Sickness funds and medical associations deplore its practice and hope that it will be restrained by professional ethics.

Quality of Care

Role of the Sickness Funds in Europe. In the past, carriers practiced utilization review only to prevent waste of their money through the venality and inefficiency of providers or the malingering of subscribers. Clinical decisions about appropriate tests and treatments were left to the medical profession and its educational and collegial institutions. The identification of good quality and the correction of poor quality were beyond the capacity of the sickness funds: their many lay employees specialized in finance; their few control doctors were not trained in the new clinical practices of all specialties. Medical associations insisted that sickness funds were limited to financial tasks, that advanced practitioners of medicine alone could evaluate the quality of care, and that the associations themselves could detect and correct poor quality.

The most dangerous malpractice could occur in the specialties practiced in hospitals. The European solution has always been closed medical staffs directed by chiefs of service. The chiefs are supposed to be picked by merit after a long preparation under supervision. The chief in turn teaches and monitors his junior staff, discharging the inadequate performers from hospital careers. The sickness funds and their subscribers are supposed to trust the quality in all hospitals admitted to insurance practice.[27]

Most doctors have worked in independent office practice, not in the structured hospitals. Although medical associations were supposed to monitor and stimulate their quality, like the sickness funds they lacked the resources and political will to cover the entire profession. The office doctors would have resisted intervention by the medical association as strenuously as they resisted control by the sickness funds. Until recently, the office doctors could practice and treat insured patients after minimum medical education, so the quality of care must have been imperfect. But unless a subscriber complains, the insurance carriers have little knowledge of individual office doctors' performance. If the sickness fund's control doctor enjoys good relations with the medical association, he might pass along the complaints and hope that the peer group devises a solution. If subscribers' complaints are common, the control doctor might investigate the practitioner, but any sanctions must be devised in collaboration with the medical association. Generally, the sickness funds still leave judgments about the quality of individual office doctors to the subscribers and the marketplace: if the patient does not like a doctor, he is free to change to another, but no insurance fund can track any resulting decline in a doctor's practice or take action.

Insurance carriers have had almost no instruments to affect the performance of the office doctors generally, except for recommending that dubious procedures be omitted from the fee schedule or priced lower. Even this step required the full cooperation of the medical associations' representatives on the joint negotiating committees that wrote the fee schedules.

The American Situation. The United States has special problems of quality assurance. Nearly all doctors have the right to admit and treat patients in a hospital. Working out of private offices elsewhere in town, large numbers of doctors with varied skills constantly enter and leave the hospital building. (In contrast, European hospitals have small, specialized, and disciplined medical staffs.) Because of weak controls over capital investment, technically advanced programs proliferate across American hospitals. Thus, many hospitals have advanced but underutilized facilities, and many doctors perform these procedures without the high volume necessary to develop expertise. In addition, as in Europe, American office doctors are free and unobserved in their private offices.

American doctors bill patients and all insurance carriers for fees for all their inpatient treatments: almost none are salaried; none route their bills through the hospital organization. In contrast, European hospitals control inpatient quality not only by means of their closed staffs and hierarchical structure but also through their trend toward full-time salaried senior staffs and their administration of much of the billing of fees.

American health insurance has been committed to pay all physicians' bills without questioning the quality of the work. All insurers—Medicare, Blue Shield, and the commercial carriers—have reimbursed any licensed doctor for any procedure, regardless of the treatment's difficulty and the doctor's training. In contrast, most European statutory health insurance systems pay for specialized procedures only when they are performed by specialists fully credentialed in that field.

During the early twentieth century, American teaching hospitals created peer review committees to review surgery. The idea was to keep up the quality of surgical teaching and exclude inept attending physicians. These peer review committees were extended to all hospitals as conditions for accreditation—first by the American College of Surgeons and then by the Joint Commission on the Accreditation of Hospitals. Until 1965, members of these committees were confined to leading members of hospital medical staffs and their mandate was restricted to the quality of hospital clinical practice. They had nothing to do with insurance reimbursement.

Medicare and Medicaid converted these committees into agencies to monitor the quality and costs of care paid for by third parties. At first, the laws merely required that all hospitals receiving Medicare and Medicaid payments be accredited by the Joint Commission. Congress soon discovered, however, that most hospitals lacked effective peer review machinery. In 1972, therefore, Congress set up outside the hospitals Professional Service Review Organizations (PSROs) consisting of local physicians with a professional staff supported by Medicare and Medicaid grants. During the 1980s, these agencies were strengthened in their independence and financial support, renamed Peer Review Organizations (PROs), and given more specific responsibilities over the cost and quality of care.

Apart from their roles in Medicare and Medicaid throughout the country, some PROs have signed contracts to monitor costs and quality for other insurance carriers' hospital claims. But since Medicare, Medicaid, and the other carriers have been preoccupied with containing costs and have been committed to respecting the professional discretion of doctors, these agencies' efforts have been oriented toward costs and their quality review has been defined by cost containment—preventing overutilization of hospital services that would unduly profit hospitals and doctors, preventing underservicing of patients that would enable hospitals to pocket unearned cash, and preventing billing for inappropriate but profitable treatments. Lacking guidelines of good clinical practice—created by the medical profession and promulgated by HCFA—the physicians governing the PSROs and the PROs did not review the clinical choices of their colleagues.[28]

During the 1970s, office doctors in several parts of the American West devised methods of attracting all the business from health insurers by processing all claims of their physician members. The arrangements—first called "foundations" and now called "Independent Practice Associations"—were the office doctors' alternative to HMOs. The insurance company or self-insured employer gives a lump sum to the association, which pays claims according to a fee schedule (much like a German *Kassenärztliche Vereinigung*). The system is highly computerized, since the governing committees warn those with practice profiles beyond the average. The computer output can be profiled by patient, so that each doctor's treatments can be related to each patient's diagnosis. Originated to control costs to insurers, the San Joaquin Medical Foundation during the 1970s experimented with use of the system to evaluate individual doctors' courses of treatment compared to an ideal course. The computer could pick out the doctors who submitted too many claims. The information about quality was used in the association's continuing education rather than to force individual doctors out of practice.

As in all evaluation and influence over quality of care, the early foundations' method was peer review by doctors over doctors. The laymen in the insurance companies were kept at arm's length.[29] The foundations suffered from limitations: most local doctors were hostile and refused to cooperate; guidelines of good practice were not backed up by enough empirical proof or by wide professional agreement. But the early foundations were among the first attempts to combine reimbursement and quality control. Moreover, they were the first attempt to review and regulate quality in office practice as well as in inpatient hospital practice.

Events began to move toward a sophisticated method of guiding quality. America more than ever during the 1970s and 1980s was the country of techno-logical advance, widespread and enthusiastic adoption of expensive new meth-ods, financing of these methods by permissive insurance, and exploding costs. Not only were the newest methods used prematurely, but large aggregate costs resulted from indiscriminate use of established and smaller-scale procedures, such as diagnostic tests.[30] Several clinical researchers documented wide variations throughout the country in the use of expensive methods without apparent clin-ical justification.[31] Medicare and other insurers questioned whether many of these treatments and expenditures were justified. The medical profession was panicked by a great increase in lawsuits over inappropriate and inept use (or omission) of technically advanced methods.

Blue Cross/Blue Shield pioneered in developing criteria and methods for paying for some but not all procedures on the basis of both the cost/benefit ratio and clinical quality. The association's matrix contract signed by the member Plan states that only "medically necessary" services will be reimbursed—the procedures must be essential for learning the diagnosis, appropriate to treat the symptoms and diagnosis of that case, in accordance with standards of good med-ical practice, and safe for that patient. Since 1977, the association has sent infor-mation to all Plans about the clinical value and appropriate use of procedures and tests. The Plan should not pay providers for procedures and tests that are still unproved, that (although established) are doubtful in usefulness, and that cannot succeed through repetition. The "medical necessity" programs can be operated by the Blues because, unlike the commercial insurance companies, they have special relations with the providers at the national level and in the localities. The standards were first created and constantly updated by joint consultations be-tween the national leadership of the Blues and the leaders of the clinical special-ties. Each Plan is supposed to confer with doctors and hospitals that deviate from the guidelines, persuade them to conform to professional norms, and (as a last resort) deny payment.[32] (One does not know the levels of enforcement across the country in this delicate area of independent doctors' clinical judgments.)

Meanwhile, researchers quite independently were discovering wide varia-tions in individual American doctors' practice styles. To reduce this clinically unjustified and possibly dangerous range, they sought methods of identifying and enforcing guidelines for the best course of testing and treatment for each diagnosis. They took advantage of the considerable research being done in the United States and Europe to identify the outcomes of various therapies, so that only effective procedures would be incorporated into practice guidelines. Unlike earlier utilization control and quality review—which examined one doctor's use of a procedure in comparison with his peers' aggregate use of that procedure—practice guidelines were decision trees wherein each result of a test or treatment would lead to a subsequent step. The United States government then invested large funds in research on outcomes and in the development of practice guidelines. Many clinical investigators and medical specialty associations worked on these guidelines. One goal was to operationalize the definition of "appropriate care" and "medically necessary treatment" for reimbursement by Medicare, the Blues, and commercial insurers.[33] But the work might yield other benefits too: if a doctor demonstrates conformity to practice guidelines, he is less likely to be sued for malpractice and can pay lower premiums for his malpractice insurance.

During the 1990s, the principal development center and several Blue Cross/Blue Shield Plans experimented with the method that might be used in health insurance in the future. Many practice guidelines in decision-tree form are stored in the Blues' computer. If the doctor intends an expensive course of tests and treatments for a Blue subscriber or proposes a procedure that is questioned on the Blues' medical necessity list, he must phone the Plan's office. A clinician (usually a nurse-employee), after asking a series of questions, obtains the diagnosis and principal intended procedure. Entering these into the computer brings the appropriate practice guideline onto the computer screen. The clinician asks questions, the doctor provides information about the case, and they agree on an immediate course of testing and treatment consistent with the guideline. (The doctor may phone again at a later stage to gain approval of the later steps.) An approved course of testing and treatment will be reimbursed in full.

This method minimizes unnecessary use of costly tests and treatments and reduces clinically inappropriate care. Thus, insurance would control both costs and quality. The questions for the future are these: Can all doctors—not just a few in a demonstration project—be persuaded (or forced) to follow guidelines administered by private carriers? Will insurers contract selectively only with those who conform? Although the leaders of medical associations helped researchers develop practice guidelines, the rank-and-file practitioners grumbled about "cookbook medicine" and protested at plenary meetings of the associations.

Managed Care. HMOs have been prepaid closed panels that have guaranteed satisfactory care for reasonable costs. Conscientious management and peer cohesion are supposed to have assured both. Subsequent arrangements with limited lists—foundations, IPAs, and PPOs—have been designed to offer insurance companies and subscribers low costs like those promised by HMOs. But they have been oriented to cost containment, not quality assurance. Any community doctor willing to conform to the fee schedule and follow the rules is welcomed to the list, since these enterprises need to widen their appeal to subscribers and must mollify the public's distate for lock-ins to limited lists.

Since each such arrangement is an organization with a name and image, it has needed to protect its reputation by refusing physicians with notorious deficiencies. But it usually has lacked any mechanism to observe and promote the clinical performance of doctors it has already accepted. Since the arrangements have been constructed to process claims within the predicted premiums, supervision has been designed to limit utilization. More thorough care might raise costs rather than limit them. Little evidence has yet been collected. But so far it shows that managed care—although clearly saving money through lower hospitalization—has neither higher nor lower quality than conventional American office practice.[34]

During the 1980s, American health economists argued that greater competition among providers would improve quality as well as lower costs. In order to maximize revenue while offering lower market prices to purchasers, providers would have to become more efficient—and efficiency improves the quality of services. This line of reasoning assumes that the purchasers are also the users and thus personally interested in the quality of care they receive. But the principal purchasers of health insurance are American employers: since their priority is reducing their labor costs, they prefer the cheapest providers. The result can be underservicing and use of less skilled providers.

After many years when recommendations for more competition revolved around lower prices and lower expenditures, a few thinkers began to recommend that competition in the market for physician services should stress quality. Purchasers of insurance (such as employers and individuals) and purchasers of provider services (such as insurance companies and self-insuring employers) should shop for those providers who can offer the best services at reasonable (not necessarily the lowest) prices. This policy can be implemented only after criteria of good care are developed, providers can be rated on outcomes, and comparable information is published about all providers.[35] HCFA took the first steps by releasing mortality rates for all American hospitals,[36] but this was far from publishing outcome measures for all medical groups and individual physicians.

Effects on Utilization and Health

What difference does it make whether the medical profession is organized in one or another form in its relations with health insurance carriers? What differences result from the way doctors are paid? Since these arrangements have great effects on the independence, morale, and incomes of the doctors themselves, the medical profession differs on these characteristics from country to country.

But tracing out the effects on clinical care and patients' health is more difficult. Doctors' clinical performance depends on many aspects of a country in addition to its insurance arrangements—such as the content and discipline of undergraduate and postgraduate medical education, the introduction of new technology and pharmaceuticals, and the style of clinical practice prevalent in the doctor's entire country and in his immediate community.[37] These traits may shape the insurance system rather than be shaped by it. For example, countries with a long tradition of interventionist and procedure-oriented clinical practice (such as Germany and the United States) develop reimbursement by fee-for-service. Countries with a long tradition of clinical restraint, by contrast, develop national health services paying doctors by capitation and salaries (as in Great Britain) or develop conservative statutory health insurance systems paying many doctors by capitation fees (as in Holland).

Another difficulty in attributing effects to organizational and reimbursement variables is the gross nature of the evidence. Whether one is comparing system differences among countries or insurance program differences within countries, the evidence is aggregate statistics about services and spending—statistics collected and organized for purposes other than ours and full of clerical errors. Governments have no need to compare their clinical services with those of other countries, so they do not invest in special data-collection efforts. Even when immense funds are spent on health services research—as in the United States—nearly all goes into secondary macroeconomic analysis of existing data and almost none is spent on interviews asking doctors why they made specific clinical and career decisions. For these reasons, much of the macrostatistical research comparing the effects of insurance and reimbursement arrangements on clinical output—such as the voluminous American comparisons of HMOs and unmanaged care—show only small differences or none at all, even when substantial differences are expected.

Employed and Independent Doctors. Once many countries were a mixture: some doctors worked for clinics owned by sickness funds, others were self-employed contractors, still others were self-employed but lacked insurance contracts. Professional training and professional norms were so weak at that time that medical practice probably differed among the three modes. But, as in the case of all organized arrangements, much depended on how the sickness funds' panels were recruited and managed. Nowadays, office practice has become standardized in nearly all countries: all licensed office doctors are self-employed and are admitted to insurance practice under the same rules. Therefore, variations in clinical practice among countries with statutory health insurance are due to causes other than their administrative relations with insurers. But no data exist to pinpoint these variations and their causes.[38] France is the only country with doctors who still work in health centers owned by sickness funds, primarily the *mutuelles*. Little information has been collected so far comparing the skills and work of these doctors with those in self-employed office practice.[39]

Without a statutory health insurance system that would standardize office doctors' contracts and working conditions, American doctors have a variety of arrangements. The number working in cohesive HMOs—the staff, group, and network models—are few, since their total market share is small. Of all American doctors in patient care (not including hospital residents and fellows):

☐   2.5 percent have full-time affiliations with a closed panel (HMO or IPA).

☐   1.9 percent have part-time contracts, earn more than half their revenue from

HMOs or IPAs, and earn the rest from fee-for-service with conventionally insured patients.

☐ 32.7 percent have part-time affiliations, earn much less than half their revenue from HMOs or IPAs (chiefly the latter), and devote most of their time to conventional fee-for-service practice.[40]

Determined to document the superiority of their preferred practice mode, the United States government and several private foundations have poured money into research comparing HMOs and conventional office practice. Certain results occur consistently: doctors in HMOs hospitalize less often for treatment and diagnostic tests; use their work time more productively; do more testing and preventive care in the office; and have slightly more visits with patients. (There are also occupational differences between doctors in HMOs and those in office practice: the former work shorter hours and earn lower net incomes).[41] Some differences in clinical performance are due to the clear policy and strong management of the HMO; some are due to the financial incentives in the fixed budget whereby the doctors share the savings. But it is hard to identify any other clear effects of the control over doctors by the insurer itself: a complete examination of the voluminous research includes contradictions and weak statistical outcomes; the numbers of doctors being compared with the conventional office practitioners are few and probably atypical; very few doctors under network-model and IPA-model arrangements have a large enough HMO practice to be significantly affected by the HMOs' norms, since the bulk of their practice is conventional.[42]

Among the conventional self-employed doctors, some have special contracts—with insurance companies, with third-party administrators, or with self-insured employers—whereby they agree to follow a fee schedule. The subscriber has the option of going to the in-plan doctor and paying only the listed cost sharing or going to any out-of-plan doctor and paying a substantial uncontrolled balance. (These are "Preferred Provider Organizations," or PPOs.) Many doctors by the 1990s had one or more PPO contracts. These arrangements had little effect on participating physicians' clinical methods and patients' health: they are designed to limit costs by limiting fees and may be very cautious about questioning frequency of utilization and doctors' choice of therapies. Moreover, the PPOs lack significant management offices close to doctors' practice sites. Even when much of a doctor's market share comes from PPOs, he may be involved in so many different PPOs and IPAs that he cannot remember and conform to the norms of any one. Therefore, the much-publicized proliferation of PPOs has had little effect on the total costs of physicians' services or their clinical styles.[43]

Units of Payment. Fee-for-service is associated with more diagnostic tests, more surgery, and more prescribing of drugs than payment by salary.[44] Many other variables in a country's predominant organization of health insurance and physician's reimbursement are associated with method of payment—either reinforcing or reducing the distinctive effects of fee-for-service. When paid by fee-for-service rather than by salary or capitation fees, doctors work longer hours and work at a faster pace. Their contacts with patients in the office are shorter in duration and more numerous.

Fee-for-service and capitation fees are usually associated with self-employed practice in offices and private clinics, although some medical staffs in nonprofit hospitals (as in Holland and Belgium) bill fees. Salary implies employment by an organization, particularly a hospital. In many countries, salary is associated with advanced specialty practice. Therefore, the complete organization of the doctor's practice, not the unit of payment alone, accounts for the clinical results.

Waiting lists for care develop in publicly financed systems (where cost containment eliminates idle capacity and limits acquisition of new technology) and in systems with salaried doctors (who try to spread out their work evenly). Deferring or denying care is rare under statutory insurance (which retains the private insurance philosophy of guaranteeing benefits to those who purchase policies); it is also rare in systems with doctors paid by fee-for-service (whose income increases with treatments and who are not bound to fixed hours).

It is not only national variations in organizations that govern outcomes independently of the theoretical incentives in units of payment. Even if doctors are paid by the same method, national differences in practice style can produce different results. German, French, and American office doctors are paid by fee-for-service, for example, but German doctors practice many short repeat visits whereas the others do not.[45]

Designation of the care-giver and the site depend on the total organization of practice, and not on the reimbursement rules alone. For example, home deliveries of babies are still more common in Holland than in the rest of Europe. The insurance system pays fees to the midwife and GP for normal home delivery in Holland. GPs and obstetricians can collect fees for hospital delivery if the case is complicated, and false diagnoses are common to satisfy patients' preferences for hospital deliveries. The system presumes the role of midwives in home care—not only in insurance reimbursement, but in the stated official preference for home delivery and in the backup in the form of insured services by the Cross Association (the voluntary association that delivers home care). Elsewhere in Europe, insurance might still pay for normal home deliveries by midwives. But clinical policy prefers hospital delivery, medical services and insurance do not back up home deliveries, and the doctors have captured the market.[46]

At times, managers of statutory health insurance systems criticize fee-for-service because of the incentives to overproduce services and perform technically advanced treatments. They must install utilization review machinery and handle disputes with the medical associations. But fee-for-service has administrative advantages over capitation and salary: it generates claims forms that record the work done, while the flat-rate methods do not.

Implications for the United States

Standing Negotiating Machinery. Organizing stable relations with the medical profession is one of the principal tasks in creating statutory health insurance. Structuring and standardizing reimbursement and the rules of practice with all providers are fundamental. Some providers will accept dictation by the health insurance carriers and by government, so long as they are paid. But the medical profession will not, because of its long history and its ideology of self-determination. In every developed country, the doctors consider themselves the exclusive experts in clinical care and patient management. They think that every financing system's responsibility is to provide them with the resources they deem necessary, and they refuse to defer to laymen. If any third-party system tries to dictate to them—as in the first decades of Germany's statutory health insurance and as in America's Medicare and Medicaid—chronic trouble results.

Therefore, every country with statutory health insurance creates standing negotiating machinery between the carriers and the medical associations. Even national health services run by governments that direct other sectors by fiat create some form of negotiation or arbitration between the Ministry of Health and the medical associations. The Americans have been unable to grasp this point. Instead they have managed reimbursement and other relations with doctors by means of unilateral congressional and state legislation, by means of unilateral decisions by insurance companies, or by means of esoteric financial formulas ultimately enacted by legislatures and insurance companies.[47] In opposition, the medical associations have pleaded for complete independence by each doctor in selecting therapies, setting his fees, and billing patients, although this is unrealistic under modern third-party payment.

In the United States, as in every other country, the negotiating machinery would settle rules of practice under long-term contracts, the fee schedule, the conversion factor, utilization review to contain costs, and (if they become feasible) practice guidelines to promote quality. If they share in the management of the health insurance system, the doctors are more willing to cooperate with the rules of practice, with cost controls, and with mandatory assignment (if it is adopted in whole or in part). Health insurance should become less conflict-ridden and less prone to lawsuits. Instead of its present overload due to involvement in all details and all disputes, Congress could enact basic principles and oversee operations.[48]

The futility of America's legislative and politicized methods is evident in quality control as well as in reimbursement. When the PROs were criticized for weak supervision of quality of care, Congress—as usual—tried to remedy the problem by enacting new legislation. In 1986, PROs were instructed to block Medicare payment of poor-quality treatment and to discipline doctors with "gross and flagrant" quality problems. Organized medicine lobbied Congress in protest, individual doctors refused to cooperate with the PROs, and the PROs (consisting of doctors) complained about their new responsibilities. A year later

Congress amended the law: now the PROs were instructed to discipline a doctor only if they could prove that the physician was "unwilling and unable" to change his behavior. On the grounds that the law could not be understood and implemented, the PROs then did nothing. Congress resumed its tinkering with these clauses in the 1990s. Quality control can be administered not by the payer's unilateral dictation but as part of joint negotiating machinery.

Standardization. Many American policy analysts argue for a free competitive market in physicians' services on several grounds. Competition for patients will reward the more efficient and better-quality doctors; the less efficient and lower-quality doctors will be forced to improve, turn to other lines of medical work, or drop out of medical practice. New forms of service delivery, clinical techniques, and financing will be introduced and rewarded. For rhetorical ammunition against government controls and the enactment of statutory health insurance, medical societies also argue for the maximum economic independence and clinical discretion of each individual doctor.

Individualism and vigorous competition once ruled the market in physicians' services, but today the trend is different. Every profession has norms of proper clinical practice, and ethics and the profession's associations define and enforce them.[49] Throughout its history, a principal program of the American Medical Association has been the elimination of unorthodox and unduly innovative therapies, called "quackery." Medical education was formalized early in the twentieth century. Postgraduate and continuing education have been expanded and made obligatory in order to standardize approved techniques and discourage others. As large third-party programs spread—including those, like Blue Shield, created in collaboration with medical societies—doctors must follow rules about allowable therapies, limits, and administrative procedure in order to be paid. Clinical therapies and forms of service delivery are remarkably similar in all developed countries.

Instead of a single all-payers market in physicians' services, the United States now has a mosaic of public and private payers who compete with each other for subscribers, refuse to cooperate with each other in reimbursing doctors and other providers, seek preferential arrangements with doctors and other providers, and try to shift providers' costs and bills onto each other, thereby lightening their own burdens and increasing their competitors'. Advocates of competition argue that this market produces innovations and efficiencies; a standardized all-payers system, they say, would lose them.

One must question whether this is true. Does the American market in physicians' services possess beneficial features that Europe and Canada lack? The most notable innovations that Americans have attributed to their less structured market are:

☐ Group practice and partnerships
☐ Prepaid multispecialty group practice combining both the insurance and the service functions—that is, HMOs

☐ Selective contracting by carriers with those doctors who conform to rules and fee schedules—that is, PPOs

But are these uniquely American inventions and do they operate successfully in the United States?

Group practice and partnerships—several doctors in the same specialty work together or a multispecialty group is formed—both vary from the original model of self-employed solo practice. In reimbursement, the group follows traditional forms of billing patients and third parties. Each doctor may retain his own fees; the group always shares costs of practice and often shares some net revenue. The United States was indeed the first country to use group practice on a large scale. For several decades, medical societies (dominated by solo practitioners) fought groups as unfair forms of competition. But enforcers of antitrust laws defended them against the medical societies. Most American office doctors now belong to groups, and they are a normal form of practice.[50]

Since groups and partnerships bill third parties in the conventional way, they are consistent with decentralized insurance markets (as in the United States), with universal health insurance and all-payers physician reimbursement (as in Europe), and even with national health insurance (as in Great Britain). After a belated start, group practices have spread in Europe: they are now a common strategy in Germany to cover expensive practice costs; most European private clinics are now run as multispecialty groups. They are created by doctors' preference and are neither helped nor hindered by the insurance and reimbursement system.

What about HMOs? As the early pages of this chapter explained, the HMO was not an invention of America's unstructured market. It was created and long survived in Europe, both under private and (in Germany) under statutory health insurance. As noted earlier, provisions in laws and contracts conceded to all licensed doctors the right to treat and bill for any patient. All subscribers could select any doctor, sickness funds could not restrict their subscribers to closed panels, and the closed panels have nearly disappeared.

America still has closed panels, because it does not yet have a universal health insurance law interfering with the lock-in. But the free competitive market has not been the secret of their success. In fact, their success has been small and has depended heavily on nonmarket help by the United States government. Their market share has remained small despite government preferences in laws (such as the requirement that all employer-paid group insurance include an HMO option), subsidies, and much publicity. The free-market choice by patients has favored traditional health insurance and traditional physician service delivery.

HMOs could survive under statutory health insurance in the United States, just as the *mutuelles'* medical groups have survived in France. But the key is an inducement to a sufficient number of patients, such as the group's waiver of cost sharing by patients and balance-billing by doctors. But this requires a statutory health insurance law that retains substantial cost sharing and balance-billing. It requires a regulated rather than a "free" market. The HMOs would merely become conventional multispecialty groups with a special appeal.

As for the third claim to innovation—the PPOs—these arrangements seem remarkable to Americans because private carriers have had so little success in restraining doctors' fees. PPOs are voluntary contracts accomplishing this without government price controls. However, it is not much of an invention. European health insurance carriers—both the sickness funds under statutory health insurance and private health insurance companies—have had such contracts for decades. Any patient may see any doctor privately and pay unregulated fees (with the help of private health insurance). Every country under statutory health insurance now is an all-payer and all-physician PPO.

A serious question is whether the American market today is implementing PPOs rather than merely offering them. Many patients and physicians are listed in PPO arrangements, but the lower cost sharing may be too small for the average patient to forgo his normal doctor in favor of a member of the limited list.[51] Doctors may be involved in so many special arrangements that they may not observe all of them.

Moreover, the less structured American market for physicians' services has many drawbacks lacking in the standardized and simpler arrangements of Europe and Canada:

☐ *Bankruptcies.* The idealized American literature about the benefits of competition omits the harsh fact that risk results in losers as well as winners. The late 1980s were a particularly competitive period when new HMOs and IPAs sought to attract subscribers with low premiums—thereby restraining actuarially required premium increases by established HMOs. Several HMOs and IPAs went bankrupt, leaving their physicians with unpaid claims and leaving their subscribers without insurance.[52]

☐ *A higher retention rate by insurance carriers to cover marketing costs.* Patients must therefore pay out-of-pocket a much larger share of physicians' costs than in any other developed country.

☐ *A larger administrative machinery to manage the market.* An entire layer of "third-party administrators" exists to relate group purchases and providers. Insurance companies must manage their own PPOs directly—a laborious task—or manage relations with stand-alone PPOs operated by laymen or doctors.

☐ *Complications.* Every payer has different rules, and the doctor in theory must understand all. In practice, he cannot and tries to avoid all contact with insurance carriers. He avoids accepting assignment for any of them, when he might do so otherwise and save the patient out-of-pocket cash and trouble. The complexity of the reimbursement system is a principal source of the American medical profession's frustration and generalized hostility toward government and insurance companies.

At present, the American medical profession and its associations have an ideological opposition to statutory health insurance and to all-payer methods of paying doctors. This is the universal posture of medical professions on the eve of enactment. In America, as elsewhere, they are the principal political opposition. But, on close inspection, the present market for American physicians' services has few advantages and many drawbacks. A statutory insurance system with negotiated all-payer reimbursement would be a great improvement. It would involve less government intervention than that experienced by the confused American "private" market at present.

Americans like to think that innovations can be produced only by decentralized markets and private enterprise. That is true in other economic sectors, and it is true in the two industrial markets in health: pharmaceutical drugs and technology. But the two principal innovations in health care finance during the 1980s were supported, tested, and implemented by government:

☐ *The diagnosis-related group (DRG).* This method of paying American hospitals under Medicare was developed by academic researchers under grants from HCFA. It was applied to reimbursement by state government regulation of all hospitals in New Jersey, aided by a demonstration grant from HCFA. It was then evaluated by civil servants in the national government. It was adopted as the Medicare method of paying all hospitals by Act of Congress.

☐ *Global budgeting.* This method of paying all hospitals under all statutory health insurance in France was designed by consultants to the Ministry of Health and tried out in a municipal hospital under demonstration grants from the national Ministry. The consultants were hired as civil servants and tested the method on other municipal hospitals. Then the national government mandated that all sickness funds pay all public and nonprofit hospitals in this manner. The French experience demonstrates how a normally standardized and highly regulated statutory health insurance scheme can innovate and experiment.[53]

Even if statutory health insurance should standardize the reimbursement of doctors in the United States, that result might not differ much from the final outcome of a free competitive market. Health services may be one of the industries where competition eventually produces identical products and competition takes the form of advertisements about images. There could still be much competition among providers for market share and reputation under statutory health insurance. They could, for example, stress the objects that count most: quality of care and pleasing the patient.

Incentives. Physicians are supposed to be professionals performing a public service, not merely businessmen maximizing their own profits. Once, in all countries, they struggled to achieve incomes comparable to those of other educated classes. Third-party payment systems include negotiated decision making that now places the entire medical profession at a very high income level. Striving for high incomes motivates many individual doctors, but it need not be the policy of the collective profession. Economic security and prosperity permit the profession to focus on its other humanitarian and scientific responsibilities.

All other developed countries must devote enormous attention to health care finance, but money alone is not the "magic bullet" of their health policy. In the United States alone, neoclassical economists have been put in charge of health policy analysis and implementation. They have tried to design arrangements whereby pecuniary incentives elicit optimum clinical and organizational response from doctors: patient and doctor would bargain over fees and then choose; the right set of fees would be calculated to elicit appropriate careers and immediate services by doctors; doctors would calculate alternative profits and would then settle on appropriate work sites; doctors would share in the monetary savings from limiting services and choosing the cheapest work sites; patients would be attracted to doctors who would save money; and so on.

The armchair theory does not work in the desired ways in actual practice, as this and other chapters report. If individual doctors are invited to maximize their incomes, they will indeed—by multiplying their procedures, by making up for low surgical volume with increased fees, by converting hospitals into money machines, by ignoring cost controls, and so on. American attempts to counter these tendencies by controls and new financial incentives produce complicated reimbursement, numerous and contradictory regulations, and much dispute.

In contrast to these vain appeals to money alone, the United States needs a style of policy analysis that will understand the complete set of economic and noneconomic incentives appropriate to a profession. Institutions must be designed that appeal to the complete set of incentives—for example, competition can be oriented to rewarding the doctors who practice the highest quality. Such a new style of health policy analysis requires a new generation of health policy analysts.

Notes

1. No systematic history has been written about the financial arrangements between all European mutual assistance funds and doctors. Nor are there any estimates about the proportions of all doctors involved or the shares of income coming from these contracts. Partial descriptions exist in a few sources, such as Jean Bennet, *La mutualité française à travers sept siècles d'histoire* (Paris: Coopérative d'Information et d'Edition Mutualiste, 1975), pp. 129–145; and Brian Abel-Smith, "The Rise and Decline of the Early HMO's: Some International Experiences," *Milbank Quarterly*, vol. 66, no. 4 (1988), pp. 694–719.

2. Frieder Naschold, *Kassenärzte und Krankenversicherungsreform* (Freiburg im Breisgau: Verlag Rombach, 1967), pp. 47–74 passim; and Maximilian

Sauerborn, "Kassenärzterecht in der Entwicklung," *Bundesarbeitsblatt,* no. 3 (April 1953), pp. 205-215.

3. The *mutualist* medical groups and health centers practicing general medicine are concentrated near big cities, particularly Paris and Lyons. France has other types of health centers, owned by municipalities, industries, and other organizations and devoted to special tasks rather than general medicine. The *mutualist* groups and many others are described in Jean Claude Seguy, *Médecine de groupe et centres de santé* (Rennes: Ecole Nationale de la Santé Publique, 1981); Dominique Brasleret, *Les centres de santé mutualiste des bouches du Rhône: Emergence d'une pratique médico-sociale originale* (Rennes: Ecole Nationale de la Santé Publique, 1984); François Steudler, *La médecine de groupe en France* (Paris: ATP INSERM, 1986); and Alain Trehony and others, "Centre de santé et médecine libérale de groupe: Aperçu statistique des pratiques médicales," *Cahiers de sociologie et de demographie médicales,* vol. 22, no. 4 (Oct.-Dec. 1982), pp. 349-366.

4. Monika Steffen, "La cogestion dans les centres de santé," *Journal d'Economie Médicale,* vol. 3, no. 2 (1985), pp. 81-96.

5. This decision was the *Kassenarzt-Entscheidung* of March 1960, discussed in Hans-Jürgen Papier, *Zulassungsbeschränkungen für Ärzte aus verfassungsrechtlicher Sicht* (Cologne: Verband der privaten Krankenversicherung, 1985).

6. The history appears in Naschold, *Kassenärzte und Krankenversicherungsreform* (see note 2, above); and in Marian Döhler, "Historische und gesundheitspolitische Aspekte im Verhältnis zwischen medizinsicher Profession und integrierten Versorgungssystemen in Deutschland," in Heinz Hauser and J. Matthias Graf von der Schulenburg (eds.), *Health Maintenance Organizations—eine Reformkonzeption für die gesetzliche Krankenversicherung in der Bundesrepublik Deutschland* (Stuttgart: Bleicher Verlag, 1987). The Hauser book explains at length why the much-admired idea of HMOs has become unfeasible in Germany and, for the same reasons, in every country with statutory health insurance.

7. The design and operations of the program appear in Hermann Levy, *National Health Insurance: A Critical Study* (Cambridge: Cambridge University Press, 1944); and R. W. Harris, *National Health Insurance in Great Britain 1911-1946* (London: Allen & Unwin, 1946). For the politics of enactment and the difficulties in administering the result see Harry Eckstein, *The English Health Service* (Cambridge, Mass.: Harvard University Press, 1958), pp. 19-29, 123-129.

8. The definition of the GP's role under the National Health Service is described in Almont Lindsey, *Socialized Medicine in England and Wales* (Chapel Hill: University of North Carolina Press, 1962), chaps. 3, 7-9.

9. Margaret C. Klem and Margaret F. McKiever, *Management and Union Health and Medical Programs* (Washington: Public Health Service, U.S. Department of Health, Education, and Welfare, 1953); Raymond Munts, *Bargaining for Health: Labor Unions, Health Insurance, and Medical Care* (Madison: University of Wisconsin Press, 1967), chaps. 1, 12-14; and George Rosen, "Contract or Lodge

Practice and Its Influence on Medical Attitudes to Health Insurance," *American Journal of Public Health,* vol. 67, no. 4 (April 1977), pp. 374-378. Rosen describes the hostility toward panels that has spread throughout the American medical profession.

10. Lawrence D. Brown, *Politics and Health Care Organization: HMO's as Federal Policy* (Washington: Brookings Institution, 1983); and Alma McMillan and others, "Medicare Enrollment in Health Maintenance Organizations," *Health Care Financing Review,* vol. 8, no. 3 (Spring 1987), pp. 87-93.

11. Philip Kissam, "Health Maintenance Organizations and the Role of Antitrust Law," *Duke Law Journal,* no. 2 (May 1978), pp. 487-541.

12. Harold Luft, *Health Maintenance Organizations: Dimensions of Performance,* 2nd ed. (New Brunswick, N.J.: Transaction Books, 1987); Peter D. Fox and LuAnn Heinen, *Determinants of HMO Success* (Ann Arbor: Health Administration Press, 1987); W. Pete Welch, "The New Structure of Individual Practice Associations," *Journal of Health Politics, Policy and Law,* vol. 12, no. 4 (Winter 1987), pp. 723-739; and S. Brian Barger and others, *The PPO Handbook* (Rockville, Md.: Aspen Systems, 1985).

13. "Physician Involvement with PPO's," *SMS Report* (of the American Medical Association), vol. 2, no. 5 (Sept. 1988), pp. 1-2; and David W. Emmons, "Changing Dimensions of Medical Practice Arrangements," *Medical Care Review,* vol. 45, no. 1 (Spring 1985), pp. 117, 127. For the numbers of subscribers covered by contracts with a PPO option see Gregory deLissovoy and others, "Preferred Provider Organizations One Year Later," *Inquiry,* vol. 24 (Summer 1987), pp. 127-135. The enthusiastic estimates of the growth in coverage fail to tell how many subscribers actually used the PPO option.

14. The legislative drafts during the late 1970s are summarized in Judith Feder and others, *Insuring the Nation's Health* (Washington: Urban Institute Press, 1981), especially chap. 5. The American public's refusal to accept lock-ins is evidenced in the many public opinion surveys summarized in Robert J. Blendon, "The Public's View of the Future of Health Care," *Journal of the American Medical Association,* vol. 259, no. 24 (June 24, 1988), p. 3588. These facts have not dampened the conviction of many American health care policy analysts that HMOs should become the normal form of financing and delivery.

15. Eugene Vayda, "Prepaid Group Practice Under Universal Health Insurance in Canada," *Medical Care,* vol. 15, no. 5 (May 1977), pp. 382-389.

16. William A. Glaser, *Health Insurance Bargaining* (New York: Gardner Press and John Wiley, 1978). Individual chapters of that book present details about the principal countries with statutory health insurance: West Germany, France, Holland, Belgium, and Switzerland.

17. Physician Payment Review Commission, *Annual Report to Congress* (Washington: Physician Payment Review Commission, 1990), p. 15; Sharon McIlrath, "Medicare Participators Gain Market Share," *American Medical News,* Sept. 7, 1990, pp. 3, 30; and Shelah Leader, "Medicare's Participating Physician Program" (Washington: American Association of Retired Persons, 1987).

18. Lyle Nelson and others, *Assignment and the Participating Physician Program* (Washington: Physician Payment Review Commission, 1989).

19. The choice between *tiers payant* and *tiers garant* is described in "Les accords du 28 décembre 1984," *M Informations* (of the Alliance Nationale des Mutualités Chrétiennes), no. 117 (Dec. 31, 1984), p. 4; and "Les accords et conventions pour 1986," *M Informations,* no. 122 (Jan. 31, 1986), p. 9. The reforms of 1986 are described in Johan Huybrechs, "L'exécution du plan de Val Duchesse," *M Informations,* no. 124 (Sept. 30, 1986), p. 9.

20. Described in William A. Glaser, *Paying the Doctor* (Baltimore: Johns Hopkins Press, 1970); and Glaser, *Paying the Hospital* (San Francisco: Jossey-Bass, 1987), chap. 11.

21. See Glaser, *Paying the Doctor* (see note 20, above), chap. 6.

22. For the negotiating procedures and the content of the agreements under both NHI and NHS see Glaser, *Health Insurance Bargaining* (see note 16, above). For a detailed summary of the negotiating methods in one country see Bradford L. Kirkman-Liff, "Cost Containment and Physician Payment Methods in the Netherlands," *Inquiry,* vol. 26, no. 4 (Winter 1989), pp. 468–482.

23. Barbara N. Armstrong, *The Health Insurance Doctor: His Role in Great Britain, Denmark and France* (Princeton: Princeton University Press, 1939), pp. 217–219.

24. Described in Gustav Heinemann and others, *Kassenarztrecht,* 4th ed. (Berlin/Wiesbaden: Engel-Verlag, 1975), the section discussing §368f of RVO; and James Hogarth, *The Payment of the General Practitioner* (Oxford: Pergamon Press, 1963), pp. 231–248. Current methods of the KVs are described in the most recent edition of Heinemann; in Marian Döhler, "Regulating the Medical Profession in Germany: The Politics of Efficiency Review" (Berlin: Wissenschaftszentrum, 1987), pp. 11–24; and in the many sources cited by Döhler.

25. For the organization and detailed operations in France see the articles by Antoinette Catrice-Lorey and Jean Marty in *Prospective et santé,* no. 34 (Summer 1985), pp. 67–72, 81–85; and Inspection générale des affaires sociales, *Tutelle et contrôle dans le domaine social: Rapport 1985/1986* (Paris: Ministère des affaires sociales, 1986), pp. 327–357.

26. Thierry Poucet, "Les mutuelles face au scandale," *Actualité-santé* (of GERM), no. 45 (Sept.–Oct. 1982), pp. 32–42.

27. I describe European hospital medical staff structures and their responsibility for quality of care in Glaser, *Paying the Hospital* (see note 20, above), chap. 11.

28. Descriptions of the PROs, a critique of their performance, and a proposal for reform appear in Institute of Medicine, *Medicare: A Strategy for Quality Assurance* (Washington: National Academy Press, 1990).

29. Richard H. Egdahl, "Foundations for Medical Care," *New England Journal of Medicine,* vol. 288, no. 10 (March 8, 1973), pp. 491–498.

30. Thomas W. Moloney and David E. Rogers, "Medical Technology: A

Different View of the Contentious Debate over Costs," *New England Journal of Medicine*, vol. 301, no. 26 (Dec. 27, 1979), pp. 1413–1419.

31. John E. Wennberg and others, special issue on medical practice variations, *Health Affairs*, vol. 3, no. 2 (Summer 1984).

32. Johanna Sonnenfeld, "The Blue Cross and Blue Shield Associations' Medical Necessity Program," *Voluntary Effort Quarterly*, vol. 3, no. 2 (June 1981), pp. 5–8; and *Medical Necessity Program* (Chicago: Blue Cross and Blue Shield Association, frequently updated).

33. Mark R. Chassin, "Standards of Care in Medicine," *Inquiry*, vol. 25 (Winter 1988), pp. 437–453 and sources cited there; Paul Tarin, "A Better Preauthorization Tool or Another Way of Saying 'Cookbook'?", *American Medical News*, April 20, 1990, pp. 13, 16–17; and Ruth E. Brown and others, *Options for Using Practice Guidelines in Reducing the Volume of Medically Unnecessary Services* (Washington: Battelle Human Affairs Research Centers, 1989). The voluminous work on clinical outcomes and its relevance for Medicare are summarized in William L. Roper and others, "Effectiveness in Health Care," *New England Journal of Medicine*, vol. 319, no. 18 (Nov. 3, 1988), pp. 1197–1202.

34. Harold S. Luft, "HMOs and the Quality of Care," *Inquiry*, vol. 25, no. 1 (Spring 1988), pp. 147–156; and Luft, *Health Maintenance Organizations* (see note 12, above), chap. 10.

35. Walter McClure, "Buying Right" (Minneapolis: Center for Policy Studies, 1988); and John K. Iglehart, "Competition and the Pursuit of Quality: A Conversation with Walter McClure," *Health Affairs*, vol. 7, no. 1 (Spring 1988), pp. 79–90.

36. Harry M. Rosen and Barbara A. Green, "The HCFA Excessive Mortality Lists," *Hospital and Health Services Administration*, vol. 32, no. 1 (Feb. 1987), pp. 119–127.

37. Some national practice styles are described in Lynn Payer, *Medicine and Culture: Varieties of Treatment in the United States, England, West Germany and France* (New York: Henry Holt and Company, 1988); and in Tavs Andersen, "Variations in Common Medical Practice: Some Economic Challenges" (Paris: Organisation for Economic Co-Operation and Development, Working Party on Social Policy, 1987).

38. The large and increasingly repetitious comparative publications about European health services describe systems and list expenditures. One can compare total expenditures on physicians' services in all countries with statutory health insurance and national health services. But the publications never describe and compare the detailed clinical services given by doctors and the outcomes for patients. More penetrating comparative data are collected and published about topics other than physicians' services, particularly the consumption of pharmaceutical drugs.

39. These comparisons are to be summarized in a forthcoming book by François Steudler.

40. My calculation from data collected in 1986 by the Socioeconomic Mon-

itoring System, American Medical Association. Related information appears in Emmons, "Changing Dimensions of Medical Practice Arrangements" (see note 13, above), pp. 101–128.

41. Luft, *Health Maintenance Organizations* (see note 12, above), especially chaps. 5–9, 15; and Harold S. Luft, "Economic Incentives and Constraints in Clinical Practice," in Linda H. Aiken and David Mechanic (eds.), *Application of Social Science to Clinical Medicine and Health Policy* (New Brunswick, N.J.: Rutgers University Press, 1986), chap. 23. Luft's book is full of wise cautions about the quality and relevance of the data for inferring the differences between HMO practice and self-employed practice in the United States.

42. An example of the weak effects of HMO rules on doctors with mixed practices is reported in Stephen H. Moore and others, "Does the Primary-Care Gatekeeper Control the Costs of Health Care? Lessons from the SAFECO Experience," *New England Journal of Medicine*, vol. 309, no. 22 (Dec. 1, 1983), pp. 1400–1404.

43. As reported in "Physician Involvement with PPO's" (see note 13, above). In California, the state where managed care is most common, office doctors who signed up reported that fees were indeed lower and volume of patients was higher. Unexpectedly, most experienced declines in their gross revenue and were unhappy to continue. But they had to continue, lest they lose patients. See "Physician Involvement in Contracting Activities," *Socioeconomic Report* (of the California Medical Association), vol. 26, no. 5 (July–Aug. 1986), pp. 1–5.

44. For a more extensive summary of these propositions and the supporting evidence in this section see my other publications: Glaser, *Paying the Doctor* (see note 20, above), especially chaps. 7–10; Glaser, *Paying the Hospital* (see note 20, above), pp. 317–319; and Glaser, "Payment Systems and Their Effects," in Aiken and Mechanic (eds.), *Application of Social Science to Clinical Medicine and Health Policy* (see note 41, above), chap. 22. Another summary of evidence is Simone Sandier, "Health Services Utilization and Physician Income Trends," *Health Care Financing Review*, 1989 Annual Supplement, pp. 36–42.

45. James DeLozier and others, *Ambulatory Care: France, Federal Republic of Germany, and United States, 1981–83*, Vital and Health Statistics, series 5, no. 5 (Washington: National Center for Health Statistics, 1989); and Payer, *Medicine and Culture* (see note 37, above).

46. The Dutch situation is described in Alberto Torres and Michael R. Reich, "The Shift from Home to Institutional Childbirth: A Comparative Study of the United Kingdom and the Netherlands," *International Journal of Health Services*, vol. 19, no. 3 (1989), pp. 405–414. For the more typical reimbursement and practice arrangements in neighboring countries see Steve Sammut, *La maternité* (Paris: CREDES, 1989).

47. For a critique of the American propensities for reimbursement by formula, for government dictation of the formulas and practice conditions, for guerrilla warfare between medical associations and government, and for the overload of executives and legislators, see William A. Glaser, "The Politics of Paying

American Physicians," *Health Affairs,* vol. 8, no. 4 (Fall 1989), pp. 129–146; and Glaser, "Designing Fee Schedules by Formulae, Politics, and Negotiations," *American Journal of Public Health,* vol. 60, no. 7 (July 1990), pp. 804–809.

48. Possible American negotiating arrangements are described in Glaser, *Health Insurance Bargaining* (see note 16, above), chap. 10.

49. Every country with statutory health insurance now experiences a mixture of competition for market share and reputation among individual doctors and standards imposed by the financing systems and by professional organizations. The present German mix is described in Hanfried H. Andersen and J.-Matthias Graf von der Schulenburg, *Konkurrenz und Kollegialität: Arzte im Wettbewerb* (Berlin: Edition Sigma, 1990). Once, in all countries, the competition among office doctors was even more intense.

50. "Changing Medical Practice Arrangements," *SMS Reports* (of the American Medical Association), vol. 2, no. 7 (Nov. 1983).

51. Howard Larkin, "AMA Survey Shows Cost Not Big Factor in Choosing Doctors," *American Medical News,* May 25, 1990, pp. 17–18; and Mike Mitka, "Patients Choose Doctors Based on Reputation, not Price, Study Says," *American Medical News,* Feb. 18, 1991, pp. 13, 14.

52. The weekly business journal *Modern Healthcare* reported the frequent bankruptcies and salvage efforts.

53. I describe the genesis of American DRGs and French global budgeting in Glaser, *Paying the Hospital* (see note 20, above), pp. 58–62, 196–197.

CHAPTER 11

Hospital Care

───────────────── **Summary** ─────────────────

Health insurance carriers pay hospitals for the care of subscribers. Rarely do they own and manage hospitals themselves. Since statutory health insurance is indispensable to the survival and modernization of hospitals, the industry becomes a principal political force for its enactment.

Statutory health insurance is usually committed to cover the operating costs of hospitals—with neither profits nor losses. Because of the complexity of hospital accounts, the rates are usually set by a neutral regulator employed by government. Germany has negotiations between the local associations of sickness funds and each individual hospital. Standard rates are set for all payers, including the privately insured. Usually the carriers pay the hospitals directly; there is virtually no cost sharing by patients.

All-inclusive per diems were long the customary method of paying hospitals. Regulators divided the approved prospective budget by the expected number of patient-days, and every carrier paid the same daily charge. The method had the virtue of simplicity and minimum dispute, but patients' bills did not reflect work, one could not estimate the costs by diagnosis and by treatment, and the hospital had no incentive to reduce length of stay. Private for-profit hospitals added itemized charges to a per diem for housing and nursing care. Private health insurance companies in all countries are accustomed to paying for some services by such charge lists.

Note: This chapter gives highlights of the relationship between hospitals and the health insurance system. Full details and documentation appear in my book *Paying the Hospital* (San Francisco: Jossey-Bass, 1987).

To contain costs and give hospitals incentives toward more efficiency, governments and their regulators have begun to impose a global budget on each hospital. The amounts are still each hospital's unique costs, not an industry-wide average. Annual increases are kept within the fiscal capacity of statutory health insurance. The carriers in France share each hospital's total according to their admissions.

Case payments averaged across the hospital industry and dictated by the payer are peculiar to American Medicare. Reimbursement of American hospitals is complicated because each private insurance carrier follows a different procedure, offers a different price, and requires different cost sharing by patients. The hospital must make up bad debts by shifting costs to the other payers. Hospital reimbursement is a chief source of administrative costs and disputes in American health care.

Capital is usually paid for by government grants or by special revolving funds, not by health insurance. Where hospitals can borrow and amortize the debt under the operating costs charged to the health insurance carriers—as in Holland and the United States—hospital managers are independent, public planning is weak, and hospital costs grow rapidly.

The sickness funds under statutory health insurance have difficulty blocking unnecessary admissions and length of stay. They lack the staff to monitor all cases, and the attending physicians insist on exercising professional judgment. Under "managed-care" arrangements, American insurers try to prevent unnecessary admissions and excessive stays. Insurers welcome new methods of reimbursement—such as global budgets in Europe and diagnosis-related groups in the United States—because they motivate hospitals to reduce overtreatment and costs.

Relations Between Sickness Funds and Hospitals

Ownership. Hospitals originated as charitable programs of churches and religious associations. When surgery and obstetrics became safer and more successful in organized settings, some physicians set up small hospitals ("private clinics") for the middle classes. Usually guilds and mutual aid associations did not need to create and manage hospitals, since their members were treated at home, at the nonprofit hospitals, or at the private clinics.

In a few countries where the hospitals had been few, underfunded, and primitive under charitable fundraising, the mutual assistance funds had to find satisfactory facilities for their subscribers. Or perhaps the country was newly settled and without social programs by churches and governments. Thus, a few sickness funds used extra cash to develop hospitals, primarily for their own members. Several examples survive today, such as the hospitals owned by the *Kupat Holim* of *Histadrut,* the labor federation of Israel. They are among the largest and best in Israel, and they are an important key to *Histadrut*'s marketing appeal.[1]

Like Israel, Spain for several decades had closed-panel statutory health insurance (the *Seguro Obligatorio d'Enfermedad,* or SOE) that employed its own doctors and built its own hospitals.[2] SOE thereby could offer better care than that in the church-owned and public hospitals. The Spanish national government for years struggled with SOE—an autonomous public corporation—to serve the entire population by allowing non-SOE subscribers to enter as paying patients. The government finally settled the controversy during the 1980s by terminating the incomplete statutory health insurance, substituting a universal national health service, and nationalizing all of SOE's hospitals. They still have the reputation as the best, and the privately insured prefer them to the private clinics.

A few European mutual assistance funds with large memberships and with large treasuries from subscription fees used extra money to construct and staff facilities. Besides the health centers described in the last chapter, a few French *mutuelles* during the twentieth century built acute-care hospitals. More often, they built facilities that were cheaper and simpler to operate than hospitals and did not duplicate the services already available from nonprofit owners and the private clinics, such as nursing homes and rehabilitation centers. The *mutuelles'* acute-care hospitals are open to their members and to any other insured patients; cost sharing is reduced or eliminated for the *mutuelles'* members.

In order to finance and fill a hospital, the *mutuelle* must be large and nationwide. The principal such owner is the *mutuelle* for French schoolteachers (MGEN). It has a few acute-care hospitals, some specialized hospitals (particularly in mental health), some centers for convalescence, and some nursing homes. Most have fewer than one hundred beds, much smaller than the nearby public acute-care hospitals.[3]

During the 1980s, several investor-owned hospital chains in the United States—Humana, the Hospital Corporation of America, and American Medical International—created their own health insurance. Instead of a carrier creating its own hospitals, the relationship was reversed. The companies thought they could fill their beds and attract more business to their affiliated medical groups.[4] These efforts were later abandoned. Not enough employers were willing to steer their workers into arrangements designed to help for-profit chains; the workers preferred traditional insurance and the employers preferred self-financing with strong controls. Nonparticipating doctors in the community resented competition from the closed financing networks and retaliated by reduced referrals to the for-profit hospitals—thereby aggravating problems that the new insurance methods were supposed to alleviate. Managing insurance strained the financial and administrative capacities of the hospital chains at a time of recession.

Third-Party Payment. Since sickness funds lack the resources and expertise to build, staff, and manage large modern hospitals, they press the hospital owners and government to modernize the existing nonprofit and municipal hospitals. The carriers are satisfied merely to pay their members' costs. Physicians press for similar recognition of their private clinics by the sickness funds.

Whether all hospitals are treated alike under the payment system—private nonprofit, municipal, and private for-profit—depends on the policies of the sickness funds and government. In Germany, for example, the sickness funds pay all hospitals by the same procedures. Since the nonprofit hospitals are not allowed to include profits in the prospective budgets that are the basis for the rates, the doctors' private clinics are not allowed to earn a profit either. The French sickness funds and government treat the hospitals quite differently. Rate regulators screen the prospective budgets of the municipal and private nonprofit hospitals and allow full reimbursement of all reasonable operating and capital costs. But the private clinics must negotiate per diem rates directly with the sickness funds, who are often very strict. Reversing the French situation, American Medicare in the past was more generous to the proprietary hospitals by allowing inclusion of a "return on equity" in their operating costs and per diem payments. Medicare's DRG payment method during the mid- and late 1980s eliminated the extra payment for the private clinics. Extra payments went to the nonprofit and municipal hospitals in the form of special supplements to the establishments with the more stressful work loads.

While doctors are often leery of direct contact with sickness funds, hospitals welcome it. The doctors prize professional and individual autonomy, but the hospitals are organizations ruled by laymen. Medical associations often oppose the enactment of statutory health insurance, while hospitals usually welcome it as a cure for their deficits and a guarantee of steadily higher revenue as utilization and costs rise. The doctors imagine that they can survive without statutory health insurance, but the hospital owners and managers know they cannot. The doctors submit many small bills to patients and prefer to collect the fees directly. The hospitals submit fewer and much larger bills, need prompt payment, prefer to avoid the delayed and incomplete payments by patients, and prefer to bill the third parties. In some countries, the doctors limit the sickness funds to the reimbursement of patients (*tiers garant*), but in every country the hospitals bill the carriers for the full amount (*tiers payant*).

Reimbursement. Indirect payment is used only in exceptional conditions. If a patient comes from a foreign country that lacks a social security reciprocity treaty with the host country, the European hospital often asks the patient for a substantial deposit at the start of hospitalization and for any unpaid balance at the end. The patient then seeks reimbursement from his carrier after returning home. This method is common in countries with many tourists and temporary migrant workers after a history of bad debts, such as Switzerland.

In a few countries, the law guarantees free choice of doctor by the patient and free entry into insurance practice by the doctor, but his private clinic does not meet the minimum quality standards for full reimbursement under the insurance system. An example is Germany, where every province has a hospital plan and approval under the plan is essential for the hospital's right to receive full direct payment by the sickness fund. In such a case, the patient's doctor can bill the KV for his full fees, but his private clinic cannot bill the sickness fund directly for its hospitalization costs. Competition among the sickness funds to please subscribers inhibits carriers from refusing all coverage. Thus, the patient pays the private clinic and gets partial reimbursement from the carrier. Political pressures from doctors and patients usually prevent the German provincial governments from excluding too many private clinics from the hospital plans.

Units of Payment

Per Diems. The daily charge has been the most common unit in paying the hospital for each inpatient's stay.[5] It has been used for over a century by most payers in almost all countries. The hospital's prospective budget for operating expenses is divided by the expected number of patient-days to derive the per diem. It is an average across all clinical services and all patients and does not accurately describe the particular costs of each patient. Billing is simple: the hospital tells each sickness fund the dates of admission and discharge for each subscriber, it counts the total number of patient-days for the week, and the sickness fund pays the multiple of days times that hospital's unique daily rate.

The per diem has long been criticized for failing to describe individual patients' costs and for giving hospitals an incentive to prolong stays. Nonetheless, carriers have found advantages in the per diem: they do not have to monitor each patient's detailed bill and can pay the hospital with minimum administrative effort.

Charge List. Just as physicians bill patients and sickness funds by itemized fee-for-service, their private clinics write a list of charges for separate hospital services. The per diem covers only nursing, food, and overhead: separate charges are calculated for tests, pharmaceuticals, use of the operating theater, physicians' fees, and amenities. The private clinics usually charge the more affluent privately insured patients according to the list rather than by an all-inclusive per diem.

For the social insurance carriers, billing by charges has the advantage of specifying exactly what services were rendered to each patient. But sickness funds do not like itemized charge lists because they do not set them: the hospital management fixes the amounts and earns profits over the costs that the sickness funds agree to cover. The German sickness funds refuse to pay charges and insist that the private clinics follow the same procedure as the nonprofit, municipal, and provincial hospital: the clinic managers submit a verified cost report and negotiate an all-inclusive daily rate that allows no profits. French law does not give the sickness funds and government the same power: the sickness funds must pay the private clinics' itemized charges, but they negotiate low annual increases in accordance with guidelines from the national government, and profits are minimized.

Every American hospital generates a list of charges for every patient, and certain items (particularly diagnostic tests and pharmaceuticals) contain substantial markups. As in other countries, the programs depending on Social Security payroll taxes and general revenue (Medicare and Medicaid) refuse to pay the charges dictated by the hospitals. Once they paid all-inclusive cost-based per diems; now they pay diagnosis-related groups. Likewise, in half the states where it has sufficient market power and support from state legislation, Blue Cross has insisted that hospitals negotiate an all-inclusive per diem calculated from cost reports. Otherwise American hospitals bill all the privately insured and the remaining Blue Cross subscribers according to their charge lists. This becomes the principal source of extra cash for the nonprofit and proprietary hospitals.[6]

Global Budgets. As the basis for calculating per diems or other payment units, hospitals have always prepared budgets of all operating costs expected during the next year. A trend in several countries is to make the approved budget the unit of payment. After the government rate regulator and the sickness funds examine it and accept the estimates of clinical work load and costs, the sickness funds pay the annual total in installments. Each hospital has a unique amount reflecting its costs. If there are several sickness funds, as in France, the hospital's global budget is collected from them according to their shares in total admissions.

Originated in countries where the Ministry of Health pays each hospital from general revenue, global budgeting has been welcomed by sickness funds and governments under statutory health insurance as the most effective instrument of cost containment. Hospitals cannot exceed the financial capacities of the system by multiplying patient-days (to earn more per diems) or by multiplying procedures (under charge lists). At first hospital managers welcome the reduction in reporting and in detailed monitoring by governments and sickness funds, but they soon fear financial squeezes in the annual totals. The sickness funds seek some new mechanism to learn whether their subscribers are being underserviced, since they no longer receive detailed bills about individual patients.

Case Payments. Statutory health insurance aims to cover the costs of caring for each patient and no more. Global budgets and per diems are calculated after detailed scrutiny of each hospital's annual operating costs. Economists and insurance actuaries have long searched for more refined methods of calculating and covering the costs of each patient in each hospital. But hospital accounts have always been kept by function (wages, heat, depreciation, and so on) or by department (surgery, medicine, pediatrics, and so on). Thus, hospital accounts have lacked the linkage with clinical diagnoses of individuals necessary to estimate the resource costs of each type of case.

Disillusioned by a method of per diems calculated from permissive cost estimates, Americans adopted a case payment method for all third parties in several states (New Jersey, Maryland, and New York) and in the national Medicare program. Diagnosis-related groups are created by computer for types of patients with similar clinical resource uses. In the state programs, the third party pays the hospital for each patient; the DRG rate blends costs in treating that case in that hospital and in all hospitals in that state. The calculations are performed by the state's rate regulators. (Medicare started with blends but now pays average national rates weighted for regional labor costs.)

The DRG payment method has been difficult to implement. It is supposed to cluster diagnoses with similar costs, and it is supposed to be weighted according to variations among costs. But reliable data have never been collected about costs by diagnosis. Therefore, calculations use imperfect surrogates of costs (such as length of stay) and other estimates. Ideally, a payment system should be simple so that payers, hospitals, government monitors, and the public can understand it. But Americans are constantly tinkering with formulas in an incessant but vain search for optimum incentives and political equity. Within only a few years, the Medicare calculations had changed from a simple plan to incomprehensible practice.[7]

There is further complication: while several other payers—notably some Blue Cross Plans and Medicaid—adopted DRGs as units of payment, their calculations differed from Medicare's and from each other's. All followed the computer clustering program that converted detailed diagnoses into the 476 basic DRGs. But all added new diagnoses appropriate to younger patients (such as neonates, substance abuse, and AIDS)—which then changed the entire structure. Even when they appear to use the same DRGs, Medicare, Blue Cross, and Medicaid give them different weights and pay different prices.

Methods of Deciding Rates

Hospital costs absorb half the revenue of statutory health insurance in nearly every country. The great problems of cost escalation that troubled all health insurance systems during the 1970s were due primarily to the modernization and expansion of hospitals. Cost containment efforts during the 1980s were directed largely at controlling the annual increases in the operating and capital costs of hospitals.

Setting rates for hospitals differs from setting physicians' fees.[8] The sickness funds and their governments aim to cover the hospitals' legitimate costs exactly, without giving surpluses or causing deficits. But the carriers know they will pay the doctors more than their practice costs—an "honorarium" is in each fee, generating each doctor's net income. The sickness funds try to drive a bargain so that the doctors' net incomes are not excessive.

Negotiation. Bilateral bargaining betweeen sickness funds and the medical association is the standard method of deciding physicians' fees. National associations of sickness funds maintain research staffs that produce reports about the costs of medical practice and the net incomes of doctors. Ultimately the decisions result from power bargaining between the two sides and do not depend completely on the accuracy of the cost data.

Negotiating rates with hospitals is a nearly impossible task for sickness funds. Since each hospital's unique costs are supposed to be the basis for its rates, the carriers cannot negotiate approximate average rates for the entire industry, as they do with the doctors. The sickness funds lack the large staffs, conversant with hospital management and hospital accounting, to estimate the probable utilization and appropriate resources for each establishment. The hospitals negotiate adversarially, kite their prospective budgets, and do not allow the sickness funds access to their books.

Negotiation is the predominant method of deciding hospital rates only in Germany. The country prefers negotiations between rival groups throughout the economy and a minimum of regulatory intervention by civil servants. The ground rules about allowable hospital costs to be covered by the daily rates are specified in the law about hospital finance and health insurance. The law requires the hospital to fill out a prospective budget and retrospective cost report accurately and then submit it to the bargaining committee of sickness funds. The policy forum that represents all payers and providers—the *Konzertierte Aktion*— every year studies the fiscal capacity of health insurance and recommends target rate increases for each health care sector, including hospitals. A bargaining meeting in each locality—consisting of the particular hospital and a committee drawn from the sickness funds—negotiates the hospital's daily rates every year and usually decides close to the KA guidelines. If the two sides deadlock, they create a special joint committee to arbitrate.

The law and guidelines govern the adequacy of the rates. Before 1972, the sickness funds were preoccupied with appeasing the doctors and gave little money to the hospitals. These establishments were underfunded in staffing and in capital. The hospital reform law of 1972 required the sickness funds to provide enough money for staffing and supplies and made capital grants the responsibility of the provincial and national governments. By a legislative transfer of short-term invalidity payments from the carriers to the employers, the sickness funds were given greater financial capacity to pay the hospitals.

Several other countries have special negotiating arrangements for certain hospital rates. Whether the outcomes are generous or stingy depends on the policies of government and those of the sickness funds. Government guidelines in France used to instruct local sickness funds to grant generous charge schedules to the private clinics, for example, but government and the sickness funds became much stricter during the 1970s and 1980s. America's Blue Cross Plans used to grant generous annual increases in hospital per diems in the states where they negotiated hospital rates. (The Plans retrieved the money by persuading the employer groups and state insurance commissioners to raise the insurance rates.) But Blue Cross became much stricter with the hospitals during the 1970s (when state insurance commissioners made rigorous hospital bargaining a condition for premium increases in individual and family policies) and during the 1980s (when employer groups insisted on stabilization of their health care fringe benefits).

Rate Regulation. The usual method under large-scale health insurance is screening of hospital budgets and setting of rates by a civil servant. The official is a disinterested neutral carrying out pertinent laws and protecting the interests of both hospitals and the health insurance taxpayers. Government employs and provides administrative support for enough specialists in hospital finance to examine all prospective budgets and cost reports for all establishments throughout the country every year. In case of questions, the regulators have the authority to visit the hospital, interview executives, and examine the books.

Until the cost containment reforms of the 1980s, the regulators (in France, Holland, several American states, and elsewhere) made the decisions without participation by the sickness funds. Now procedures have been expanded, since the insurance carrier staffs in particular localities can provide insights into the individual hospital unknown to the busy desk-bound civil servants. The sickness funds are clearly interested parties, since it is they who will pay the rates. The hospitals in several countries now are expected to send their prospective budgets to the local offices of the sickness funds as well as to the regulatory agency. The sickness fund may then send a memo to the regulators, if the fund's managers think utilization has been predicted too high or if the lines in the budget (particularly the numbers of employees) seem excessive.

Payer Dictation. Social insurance funds cannot dictate what they will pay for patient care. Since the health insurance law or hospital finance law guarantees that the carriers must cover the hospitals' costs, the rates must be set either by a neutral civil servant or by bilateral negotiation.

Under some private insurance contracts, such as those in the United States, the carrier promises to pay a fixed amount. But the agreement is made with the subscriber, not with the hospital. The hospital is left free to charge the subscriber whatever it wishes—equal to or higher than the indemnity payment. The American hospital every day has so many patients covered by different commercial insurance arrangements that it cannot keep track of their indemnity benefits. So it presents its bill to the patient upon discharge for payment in full; or it bills the insurance company, receives partial payment of the total, and then bills the patient for the rest. Each hospital must maintain a considerable collection apparatus,[9] a department nearly obsolete in other countries. One result is that American patients pay out-of-pocket nearly 10 percent of all inpatient hospital operating revenue—the highest of any developed country.[10] Another result is a considerable amount of uncollected bills—perhaps as much as 5 percent of the total liability of those with third-party coverage.

Payer dictation of the *hospital's* receipts occurs not under insurance but under government grants of global budgets. Examples are Great Britain, Canada, and Sweden. Money for the operating costs of all hospitals—both private nonprofit and governmentally owned—is a part of the Ministry of Health's annual budget. The Ministry must live within its limits and distributes the appropriation among the hospitals, each with individual limits.

America's Medicare has been a government-managed insurance program that also appears to pay hospitals by governmentally dictated rates. Until the mid-1980s, the law specified the allowable costs in each hospital's budget and paid the resulting per diem. The payer's authority, however, was exercised permissively: the law required Medicare to cover many costs that the hospital could raise at its discretion, the hospital often substituted new operating budgets during the year, and the per diems were frequently increased.

Medicare's DRG payment system was supposed to impose true prospectivity and budgetary discipline. The Congress and the Health Care Financing Administration would calculate the cost base and the formulas; hospitals would work within the revenue. Utilization control would prevent extra billing, such as excessive numbers of outlier days. The method was phased in generously during the mid-1980s but later became stricter. The hospital industry evaded the controls by moving much of its Medicare work into outpatient departments (paid for by permissive cost pass-through methods). The hospital industry barraged Congress with pressures to ease the inpatient DRG limits. The system proved not to be simple governmental dictation in practice, like the direct power over hospital budgets exercised by Canadian provinces. Instead it involved laborious and contentious political log-rolling in a responsive Congress—limited only by the fiscal capacity of the Hospital Insurance Trust Fund.

Hospital Dictation. Every hospital manager would like to charge whatever he thinks he needs. He can succeed when he faces customers with sufficient funds and weak bargaining power, such as individual patients. But the manager cannot dictate rates to third-party payers: the sickness funds must operate within the limits of payroll taxes enacted by Parliament; private insurers must operate within the limits of premiums regulated by government; all third parties must distribute their limited revenue among other providers. Thus, hospital charges are limited by rate regulators or by collective bargaining with the payers.

Hospitals never can persuade any commercial insurance company to cover potentially unlimited charges in full. If the insurance company makes a paid-in-full promise to its subscribers—even if the premiums are very high and the subscribers are rich—the company may discuss the rates with each hospital, either by phone or by mail. More often, the private insurance companies in the United States and Europe guarantee only cash indemnity payments that the subscriber can assign to the hospital. The patient must pay any extra amounts to the hospital out-of-pocket. Knowing that the patient must pay, the hospital may restrain its rates. A very rich person, of course, is free to patronize a very expensive private clinic and pay more than his insurance coverage.

In the United States, one must distinguish between the charges officially posted by the hospital and the charges actually collected. In order to get business in a competitive market, some hospitals agree to discounts. This practice is common among the several dozen Blue Cross Plans that pay charges rather than per diems. Discounts may be offered for the business of very large HMOs. Discounts are sought by self-insured employer groups (who press hospitals directly or through third-party administrators) and by commercial insurance carriers (who offer PPO options to subscribers in the hope that the patients will go to doctors who observe fee schedules and to hospitals that offer discounts).

In actual practice, an insurance carrier must have a large market share in order to exact discounts from a hospital. Usually Blue Cross alone is significant; occasionally a managed-care firm with several employer group accounts (such as the CIGNA Corporation) has enough market share to gain bargaining power. Most insurers have too few patients in that hospital, however, and the carriers refuse to join in collective bargaining. HMOs and PPOs save hospitalization costs by minimizing admissions, thereby reducing their leverage in the inpatient market. Their savings do not come from lower charges.[11] Trying to make up shortfalls that they blame on Medicare, American hospitals are increasingly reluctant to give discounts to anyone. But if it does take HMO or PPO business, a hospital gains administrative advantages: prompt and direct payment (*tiers payant*) and a more predictable cash flow.

Capital. Whether capital is included in operating costs and whether it is paid for by health insurance carriers are arrangements that have evolved over time and now differ among countries.[12] In the past, owners of nonprofit and governmental hospitals raised charitable donations and tax revenues for both operating and capital costs. When mutual assistance funds and governments began to pay per diems, it was assumed that owners and governments would continue to pay for building construction, building maintenance, and durable equipment. As modern cost accounting developed during the twentieth century, it included "depreciation" and purchase of disposable materials, and hospital managers calculated them in the per diems charged to carriers. Construction and new equipment became more expensive and outstripped charitable donations and government grants, and managers of private clinics and nonprofit hospitals tried to include them in operating costs chargeable to third parties.

Disposable equipment and supplies are included in operating budgets in all countries, and they are covered by health insurance carriers. If the prospective budget includes a "depreciation" line, some or all of it is used for small equipment. All countries with government-financed health services—such as Britain, Canada, and Sweden—pay for construction and heavy equipment through public grants to nonprofit hospitals (as in Canada) as well as to the publicly owned. Countries with health insurance have evolved in different directions:

☐ *Government grants.* In Germany, hospitals receive government grants; other operating costs are covered by the sickness funds. The grants are made pursuant to provincial plans. The sickness funds have sought to participate in planning decisions but have not succeeded.

☐ *Loans from revolving funds.* In France, such funds are maintained by the government and the sickness funds. Amortization is an operating cost payable by the carriers. The sickness funds' opinion is sought when the regulators approve the hospital's prospective operating cost. But planning is primarily the function of government.

☐ *Borrowing on the capital market.* Hospitals may borrow money, include debt service in the operating budgets, and retrieve all costs from the sickness funds. Examples are the statutory health insurance systems of Holland and the United States (that is, Medicare) and America's private health insurance system. Decisions about new construction and new equipment are made entirely by hospital managers. Approvals are obtained from lenders and not from planners. Insurance carriers have no voice in capital decisions.

☐ *Mixed methods.* Some hospitals rely on government grants, but private clinics must borrow and amortize the loans under operating revenue charged to the insurance carriers. An example is Switzerland.

Unless government owns and finances hospitals—as under a national health service—the planning of hospital services is weak. If it exists, it is a task of government and the health insurance carriers have little place. The sickness funds can only influence the operating budgets and utilization of individual hospitals one by one. They cannot shape the system as a whole.

Utilization Control

Sickness funds have long had machinery to prevent unnecessary admissions and prolonged stays.[13] The goals have been to prevent waste and venal overutilization by hospitals and doctors. But the controls have been weak in practice, since they depend on the control doctors employed by the sickness funds. Both in Europe and the United States, the control doctors and the sickness funds defer to the patient's attending physician: he is supposed to understand the patient's condition best, he has been selected by the patient, and his clinical credentials usually surpass those of the control doctor. The control doctors are too few and too busy; most of their time is devoted to certifying persons for disability cash benefits.

Admissions. In theory, the decision to hospitalize in France, Holland, and several other countries is not made by the attending specialist himself. He recommends to the sickness fund's control doctor that a patient be hospitalized, and the control doctor orders the hospitalization.[14] But the system never works this way. The attending specialist and patient always consider admission to be urgent, the patient is admitted before the busy control doctor can study the papers, and the attending specialist can always give clinically plausible reasons for hospitalization. Since the control doctor shrinks from ordering the sickness fund to refuse coverage, he approves automatically and (usually) retroactively.

To eliminate incentives for excessive lengths of stay, some countries have abandoned per diem units of payment in favor of global budgets and other flat rates. While case payments (DRGs and the like) induce a hospital to conserve money by reducing the length of stay, they reward the hospital for more admissions of profitable diagnoses and fewer admissions of diagnoses that it can treat less profitably. But such a configuration of admissions may contradict the clinical needs of the hospital's catchment area. So the law that adopted DRGs for American Medicare also created one Peer Review Organization (PRO) in each area to monitor hospitals—primarily to prevent unnecessary admissions of profitable cases. Governed by local physicians and supported by a professional staff, the autonomous PRO is Medicare's counterpart to a control doctor employed by the third party. Like the control doctors, the American PROs have been overloaded with many tasks, have varied in performance across the country, have not challenged attending doctors often, and have not found substantial numbers of unnecessary admissions and premature discharges. Their existence may have a beneficial "sentinel effect," however, reminding hospitals and doctors to be careful.[15] The Medicare payment system itself—with its low annual rate increase—has persuaded hospital managers to avoid unnecessary inpatient admissions and to substitute ambulatory care, lest the hospital risk losses from the inpatient DRG payment.

American private insurers have strengthened their vigilance over unnecessary admissions that would raise their costs. The Blue Cross Plans, created by the hospital industry, once deferred to the judgments of doctors and hospital managers with respect to admissions. The payment system had incentives to hospitalize: Blue Shield paid for physicians' services inside but rarely outside the hospital. Blue Cross often paid for several short stays to test and treat the same case. Hospital costs and Blue Cross rates rose rapidly during the 1970s. State insurance commissioners (as in Pennsylvania) insisted that Blue Cross bargain more strictly with hospitals as a condition for increased rates for family policies. Commercial insurance companies offered to cover group hospitalization contracts for less money than Blue Cross. Blue Cross and Blue Shield then redesigned their financial incentives, covering physicians' fees in hospital outpatient work and in private offices. Blue Cross Plans (starting in New York) pressed hospitals to expand their capacity to perform same-day surgery, other care in an ambulatory mode, and convalescence at home. Many Plans offered to pay for second surgical opinions.[16]

The commercial insurers in the United States, by contrast, for many years depended on the price-sensitive consumer to judge the necessity of hospitalization: the carriers paid fixed daily amounts; the subscriber paid the rest out-of-pocket. In the competition for group hospitalization contracts and family policies, the commercial carriers had to match the Blues' paid-in-full hospital service benefits but also had to charge the subscribers less. The commercial insurers could not easily control hospitals' admissions and charges. Each was oriented to selling policies to employers and individuals, collecting premiums, and paying cash benefits. Each operated out of national headquarters; unlike Blue Cross, it lacked regional benefit offices that could confer with hospitals. For a while during the 1970s, the Health Insurance Association of America advocated state regulation of hospital rates, but this position contradicted the carriers' conservative competitive ideology and succumbed to the nationwide trend to deregulate the economy.

A free-market solution arose during the 1980s. Entrepreneurs offered "managed-care" arrangements to insurance companies and to self-insured employers. In return for a fee, these preferred provider organizations (PPOs) and third-party administrators (TPAs) locate hospitals and office doctors who treat the carrier's subscribers for fees lower than their normal rates. Some PPOs and TPAs screen the carrier's claims in order to steer tests and treatments into ambulatory (rather than inpatient) modes and to reduce stays. A few large carriers have created their own managed-care departments and take advantage of modern computerization and telecommunication to monitor and negotiate with hospitals throughout the country.[17] Although these arrangements are much discussed by Americans, it is a mystery how they operate in practice.

Health maintenance organizations are a different matter. These arrangements control both the working environment and the referral decisions of their physicians. Unnecessary hospitalization reduces the revenue available from the subscribers' fixed capitation payment. "Staff-model" and "group-model" HMOs have managers who screen hospital referrals. "Staff," "group," and "network" models build up the participating doctors' health centers and offices so that most tests and many treatments can be performed there. As a result, HMOs have much lower hospitalization rates than conventional insurance—particularly for less serious short-stay cases.[18] But such disciplined HMOs enroll barely 7 percent of the American population and affect few hospital markets.

Past European hospital reimbursement systems had limited authority to affect admissions. The rate regulators who approved the prospective budgets of hospitals scrutinized the hospitals' predicted number of patient-days but had little evidence to challenge them. They had no authority to order substantial reductions in the predictions of admissions or patient-days. Paid by per diems, hospitals had no incentive to reduce volume. Europe had more admissions and longer stays than Britain and North America.

The payment reforms in France and Holland during the 1980s—mentioned earlier in this chapter—introduced the sickness funds as reviewers of utilization. The government rate regulators were specialists in finance, they had insufficient understanding of each hospital's patient management, and they were too busy to investigate thoroughly. Thus, at the start of each year's cycle in rate setting, the local office of the principal sickness fund gets the hospital's prospective budget, examines the predictions about admissions and stays, and negotiates with the hospital. If the sickness fund reports to the regulator that the predicted admissions, stays, and budget are excessive, the regulator can enforce cuts.

Length of Stay. The control doctors employed by European sickness funds have more leverage over excessive stays than over initial admissions. The hospitals in several countries must renew the guarantees provided by the sickness funds upon admission. As the twentieth day approaches for a patient in a French hospital, for example, the establishment must notify the sickness fund of any intent to keep the patient longer; and the extension must be supported by the service chief's explanation. The German control doctor reviews the records of a hospital whenever he visits one, asks for justification of long stays, and may press for discharge.

The per diem provides financial incentives to keep beds full and to profit from the late stages of a prolonged stay. A reason for the adoption of flat-rate payment methods—such as the French global budget and the American DRG— has been to give the hospital the incentive to shorten stays. The sickness fund's control doctor need no longer argue with the chiefs of service. Even before this reform, the French calibrated the per diem to reduce the incentive for prolonging the stay for convalescing inpatients: after the twentieth day, the control doctor could recommend the full or a reduced daily rate for a specific number of additional days.

An important feature of managed-care arrangements in the United States during the 1980s is limitation on length of stay. The office may preauthorize admission for a specific number of days for that diagnosis. The approved length is usually the peer average in that region. The Blue Cross Plan's staff has long monitored length of stay in its area; the PRO is supposed to do the same for Medicare; and the advent of PPOs finally provided such a capability for the commercial insurance companies. Programs vary with respect to how quickly they notice and challenge excessive stays, but no research has been done about implementation in practice. The managed-care staff must tread carefully: it needs the most widespread participation of hospitals and doctors in order to expand its own market, unnecessary hospital days are an important cause of financial loss, and length of stay is one of the few costs it can really control. Although they are logical in theory, controls antagonize doctors.

Effects on Utilization and Health

What difference does it make, for medical care and patient outcomes, if the health insurance system has one or another relationship to hospitals and pays them by one or another method? Since I have discussed effects in detail elsewhere,[19] the following paragraphs summarize a few highlights.

Universal statutory health insurance has expanded access by the population in every country—and it has made services equal. At the beginning of the twentieth century, hospital and physician services were socially unequal—the rich had better care in private clinics—but the nonprofit and public hospitals were improved by the great increase in funds and all social classes now patronize the same facilities. The rich can still purchase private health insurance and receive amenities—private rooms and special attention by the chiefs of service in return for private fees—but otherwise all classes now get the same care. (If, as in the United States, health insurance is not universal and standardized, hospital access and services still vary by social class and the public hospital for indigent care survives.) Universal statutory health insurance spreads coverage and funding throughout the country. Rural areas and small towns that once had only primitive hospitals or none at all now have modern care. Specialist physicians who once clustered in cities now spread throughout the country.[20]

During the phase when statutory health insurance expands in coverage and cash, the hospital sector modernizes throughout the country and grows in underserved regions. Eventually costs must be limited within the fiscal capacity of the payroll taxes and public subsidies and—since it is the biggest share of all health care spending and since hospital managers are more cooperative than medical associations—the hospital sector becomes the first target of cost containment. Under statutory health insurance, the effort tries to make the hospitals more efficient. It never denies services to patients or creates waiting lists: statutory health insurance guarantees to every subscriber prompt necessary services prescribed by doctors; the sickness funds lack any instruments to force the hospitals to reduce or close their clinical services. Sickness funds in several countries have added staff members who can monitor the quality and necessity of hospitals' programs, so they can advise the rate regulators about the hospitals' prospective budgets, and this new role might improve the hospitals' performance and the patients' satisfaction. Old-fashioned utilization review was oriented toward detecting cost outliers and did not affect the general frequency and quality of care.

All-payer methods of paying hospitals are universal in all developed countries except the United States. Rate regulators and joint negotiating committees set a standard rate for each hospital, since the rate covers the hospital's costs (no more and no less) and since it charges all users for a standard product. All-payer reimbursement is one of the methods to ensure that all persons get identical care and the hospital gets enough money to carry out its clinical plans. If different social groups belong to different carriers, and if the carriers pay different rates to the hospital—as in the United States—the groups do not get the same access and services.

Paying the hospital by a particular unit—such as per diems, charges, global budgets, or case payments—does not have inevitable results for patient care and costs. It depends on how each is administered and the type of prospective and concurrent review applied by rate regulators and carriers. Once it was assumed that per diems always prolong stays unnecessarily, for example, but European hospitals using per diems have been steadily reducing stays. Global budgeting can be either strict or generous, providing the hospital with few or many resources. Like fee-for-service, charge lists may be an incentive to the overprescribing of tests and drugs. But this assumes that the method of paying the hospital organization affects the prescribing doctor, whose income depends on his own fees and not on hospital charges.

The benefit structure of insurance and the methods of reimbursing doctors facilitate or hinder certain reforms in site of care. For example:

☐   Many countries have too many hospital beds and too many admissions. But it is difficult to transfer clinical work to the outpatient department, since most European health insurance programs do not pay enough (or do not pay at all) for hospital outpatient care. In contrast, America's Medicare Part B and Blue Cross pay very generously for outpatient surgery and other expensive outpatient work. Since hospitals are squeezed by inpatient DRG rates for simple procedures, American hospitals transfer much work to their outpatient departments.

☐   In much of Europe elderly patients with prolonged stays fill up the acutecare beds, preventing a reduction in the excessive numbers of beds. But they resist transfer to nursing homes, since statutory health insurance requires them to share room-and-board costs. The more expensive acute-care hospitalization is covered in full.

Implications for the United States

The American hospital has a number of problems due to its health insurance system. Countries with universal statutory health insurance lack these problems.

As noted in Chapter Three, a substantial fraction of the American population has never had health insurance. Therefore, they lack primary physicians. Even persons with Medicaid attract no interest by office doctors. If they need care, they go to the outpatient departments or emergency rooms of public and nonprofit hospitals. In a survey conducted in 1982, about 10 percent of the entire American population said they depended on the hospital as their principal source of care.[21] But these parts of acute-care hospitals are not set up to deliver primary care. These patients are principal sources of the overload, bad debts, and deficits that afflict America's urban hospitals.[22]

Because of self-referred patients' lack of primary care, the American urban hospital has many cases that are rare in other developed countries, such as the care of disabled neonates. Pediatrics has diminished in European hospitals, but it is a large and technically advanced part of the American urban hospital. It is also an important source of bad debts and deficits.

American hospitals try to cover their bad debts by shifting the costs to other payers—particularly the privately insured who pay charges, a method inconceivable under statutory health insurance in other countries.[23] An invitation to deviousness and dispute, the method makes the chief financial officer an important and well-paid part of American hospital management. It is possible only if a hospital has few bad debts and many private payers. If a hospital has many bad debts and few private payers—a combination that intensifies as the uninsured poor cluster there—the hospital declines, may go bankrupt, and closes, a spiral that is nearly impossible under statutory health insurance.[24]

To protect themselves from this fate, many American hospitals try to avoid all patients lacking sufficient insurance. For-profit hospitals and the smaller nonprofit establishments close their emergency rooms, a common entry point for the uninsured. They try to transfer uninsured patients to the public hospitals, touching off indignant exposés by the mass media and congressional committees.[25] This never occurs in countries with statutory health insurance, since all patients are fully covered at the standard rates.

American hospital management is complicated—not only in order to cope with bad debts and collect from slow payers, but also to keep track of the third parties. Every other country with statutory health insurance has standardized reimbursement of hospitals in order to facilitate budgeting, to make sure that costs are covered, to simplify rate determination, and to necessitate no more than a small administrative office in the hospital. In the United States, the opposite situation prevails: each insurance carrier pays the same hospital by different rules, each tries to underpay while shifting costs to its competitors, a large administrative capacity is required in each hospital, the hospital's managers conceal their manipulation and financial outcomes, many disputes and complaints result, and hardly anyone understands the country's hospital finance. American hospital finance cannot be stabilized without creation of all-payer reimbursement with sufficient revenue.

Notes

1. The *Kupat Holim* and its hospitals are described in Theodor Grushka, *Health Services in Israel*, rev. ed. (Jerusalem: Ministry of Health, 1968); and Richard F. Strongwater and David Rosenbach, "Medical Care Under the Administration of a National Health Insurance," *Journal of Family Practice*, vol. 17, no. 2 (1983), pp. 339–341.

2. SOE and its hospitals are described in Enrique Serrano Guirado, *El Seguro de Enfermedad y sus Problemas* (Madrid: Instituto de Estudios Politicos, 1950); and Manuel Alonso Olea, *Instituciones de Seguridad Social* (Madrid: Editorial Civitas, early editions).

3. The hospitals and other facilities owned and managed by MGEN and other *mutuelles* are described in *Les formes complémentaires de la protection sociale* (Paris: Inspection Générale des Affaires Sociales, 1975), pp. 233–249.

4. Jon Gabel and others, "The Emergence and Future of PPO's," *Journal of Health Politics, Policy and Law*, vol. 11, no. 2 (Summer 1986), pp. 316–318.

5. The units of payment are described in detail in William A. Glaser, *Paying the Hospital* (San Francisco: Jossey-Bass, 1987), chap. 4.

6. For an explanation of how American hospitals calculate their charge lists see Howard J. Berman and Lewis E. Weeks, *The Financial Management of Hospitals*, 6th ed. (Ann Arbor, Mich.: Health Administration Press, 1986), chap. 8; and Bruce R. Neumann and others, *Financial Management*, 2nd ed. (Owings Mills, Md.: AUPHA Press, 1988), chap. 11. Hospital payment by Blue Cross and commercial insurers before DRGs is described in William O. Cleverley (ed.), *Handbook of Health Care Accounting and Finance* (Rockville, Md.: Aspen Systems, 1982), chaps. 31, 33.

7. Compare the original design in Paul L. Grimaldi and Julie A. Micheletti, *DRG Update: Medicare's Prospective Payment Plan*, and the change after

only a few years in Grimaldi, *Prospective Payment: The Definitive Guide to Reimbursement* (both Chicago: Pluribus Press, 1983 and 1985). The annual changes thereafter are summarized in the annual reports of the Prospective Payment Assessment Commission.

8. Methods of deciding rates are described in detail in Glaser, *Paying the Hospital* (see note 5, above), chaps. 6–8.

9. Allan J. Zlimen, "Collection Practices," in Cleverley, *Handbook of Health Care Accounting and Finance* (see note 6, above), chap. 51.

10. Unpublished data from the Office of National Cost Estimates, Health Care Financing Administration.

11. *Hospital Contracting in Group Practice HMO's* (Washington: Group Health Association of America, 1981); and John E. Kralewski and others, "HMO-Hospital Relationships: An Exploratory Study," *Health Care Management Review*, vol. 8, no. 2 (Spring 1983), pp. 27–36. The great variety of price and non-price relations between PPOs and hospitals are summarized in S. Brian Barger and others, *The PPO Handbook* (Rockville, Md.: Aspen Systems, 1985).

12. The various arrangements are described in detail in Glaser, *Paying the Hospital* (see note 5, above), chap. 9.

13. Utilization control is described in detail in Glaser, *Paying the Hospital*, pp. 333–340.

14. The French control doctor's prior approval and his more effective powers in monitoring prolongation of stays are described in Jean Delmas, *Guide du praticien dans ses rapports avec le médecin-conseil de la Sécurité sociale* (Paris: J. B. Baillière, 1984), pp. 9–26. Approval of hospitalization, thermal cures, and disability allowances by the control doctor in Germany are described in Erich-Michel Simon, *Le contrôle médical de l'assurance-maladie dans la République Fédérale Allemande* (Strasbourg: Université Louis Pasteur, Faculté de Médecine de Strasbourg, 1971), pt. 2 passim.

15. *The Utilization and Quality Control Peer Review Organization (PRO) Program* (Washington: Office of Inspector General, Department of Health and Human Services, 1988); and Institute of Medicine, *Medicare: A Strategy for Quality Assurance* (Washington: National Academy Press, 1990).

16. All methods by the Blues, commercial insurers, and HMOs are described and their effects estimated in Bradford H. Gray and Marilyn J. Field (eds.), *Controlling Costs and Changing Patient Care? The Role of Utilization Management* (Washington: Institute of Medicine Committee on Utilization Management by Third Parties, National Academy Press, 1989). The various preadmission controls and other cost containment efforts by the Blues are described and evaluated in Richard Scheffler, James O. Gibbs, and Dolores Gurnick, *The Impact of Medicare's Prospective Payment System and Private Sector Initiatives: Blue Cross Experience 1980–1986* (Chicago: Blue Cross and Blue Shield Association, 1988), pp. 32–43, 131–147.

17. Jon Gabel and others, "The Commercial Health Insurance Industry in Transition," *Health Affairs*, vol. 6, no. 3 (Fall 1987), pp. 46–60; and Peter R.

Kongstvedt (ed.), *The Managed Care Handbook* (Rockville, Md.: Aspen Publications, 1989), especially chaps. 8, 10. Current events are described in the biweekly newsletter *Managed Care Report.*

18. Harold S. Luft, *Health Maintenance Organizations: Dimensions of Performance,* 2nd ed. (New Brunswick: Transaction Books, 1987), chap. 5.

19. Glaser, *Paying the Hospital* (see note 5, above), especially chap. 13.

20. While basic services are now available throughout small towns and rural areas, medicine has become more technically advanced, the number of specialists has grown, urban populations have increased, and therefore the urban concentration of *expensive* services has intensified. See Bui Dang Ha Doan, *Les médecins en France* (Paris: Centre de sociologie et de démographie médicales, 1984), chaps. 4–5.

21. Lu Ann Aday and others, *Access to Medical Care in the U.S.: Who Has It, Who Doesn't* (Chicago: Pluribus Press, 1984), chaps. 2–4; and Charlotte Muller, "Review of Twenty Years of Research on Medical Care Utilization," *Health Services Research,* vol. 21, no. 2 (pt. 1) (June 1986), pp. 131–135. The heavy reliance of uninsured expectant mothers on hospital clinics is reported in Lois A. Fingerhut and others, "Delayed Prenatal Care and Place of First Visit: Differences by Health Insurance and Education," *Family Planning Perspectives,* vol. 19, no. 5 (Sept.–Oct. 1987), pp. 212–214, 234.

22. The deficits from bad debts in the outpatient department and after inpatient hospitalization are documented in Jack Hadley and Judith Feder, *Hospitals' Financial Status and Care to the Poor in 1980* and *Cutbacks, Recession and Care to the Poor* (Washington: Urban Institute, 1983).

23. For a comparison with European methods see William A. Glaser, "Juggling Multiple Payers," *Inquiry,* vol. 21, no. 2 (Summer 1984), pp. 178–188. For a guide to American cost shifting see Donald F. Beck, *Principles of Reimbursement in Health Care* (Rockville, Md.: Aspen Systems, 1984).

24. Alan Sager, "Why Urban Voluntary Hospitals Close," *Health Services Research,* vol. 18, no. 3 (Fall 1982), pp. 451–481.

25. *Equal Access to Health Care: Patient Dumping* (Washington: Committee on Government Operations, U.S. House of Representatives, 100th Congress, 2nd Session, House Report 100-6531, 1988).

CHAPTER 12

Pharmaceutical Drugs

──────────────── **Summary** ────────────────

In the early years, pharmaceuticals were often dispensed by office doctors and fit into health insurance as one of many treatments. But the creation of pharmaceuticals has become a large and powerful multinational industry, the service providers have diversified, the relations of creators and providers with governments and insurance carriers have become complex and volatile, and countries vary in the management of drug benefits under insurance.

Some characteristics of statutory health insurance, such as the payment of doctors, are remarkably similar across many countries. All countries are concerned about the costs of pharmaceuticals, but their responses differ widely. Regardless of insurance arrangement, all governments in developed countries regulate the drug market to protect the public from dangerous products and fraud. European governments are becoming more alike in their requirements for testing and licensing. Every country maintains a formulary of drugs licensed for prescription by doctors and for sale in the private market. Health insurance carriers reimburse for some or all, depending on methods peculiar to each country.

To protect the public and the health insurance system from excessive earnings by a politically unpopular industry, some countries regulate the prices of all pharmaceutical drugs. Their methods and strictness vary. Estimating the costs and fair prices for each drug in each country is very difficult, since the companies are multinational.

Statutory health insurance once paid for any drug prescribed by a doctor from the national formulary, just as it paid for all exercises of professional clinical discretion. But national formularies include many duplicative and less effec-

283

tive drugs, as well as simple remedies for everyday comfort, and total costs have been excessive. Thus, several statutory health insurance systems have adopted limited lists of cost-effective drugs appropriate to acute care. The remaining drugs may still be prescribed by doctors and paid for by patients, either out-of-pocket or with private health insurance. A considerable decision-making machinery creates and updates the limited lists.

Payment by health insurance carriers varies from country to country. Some pay whatever prices are set by government price controls; the social insurance carriers may obtain discounts while private insurance does not. If no general price controls exist, the Parliament and the finance officers for the statutory health insurance system develop special methodologies for fixing the prices paid by the sickness funds. They do not use the methods used for deciding the reimbursement of doctors and hospitals—that is, negotiations with the industry or cost-based regulation by civil servants.

In some countries, such as Holland and Germany, reimbursement distinguishes between the dispenser and the producer. The sickness funds contract with pharmacists and dispensing general practitioners, and the dispensers are paid for their work. Fees for their prescriptions depend on the prices of the products.

Statutory health insurance once paid for drugs in full. Now user charges are common. The precise formulas vary among countries. The motives are to shift a portion of costs to consumers, discourage overprescribing by doctors, discourage waste of drugs by patients, and press the pharmaceutical industry to limit prices. A recent trend is differential cost sharing, so patients and doctors prefer generic substitutes. Cost sharing may have limited effects on prescribing and on consumption: many of the heaviest users are exempt.

Statistical utilization review is often used to detect and discourage doctors who prescribe far more drugs than their peers. However, as in utilization review of physicians' practice styles, sickness funds are often reluctant to challenge doctors' professional decisions. Utilization review is directed at providers, not at the overconsuming patient who presses doctors for prescriptions. Countries vary widely in national propensities to prescribe and consume drugs.

Private health insurance in Europe and the United States has recently added drug benefits. Because the carriers are lucrative markets, they win agreements with pharmacists throughout the country. Modern telecommunication makes possible the management of a large and decentralized market. The private carriers avoid negotiating with medical associations and reviewing each doctor's pharmaceutical choices.

Evolution of Provider Roles

Several centuries ago, the providers of medical care were:

☐   Physicians, who theorized about the internal states of sick people, diagnosed diseases and distempers, and prescribed remedies. Some applied remedies themselves, usually treatments other than drugs.

☐ Surgeons, who treated injuries and structural abnormalities by manipulating and cutting.

☐ Apothecaries, who mixed medicine from powders and liquids. They earned income from sales. By claiming he had invented a secret wonder drug, the apothecary captured the market from his competitors. Since the methods of physicians were few, feared, and ineffective (blood-letting, blistering, cupping, enemas), the public desperately hoped that a particular apothecary had discovered a miracle cure. Physicians and surgeons had no shops, but most apothecaries did.

Gradually the roles of physician and apothecary overlapped. Some physicians mixed and supplied medicines in addition to their usual treatments. Many apothecaries became general practitioners for the general public. Not all apothecaries became doctors, though. Some became large-scale manufacturers; others became merchants selling nonmedical goods as well as continuing to mix and dispense drugs.

During the nineteenth and early twentieth centuries, sickness funds began to pay for pharmaceuticals, since they were at least as successful as other medical interventions. The carriers had to cover the different forms of delivery:

☐ General practitioners in several countries were paid a capitation fee for every person on each list of subscribers. If the GP prepared and dispensed drugs and did not merely prescribe them, the sickness fund paid him an extra capitation fee. These arrangements survive today in a few communities in the Netherlands.

☐ If GPs and specialists were paid by fee-for-service, some early fee schedules included global fees for prescribing, mixing, and delivering each medicine. These fees were later divided: a fee to the doctor for writing the prescription and a separate fee to the pharmacist for mixing each product.

☐ If the sickness fund employed and housed doctors in a health center, it also maintained a pharmacy there. These arrangements survive today in many Belgian and French *mutuelles*.[1]

☐ When sickness funds began paying the hospital, the comprehensive daily rate was supposed to cover the costs of the pharmacy as well as all other clinical services.

Rapidly, the creation of drugs became rationalized and their production and distribution became industrialized. Pharmaceuticals became more effective, more dangerous, and more profitable. Unlike health care providers, the managers of the drug industry were not churchmen and doctors dedicated to the principles of religion and professionalism; they were businessmen.[2]

Government Regulation

Quality assessment of other medical services is left to the education, conscience, and peer review of doctors. Government and sickness funds accept the judgments of doctors—either the patient's attending physician or the doctors they themselves employ. Government ensures a minimum general level of safety by examining and licensing doctors and hospitals. Individual pharmaceutical products may be unsafe or have serious side effects. To protect the patient and discourage exaggerated marketing claims, governments impose upon individual products investigation, licensing, and warning labels.

Approvals for Drugs. Nearly every country has safety regulations for drugs, some going back for centuries.[3] The administrative procedures and speed for investigating and approving vary among countries. Every nation can set its own minimum standards for approval, but all have gotten stricter and have become more alike since World War II—because of wider scientific awareness of delayed side effects, international publicity of sensations like the thalidomide scandal, and the harmonizing efforts of international scientific committees. Besides safety, efficacy has recently been added to the criteria for approval. A drug must not only be relatively safe or have limited side effects, but it must accomplish substantial therapeutic goals.

Until the 1980s, each country adopted its own regulatory goals and methods. The drug market—like all medical services and medical financing—was confined to the individual country. A drug sold by a multinational company had to satisfy different investigations and criteria in order to be sold in each one.[4] During the 1970s, the European Economic Community (EEC) issued directives to harmonize member countries' rules about licensing and marketing drugs. These efforts accelerated during the 1980s, when the EEC decided to unify its economy by 1992. Other medical services remain national, tied to their health regulations and social security financing, but pharmaceuticals are a typical multinational industry that can sell and manufacture freely throughout the continent. Thus, the EEC has set up special committees to explore standardization in manufacturing, testing, and approving drugs. (Countries outside the Common Market will continue with their own rules.) The EEC has engaged in long and complex negotiations to reconcile the objective of a unified continent-wide pharmaceutical market with the diversity of prices and reimbursement rules that each country retains in its statutory health insurance.[5]

National Formularies. Every country issues a formulary of approved drugs. Usually it is published by the Ministry of Health or the government agency that administers the investigations and approvals. Formularies used to be informal and published by many individuals and organizations; now they are standardized and official. Formularies used to be instructions to apothecaries about how to mix drugs; now they are lists and scientific explanations of the standard products from drug companies. Usually they contain the ingredients for a generic mixture, several brand names available, indications for which each is prescribed, recommended use, possible side effects, and (sometimes) references to the literature. The formulary often states whether a doctor's prescription is required for purchase under the country's law. (Sometimes these are called "national official compendia." Some administrators use the word "formulary" for what I describe later as "limited lists"—the items reimbursed by statutory health insurance.)

Drug companies and doctors can ask for additions to the formulary. A special committee of scientists, pharmacologists, physicians, and others usually oversees, corrects, and modernizes the volume; officially, it is usually an advisory committee to the official (such as the Minister of Health) who issues amendments and new editions as government regulations. Since doctors or hospitals cannot in their ordinary practice prescribe a drug not in the formulary, omitted drugs are not covered by NHI. (In practice, teaching hospitals perform unlisted experimental therapies whose purchase costs are mixed into their full budgets covered by the sickness funds.)

As the volume and complexity of pharmaceuticals grow, licensing regulators have greater difficulty keeping up. In theory, they should be dropping obsolete and ineffective drugs from the formulary. The scientific knowledge needed to classify a drug as "ineffective" is ambiguous, however, and the drug companies resist the banning of established products. Since most regulatory agencies lack the personnel and budget to perform this troublesome part of the job, a great deal of expensive ineffective prescribing probably results.

General Price Controls

The final price of a drug is the sum of three parts: the producer's price, the wholesaler's markup, and the seller's markup. Each part covers both costs and profits. If a government in some fashion regulates drug prices, it might limit separately the producer, or the wholesaler, or the seller. Or it might simply limit the final sales price.[6] General price controls are designed to protect the entire population, regardless of payer. If they do not exist, each payer must fend for itself. Whether a country's drug prices are controlled by a government makes a great difference to the health insurance system.

A national government has limited jurisdiction. The seller and (usually) the wholesaler are citizens located within its boundaries and subject to its laws. But the manufacturer may be foreign, not directly controllable, and immune from disclosure requirements. If the government tries to limit the volatile producer prices when nearly all production is foreign, it may set the price equal to the wholesale price in the country of origin plus a fixed markup for the importer. The country with the strictest price controls, Belgium, uses this method. The European Federation of Pharmaceutical Industries' Associations responds with lawsuits alleging that such price regulations violate the Common Market's directives about the free flow of goods without interference with pricing.

Some national governments impose direct price controls. The targets vary: the producer's price, the wholesale markup, or the retail markup. Some methods accept the producer's legal right (or practical ability) to dictate his own price, and the control falls on the markups. Some limit producer prices by requiring a complete filing of all and cutting back those that seem to reap excessive profits.

General price surveillance is part of a tradition in some countries (such as France) allowing government to prevent hardships and profiteering in essential commodities and services. While nearly all other items were eventually decontrolled after World War II, drugs never were—on the grounds that they were essential to human survival and could yield excessive profits. In a few countries (such as Belgium and Italy), price controls were instituted on the pharmaceutical industry alone during the 1950s and 1960s as the first concerted policy to control health care costs. The first visible cost explosion to bother European policymakers was the great increase in drug expenditures—both in aggregate consumption and in unit prices—and the drug companies' rapidly increasing share of NHI. So, to protect the NHI accounts, unit prices were controlled by government. Doctors and hospitals normally resist cost containment laws since they are the targets; but they were happy to see the drug companies limited, lest the companies end up with all the money.[7]

Usually drug prices are monitored by the government agency in charge of all the price surveillance laws (such as the Ministry of Economic Affairs) and not by the agencies that administer drug safety approval and health insurance (such as the Ministries of Health and Labor). The sickness funds under NHI will not pay more than these official prices and often try to pay less.

Several developed countries have no general price controls on pharmaceuticals—for example, Germany and the United States. These are the home bases of the multinational firms. The companies contribute to the countries' economies, the firms have considerable political influence (because of high employment and financial contributions to political parties), and the countries in general prefer free markets. But there can be important exceptions: Switzerland controls prices in many sectors, lest inflation jeopardize its overriding role in international finance, and therefore it controls the prices of its powerful drug industry. Some countries with price controls keep them regardless of the political complexion of the government-of-the-day. The drug companies there are politically weak and unpopular. On the other hand, some governments ease controls, as in France in 1980.

The law may require the government to raise retail drug prices as the drug companies' costs rise. This policy, however, is difficult to implement: the pharmaceutical firms try not to reveal their full accounts to regulators, tax returns are privileged against disclosure to price regulators, and (even if the accounts were available) a multinational firm's research costs, manufacturing costs, and profits cannot easily be allocated to each national market. Some governments (as in France during the 1970s) are obligated by law to estimate the average annual increases in manufacturing and research costs and automatically announce an across-the-board percentage increase in retail prices once or twice a year. If they have discretion, governments are in no hurry to raise unit prices—they think the companies earn large incomes from rapidly rising utilization and from sales in the many developed and underdeveloped countries without price controls. After years of complaint by the national pharmaceutical manufacturers' association, such a government grudgingly raises prices if the controls seem to be squeezing the research capabilities and employment of domestic manufacturers. Such a government will be unsympathetic to a company that imports and resells finished products.[8]

Coverage Under Statutory Health Insurance

Limited Lists. In the past, national health insurance systems paid in full or in part for every drug prescribed by a doctor from the national formulary. If the drug was in the formulary, it was a legitimate treatment that a doctor could choose—like any test or therapy listed in the official fee schedule—and the insurance system pledged to pay for all recognized treatments. But during the 1960s and 1970s all expenditures rose rapidly, health expenditures were rising, new methods of cost containment were applied to all sectors by the sickness funds, and the carriers sought to apply to drugs more specific measures than governments' general price controls.

A common problem was the excessive size and generosity of the national formularies. The licensing agencies were allowing new pharmaceuticals that duplicated existing drugs and some that were not fully established as effective; many obsolete and marginally effective drugs were allowed to stay. In a few countries (particularly Germany) the formulary listed a large number of drugs from all schools of medicine (homeopathy, herbal medicine, and so on) and included simple over-the-counter remedies. The simple drugs were supposed to be bought by the public as costs of everyday life (such as aspirin, cough medicine, and laxatives), but if a doctor prescribed them, the sickness funds were obligated to pay.

Therefore, several countries during the late 1970s and 1980s adopted "limited lists" indicating the drugs that—when prescribed by a doctor—were chargeable to statutory health insurance.[9] As part of its package of cost containment laws in 1977 and 1983, the German government issued a "negative list" of simple medications for minor illnesses that would no longer be reimbursed from statutory insurance. As in many fundamental policy changes, the German reform was debated for many years. Since it could not be left to negotiations between the sickness funds and the powerful pharmaceutical industry, it required an amendment to the *Reichsversicherungsordnung* by Parliament. The excluded items remain in the national formulary, can still be prescribed by the doctor, and can be paid for by the patient out-of-pocket or with the help of private insurance.

Among the countries with statutory health insurance, Holland has developed the most extensive methods for creating a limited list. The responsibility is not left with the sickness funds alone, since they lack the staffing and political force to reduce coverage of the national formulary in the face of the drug industry. The decisions are made through the staffing and inclusive committee structure of the *Ziekenfondsraad.* The council since 1949 has included a committee (the *Centrale Medisch Pharmaceutische Commissie,* or CMPC) that has long offered expert judgments about drug benefits and, during the 1980s, acquired considerable new authority.

The CMPC consists of representation from the national associations of sickness funds, physicians, pharmacists, and dentists. It includes leading professors in the health sciences and in pharmacology and is supported by a large staff and research office located in the *Ziekenfondsraad.* Every year since 1982 it issues a volume that expands the descriptions in the national formulary, evaluates drugs' efficacy and side effects, points out duplications, and places many drugs on a negative list that should not be reimbursed by the sickness funds.[10] The negative list includes drugs that are unsafe or ineffective, simple everyday self-medications, and (in order to press companies to reduce prices) drugs that are excessively expensive in the light of resource costs and alternatives in the market. Like all recommendations from the committee, the annual edition is discussed by the full *Ziekenfondsraad.* Any protests by drug companies can be considered both by the CMPC and by the full council. Government then accepts and enforces the council's recommendations. The volume warns the prescribing doctor and the dispensing pharmacist that the doctor may prescribe a drug on the negative list, but the provider must bill the patient in full.

The limited lists apply to ambulatory care. The hospitals may use any drug from the national formulary—neither government nor the sickness funds know what they do, since drug costs are aggregated in the hospital's cost reports and prospective budgets. The chiefs of service and hospital managers have clinical motives to use the most effective and safest drugs, and they have financial motives to use the least costly. The hospital can save money by bulk purchasing of the minimum number of drugs and by not having to stock a number of rarely prescribed items. A large hospital in Europe or the United States may design its own short formulary to cover all its needs; it may even persuade (or order) its doctors and pharmacists to prescribe from that list. However, this limitation may not be possible in a teaching hospital committed to the newest innovations, or in an establishment (like a European private clinic or an open-staff American hospital) where the doctors are more exposed to salesmen from the drug industry.

Prices Paid by Sickness Funds. Prospective reimbursement under national health insurance applies to the prices of drugs as well as to the rates of doctors, hospitals, and other providers. In all cases, the prices and rates are fixed at the start of the year and are printed. Like the fee schedule applying to all doctors, the price for each drug is standard for all manufacturers and retailers. Usually the price list is the same throughout the country. The price list is usually set simply—without the elaborate negotiation for doctors' fees or the financial investigation used in hospital rate regulation. In countries with official prices controlled or influenced by government (the arrangement mentioned earlier), the sickness funds and all private payers may be bound to pay these prices in full.

But because of discounts, the sickness funds might be required to pay less—perhaps 7 to 10 percent less. Payment in full is expected of privately insured and self-pay patients. Pharmacists and retailers cannot extra-bill socially insured patients. Other payers, such as social welfare offices, may press drug companies and retailers to agree to even bigger discounts.

If no government price controls exist as a benchmark and the sickness funds do not negotiate prices with the drug industry, each company in theory could set its producer prices unilaterally—as all health providers could long ago. However, a drug company has never been unconstrained: it sells some of its products in markets with price controls; in the less controlled countries, it cannot exceed the prices of its competitors by too much—lest it lose the privately insured and self-pay customers, lest the sickness funds steer doctors and pharmacists to the less expensive substitutes. If the drug companies raise prices and profits too high, the sickness funds and political Left will press for statutory price controls. Across the several national markets, each company follows a complicated pricing and sales strategy for each product, a strategy that varies over the product's life cycle.[11]

Imposing firm controls over a volatile market and over a powerful industry is protracted and difficult, as German experience shows. While German sickness funds negotiate physicians' fees and hospital rates strictly, they have allowed the drug companies to set the basic producer prices. Until 1989, the only restraint on the final sales price was limited government regulation of the markups by wholesalers and pharmacists. Drug costs rose rapidly during the 1960s, both unit prices and total utilization seemed high, and drug costs absorbed a large proportion (nearly 20 percent) of all statutory insurance spending. The Germans conducted several research projects comparing their experiences with those of countries that had price regulation, utilization review, and oligopsonistic or monopsonistic purchasing.[12]

Direct price controls could not be enacted by Parliament over such a powerful industry. Nor would the drug industry agree to creation of a bilateral negotiating system with the sickness funds. Since the companies were multinational, an exclusively German negotiating system (appropriate for doctors, dentists, and hospitals) could not easily be crafted. The cost control laws of 1977 and later, as well as a special pharmaceuticals marketing law, introduced other measures:

☐ Many drugs were placed on a "negative list," removed from social insurance coverage, and left to the free market.

☐ Within the *Konzertierte Aktion* (described in Chapters Ten and Eighteen), the sickness funds and the national associations of doctors and dentists agreed on annual targets for total drug spending. The provincial associations of doctors and dentists then tried to persuade their members to prescribe within the limits. But the drug industry was not involved in these guidelines at all and remained free to increase its producer prices. If the target was

exceeded, it was not the sickness funds' drug payments that were prorated
downward: it was the fees billed by doctors for writing prescriptions.

☐   A special commission was created to publish information about the market
(the *Transparenzkommission am Bundesgesundheitsamt*). It consisted of
representatives from the sickness funds, doctors and dentists in insurance
practice, drug companies, and consumer groups. It published lists of prices
and properties of drugs. The hope was that doctors and dentists would voluntarily prescribe cheaper drugs. But each drug company remained free to
press doctors to prescribe its more expensive drugs and its new products.

☐   As part of the effort to disseminate the facts about the once mysterious drug
industry and drug market, the national associations of sickness funds used
their positions in the commission to compel disclosure, expanded their research staffs, and published much about pharmaceuticals.[13]

None of these methods controlled prices and volume, and the German
government finally had to act more directly. Parliament in late 1988 enacted a
"prudent purchaser" method, rather than the across-the-board price controls Germany had always avoided. The cheapest of all the competing products is the
"reference price." For each diagnosis, the sickness fund pays the pharmacist only
the reference price. The prescribing doctor, the pharmacist, and the patient may
agree on a more expensive drug, but the patient must pay the balance out-of-
pocket. For the first time, German statutory health insurance allows extra-billing.
To attract subscribers, commercial insurance companies and the *Ersatzkassen*
offer to cover more than the reference prices.

Role of the Physician. Prescribing drugs has always been an integral part
of the doctor's ambulatory care. In several countries, such as France, writing a
prescription has been covered by the fee for the office visit and home visit. The
fee schedule negotiated between the sickness fund and medical association makes
this clear.

German health insurance has had a tradition of itemizing and pricing all
procedures in each visit, rather than paying an all-inclusive fee. Therefore, the
sickness fund pays the office doctor for writing a prescription. All the separate
acts are listed on the quarterly bill the doctor sends the sickness fund for that
patient (the *Krankenschein*). If the patient needs a renewal of the prescription,
the doctor adds a renewal fee to the quarterly bill but does not add any other
charges.

In the many countries without this detailed method, the office doctor may
bill the sickness fund the full fee for an office visit even though the patient has
merely visited briefly or telephoned for a renewal. Such payment is one of the
more common problems in controlling the costs of ambulatory care.

All Dutch general practitioners are paid by capitation fees under statutory
health insurance; there are no individual fees for writing prescriptions or performing other procedures. Once many GPs dispensed drugs and not merely pre-

scribed them, but dispensing has steadily shifted to the increasing number of pharmacists. Almost one thousand GPs (one-sixth of the total) still dispense drugs—either because no pharmacist works in the area or because the GP is a veteran who retains this right until retirement. Dispensing GPs are no longer being licensed; eventually none will remain.

Like every GP, the Dutch dispensing GP is paid a capitation fee by the sickness funds for every subscriber on his list. The dispensing GP's capitation fee combines the average overhead costs of all Dutch office-based pharmacies plus the standard capitation fee for clinical care. The capitation fee is negotiated by the sickness funds and a committee of dispensing GPs from the national medical association, and it is approved by the regulatory commission for health care prices under social insurance (COTG).

In addition to capitation fees, the Dutch sickness funds pay the dispensing GP and the independent pharmacist the officially listed wholesale price for each medication the GP and pharmacist dispense. Neither provider is supposed to earn profits from markups over costs; their respective capitation fees include the honoraria (that is, the amounts intended for net income). In practice, the highly competitive drug companies often grant the dispensing GPs and the pharmacists discounts to reward bulk purchasing or induce use of that product. The secret windfall profits displease the sickness funds and COTG—since the insurance system does not save—but they please the doctors and pharmacists.

Role of the Pharmacist. In most countries, the traditional distinction between "apothecary" and "druggist" has disappeared. The modern pharmacist is a businessman who sells both medicines and other products in his shop. Most medicines have been mixed and packaged by the manufacturing companies; the pharmacist merely sells to the customer whatever the patient's personal physician has prescribed in writing or by telephone. The sales price per unit paid for by the sickness fund includes a markup over the wholesale price for the pharmacist's personal income and business costs. The markup is limited to a particular percentage or a flat amount—either by general government price controls, by special government regulations about statutory health insurance, or by negotiations between sickness funds and the professional association of pharmacists. Governments and sickness funds cannot easily limit the producer's prices. And if the pharmacists could set their own markups, the insurance system would be paying high profits to both the manufacturers and the distributors.

In a few European countries (such as West Germany and the Netherlands), the traditional role of "apothecary" survives. Laws forbid the apothecary shops to sell nonmedical products. Druggists are forbidden to dispense prescription drugs, as well, but they can sell the many over-the-counter remedies. Special sickness fund retainers to apothecaries have disappeared, and the pharmacist bills the sickness funds for each item sold: the wholesale price he paid plus the standard retail markup set by the general price regulation law. The prices of pharmaceuticals are high enough in Germany (and the patients' appetite for drugs is large enough) that the apothecary can earn a sufficient gross income from sales to cover merchandise, wages, rent, other costs, and profits.

The primary care role in Dutch cities is split between full-time general practitioners and full-time pharmacists. Traditionally Dutch primary care has been reimbursed by capitation rather than by the fee-for-service method (which supposedly encourages excessively technical care and fleeting doctor-patient contacts). Thus, the health insurance system has mimicked general practice in organizing and paying for pharmaceuticals. Every pharmacist has a list of insured persons who order all prescription drugs from him. The several GPs in the area forward their prescriptions to each subscriber's permanent pharmacist. For his work, the pharmacist is paid:

☐   A capitation fee for every subscriber on his list. It is set by annual negotiations between the national associations of sickness funds and pharmacists and is approved by COTG. The fee covers the average Dutch pharmacist's net income, overhead costs, and pension premium. Longer lists of subscribers yield larger gross incomes from capitation fees. The fee is higher for each of the first five thousand subscribers, lower for each additional person.
☐   The wholesale cost of each item dispensed.
☐   A delivery fee for each item dispensed. It is set by annual negotiations and is supposed to cover processing costs and labor. The delivery fee relates to units of each item dispensed—for example, f. 2.58 for every ten tablets dispensed of one item, for every six ounces dispensed of another item. More output yields larger revenue from this source.

Several reformers have criticized the traditional Dutch methods. Each pharmacist should be paid according to his own true costs, they say, rather than by national average capitation and delivery fees. Each pharmacist should be paid according to his own work, rather than by capitation fees collected for persons on a list who may generate little work. Patients should be free to go to any pharmacist, not be tied to one. If a pharmacist obtains a lower wholesale price, he should not pocket it. If the market were more competitive, he would have an incentive to pay his suppliers less and quote lower prices to payers, the reformers say. But the sickness funds fear a free market will generate more sales and prescriptions—that too many new persons will enter pharmacy. The sickness funds and the current practitioners prefer the present method of limiting the entry of pharmacists into practice: if each pharmacist is fully employed, he will not press the drug companies, doctors, and patients to increase consumption and sales; he will cooperate with any public policies to dispense generically.

At one time, apothecaries were independent practitioners supplying hospitals as well as ambulatory patients. Dispensing within the hospital has become so complex, voluminous, and quality-conscious that every hospital of moderate and large size now employs one or several full-time salaried pharmacists. Their salaries are mixed into the hospital budget, distributed among the sick funds in the all-inclusive daily charge.

Reimbursement in Full or Patient Cost Sharing. During the early years of statutory health insurance, supplying drugs was a principal therapy. Therefore, the sickness funds covered them in full—either by maintaining their own pharmacies, paying the dispensing physician in full, or paying the pharmacists' full charges. But after World War II, every government and the sickness funds decided that pharmaceutical benefits were particularly troublesome: utilization, unit prices, and total costs rose too fast. Besides, the drug companies were thought to profiteer by setting excessive prices, by producing unnecessary "me-too" drugs, and by pressing doctors to overprescribe. Doctors were motivated to overprescribe by the fee-for-service system; pharmacists had an incentive to supply the more expensive items by cost-plus reimbursement and under-the-table subsidies by the drug companies; and patients wasted many drugs because they felt the drugs were "free."

By now, every country with statutory health insurance or a national health service requires some form of cost sharing by the patient:[14]

☐ *Prescription charge.* Here the patient pays a fixed amount for an entire prescription written by a doctor and filled by a pharmacist, regardless of the number of items bought. A method that appears easy to administer, it has been adopted by Holland, the British National Health Service, and several other countries.
☐ *Copayment.* Here the patient pays a fixed amount for each medication regardless of its cost. Leading examples have been West Germany and American private health insurance.
☐ *Coinsurance.* Here the patient pays a fixed percentage of the total cost. Examples are Belgium, Denmark, Italy, and (after 1990) Germany.

Often these rules are not applied uniformly, since the purpose is to promote economy and efficiency, not increase the hardships that social insurance was supposed to alleviate. Several variations are possible:

☐ A common practice is to exempt the poor from all pharmaceutical cost sharing. Countries vary in the location of the income threshold: many British are exempt, but only a few Dutch. Because income is difficult to verify, some countries use proxies—such as whether the person receives social welfare benefits, as in Belgium.
☐ Another common practice is to exempt cost sharing by old-age pensioners. Examples are Australia and Britain.
☐ Drugs are classified by the severity of the illness they treat. Cost sharing is eliminated or reduced for the drugs prescribed for the most serious diseases in France and Belgium.

☐   If a country has different sickness funds for different occupations and certain
    groups are thought very vulnerable or very poor, they will have lower cost
    sharing or none at all. For example, the regime for French miners does not
    require the same cost-sharing rate as the other regimes.

☐   If the country imposed cost sharing reluctantly, it may limit the total out-
    of-pocket for the year, since the heavy users are thought medically and ec-
    onomically vulnerable. When Holland introduced a f. 2.5 prescription
    charge per item in 1983, it limited total out-of-pocket spending for the entire
    family to f. 125 per year. After a family has reached the limit, the sickness
    fund pays all costs.

At the time the patient receives the drug from the pharmacist, he makes whatever
payment is required by the country's rules. The pharmacist then bills the patient's sickness fund for the balance, calculating the total according to that country's rules about wholesale costs and retailer markup.

There are several motives for adopting and designing cost sharing:

☐   To divide total pharmaceutical spending between the overburdened sickness
    funds and the users ("cost shifting")
☐   To discourage patients from asking doctors for too many original prescrip-
    tions and renewals
☐   To remind doctors to be economical
☐   To motivate patients to ask pharmacists to supply less expensive substitutes
    where the doctor's prescription allows it
☐   To discourage patients from wasting drugs

Charges become part of the normal arrangements in every country, and
populations come to take them for granted. When they are first introduced or
significantly increased, every country shows an initial drop in the annual rate of
increase in consumption and then the normal rate resumes.[15] Patient cost sharing
for drugs as well as for the rest of health care is usually too small to have important permanent effects. In practice, therefore, charges are merely a method of
shifting costs from the sickness funds to the user.

Certain methods of cost sharing are ineffective and even counterproductive. For example, a common method is a flat charge for each prescription. A
common response by the doctor is to enter more medicines on each prescription.
In a country with this method of cost sharing, therefore, the annual number of
prescriptions drops but annual spending remains the same or (because of waste)
increases.[16]

Coinsurance may be replacing copayments. The copayments of 2 DM and
3 DM per medication seemed too small in prosperous West Germany, for example, and drug consumption steadily mounted, particularly for the new and expensive drugs. So a percentage of the price was substituted during the 1990s.

Cost sharing is sometimes difficult to enforce. The waiver for low-income persons requires evidence of each person's income. The tax collection agency refuses to release this privileged information. The sickness funds know only about earnings and pensions, not about total income. Doctors and pharmacists refuse to investigate and certify the income levels of their clients. Some apparently formidable cost-sharing requirements—such as the British NHS prescription charges—are dead letters because most patients (three-fourths of the British) "self-certify" that they are poor and therefore exempt.

Competition among providers in pharmaceuticals—as in all other areas of health—can undermine well-crafted incentives to deter waste. For example, statutory insurance in French ambulatory care has required reimbursement of the patient and not direct payment by sickness funds to the provider. The need to lay out cash, it was thought, would deter unnecessary utilization. But the *mutuelles* have not required this step for their subscribers using their own doctors and pharmacies: the *mutuelles* billed the subscriber's sickness fund and might not even collect the patient's cost sharing. The self-employed pharmacists feared that the *mutuelles* could expand their pharmacies by offering the same arrangements to the general public. Since 1975, they too have banded together in a contract with CNAMTS, allowing them to bill the sickness fund and charge the patient only for the statutory cost sharing. The pharmacists bill quickly and obtain rapid reimbursement with the help of a computerized system (*Santé Pharma*). Pharmaceuticals became the first sector in French ambulatory care to abandon *tiers garant* and adopt *tiers payant*.[17] The method is believed to be one of several reasons for the high levels of utilization and costs in French prescription drugs.

Utilization Review. It has long been known that pharmaceutical spending both generally and also under statutory health insurance varies substantially among developed countries, even though clinical medicine and the populations' health problems are much alike. Several recent research projects have identified cross-national variations in utilization and unit prices.[18] Countries spend more on pharmaceuticals if:

☐ The public and the medical profession have a consumer culture and a style of medical practice in favor of science and active treatment. For example: France, Italy, Japan, and Germany in contrast to Holland, Britain, and Scandinavia.

☐ Both general practitioners and specialists are paid by fee-for-service and collect fees for writing prescriptions.[19]

☐ Their drug companies have enough influence to require prescribing by brand name and to discourage or prevent pharmacists from substituting cheaper brands and generics.

The importance of utilization in determining total costs is underscored by a comparison of Belgium and the Netherlands. Belgium's strict government price controls give it the lowest unit prices of any country with statutory health insurance, lower than neighboring Holland's. But because Belgium's utilization is so much higher than Holland's, its per capita pharmaceutical costs are higher.[20]

The health insurance system has little leverage to induce consumers to seek the minimum necessary over-the-counter and prescription drugs or to persuade the medical profession to prescribe economically. Consumer groups and the Ministry of Health may urge patients and doctors to be more cautious, but meanwhile the faith in cures survives and drug advertising grows. The sickness funds also have little leverage over the prescribing by doctors and the dispensing by pharmacists, since those decisions depend on more general public health laws.

The sickness funds that create statistical profiles and perform utilization review over clinical work—described in Chapter Ten—try to use the same methods to monitor physicians' prescribing of drugs. Separate profiles are created for number of prescriptions and average cost per prescription. If a doctor greatly exceeds the average for his peers, the control doctor from the sickness fund urges him to cut back. A German *Kassenärztliche Vereinigung* may reduce payments for his bills for writing prescriptions. The method restrains excess over the average but not the average itself. Several countries with utilization review have substantial levels of drug consumption.

In countries where GPs are paid by capitation fees—such as Dutch statutory health insurance and the British National Health Service—prescriptions are quantifiable items; so statistical profiles and utilization review are employed there too.

Utilization review profiles for drug prescribing are more difficult to construct accurately than the profiles for procedures actually performed and billed by the doctors. They depend on claims forms filled out by pharmacists and might combine all information necessary to collect payment but no more—the doctor's ID number, the drug, the dosage, the cost, and the pharmacist's ID number. A profile of one doctor must be constructed from all the bills submitted by all pharmacists. In practice, profiles are used at present to detect the doctor who causes the system unusually high costs, rather than to detect different prescribing patterns. Utilization review is still far from the capability to detect appropriate and inappropriate prescribing behavior for each patient diagnosis.

Where it is attempted, utilization review inhibits the prescribing doctor but not the patient. The computer could generate profiles of subscribers with much higher-than-average drug consumption. Under fee-for-service systems and in highly competitive medical markets (as in Belgium), such patients shop until they find a doctor willing to prescribe what they want. This defeats policies to restrain overprescribing. But statistical profiles of patients are rarely calculated, and utilization review is not applied to them. The sickness funds themselves compete for subscribers and do not want to antagonize any. Even if the sickness funds wanted to detect overconsumers, the task would be impossible at present—profiles would have to be constructed for millions of persons. Because of these inhibitions and technical difficulties, the cost-sharing requirements are the only practical restraint upon patients.

Traditionally, physicians prescribed at their discretion whatever drugs were recognized. Utilization review was a retrospective method to identify the prescribers of excessive numbers of units. The progress of pharmaceutical science has produced a new problem: expensive new drugs that are not prescribed in large numbers but can still total substantial amounts of money. France in 1991 became the first country to apply prospective screening to any form of clinical practice and to pharmaceuticals in particular. To prescribe a few very expensive drugs, the physician must obtain prior approval from the sickness fund's control doctor.

Bulk Purchases. One might think that a sickness fund could contain costs and simplify the administration by merely buying and distributing all the drugs itself. This is never done on a national scale under statutory health insurance, however, and rarely even under Treasury-financed and government-administered national health services.[21] (I say "rarely," rather than "never," because Sweden's pharmacies are managed and supplied by an autonomous public corporation that negotiates prices with the manufacturers.) Statutory and private insurance employs in pharmaceutical dispensing the same model of small self-employed business as the one used for the rest of primary care: business corporations produce the supplies, and self-employed pharmacists purchase and distribute them on prescription from the self-employed doctors. A few sickness funds in Belgium and France have their own pharmacies and therefore buy and use batches of drugs, but their market shares are small. In the United States, staff-model HMOs, group-model HMOs, and certain state Medicaid programs buy and use batches of drugs, but these are exceptions and constitute a small part of the American market.

The fact that the pharmacists are independent entrepreneurs means they can stock and dispense what they prefer (when the prescription allows an option). If the branded drugs are more profitable, pharmacists refuse to cooperate voluntarily with the governments' and sickness funds' preference to substitute generic drugs. The "reference price" reform in Germany in 1988 was designed to give the patient a financial incentive to request generic drugs from pharmacists.

Private Pharmaceutical Insurance

Europe. In countries with social health insurance, private coverage of drug benefits simply follows the same procedures for drug benefits as those for basic statutory benefits. The extra cash in private health insurance goes into more generous payments to doctors (particularly specialists) and extra benefits in hospitalization (such as charges for first-class rooms). If the government regulates pharmaceutical prices and sets other rules, these apply to the privately insured as well as to everyone else. The pharmacist follows the standard rules and prices of statutory insurance for nearly all his business, and he usually follows them also for the small number of claims forms destined for private health insurance companies. A private carrier may be more generous in coverage of products than the sickness funds' limited list. For such items, usually the patient pays the pharmacist (as would any socially insured person for a negative-list item) and is reimbursed by his private insurer.

United States. America is the one country where nearly all health insurance is private, there is no massive social insurance program to set benchmark prices, and the national government's role in pharmaceuticals is limited to verifying safety and effectiveness. The only public third-party program with a large market share in ambulatory drug coverage—Medicaid—has not been able to enforce its price rules on pharmacists and on the drug industry generally,[22] and only a few pharmacies cooperate. Therefore, American private health insurance has a problem in limiting the numbers and prices of drugs.

The very competitive, well-financed, and worldwide pharmaceutical industry produces a large number of drugs for the same diagnosis. The winner in the competitive race for a new discovery patents the formula, copyrights its brand name, and obtains a license for sale in the United States from the Food and Drug Administration (FDA). The apparent losers do not give up in the American market: they patent slight variations in the formula ("me-too" drugs), copyright their own brand names, and submit evidence to FDA that their products are safe and effective for the same uses. Competition in America then moves to the marketplace: the drug companies send salesmen, advertisements, and samples to persuade doctors to prescribe by brand name; they urge the pharmacists to prefer their brands in case the prescribing doctor authorizes substitutions.[23]

There then ensues a struggle between insurance carriers and drug companies, each trying to influence doctors and pharmacists. The carriers and manufacturers never negotiate directly. The United States government never intervenes in this competitive market. The carriers urge methods that will reduce costs: the doctor should prescribe generically or allow the pharmacist to substitute; the pharmacist should substitute generically if the doctor's prescription gives him discretion; the patient should prefer generic to branded drugs.

Without government price controls and without national health insurance price lists, the many American insurance carriers need guidelines about reasonable prices. The pharmaceutical manufacturers associations and the pharmacists' professional associations are prevented by the antitrust laws from producing industry-wide price lists. Thus everyone relies on catalogues published privately every year for the country's pharmacists; they list all prescription and nonprescription drugs currently on the market, along with their "average wholesale prices" (AWP).[24]

Blue Cross and Blue Shield. For many years, some Plans offered drug benefits in their catch-all major medical contracts. Unlike hospital benefits (but like physician benefits), the method was *tiers garant* and indemnity: the patient bought the drug from the pharmacist, paid in full, sent the receipt to the Plan, and the Plan paid him whatever percentages of the AWP and the pharmacist's dispensing fee were specified by the patient's policy. Blue Cross and Blue Shield

Plans in many states during the 1950s and 1960s developed staffs capable of designing payment proposals and signing "participant physician" agreements with many doctors—and several Plans followed the same procedure with pharmacists. So did the administrators of union group insurance plans in Michigan and California.[25] A disadvantage to the Plan was the high administrative cost in an indemnity system with small claims. A disadvantage to the patient (but a windfall for the Plan) was forgetting to send in receipts.

When commercial insurance companies entered the Blues' group market during the 1970s, wider drug coverage with easy administration was one of their offers. Taking advantage of telecommunications, they offered a *tiers payant* system with minimum cost sharing and greater degrees of third-party standardization and coverage than in the design of their insurance for hospitals and doctors. The Blues had to match the competition by improving their own coverage and by paying participating pharmacists directly. Because each Blue Cross/Blue Shield Plan develops its own packages and methods (and employers vary in attitudes toward drug benefits), the Blues have a great variety of arrangements across the United States. Each Plan develops its own schemes, sells each (if possible) to several employed groups, and signs up "participating pharmacists" to fill the prescriptions from this and all of its drug reimbursement programs. Some Blue Cross/Blue Shield Plans discuss terms to ensure that enough pharmacists will cooperate; others merely fix the rules and rates and assume the pharmacists depend too much on the Blues' business to refuse. The arrangement is entirely between the Plan, the patient, and the pharmacist; it does not involve the physician, the pharmaceutical manufacturer, or the wholesaler.[26]

An increasingly common Blue Cross/Blue Shield arrangement consists of the following elements:

☐ Dispensing fee paid by the Plan to the pharmacist for each medication filled. This is a flat fee set by the Plan, not a percentage of AWP. The percentage would be an incentive to avoid generics and fill each prescription with the most expensive branded drugs. The flat fee is an incentive to use generics, since the pharmacist can maintain a less expensive inventory.

☐ Reimbursement to the pharmacist for each prescription by the product's AWP less a percentage discount. The pharmacist has an incentive to use generics or "me-too" drugs, since the numerous (and very competitive) generic and "me-too" manufacturers offer him prices considerably lower than their discounted AWP. Wholesalers of a widely prescribed and well-known branded drug are under little pressure to discount their AWP. Some Blue Cross/Blue Shield Plans offer to pay a "maximum allowable cost" for a category of drugs. This gives the pharmacist an incentive to dispense a generic and buy the cheapest one in the group.

☐ Copayment that the patient must pay the pharmacist. The size of the copayment determines the cost of the contract and the premiums of the employed group: the higher the copayments, the lower the premiums. Blue Cross/Blue

Shield Plans increasingly craft the copayments to motivate generic substitution: the patient's copayment is lower for a generic drug (about $2 or $3) than for a branded drug ($5 or more).

The patient takes his ID card and physician's prescription to the participating pharmacist, pays his copayment, and allows the pharmacist to feed the card into his computer. The Blue Cross/Blue Shield Plan records all such purchases in its home office and pays the pharmacist for all materials costs and dispensing fees every few weeks. Blue Cross/Blue Shield of Western New York does the claims processing work for itself and a half dozen other Plans throughout the country. (Although the Blues pioneered the new drug benefits, their processing of claims by telecommunications followed the innovations of the commercial sector, to be described in the next section.

If a patient insists on going to a nonparticipating pharmacist, he follows the old-fashioned sequence. He pays the pharmacist in full and is reimbursed by his Plan the amount it would have paid a participating pharmacist (minus the copayment or minus substantial coinsurance). The patient loses money in the pharmacist's extra-billing. Since patients lose money to nonparticipating pharmacists that they save as participants, there is no reason not to go to the latter. Lest they lose business, nearly all pharmacists participate.[27]

Commercial Insurance. When the carriers offered drug insurance on a large scale, they emulated the Blue Cross/Blue Shield benefits: the pharmacists received their acquisiton costs plus a dispensing fee; premiums paid by employers varied according to copayments paid by patients. The Blue Cross/Blue Shield drug benefits varied among the Plans, but the commercial insurance industry—consisting of centralized national carriers—created competing national benefit packages, each with options for the purchaser depending on copayments. While the insurance companies could underwrite insurance, they could not administer relations with pharmacies and could not administer claims since, unlike the Blues, they lacked regional offices. As in their relations with physicians, the commercial insurance companies needed local representatives.

Youthful entrepreneurs then arose to represent health insurers in the tedious work of negotiating with individual pharmacists and processing patient claims. Originating during the 1960s and specializing in pharmaceuticals, they were the precursors of the third-party administrators who offered to manage all health care reimbursement for insurance companies and self-insured groups during the 1980s. Arising in the West, these firms (such as Pharmaceutical Card System, Inc., or PCS) managed drug insurance throughout the country. Some management firms were set up by pharmacists themselves and became nationwide operations (such as Paid Prescriptions).

The spread of these arrangements illustrates how small-scale market relations cannot operate any sector of health care finance. Operating a market by means of millions of localized relations cannot succeed when services like drugs are standardized on a national and even international scale and when the financing depends on large pools such as nationwide or statewide health insurance. The American catalogues of wholesale prices (AWP) for all prescription and nonprescription drugs recommended by each manufacturer provide the acquisition costs to be reimbursed. Within each locality, the management firm discusses the economics of pharmacy operations with several pharmacists, and it proposes AWP minus a discount plus a dispensing fee. The management firm signs up enough participating pharmacists to cover the purchases by the subscribers of the insurance carriers. The management firm then sells its package to as many health insurance companies as it can: each carrier agrees to pay for all wholesale drug costs, pharmacists' markups, and the management's own markup for administration and profit. (The management company charges the carrier a small amount per prescription (such as $0.75), but huge volume from all carriers can produce large and growing earnings.)

The insurance company then sells drug benefit coverage to its groups and individual policyholders at premiums that will cover the operation. The insurance company can offer these policies only in those parts of the country where the management firm has participating pharmacists. But by the late 1980s, coverage had become very extensive: 145 million persons had coverage for prescriptions under employer-sponsored major medical plans. PCS in 1988 alone administered benefits for 18 million of them: PCS was the manager on behalf of 100,000 self-financed plans, 200 insurance companies, 40 Blue Cross and Blue Shield Plans, and more than 50 HMOs.

The health insurance carrier administers its own hospital and physician claims but turns all drug claims administration over to the management firm. Some management firms are subsidiaries of individual insurance companies and work exclusively for them, but the larger ones (such as PCS) handle the business of many carriers in a standardized manner. The insurance company distributes to its drug benefits subscribers an ID card issued by the management firm. The subscriber takes the doctor's prescription and his ID card to a participating pharmacist, pays the pharmacist the copayment or coinsurance required by his policy and indicated on his card, and receives the drug. The pharmacist bills the management firm's central office for the wholesale cost and his markup (less the subscriber's cost sharing). Some systems are now centralized and computerized: PCS, for example, has signed up over 90 percent of all the drugstores in the United States; all the billing and payment is done through PCS headquarters in Scottsdale, Arizona; and all are joined by telecommunications.

Drug benefits were once thought to be unmanageable and uninsurable because of the many small claims, the uncontrollable pricing of the drug companies, the central role of nonphysicians (the pharmacists), the possibility of provider-induced demand (by pharmacists and drug companies), and the possibility of adverse selection and moral hazard by subscribers. The ingenious administrative arrangements described above have solved the tasks of managerial efficiency and standardization in the normally unstructured and chaotic American health care market. But the system requires enough subscribers. Once nearly all ambulatory prescription drugs were paid out-of-pocket. Drug benefits insurance has been growing and by 1990 covered over one-third of all ambulatory prescription drug costs.[28] (Some of this money is recovered from Blue Cross/Blue Shield Plans and from insurance companies who offer reimbursement of drugs under their major medical policies.)

One might think an HMO could limit its use of drugs to the most efficacious and thereby control its costs. Staff-model and group-model HMOs employ both the ambulatory-care doctors and pharmacists, they operate the pharmacies, and they purchase the drugs in bulk. But coverage of all drugs licensed by FDA and prescribed at physicians' discretion is so deeply ingrained in the United States that remarkably few HMOs have ever had formularies, have ever used their full bargaining power to purchase selectively, or have ever regulated the prescribing of their own doctors.[29]

Effects on Utilization and Health

Pharmaceuticals can improve patients' health, longevity, and moods. Some can substitute for more unpleasant and more expensive treatments, such as surgery and prolonged hospitalization.[30] Do the forms of insurance reimbursement make any difference in promoting or inhibiting the beneficial effects of drugs? Do they accentuate or limit the undesirable side effects?

Several important sources of cross-national variations in drug prescribing and drug consumption are completely independent of differences in insurance reimbursement. In particular, national styles of practice differ: some countries prescribe and consume far more drugs than others with similar statutory health insurance coverage. France, for example, is a higher user than its neighbors.[31] But variations in practice style—in drug prescribing as in acute-care treatments—are as wide within as among countries.[32]

Drugs cannot be reimbursed by insurance before they are fully licensed by regulatory agencies as safe and effective. At one time, countries with similar statutory health insurance coverage of licensed drugs varied in the strictness of regulation for safety and effectiveness. A few (like Germany) allowed drugs on the insurance and self-pay market after mere basic testing for safety but might pull them off if trouble arose. Other countries insisted on stricter and longer testing and would then license the survivors once and for all. More drugs would be marketed in the first type of country, and they would have longer periods of earnings before the patents expired. In the second type of country (such as the United States), drug companies and patients (particularly victims of cancer and AIDS) complain about bureaucratic "regulatory lags" that deprive the companies of deserved profits, deprive victims of miraculous cures, and discourage research and innovation in that country's industry.[33] As Europe unified during the 1980s and 1990s, these regulatory differences were reduced.

The rules of health insurance systems affect the structure of the industry, the number and types of drugs on the market, and the frequency of prescribing. Limited lists are recent developments designed to control costs: statutory health insurance will only cover the most cost-effective remedies. No one has yet studied the effects of the limited lists, but I suspect they benefit the original branded drugs and exclude the clinically unnecessary "me-too" creations that the other companies develop and patent in order to win shares of the market. In competitive countries without limited lists, such as the United States, some of the new research of drug companies is devoted to creation of "me-too" drugs for the market.[34] Limited lists force drug companies to use their research capacities for true clinical innovations.

Health insurance—both statutory and private—covers the research and development costs of the producers and guarantees the livelihood of dispensing pharmacists. The principal licensed drugs are covered—and if there is no limited list, all are covered. Reimbursement steadily rises as the costs of new drugs rise. As a result, health insurance has fully guaranteed the creation and widespread sales of all new drugs for decades. Insofar as pharmaceuticals promote health, statutory health insurance has financed it. But prices paid by the health insurance system vary from country to country. In the least controlled countries, such as Germany, the pharmaceutical industry has had plenty of cash for research and development, and the products are sold everywhere else in the world. But in some countries, conservatives grumble that the health insurance prices are not high enough to finance their drug industries' continued innovation.[35]

If too much drug prescribing jeopardizes health, statutory health insurance has financed that too. Prescribing has long been left to the discretion of the doctor as one of his fundamental clinical prerogatives. The system automatically pays the pharmacist his dispensing fee, and he welcomes high volume. Until the introduction of stricter cost controls during the 1980s, there has been very little utilization review to detect doctors who prescribe far more than their peers or to detect patients who present an unusually large number of prescriptions. As Chapter Ten reported, utilization review and quality control over all of physicians' ambulatory care have been lax. The limited monitoring of prescriptions by sickness funds in the past was designed only to detect the submission of fraudulent bills by dispensing physicians and pharmacists. In addition to the statistical profiles now being constructed and analyzed in many countries to detect and caution ambulatory-care physicians who submit an unusually large number of claims, the statistical staffs have now begun similar profiles for physicians' drug prescriptions.

Despite the presence of other determinants of cross-national variations in drug consumption—culture, practice style, safety regulations, limited lists, and utilization review—some features of drug reimbursement may influence the volume. Drug prescribing by doctors is higher in those countries (such as France and Germany) where the fee-for-service system pays the doctor a separate fee for writing a prescription or a complete fee for an office or telephone visit when the patient merely obtained a prescription. Payment of fees in this form may be an incentive to enter fewer doses on each prescription and encourage the patient to renew later.[36] Reimbursement systems that pay pharmacists itemized dispensing fees rather than global amounts (for example, France and Germany rather than Holland) also encourage a national prescribing style—with small doses on each prescription, many renewals, and higher total consumption in the long run. If an insurance system pays doctors by fee-for-service, allows them to dispense as well as prescribe, and pays them the full reimbursement for dispensing by pharmacists—as in Switzerland—the result is higher pharmaceutical costs than if the medical and pharmacist roles are separated.

Cost sharing by patients is thought to restrain overprescribing and overconsumption of pharmaceutical drugs, and now all countries have it. Subscribers soon take the cost sharing for granted, however, and the historic levels of consumption persist. Even a *tiers garant* system wherein the patient pays the pharmacist in full at first does not reduce consumption below the levels of *tiers payant* systems in the face of custom—for example, French health insurance for many years had *tiers garant* and high consumption. Cost sharing may reduce waste rather than consumption: the patient orders only what he needs, but he consumes all that he obtains.

Implications for the United States

Proposing pharmaceutical benefits for a future American national health insurance plan was once very difficult, since few private or public models existed and they were diverse. At best, one could present a catalogue of options and policymakers had little guidance.[37] At first sight, insurance reimbursement in the United States today seems just as diverse as in the past, as disorganized as the markets for physicians and hospitals, and lacking any precedents for national health insurance.

Actually, American ambulatory drug insurance may be on the verge of rationalization and standardization beyond the forms of coverage and reimbursement for physicians and hospitals. Coverage is growing. Elements are already becoming common: the doctor prescribes the drug; the patient has free choice of participating pharmacist; all pharmacists participate and deal with all payers. The pharmacist is then paid his acquisition costs based on the AWP from universally used catalogues; he is paid a flat dispensing fee; he reads the patient's prescription drug card into a standard computer terminal communicating with one or more central offices that administer claims for many insurance carriers. The patient pays a copayment; the claims management office pays the pharmacist in lump-sum installments for all his claims; and the office bills the patients' insurance carriers. While doctors resist standardization and direct payment by carriers and claims managers, pharmacists welcome it: it is much cheaper and simpler if they maintain a single computer terminal with standard software communicating with all payers.

A principal controversy will be whether any future American statutory health insurance pays for all licensed drugs (as at present) or uses a limited list. Politically powerful drug industries (as in Germany) can block enactment of a limited list, but a determined government (as in Switzerland) can overrule a powerful drug industry and impose a limited list for health insurance. Unwilling to cooperate with restrictions on their clinical freedom in acute care, American doctors might not mind limits on the drug companies. Pharmacists should welcome limited lists, since then they could maintain smaller inventories and rent smaller facilities.

In all countries with statutory health insurance—with a few variations—benefits and reimbursement are standardized across all payers. All benefits are covered and paid for in this fashion, including pharmaceutical drugs. A few Europeans now have second thoughts, however, and suggest two-tier designs: basic benefits would be standardized and financed by social security payroll taxes; variable universal benefits, optional benefits, or both would be covered by a second tier of health insurance financed by premiums. Cautious about enacting full-scale statutory health insurance, the Americans might opt for a two-tier design. Pharmaceuticals might be a benefit in the more flexible second tier: carriers could offer competing policies charging lower premiums for higher co-payments and offering a varying mix of drugs. The policies might resemble each other after the competitive market operates for a while—a common outcome of competitive shakedowns. The definition of benefits, claims administration, and reimbursement would become standardized in accordance with the trends I have described. The drawback of such discretion and competition in drug insurance would be the elimination of any financial redistribution: the healthier risks would pick the low-premium options; the heavier users of drugs would pick the high-benefit options but might not be able to afford the high premiums.

Perhaps drug insurance should not be as redistributive as acute-care insurance. Perhaps drug reimbursement should not be conceived and financed in the same way as acute-care payments. Over-the-counter nonprescription drugs are deemed part of the person's living standard and are always a consumer expense. Perhaps routine prescription drugs are so predictable that they too should be a regular consumer expense. Drug benefits as part of statutory health insurance would then be reserved for the very large and unusual claims that are insurable risks.[38] Therefore, the pharmaceutical part of statutory health insurance would have a much higher deductible than the other parts. Besides the premiums and payroll taxes that people pay for their current drug insurance, they would pay a compulsory levy to cover the elderly (much like Medicare Part A today), whereby they would finance their own likely increase in drug use when they no longer had the income to cover it.

Even before enacting statutory drug insurance, Americans are thinking about the design of utilization review and quality assurance in pharmaceutical reimbursement.[39] The telecommunication systems now being developed for claims administration can be invaluable. They can generate nationwide statistical systems capable of generalizing about the consumption of every drug, creating prescribing profiles of all doctors, and creating consumption profiles of all insured patients. By interacting with the data base when the patient presents a new prescription, the pharmacist can detect problems that have escaped doctors and patients in the modern age of advanced pharmaceuticals—namely, the consumption of excessive amounts and incompatible combinations. The system can implement standing orders by doctors and payers to substitute appropriate generics for branded drugs. By the time it is fully operational during the 1990s, the PCS telecommunication system will process 25 percent of all American retail prescriptions.

A fundamental lesson for the United States is that reforms in pharmaceutical drug coverage—as in all other sectors of statutory health insurance—depend on democratic politics. The payers, consumers, drug manufacturers, pharmacists, and political parties enter with different aims. Major changes in lists, prices, and utilization control require determined political leadership. An example of a prolonged struggle and modest outcome is the reform in pharmaceutical drug coverage in West Germany during the 1980s.[40]

Notes

1. Inspection Générale des Affaires Sociales, *Les formes complémentaires de la protection sociale* (Paris: Ministère de la Santé and Ministère du Travail, 1975), pp. 239-249; and Jean Benhamou and Alliette Levecque, *La mutualité* (Paris: Presses Universitaires de France, 1983), pp. 84-88, 90-91.

2. For overviews of the worldwide drug industry see M. L. Burstall and others, *Multinational Enterprises, Governments and Technology: Pharmaceutical Industry* (Paris: Organisation for Economic Co-Operation and Development, 1981); Robert Chew and others, *Pharmaceuticals in Seven Nations* (London: Office of Health Economics, 1985), and *The Consumer and Pharmaceutical Products in the EEC*, 2 vols. (Brussels: Bureau Européen des Unions de Consommateurs, 1984 and 1986). For a history of the occupation of pharmacist—including much about reimbursement in the past—see Glenn Sonnedecker, *Kremer's and Urdang's History of Pharmacy*, 4th ed. (Philadelphia: Lippincott, 1976).

3. For the history and the current situation see Philip R. Lee and Jessica Herzstein, "International Drug Regulation," *American Review of Public Health*, vol. 7 (1986), pp. 217-235 and sources cited.

4. National regulations before the unifying pressures from the Common Market are summarized in Graham Dukes, *The Effects of Drug Regulation* (Lancaster: MTP Press, 1985); William M. Wardell (ed.), *Controlling the Use of Therapeutic Drugs: An International Comparison* (Washington: American Enterprise Institute for Public Policy Research, 1978); *National Drug Policies* (Copenhagen: World Health Organization Regional Office for Europe, 1979), chaps. 2, 9-10; and Frans G. van Andel, "The Legal Mandate of Drug Registration Authorities in Theory and Practice," *Health Policy*, vol. 4 (1985), pp. 231-246.

5. The negotiations have been described regularly in the newsletter *SCRIP: World Pharmaceutical News.*

6. For a description of how governments regulate drug prices and how health insurance systems decide their purchase prices, see *World Drug Market Manual* (London: IMSWorld, constantly updated), especially vols. 1 and 3.

7. As a result of these controls—and the cost explosion in other sectors— the proportion of all health care expenditures devoted to drugs has steadily diminished. See A. Griffiths and Z. Bankowski (eds.), *Economics and Health Policy* (Geneva: Council for International Organizations of Medical Sciences, 1980), p. 120; and Brian Abel-Smith and P. Grandjeat, *Pharmaceutical Consumption* (Brussels: Commission of the European Communities, 1978), pp. 12–16.

8. Price policies of governments are summarized in G. Adriaenssens and H. Sermeus, *Drug Prices and Drug Reimbursement in Europe* (Brussels: Bureau Européen des Unions de Consommateurs, 1987); and Abel-Smith and Grandjeat, *Pharmaceutical Consumption* (see note 7, above); pp. 44–57. The many difficulties in estimating the costs of each company for each product within each country are summarized in Flora M. Haaijer-Ruskamp and M.N.G. Dukes, *Drugs and Money* (Copenhagen: World Health Organization Regional Office for Europe, 1986), pp. 13–20.

9. Limited lists are described in Haaijer-Ruskamp and Dukes, *Drugs and Money* (see note 8, above), pp. 26–28; and in Tony Smith, "Limited Lists of Drugs: Lessons from Abroad," *British Medical Journal*, vol. 290 (Feb. 16, 1985), pp. 532–534. Limited lists are more common under Treasury-based health financing arrangements (such as those described by Smith) than under health insurance (such as the countries described in this book).

10. This volume is the *Farmacotherapeutisch Kompas* (Amstelveen: Ziekenfondsraad, annual).

11. Explained in Klaus von Grebmer, *Pharmaceutical Prices: A Continental View* (London: Office of Health Economics, 1978).

12. See, for example, Fritz Kastner, *Volume and Cost of the Supply of Medicaments* (Geneva: International Social Security Association, 1974); and Romuald K. Schicke, "The Pharmaceutical Market and Prescription Drugs in the Federal Republic of Germany: Cross-National Comparisons," *International Journal of Health Services*, vol. 3, no. 2 (1973), pp. 223–236 and sources cited. German levels of drug expenditures are compared with those of other countries in Robert J. Maxwell, *Health and Wealth* (Lexington, Mass.: Lexington Books, 1981), pp. 71–72, 77–79.

13. For example, the *GKV-Arzneimittelindex* research program of the Wissenschaftliches Institut der Ortskrankenkassen in Bonn.

14. For details see the survey reported in L. Lebeer, *Cost-Sharing by Persons Receiving Health Care Under Sickness Insurance*, report to the Twenty-first General Assembly (Geneva: International Social Security Association, 1983), pp. 18–19, 43–44; and in Gunther Janssen, "Patient Participation in the Cost of

Pharmaceuticals, Hospital Care, and Medical Treatment" (Geneva: Association Internationale de la Mutualité, 1984).

15. See Haaijer-Ruskamp and Dukes, *Drugs and Money* (see note 8, above), pp. 28–30 and sources cited. The result is apparently invariant: it was repeated after publication of *Drugs and Money* by the increases in charges in West Germany. The only exception was found in the Rand insurance experiment conducted in America—atypical for reasons given by Haaijer-Ruskamp and Dukes and possibly superseded had the Rand experiment been a real-life long-term program.

16. Ibid.

17. Patrick Sailly and others, "Assurance maladie: La protection complémentaire maladie à l'ordre du jour," *L'Argus*, March 28, 1986, pp. 774–779.

18. For example, refer to Abel-Smith and Grandjeat, *Pharmaceutical Consumption* (see note 7, above); Antonio Brenna and others, *Comparaison des prix pharmaceutiques dans les pays de la C.E.E.* (Paris: Centre de Recherche pour l'Etude et l'Observation des Conditions de Vie, 1981); and Lynn Payer, *Medicine and Culture* (New York: Henry Holt and Company, 1988), and sources cited.

19. See Abel-Smith and Grandjeat, *Pharmaceutical Consumption* (see note 7, above). Besides differing in the total volume of prescribing, the medical professions of Europe show some differences in what they prescribe for the same diagnosis: Bernie O'Brien, *Patterns of European Diagnosis and Prescribing* (London: Office of Health Economics, 1984).

20. J. P. Heesters and Jos Kesenne, "Le financement des soins de santé en Belgique et aux Pays-Bas," *M Informations* (of the Alliance Nationale des Mutualités Chrétiennes), vol. 3, no. 11 (1985), pp. 18–19, 42–43, 49–50.

21. Pharmaceutical distribution, screening, and reimbursement arrangements in many developed countries are described in Wardell, *Controlling the Use of Therapeutic Drugs* (see note 4, above); Albert I. Wertheimer (ed.), *Proceedings of the International Conference on Drug and Pharmaceutical Services Reimbursement* (Washington: National Center for Health Services Research, 1977); and *World Drug Market Manual* (see note 6, above).

22. See Jean Paul Gagnon and Raymond Jang, *Federal Control of Pharmaceutical Costs: The MAC Experience* (New York: Health Issues/Roche Laboratories, 1979); and Milton Silverman and others, *Pills and the Public Purse* (Berkeley: University of California Press, 1981), pp. 86–88, 175–176. As the new third-party methods limited pharmacies' acquisition costs and made pharmacies more efficient, however, some discovered they could profit under the Medicaid reimbursement ceilings; see Richard P. Kusserow, *Changes to Medicaid Prescription Drug Program Could Save Millions* (Washington: Office of Inspector General, U.S. Department of Health and Human Services, 1984).

23. The creation, manufacturing, regulation, and selling of pharmaceutical drugs in the United States are described in Milton Silverman and Philip R. Lee, *Pills, Profits and Politics* (Berkeley: University of California Press, 1974).

24. *Drug Topics Red Book* (Oradell, N.J.: Medical Economics, annual); and *American Druggist Blue Book* (New York: Hearst Corporation, annual).

25. The drug programs of the 1950s and 1960s are described in J. F. Follmann, *Medical Care and Health Insurance* (Homewood, Ill.: Richard D. Irwin, 1963), chap. 11.

26. For a description of Blue Cross/Blue Shield drug benefits just before the advent of claims processing by telecommunications, see Silverman and others, *Pills and the Public Purse* (see note 22, above), pp. 176–178.

27. The bewildering variety of reimbursement methods for prescription drugs today is summarized in articles by Vincent Gardner, Stephen Schondelmeyer, and James Richards in *Final Report of the APhA Pharmacy Commission on Third Party Programs* (Washington: American Pharmaceutical Association, 1986). The early years of the commercial insurers' organized national drug benefits programs are described in *Pharmaceutical Payment Programs* (Washington: Pharmaceutical Manufacturers Association, 1973), pp. 22–26, 137–139; see also *A Course in Group Life and Health Insurance*, rev. ed. (Washington: Health Insurance Association of America, 1985), pt. A, pp. 76–78, and pt. B, pp. 111–112.

28. Stephen W. Schondelmeyer and Joseph Thomas III, "Trends in Retail Prescription Expenditures," *Health Affairs*, vol. 9, no. 3 (Fall 1990), p. 137.

29. Silverman and others, *Pills and the Public Purse* (see note 22, above), pp. 178–180; and Karen Southwick, "HMO's and Drugmakers Tangle over Slashing Costs," *Managed Health Care*, Aug. 14, 1989, pp. 1, 27. Several more diligent HMO in-house pharmacies are described in S. J. Miller, "A Survey of Nationwide Health Maintenance Organization Prescription Benefit Programs" (master's thesis, University of Maryland, 1985).

30. Documented in many sources, such as the series published by the Pharmaceutical Manufacturers Association, Washington, 1984.

31. Comparisons in national attitudes toward drug consumption (shared by doctors and patients) appear throughout Payer, *Medicine and Culture* (see note 18, above) and the many sources cited. For a discussion of the wide differences among European countries in aggregate average prescribing frequencies, see Abel-Smith and Grandjeat, *Pharmaceutical Consumption* (see note 7, above), especially pp. 25–26; and O'Brien, *Patterns of European Diagnosis and Prescribing* (see note 19, above).

32. Poppe Siderius, "European Studies of Drug Consumption," in David Alan Ehrlich (ed.), *The Health Care Cost Explosion: Which Way Now?* (Bern: Hans Huber, 1975), pp. 139–145.

33. See Dukes, *The Effects of Drug Regulation* (see note 4, above), pp. 21–30, and many attacks by the American drug industry on the Food and Drug Administration, such as Henry G. Grabowski, *Drug Regulation and Innovation* (Washington: American Enterprise Institute for Public Policy Research, 1976). Grabowski compares FDA unfavorably with Europe's more permissive regulators.

34. Silverman and Lee, *Pills, Profits and Politics* (see note 23, above), pp. 4–5, 39–43. The smaller market share by patented and brand-name "me-too"

drugs in Europe is evident in Otto H. Nowotny and George Teeling Smith, *L'industrie pharmaceutique en Europe occidentale* (Brussels: European Federation of Pharmaceutical Industries' Associations, 1981), pp. 21–23. Another reason for the development of "me-too" drugs is to enable a company to recover some of the costs of research and development when it has lost the race to patent and market a major drug.

35. Hansruedi Sutter, *La réglementation du prix des médicaments: Ses effets sur les dépenses de santé en Suisse* (Basel: Pharma Information, 1982); and *Rapport du Comité des Sages* (Paris: Etats Généraux de la Sécurité Sociale, 1987), pp. 55–56.

36. Abel-Smith and Grandjeat, *Pharmaceutical Consumption* (see note 7, above), pp. 25–26.

37. See, for example, Milton Silverman and Mia Lydecker, *Drug Coverage Under National Health Insurance: The Policy Options*, DHEW Publication (HRA) 77-3189 (Washington: National Center for Health Services Research, 1977).

38. Robert G. Evans and M. F. Williamson, *Extending Canadian Health Insurance: Options for Pharmacare and Denticare* (Toronto: University of Toronto Press, 1978), pp. 47–49.

39. See, for example, Duane M. Kirking, "Drug Utilization Review: A Component of Drug Quality Assurance," in *Final Report of the APhA Pharmacy Commission on Third Party Programs* (see note 27, above), pp. 81–91.

40. Philip Manow-Borgwardt, *Neokorporatistische Gesundheitspolitik? Die Festbetragsregelung des Gesundheitsreformgesetzes* (Berlin: Wissenschaftszentrum, 1991).

CHAPTER 13

Dentistry Services

———————————— **Summary** ————————————

Once dental care was part of public health; it was delivered primarily to school-children by salaried dentists. Dental care was covered by statutory health insurance only if it involved serious surgery. After World War II, dentistry was recognized as part of primary care and was added to both statutory and private health insurance in nearly all countries.

The list of dental benefits has become much the same, but the design of reimbursement varies among countries. Many require less cost sharing for children (or none at all), while adult patients must pay something. Some apply the same cost-sharing rules as in acute-care health insurance; others require more in dentistry. In a few countries, such as Germany, health insurance carriers compete for subscribers by offering more generous benefits, and these may include more dental procedures and less cost sharing by patients.

At one time, health insurance carriers in a few countries (such as France and Belgium) delivered care at their own health centers. Some centers still employ salaried dentists for their own or any other insured persons. But the dental profession now prefers the medical model: the dentists are self-employed and may treat all patients under statutory and private dental insurance. Once dentists prospered, since they were few and demand was high. But surpluses of dentists now seem imminent because of improvements in the public's dental health.

Dentistry is reimbursed by the same procedures as in acute care. The dental association and the health insurance carriers negotiate a contract, a fee schedule, and the monetary conversion factor. The individual dentist follows the fee schedule and its rules when he bills the carrier (in the service benefits schemes of

Holland and Germany) or when he bills the patient (in the cash benefits schemes of France and Belgium).

Cost sharing by patients is required for several reasons. Dental benefits were added in a period when government and carriers needed to contain costs, and cost sharing permitted the addition of benefits without the cost explosion that occurred in earlier stages of insurance expansion. Patients may be deterred from making clinically unnecessary visits and dentists may be deterred from giving unnecessary treatments—both hazards in dental insurance. Cost sharing and legally authorized extra-billing enable the patient to select a cosmetically pleasing but more expensive form of the care covered by the basic insurance.

The cost-sharing rules are now being designed to encourage preventive dentistry. Since periodic checkups and preventive care reduce the likelihood of future treatments, the patient need not pay for them. But cost sharing—sometimes substantial—is required for fillings, extractions, and prostheses. The method is used in statutory dental insurance in Germany and Holland and in much private dental insurance in the United States.

Dentistry provides a niche for private health insurance. It may cover the cost sharing required under statutory health insurance, as in France. It may become the carrier for the special regimes for the self-employed, as in France and Belgium. It may cover the entire population, if a publicly financed arrangement for the population is confined to acute care and omits dentistry, as in Canada. Recently there have been proposals to redesign health insurance into a two-tier scheme in all countries providing a large voluntary dental market for the private carriers.

Early Dental Care Financing

When health insurance originates and spreads—at first through nonprofit voluntary funds and later under law—it is designed for acute medical care by doctors and hospitals. Painful oral conditions that require surgery are covered under maxillofacial surgery performed by physicians or by dentists qualified in oral surgery. Some early laws covered extractions as well. A few early laws paid for prostheses (including dentures) to remedy the effects of surgery and handicaps. But other less serious dental conditions were omitted from the early health insurance laws and left to the private consumer market: individuals were expected to pay in full privately for fillings and routine dentistry.

So long as routine dentistry was not considered as urgent as acute-care health services and was not covered by statutory health insurance, dental care was underdeveloped. Cavities, periodontal disease, and edentulousness were widespread in Europe, particularly among the poor. Only the rich patronized dentists substantially; class differences were far more marked in dental than in somatic health. Because of the low demand, every European country had more doctors than dentists—usually three or four times as many. As in all free medical markets, the dentists clustered in the cities where the paying patients lived.[1]

Public Dental Programs

Universal access to routine dentistry originated before World War II as a form of preventive medicine. It was provided and paid for like the rest of preventive medicine (that is, by salaried employees of local or higher governments) and not like statutory health insurance for acute care (that is, not by office practitioners receiving fees or by hospital staffs receiving salaries). Like much of preventive medicine, the benefits were targeted to specific groups and were not universally available. Special programs were installed in the primary schools of nearly every country to detect problems and teach dental care. In some countries, these salaried public dentists treated the defects they discovered; in others, they referred the children to private dentists. The organization and salaried remuneration of the public programs made it possible to use dental nurses and other dental auxiliaries in delivering care, as well as using dentists.[2]

After World War II, the definition of primary care was broadened in all countries and the value of dentistry was recognized. Periodontal disease and edentulousness were seen to damage comfort, nutrition, and general health. General practitioner care was incomplete without dental fitness through preventive dentistry.

The British National Health Service committed itself to all forms of dentistry from the start as part of its philosophy of complete primary care and preventive medicine. Because it was universal in its access rules and commitments, it could not add dentistry slowly and incrementally, as statutory health insurance could. But the prior dental neglect and, therefore, the demand for dental care under NHS proved far greater than any predictions. The dentists refused to accept the payment arrangements that would have enabled NHS to operate like a school dental service—namely, salaries (like hospital consultants) or capitation fees (like general practitioners). The government needed the cooperation of the dentists to deliver its promises of universal access, and the dentists insisted on payment that makes this sector of NHS work like NHI—that is, fees for individual services. From the start of the NHS, Britain's few dentists were swamped with work, learned to work very rapidly, and prospered.[3]

Statutory Health Insurance Coverage

Adding Dental Benefits to Insurance. By the 1980s, all statutory health insurance programs covered dentistry. Although one easily presumes that it is "natural" to include it, adding what was long considered a private consumer service provided by a nonphysician required a gradual redefinition of health care. The evolution varied among countries: in some, oral surgery and extractions were long established, since they were included in the earliest health insurance statutes; in other countries, dentistry had to be added to fully developed acute-care coverage for the first time.[4]

France was a country where the first statute in 1930 included dental surgery and extractions. Dental prostheses were paid for if approved by a special committee. Dental benefits were added to the law from time to time, particularly during the 1960s and 1970s. At the same time, more groups in the population were being added as beneficiaries. Therefore, dental coverage in the population rapidly grew.

Germany had a unique history in that dental coverage was expanded by judicial decisions, not by legislative amendments. That dentistry was a form of medical care was established by the inclusion of extractions and dentures in the list of benefits in the law of 1911. The law stated that the purpose of insurance was the diagnosis and treatment of "sickness." After a series of lawsuits brought by dental associations, the courts held that dental deficiencies were "sicknesses" and that a series of special and routine dental treatments were fully reimbursable by the sickness funds—exactly like the services of doctors. Only dentures are not fully covered. The result is the most comprehensive of all national coverages and high incomes for the German dentists.

Benefits Covered at Present. Some countries include in the health insurance package covered by payroll taxes certain dental benefits but not others. Such a boundary cannot be maintained in the somatic benefits under basic health insurance: benefits have been steadily added to include whatever doctors do. And probably the boundary cannot be long maintained in statutory dental insurance. An illustration is the experience of the Netherlands. From the start of obligatory health insurance until 1972, the benefits included basic dentistry (fillings, extractions, and checkups) but not crowns and dentures. During the 1970s, it was decided in Holland and elsewhere that lifelong dental health depended on thorough early treatment. Many additional benefits were offered to Dutch children and teenagers under insurance. The adults and the dentists pressed to make crowns and dentures universal benefits, and so they were during the 1980s. Benefits were expanded despite a national financial crisis in social security and health insurance. The unavoidable compromise—as a later page will explain—was to require substantial cost sharing for the new adult benefits, an unusual deviation from the paid-in-full customs of Dutch health insurance.[5]

Switzerland demonstrates another approach: complete separation between medical and dental insurance. Subscriber premiums and the *Bund* subsidy enable the sickness funds to cover acute-care services of doctors and hospitals. But dental insurance is sold by the sickness funds as a separate policy. It is expensive, though, since the *Bund* offers no subsidy and employers pay no premiums. Few people buy it.

Separation of medical and dental insurance is more feasible in Switzerland than in the countries with more comprehensive and more generously financed health insurance. But the two programs are never fully united in any country. Since patients and dentists have discretion in defining benefits (such as the quality of dentures) and since dentistry has more cost sharing authorized by law, dentistry overlaps both social and private financing. Some proponents of an orderly two-tier insurance system recommend that statutory health insurance be restricted to medical services and that all adult dentistry be assigned to a private voluntary sector, giving private health insurance an important niche. Social insurance would save money, dentists would no longer collect excessive total payments from both sickness funds and adult patients, and the responsibilities of dentist and patient would become clear, they say.[6]

By the 1990s, unusually complete statutory health insurance systems cover a considerable range of benefits (conservation, dental surgery, prostheses, periodontal, and orthodontic) with no more cost sharing than is required for somatic benefits. The example of this exceptional generosity is Germany; the need to contain costs led in 1989 to increased cost sharing but not to elimination of any benefits. France covers all these benefits with the standard acute-care cost-sharing rates, but it allows dentists to extra-bill patients substantially. Some countries (such as Belgium) cover the aforementioned benefits, but not periodontal work. A few (like Holland) cover some (but not all) of these benefits and require higher cost sharing than that used in somatic services. The Treasury-supported national health services of Britain, Scandinavia, and Eastern Europe officially have maximum benefits and minimum cost sharing. But because of scarcities of funds and services—for example, in orthodontics—free care is guaranteed in the latter countries only for medically necessary cases, either by regulation or by waiting lists.[7]

The basic benefits are listed in the health insurance statute. All insured persons are entitled to receive them, and their providers are paid by the sickness funds. The carrier may offer additional benefits under the basic coverage or under private supplementary policies. Optional benefits become one of the tactics in competitive health insurance markets, such as Germany. The prosperous sickness funds there try to attract more members not by quoting lower premiums but by offering additional benefits, such as dentures and crowns. The extra cash in a German sickness fund's accounts varies around the country, according to the incomes of subscribers and the costs of medical care. In provinces where a sickness fund is especially prosperous, it will offer dentures and crowns with less or no cost sharing by patients. Less prosperous sickness funds cannot risk omitting dentures and crowns in their advertising, but they may be able to afford only one-third of the cost.

Providers

Dentistry involves several different services: diagnosis, treatment, health teaching, and other preventive work. Health teaching is performed with groups as well as with individual patients. Public health care—such as the dental services for schoolchildren—is delivered by salaried teams of dentists and paradentals.[8]

Statutory health insurance in every country has adopted for medical services the model of the self-employed doctor who manages an office, employs helpers, and charges fees to cover costs and net income. Dental coverage has mimicked the medical model: it covers tests and treatments for trauma and illness, and it pays self-employed dentists to provide specific services. It does not pay teams; the dentist is free to use his revenue to pay paradental employees.

When some sickness funds created health centers a century ago, they employed dentists as well as general medical practitioners and pharmacists. Like the doctors, the dentists were salaried full-timers or part-timers. The equipment, like the rest of the health center, was owned by the sickness fund. These arrangements survive today in the *mutuelles* of Belgium and France. The arrangement is identical with the one for physicians and pharmacists. A subscriber to the *mutuelle* may use the dentist in the health center. He avoids any cash payment and might not be billed any statutory cost sharing. The *mutuelle* recovers its costs by billing the main financing system (in France, CNAMTS or a special regime) according to the dental fee schedule. Any other member of the public may use the dentist at the health center, but he is billed the full official fee and must recover the official reimbursement (less the cost sharing) from his sickness fund. Usually nonmembers of *mutuelles* go to the ordinary office dentists rather than to the health centers.[9]

During the years of closed medical panels, some countries (such as Germany) limited the numbers of physicians admitted to ambulatory insurance practice. Pressures from the medical association have since eliminated quotas and entry procedures. The only survival in primary medical care is the limitation on the number of Dutch pharmacists in insurance practice. The dental associations—like the medical associations—now insist that all licensed dentists have the right to practice in any part of the country under insurance.

During the first decades of coverage under statutory health insurance, the problem was a shortage rather than a surplus of dentists. In previous years, when patients had to pay out-of-pocket and dental health was not publicized, utilization was low. As treatments and dentists' incomes rose under social insurance, dental school enrollment grew and new schools were created. But unlike the steady increase in medical utilization—because of the aging of the population and the survival of the disabled—dental demand does not grow indefinitely and may even decline. After the initial period of catchup by newly insured patients, utilization stabilizes. Fluoridation may soon cause a decline in dental disease. Leaders of the dental profession and the sickness funds now fear results from a surplus of dentists:[10] too many had been hastily trained and were doing poor work; if dentists had too few patients they would extra-bill in violation of the reimbursement rules and would treat healthy teeth. But the law allowed every licensed dentist to treat socially insured patients.

So far, only one country has mustered the political power to revoke this right—Holland, which had a tradition of limiting entry to primary-care insurance practice and needed to solve a financing crisis. In 1984, Holland limited entry of new dentists into insurance practice if the result would be more than one dentist for every 3,250 subscribers under statutory health insurance. All dentists may practice in Holland's large private market.

If a country cannot limit the supply of licensed providers in insurance practice, it may try to limit the numbers getting licenses in the first place. The Ministries of Health and Education in Germany, Holland, and several other countries have used their powers to reduce supply: they have closed dental schools (particularly the low-quality ones) and have reduced the size of graduating classes. (The Ministries have not yet become bold enough to cut back the medical schools in like fashion.)

Paying the Dentist

Reimbursement of the office dentist follows the same methods as paying the general medical practitioners and medical specialist. A fee schedule lists the benefits and their relative values. Joint committees from the sickness funds and dental associations periodically revise it completely and, in between, keep it up to date. Every year, the sickness funds and the dental association negotiate the "conversion factor" giving a financial value to every procedure in the fee schedule. The fee is supposed to cover the practice costs and net income of the country's average dentist, but the figures result from power bargaining. The negotiators still lack the data about practice costs and average incomes that have accumulated for doctors—partly because the dental associations have not yet built up research staff and partly because dentists do not cooperate with researchers.

Since every country applies to dentistry the decision-making methods originating in medicine, Germany has a dental counterpart of its unique reimbursement system. Nationwide negotiations occur between a bargaining team from the national associations of sickness funds and specially constituted National Association of Dentists in Insurance Practice (the *Kassenzahnärztliche Bundesvereinigung*). They create a framework contract and the fee schedule. The actual financial values and supplementary administrative arrangements are settled in each province by a bargaining team from the sickness funds and the provincial dentists (a *Kassenzahnärztliche Vereinigung*, or KZV).

Claims are administered in every country by the same procedure as the one used in medicine. In several (such as Holland), the dentist bills the sickness funds directly. In France and Belgium, the patient pays the dentist, receives a receipt, and is reimbursed by the sickness fund. In Germany, the KZVs administer the dentists' claims and use money sent them in aggregate installments by the sickness funds.

If a population is very conscious of dental health and cost sharing is low, total national spending on dentistry is high and the incomes of dentists may exceed those of doctors. An example is West Germany. Around 1985, patient out-of-pockets in all of dentistry were only about 12.9 percent in Germany and much higher—between 25 and 70 percent—in other developed countries. Dentistry consumed about 1.06 percent of the gross national product in Germany, but 0.73 percent or less elsewhere. Dentistry absorbed almost 14 percent of all health care spending in Germany, and much lower proportions elsewhere.[11] Because of the efficient organization of work in dental practice and because of generous fees under statutory health insurance, the average German self-employed dentist earns more than the average office doctor.[12] Dentists were the first health professionals to take advantage of the right of free movement in the European Economic Community—by transferring from the tightening Dutch market to Germany.

Patient Cost Sharing

Rates of Cost Sharing. Statutory health insurance originated to cover acute care, and resources have been used primarily to pay doctors and hospitals. In some countries, third-party payment is complete. In other countries, such as France and Belgium, patients are expected to bear coinsurance—25 percent of every fee, for example—as Chapter Ten explained. In these countries, the identical coinsurance rates apply to every basic dental service, such as fillings and extractions. The reasons are the same as those for cost sharing in medical services:

☐ *Utilization control.* Patients would be deterred from unnecessary visits. Dentists would hesitate before performing complex treatments.
☐ *Cost shifting.* Instead of burdening the payroll taxes and government subsidies, health care costs would be shifted in part to the users.

In most countries, cost-sharing rates are higher for some dental benefits than for others. This is true for several reasons:

☐ The benefits with higher cost sharing—crowns, dentures, and the like—have been added after the bulk of medical and basic dental services were in place. By the 1970s, cost containment became urgent. Therefore, instead of refusing to add these benefits to statutory health insurance, there was a compromise: they were added at less than full reimbursement.
☐ Several dental benefits—particularly crowns and dentures—serve cosmetic appearance and comfort as well as medical need. Dentists can provide technically adequate versions at minimum cost, but patients prefer something better. Society should not bear a personal consumption purchase. Thus, the statutory program pays an "allowance" equal to the cost of the basic service plus the dentist's honorarium. The patient and dentist are left free to select a more pleasing product and can negotiate any extra payment by the patient.

Extra-Billing over the Fee Schedule. Health insurance systems that pay doctors directly for services do not allow extra-billing of the patient. The same rules once automatically applied to the basic services of dentists—as in Germany and the Netherlands. The commitments to pay in full and to win the cooperation of all the country's dentists required German and Dutch sickness funds to concede high fees and set aside enough money in the health insurance budgets. But Germany in the late 1980s was forced to change this traditional arrangement: the costs of health insurance needed to be controlled; the dental association had not cooperated as well as the medical and hospital associations in fixing and implementing expenditure caps; utilization rates by the public were high; the German population was prosperous enough to pay cash; and the junior partner in the governing coalition (the Free Democratic Party) had always opposed third-party payment-in-full. Thus, Parliament in late 1988 enacted a controversial law requiring patients to share between 25 and 40 percent of dental claims. But extra-billing at the discretion of the dentist is still not allowed.

Preventing extra-billing is much more difficult in a *tiers garant* system, wherein the patient pays the provider and is reimbursed by the sickness fund according to the official fee schedule. After decades of complaints by French patients that doctors were extra-billing so much that they were not getting their money's worth from their payroll taxes, the de Gaulle government forced the medical profession to follow the fee schedule in the charges. But such controls have never been imposed on French dentists for several reasons: if extra-billing is tolerated, payment from the sickness funds can be kept down. Moreover, since most dental bills are low and dental extra-billing is small, monitoring the bills is cumbersome and expensive. Dentistry has a weaker professional organization than medicine, and dentists are notoriously uncooperative with their own associations. After several struggles, the Belgian government and sickness funds never succeeded in banning extra-billing by the doctors and avoided an even less promising battle with the dentists.

France allows extra-billing because costs for the same procedure can be variable for legitimate reasons and the patient can elect and share the higher costs. In contrast to the standardized nature of much medical practice, dentistry can be performed with materials varying in quality and cosmetic appearance. French health insurance pays for dental work of minimum quality. The patient can choose something better but must pay the dentist's extra charges himself. In prostheses—the chief source of extra-billing—the dentist and patient sign and the patient keeps a form specifying the procedure, the dentist's full charge, and the sickness fund's reimbursement. The form tells whether the patient obtained the advice of the sickness fund. The entire procedure is prescribed by the contract negotiated between the sickness funds and the national dental association. Disputes are resolved by the joint utilization review committee representing the sickness funds and dentists in each locality.

The considerable amounts of recorded and unrecorded extra-billing (plus the official cost sharing) mean that half of dental claims are now paid for out-of-pocket: 38.5 percent is covered by statutory health insurance and 9.8 percent by the *mutuelles*. Out-of-pockets decreased during the 1970s but increased during the 1980s. (In contrast, over two-thirds of all French physicians' claims are covered by statutory health insurance and most of the rest—the official cost sharing—is covered by the *mutuelles*.)[13] The Socialist government of the 1980s hoped to improve dental practice and protect subscribers from capricious extra-billing by increasing its share of the fees, but cost containment prevented a change.

Motivating Preventive Dentistry. The Netherlands now deviates from its medical insurance model by offering different coverages and requiring different official cost sharing from different beneficiaries. Until the 1970s, Holland provided the same benefits without charge in both medical and dental care to all age groups. But a belief spread in all countries that children should have special protection, since early care will guarantee lifelong dental health. Children under nineteen years were then offered benefits—such as orthodontics and crowns—not available to adults. During the 1980s, these benefits were extended to all persons under statutory health insurance. But since the accounts could not afford the full costs, cost sharing was introduced for the first time in Dutch health insurance. Children are not charged lest they be deterred from seeking timely care. Persons over nineteen, however, are charged. The fee depends on estimates of the total dental insurance accounts during the coming year: if utilization is expected to be high and expensive, charges are raised to enable the dental accounts to break even from all their revenue sources. Dutch dentistry became one of the first sectors in health insurance anywhere with global budgeting and fine-tuning of certain variables (whether premiums, charges, or provider fees) in order to keep aggregate expenditures within targets.[14]

Two common problems in acute care and health insurance are motivating patients to seek preventive care and rewarding doctors for giving it. The need is great in dentistry: patients who obtain periodic examinations and prophylaxis incur fewer of the serious conditions that burden them and account for much of the costs of dental insurance. Dentists welcome such visits since their profession believes in prophylaxis and the program increases business. A trend in many countries now—in statutory health insurance in Holland and Germany, in publicly financed dentistry in Sweden, and in some private American dental insurance—is to use differential cost sharing that rewards the conscientious and penalizes the neglectful. The scheme is called "bonus malus." For example, Dutch dental insurance reduces cost sharing for adult patients who are "dentally fit." The Dutch patient obtains a special claims form (a *sanieringskaart*) from his sickness fund. The dentist enters his treatments, certifies that the patient is now "dentally fit," and uses the form to bill the sickness fund. A new form must be issued and used every six months.

When Germany introduced cost sharing by patients for the first time in 1989, it adopted the bonus-malus variations. Cost-sharing rates are higher for the more expensive treatments than for the simpler ones: up to 60 percent is paid by the patient. If the patient goes to his dentist regularly for examinations and prophylaxis, his sickness fund pays 10 percent more of each treatment fee. If he has gone regularly for ten years, the sickness fund pays 15 percent more.

Denial of benefits may be used as a financial sanction against neglect. Under Belgian statutory health insurance, for example, dentures are covered only for persons over fifty years. If someone under that age needs dentures, it is presumed that he failed to use the diagnostic and therapeutic services available under dental coverage. Therefore, his coinsurance for dentures is 100 percent, not the

Belgian norm of 25 percent. After the age of fifty, loss of teeth can be due to aging rather than neglect, so dentures are covered.

Private Health Insurance

Supplementary Arrangements. In some countries (such as Germany now and Holland in the past), the rich must rely on private companies for all insurance, including full coverage of dentistry. In the social insurance regimes for the self-employed (as in France and Belgium) private companies can be the carriers. In both these arrangements, the private carriers have higher revenue and lower somatic-care costs than the sickness funds, and they can afford more generous dental coverage.

Because so many statutory health insurance systems require considerable cost sharing, tolerate extra-billing, and omit certain benefits, the private health insurance industry finds a niche for policies that supplement social insurance. Dentistry is the principal source of cost sharing in most countries and could become the principal argument for supplementary coverage. But much of the public is still apathetic about dentistry and is resigned to giving the dentist extra cash. When a population becomes more interested in dentistry (as in Germany), it presses the social insurance sector to improve the coverage and reduce its cost sharing. If some sickness funds have enough cash to offer better dental benefits, persons may transfer to them rather than buy a supplementary private dental policy. An example of such movements to carriers with better dental benefits under the basic payroll tax is the increased membership in Germany's *Ersatzkassen.*

If a statutory health insurance or national health service omits dentistry completely, the only third-party coverage must be private. One of the few examples is Canada. The only niches for private health insurance in Canada are dentistry,[15] auto accidents, and work accidents. If subscribers paid the premiums themselves, they might prefer to self-insure and pay dental claims when they arise, thereby saving the extra loadings to support the insurance companies. But much of the Canadian market is sold through employer-paid groups involving a complete set of fringe benefits.

All countries with statutory health insurance have fee schedules of dental benefits, usually negotiated between dental associations and sickness funds. Since private insurance supplements social insurance by covering the cost sharing or by covering in full those not obligatorily insured—in dentistry as well as in medical care—the private insurers use both the medical and dental fee schedules in social insurance as their benchmarks for calculating their own payments. If a private carrier opposes provider extra-billing—as do the French *mutuelles*—it will reimburse only the official cost sharing not covered by the social insurance funds. The French *mutuelles* administer the claims of office dentists as they do those of office doctors: the subscriber pays the dentist in full, the *mutuelle* reimburses the subscriber in full (including the amount of the coinsurance), and the *mutuelle* bills the social security *caisse* for the officially reimbursed amount.

Private supplementary insurance may offer to cover more than the statutory cost sharing if it caters to upper-class subscribers. Dentists extra-bill the rich on the grounds that the rich demand more time-consuming work, seek better materials, and can afford higher-priced providers. Willingness to cover more expensive dentistry is part of the image-making and sales strategy of private dental insurance. But the companies cannot afford to guarantee payment in full, since dentists have a reputation for overcharging and private insurance has to keep premiums reasonable. Therefore, subscribers bear more of the extra-billing by dentists. Patients are expected to shop in order to keep down their out-of-pocket payments.

Actuarial calculations in dental insurance differ from those in medical insurance. The elderly use medicine more but use dentistry less. German and Swiss private health insurance companies calculate age-of-entry level premiums for dental as well as for medical insurance, but they follow different principles in covering expected lifetime costs. As age of enrollment increases, medical premiums rise substantially but dental premiums do not.

The United States. A completely private system has no public model for the specification of benefits—either as a supplementary or substitute carrier—or for the payment of providers. America's one statutory health insurance program, Medicare, has no dental benefits. America's public and private health insurance has been preoccupied with medical care; until recently, basic nonsurgical dentistry was ignored. Dental problems did not threaten life or generate catastrophic bills. The dental profession did not press for organized prepayment.

Significant dental insurance programs arose during the 1950s—pushed by unions creating their own comprehensive health insurance or pressing employers for fringe benefits.[16] Dental insurance gradually increased in coverage: when employer group contracts expanded benefits during the 1970s and early 1980s, dentistry, pharmaceuticals, and mental care were the favorite additions. By 1986, about 40 percent of the American population had some sort of dental coverage, nearly all through groups. Since Blue Cross and Blue Shield have always been oriented to hospital and medical services, they have only about 15 percent of the dental business—that is, about 6 percent of the American population. By the late 1980s, nearly every dentist had some insured patients; three-quarters reported that over half their patients had some sort of coverage, but the mix of insured and uninsured varied widely among dentists. Since every dental policy requires cost sharing, considerably less than 40 percent of American dental expenditure is insured.[17]

The proportion of costs covered by insurance is not merely less than 40 percent but considerably less. Of the $32.8 billion spent on dental care in 1987, only 36.9 percent was paid by private insurance and 61.0 percent was out-of-pocket.[18] Because of the widespread confusion about insurance in the United

States, I suspect that many people belong to groups with dental benefits but do not realize it. They think their health insurance covers only medical care and do not use the dental coverage.

Calculating dentists' fees is always problematic. Americans do not use fee schedules, and payments by a public program are not available as a benchmark. (Medicaid covers dentistry in some states, but few dentists participate and the bulk of the profession would not accept Medicaid rates.) If a carrier has many contracts in the region and a sufficient data base from claims, it often tries to calculate a "reasonable charge." After rank-ordering all the bills for each procedure by size of charge, it picks a percentile (such as the 70th) as the "reasonable charge" it might cover (less whatever coinsurance it requires of the patient). Patients are free to use more expensive dentists and pay the additional cost out-of-pocket. The alternative method by a carrier is issuance of an indemnity schedule: for each procedure, the patient must pay the dentist's bill and can then collect the standard reimbursement from the carrier. The indemnity method makes unnecessary the calculation of a "reasonable charge" from all the claims in a region. The American carrier can offer more generous reimbursement if the employer offers higher premiums. Many groups now are contributory, particularly for family coverage.

Under medical insurance—both in European social security and in the American private system—the carrier accepts the physician's decisions and pays after completion of the work. But third parties and government have less trust in dentists. For expensive courses of treatment, such as orthodontics, some American dental insurance carriers require prior approval. Before the dentist proceeds and before the patient is reimbursed, the dentist must file a "treatment plan" in advance and the carrier must approve. The method restrains unnecessary work and overcharging; it is supposed to protect quality.

Effects on Utilization and Health

Dental health has steadily improved in all developed countries. The decline of edentulousness, toothaches, and caries is self-evident. Once complaints about dental problems were common; now they have almost disappeared. The improvement appears in the data gathered unsystematically by many countries.[19] But it is impossible to weight the many causes since they have operated simultaneously: improved nutrition, better self-care, public health programs (particularly fluoridation of the drinking water), more and better-trained dental personnel, better technology, public dental services, and access through third-party financing.

Cross-national comparisons of the effects of different financing arrangements on utilization and health have been hindered by the fact that systematic collection of standardized data across many countries has begun only recently.[20] Even within one country, systematic data are rarely collected about dental health and dental financing, and therefore one cannot infer the effects of different financing methods. When important innovations are adopted, such as bonus-malus cost sharing by patients, they are not accompanied by evaluation studies.

Insurance provides access for more people, but it does not automatically increase utilization and dental health, because of the persistence of old habits. The better educated have always used dental services more often than the less educated, even without insurance, and they still do. Therefore, the first extensive research about financing and utilization in several individual countries shows that the new programs of universal coverage do not automatically result in universal utilization and equality in dental health. Although the poor are less frequent users, they are not so much cheaper to the program: because of neglect, they present more expensive problems to the dentist.[21] Perhaps in the long run, class differences will diminish.

The first studies of dental insurance in several countries showed that early dental insurance reinforced traditional practices. Dentists were restoring and replacing teeth and were devoting little attention to prevention,[22] much like the acute-care orientation of doctors and the rewards for acute care in medical care insurance. For this reason, the new trend is to provide financial incentives for periodic preventive visits by the dentally healthy patient—for example, minimum or no cost sharing for examinations and prophylaxis, followed by bonus-malus cost sharing—but the effects are not yet known.

Dental insurance is traditional in that it pays the solo dentist full fees to do all the work himself and does not pay the complete team. Possibly more than in medicine, the dentist could share tasks with auxiliaries, but dental insurance does not encourage cost-effective team reimbursement.[23] To gain the cooperation of the practitioners, dental insurance—like health insurance generally—tends to preserve the status quo. Government agencies that employ both salaried dentists and salaried paradentals give the latter great responsibilities, but the dental associations usually block the dental centers from practicing under statutory dental insurance.

Implications for the United States

In a completely private market, one can choose among completely different models. When Americans debated the creation of a traditional acute-care statutory health insurance law during the 1970s, they assumed that dentistry would be included in a traditional insurance form (as it had been in Europe): treatments would be listed, the patient would visit the dentist when he needed treatment, and the patient would contribute a deductible and coinsurance, as in acute care.[24]

But most dental episodes do not constitute large insurable risks occurring randomly and unexpectedly throughout a population. Most dental care consists of small claims that occur regularly—as in the case of most ambulatory pharmaceutical purchases described in the last chapter. Such small dental claims are uneconomic to insure. They might be considered a routine consumer expense, best left to family budgets, and excluded from insurance by a large deductible. Then dental insurance would cover only the large random events.

The need for expensive dental care might not fit the insurance model either. Poor oral health and regular preventive dentistry are outcomes of lifestyle and vary by social class. As populations are protected by fluoridation, become more careful about dental health, and use their own cash or third-party coverage to consult dentists earlier, expensive dental problems become less common and result from neglect. Insurance would redistribute resources from the more to the less conscientious persons—provided that the less conscientious go at all. (Universal financing for a prepayment system for preventive services used primarily by the more educated and underused by the less educated would transfer resources from the poor to the rich.)

Early statutory health insurance and early private health insurance used deductibles and coinsurance to prevent moral hazard and overutilization. But the new trend is to redefine dental insurance as prepayment for preventive dentistry: if someone is covered, he should visit the dentist regularly even if he has no complaints. To encourage regular examination and prophylaxis, some European social insurance (and much American private insurance) reverse acute-care practice, eliminate deductibles and coinsurance for periodic checkups, and impose coinsurance and copayments as penalties on the more expensive dental claims. Carriers also preserve substantial cost sharing by patients in the more expensive claims in both Europe and the United States because they must rely on patients to prevent fraud and overtreatment by dentists. Unlike their relations with doctors, the carriers have no statistical utilization review or utilization control over the private office dentists. Not even the dental associations have influence over the practitioners.

If much of dental insurance is becoming prepayment for preventive medicine, a problem is marketing it. No country has been able to sell large numbers of voluntary dental policies. Among the dentally conscious upper and middle classes, every private market for individual enrollment is overwhelmed by adverse selection.[25] The lower classes neglect prepayment opportunities and preventive self-care. Thus, the usual method is obligatory prepayment for all. Compulsory coverage and taxation are included under statutory health insurance in developed countries. The American method is to include the new type of dental coverage in employer group coverage that the individual subscriber does not buy. But since American group coverage is often restricted to acute care and omits the poor, many Americans lack dental benefits. And these are precisely the people who will not buy them privately.

Some proposals for two-tier social health insurance try to build up the importance of the second tier by excluding certain benefits from the first obligatory tier. The public could buy private insurance covering these benefits or could self-insure. Holland's Dekker Commission—as noted earlier in this chapter— proposed reserving dentistry as well as pharmaceutical drugs for the second tier. But in view of past experience, there is little likelihood of widespread prepayment or adequate self-insurance, particularly among the poor. If Americans, as well as others, wish to organize universal prepayment and make their countries preventive-minded, obligatory financing is inescapable. Probably the public planning of service delivery is inescapable too. Appealing to "market forces" and pecuniary "patient incentives" to produce an "efficient" dental care sector is beside the point.[26]

Since dental services are used unequally by different social classes—with or without dental insurance and public dental services—American statutory insurance should be accompanied by public education and case finding targeted at the low-using classes. This requires policy research about the behavior of different social classes—in dentistry and in other health sectors—that differs from the current American econometric style that generalizes about the monolithic Average Patient and the entire market.[27]

Notes

1. For a history of dental practice see Walter A. Hoffmann-Axthelm, *History of Dentistry* (Chicago: Quintessence, 1981).

2. Dentistry still depends heavily on organized public services with salaried dentists and salaried auxiliaries, according to J. Kostlan, *Oral Health Services in Europe* (Copenhagen: World Health Organization Regional Office for Europe, 1979), and John J. Ingle and Patricia Blair (eds.), *International Dental Care Delivery Systems* (Cambridge, Mass.: Ballinger, 1978).

3. For the sometimes tumultuous early history of the British dental services see Almont Lindsey, *Socialized Medicine in England and Wales* (Chapel Hill: University of North Carolina Press, 1962), especially chap. 15.

4. The evolution of dental insurance coverage during the decade after World War II is summarized in *The Cost of Medical Care* (Geneva: International Labour Office, 1959), pp. 63–68, 125–130, 150–151. The present situation is described in *Financing of Dental Care in Europe*, 2 vols. (Copenhagen: World Health Organization Regional Office for Europe, 1986 and 1990), and F. J. Oldiges, *The Relationship Between Dental Care and Sickness Insurance*, report to the Twenty-first General Assembly (Geneva: International Social Security Association, 1983).

5. *Tandheelkundige hulp in de ziekenfondsverzekering* (Amstelveen: Ziekenfondsraad, 1978) describes the situation just before adoption of the different classes of cost sharing.

6. Proposed by the Dekker Commission (assigned the task of restructuring Dutch health insurance). See Commissie Structuur en Financiering Gezondheidszorg, *Bereidheid tot verandering* (The Hague: Distributiecentrum Overheidspublikaties, 1987), pp. 12, 52, 54, 211–214.

7. *The Basic Fact Sheets* (London: Fédération Dentaire Internationale, frequently updated).

8. The work of these salaried dental teams in several countries is described in Robert Kudrle, "The Implications of Foreign Dental Coverage for U.S. National Health Insurance," *Journal of Health Politics, Policy and Law*, vol. 5,

no. 4 (Winter 1981), pp. 653–689; and Kostlan, *Oral Health Services in Europe* (see note 2, above).

9. In the national contract for dentistry—like the one for doctors—CNAMTS and the other social insurance *caisses* agree not to provide dental services to subscribers by creating health centers with salaried dentists. But they can create dental health facilities. The dentists are typical private practitioners, not salaried employees, and they merely take advantage of the *caisses's* investments by renting offices. Patients may freely choose between office dentists and health center dentists. The centers (part of the sickness funds' *action sanitaire et sociale*) are described in Marcel Gaspard, *Economie, médecine, et chirurgie dentaire* (Paris: Economica, 1980), pp. 255–285. The *mutuelles* can continue to operate their health centers with salaried dentists and doctors.

10. One result has been research by the European Regional Organization of the International Dental Federation to estimate the supply and demand for decades to come. Ministries of Health in member countries have created capabilities in dental manpower planning, a subject they had previously ignored.

11. See Markus Schneider and others, *Gesundheitssysteme im internationalen Vergleich*, 2nd ed. (Bonn: Bundesministerium für Arbeit und Sozialordnung, 1990), pp. 57, 159, 357.

12. Romuald Schicke, *Soziale Sicherung und Gesundheitswesen* (Stuttgart: Verlag W. Kohlhammer, 1978), pp. 147–148.

13. Dental coverage in 1988 is summarized in Jean-Pierre Gallet, *L'exercice libéral de la chirurgie dentaire* (Paris: CREDES, 1989), p. 3. Medical and dental coverages are compared in *Le secteur libéral des professions de santé en 1984*, Carnets Statistiques no. 20 (Paris: CNAMTS, 1985), p. 131.

14. For the previous structure of benefits and the plans for the reforms during the 1980s see *Tandheelkundige hulp in de ziekenfondsverzekering* and *Toekomstige tandheelkundige voorzieningen* (Amstelveen: Ziekenfondsraad, 1978, 1982, and 1984).

15. The mosaic of private and public programs in Canada is described in R. G. Evans and M. F. Williamson, *Extending Canadian Health Insurance: Options for Pharmacare and Denticare* (Toronto: University of Toronto Press, 1978), chap. 4.

16. See J. F. Follmann, *Medical Care and Health Insurance* (Homewood, Ill.: Richard D. Irwin, 1963), chap. 12; and Helen Avnet and Mata Nikias, *Insured Dental Care* (New York: Group Health Dental Insurance, 1967), chap. 1.

17. For numbers of subscribers see *Source Book of Health Insurance Data: 1988 Update* (Washington: Health Insurance Association of America, 1988), p. 8. For numbers of dentists with insured patients see Belinda Wilson, "Dental Fees: National and Regional Survey," *Dental Management*, vol. 29, no. 2 (Feb. 1989), p. 26. Shares of expenditures are being calculated from the 1987 National Medical Expenditure Survey by the Division of Intramural Research, National Center for Health Services Research, Rockville, Maryland.

18. Unpublished data from the Division of National Cost Estimates, Of-

fice of the Actuary, Health Care Financing Administration, U.S. Department of Health and Human Services.

19. Ingle and Blair, *International Dental Care Delivery Systems* (see note 2, above).

20. *Country Profiles on Oral Health in Europe* (Cophenhagen: World Health Organization Regional Office for Europe, 1986).

21. World Health Organization, *Oral Health Care Systems* (London: Quintessence, 1985), chaps. 7–8.

22. Ibid., p. 208; see also *Financing of Dental Care in Europe* (see note 4, above), vol. 2, pp. 20–22.

23. World Health Organization, *Oral Health Care Systems* (see note 21, above), pp. 80–84.

24. Robert T. Kudrle, "Dental Care," in Judith Feder and others (eds.), *National Health Insurance: Conflicting Goals and Policy Choices* (Washington: Urban Institute, 1980), chap. 12; and Paul J. Feldstein, *Financing Dental Care: An Economic Analysis* (Lexington, Mass.: Lexington Books, 1973), chap. 6.

25. Douglas A. Conrad and others, "Adverse Selection Within Dental Insurance Markets," *Advances in Health Economics and Health Services Research*, vol. 6 (1985), pp. 171–190.

26. As in Feldstein, *Financing Dental Care* (see note 24, above); and Robert T. Kudrle and Lawrence Meskin (eds.), *Reducing the Cost of Dental Care* (Minneapolis: University of Minnesota Press, 1983), especially chap. 1.

27. Summarized in David Grembowski and others, "The Structure and Function of Dental-Care Markets: A Review and Agenda for Research," *Medical Care*, vol. 16, no. 2 (Feb. 1988), pp. 132–147. A new generation of more sophisticated dental policy researchers is examining the differential effects of insurance on utilization by social class. See, for example, Douglas Conrad and others, "Dental Care Demand: Insurance Effects and Plan Design," *Health Services Research*, vol. 22, no. 3 (Aug. 1987), pp. 341–367.

CHAPTER 14

Mental Health Services

─────────────────────────── **Summary** ───────────────────────────

When mental care was custodial, it had no place in health insurance. But as
psychopharmacological and surgical treatments became effective after World War
II and patients seemed curable, psychiatry seemed to fit an insurable medical
model. Statutory health insurance now covers hospital stays other than lifelong
institutionalization, and the method is the same as the one used for acute-care
hospitalization. Short-stay psychiatric hospitalization is often a service in a
general hospital; the prospective budget and per diems for all services are set by
regulators and paid by carriers. Psychiatric and internal medicine services are
covered in the same fashion. Special psychiatric hospitals—with short-stay and
long-stay patients—are regulated and reimbursed like other special hospitals.
Holland in addition has a special statutory insurance program funded by payroll
taxes and designed for the permanently institutionalized.

Psychiatrists have long been salaried employees of hospitals and governments, receiving any insurance money indirectly. They have long received private
out-of-pocket fees from ambulatory patients. Slowly they were added to the fee
schedules of the medical profession, as the efficiency of treatments improved and
insured patients began to visit them. At first, neurosurgical and neurological
interventions were itemized and paid for. Eventually fee schedules added office
visits for analytic therapy.

Psychiatrists have long struggled for professional recognition within medical associations, whose tariff committees wield powerful influence over the relative values among procedures, the relative shares of insurance revenue among
specialties, and relative incomes. Slowly the psychiatrists have improved their
social insurance reimbursement under fee-for-service in some countries (such as

France and Holland), but not in others. Unlike other doctors, few psychiatrists can earn their entire incomes from statutory health insurance.

Patients are required to pay higher rates of cost sharing for mental than for acute-care services. One motive is to discourage unnecessary visits, which are thought to be more common in mental health than in other sectors. Cost sharing also enables government and the carriers to limit the additional costs to the system from the recent addition of mental health benefits. To prevent unnecessary utilization, benefits are limited to a maximum number of hospital days and a maximum number of office visits.

Private health insurance in Europe could insure for cost sharing and offer extra benefits. But the European carriers hesitate, since they think mental health insurance is vulnerable to adverse selection and moral hazard. A few European social insurance carriers, such as the French, create and manage their own inpatient and outpatient mental services. These carriers avoid waste by employing and directing the providers.

Mental health is a widespread benefit in American private health insurance. Many subscribers use it, and employer groups are pressed to cover it. Many state governments require that all insurance cover it. Utilization is high and providers prosper. As in European statutory health insurance, private American insurance tries to prevent excessive use by imposing cost sharing, by limiting hospital days, and by limiting the number of office visits.

Early Mental Health Financing

For centuries, the public policy problem in mental health was to isolate and maintain the insane poor. Governments throughout Europe and North America created large mental hospitals and paid for them from their social welfare budgets. Some mentally disturbed with families were maintained at home at the families' expense. A few churches and local governments provided services from their welfare budgets.[1] The mutual assistance funds and statutory health insurance covered somatic and not mental illness. The physicians and others who treated the hospitalized and the ambulatory mental cases were paid by government and by charitable organizations, not by insurance.

Psychopharmacological innovations after World War II created new treatment modes: short hospital stays followed by restoration to the family and work; ambulatory care while the patient continued in his other social roles. This made possible the integration of mental care financing into statutory health insurance. The patient had coverage under health insurance, either as a worker or as a dependent. Services were given by a physician. Treatments resembled the medical model, since they involved drugs, surgery, electronic diagnostic testing, and electroshock treatment.

Paying for Hospital Care

Short Psychiatric Stays. Before World War II, private ambulatory and institutional care in psychiatry developed for the middle classes. The evolution was much like the change in acute-care hospitalization for diseases during the nineteenth century: the public and charitable hospitals had been warehouses for the poor, but the innovations in acute care necessitated inpatient facilities appropriate to the middle classes. During the twentieth century, the middle classes began to go to neurologists and psychiatrists and the doctors created private clinics. But the patients had to pay for ambulatory and inpatient care completely out-of-pocket, since even private insurance did not yet cover mental health.

During the twentieth century, general hospitals modernized to accommodate persons covered by statutory health insurance and private insurance. After World War II, in all countries, they added psychiatric services to accommodate short-stay patients. Statutory health insurance was expanded to cover patients referred to the psychiatric service.

Instead of a single average daily charge for all patients, French public hospitals—particularly the large ones—had different daily charges for the principal clinical services. One per diem covered the costs of the psychiatric service; others were paid by the sickness funds to cover the inpatients in other clinical services. The psychiatric daily charge was usually lower, since that service had less equipment, fewer employees, and lower operating costs.[2]

Private psychiatric clinics remained important and still are a significant proportion of all private clinics in several European countries. In France, for example, they operate over a quarter of all private clinic beds.[3] Several have contracts as the principal psychiatric facilities for the governments of their *départements*, and several offer community mental health services such as day hospital care. When statutory health insurance was extended to psychiatric hospitalization, it paid for short and extended stays in the private clinics. The sickness funds paid according to the method used for private clinics in each country: a per diem plus itemized charges and the doctors' fees in France; an inclusive per diem plus the doctors' fees in Germany.

Long Stays. After World War II, Europe tried to abolish or reform its asylums. Europe had many specialized hospitals: some were psychiatric; others were devoted to tuberculosis, rheumatism, ophthalmology, thermal cures, and so on. Some psychiatric hospitals were newly built by government or were converted from the asylums; some were private clinics; and some clinics (as in France) had contracts with local governments to save the communes from having to construct new local public psychiatric hospitals. The psychiatric patients in the extended-care specialized hospitals might stay for over a year.

Statutory health insurance covered long stays in all special hospitals as well as the shorter stays in acute care and psychiatry. Rate regulators (as in France) or sickness fund negotiators (as in Germany) screened the public psychiatric hospital's prospective budget in the usual way and agreed on an inclusive per diem or global budget.[4]

Permanent Institutionalization. Residential establishments for the permanently institutionalized do not seem to fit the health insurance methods designed for curable and short-stay illnesses and injuries. Holland's AWBZ is the one exception—statutory long-term care insurance designed in large part to pay for the permanently institutionalized. Custodial institutions for the mentally handicapped and mentally ill no longer need be supported by charitable fundraising or by government subsidies. Since the enactment of AWBZ in 1968, it pays for these indefinitely hospitalized persons by the same procedure as the statutory acute-care health insurance system's payment for persons spending less than a year in acute-care and extended-care hospitals. The long-stay establishment submits a prospective budget and retrospective cost report to the rate-regulation agency (COTG), which then issues an all-inclusive per diem rate covering average costs for all long-stay patients. For each patient, the establishment bills that person's sickness fund, which pays the per diems from its AWBZ revenue. Over one-third of all AWBZ expenditures is devoted to persons in establishments for the mentally handicapped and mentally ill. In addition, AWBZ pays for a large number of elderly persons in nursing homes who, in the past, might have been consigned to mental hospitals.[5]

Paying the Psychiatrist

Salaries. Until recently, most psychiatrists were salaried government employees. They worked in the large mental hospitals, managing the installations, treating patients, and evaluating them for discharge. Some worked as government employees in the community, evaluating patients for voluntary or involuntary hospitalization and providing some treatment. In all countries today, many psychiatrists continue to be full-time salaried.

Some sickness funds with health centers have added mental health care. An example is the *mutuelles* of France. In particular, the *mutuelle* for schoolteachers (MGEN) has pioneered mental health care in France, as well as operating its own inpatient services. These health centers and day hospitals employ psychiatrists on full-time or part-time salaries.[6]

Neurosurgeons and neurologists have long been affiliated with European hospitals and have collected small salaries for part-time work. As psychiatry became a recognized service in the acute-care general hospital in many countries, psychiatrists were paid part-time salaries. When all the chiefs of service in general hospitals—such as in France and Germany—became full-time salaried, the neurosurgeons, neurologists, and psychiatrists received full-time salaries too. The neurosurgeons could negotiate salaries as high as the more glamorous and more affluent specialties (such as surgery), since salaries covered income forgone from private fee-for-service practice. Since the psychiatrists earned less in their complete practices before, their full-time salaries have been lower.

Private Fees. The private psychiatric clinics were important to the psychiatrists as the source of most of their income. Until the 1970s, in psychiatry as well as in other specialties, hospital chiefs of service earned only small salaries from hospital budgets and got most of their income from private fees and their private clinics. The chiefs served in the public hospital during the morning and in their private clinics the rest of the day. The chiefs in psychiatry as well as in other clinical specialties operated such short-stay private clinics for middle-class paying patients. Many other psychiatrists operated private clinics too. They still rely on them today, because fee-for-service practice under statutory health insurance has never become remunerative enough.

Fees from Social Insurance. Fee schedules are designed to pay for office visits, home visits, and a long list of specific procedures. A physician can bill for surgical and other technical acts in mental care if they appear to fall within his specialty. Neurosurgeons and neurologists have always been able to perform these tasks and bill the sickness funds.

Problems of recognition and adequate remuneration long beset psychiatrist physicians. As licensed doctors, they could treat and bill at least as general practitioners. But in countries like France, where a specialist's office visit is paid at a higher rate and specialized acts are restricted to specialists, the psychiatrists for a while were not recognized as specialists by the licensing and insurance authorities. Eventually they were and could then collect the specialist's higher rates for office visits.

During the 1950s in all European countries, the problem was insufficient earnings from office visits. When psychiatrists analyzed rather than treated patients technically, they organized their day as a series of fifty-minute office visits. The other cognitive specialties—such as internal medicine and pediatrics—conducted several office visits per hour, performed itemized technical acts, and therefore earned from social insurance far more than the psychiatrists. The payment system perpetuated European psychiatry's technical and procedure orientation and retarded the growth of analysis.[7] Analytically oriented psychiatrists depended on private practice long after all other doctors earned most of their income from statutory health insurance.

It was not merely sickness funds and governments that were skeptical of the work of psychiatrists and the insurability of mental illness. A principal barrier was the marginal position of analytic psychiatry in the European medical profession. Medical practice and medical associations were dominated by the technical specialties, particularly surgery. The tariff committees within the medical associations and the joint fee-schedule committees with the sickness funds have always been dominated by the technical specialties. During the 1940s and 1950s, they grudgingly allowed analytic psychiatrists to bill as specialists. During the 1950s and 1960s, the general practitioners and the other cognitive specialties (internal medicine and pediatrics) expanded their influence within medical associations and obtained support of the tariff committees for higher fees from the health insurance system. Analytic psychiatry gained such support within the medical profession only much later in some countries (as in France and Holland) and never to this day in others.[8]

The financial solution for analytic psychiatry eventually was a special fee for the analytic hour. In 1988 in France, for example, the fee for an office visit was 85 F for a general practitioner, 125 F for a specialist, and 195 F for a psychiatrist. The annual increases during the last decade have been higher for the psychiatrists than for the others. But since other doctors have more visits per hour and can perform technical acts, their total incomes are higher. Average gross earnings from French statutory health insurance in 1985 were 413,000 F for general practitioners, 706,000 F for all specialists, and 365,000 F for psychiatrists.[9] Most psychiatrists continue to rely on salaried jobs for much of their income.

Community Services

Traditional health insurance is accustomed to pay fees to doctors, dentists, pharmacists, and several other providers. And it is accustomed to pay daily rates, charges, or global budgets to short-stay or extended-stay inpatient hospitals. But health insurance has never devised a method of paying a multidisciplinary team like those in modern mental health. As noted in Chapter Fifteen on long-term care, health insurance has always paid persons credentialed in health care and has never paid for those providing social and personal support for the socially disabled.

A trend in many countries has been community mental health care. In some, it is managed and paid for by local governments. In others, it is managed by nonprofit associations or private entrepreneurs and paid for by patients out-of-pocket. The interdisciplinary teams receive salaries from the local government or from the private owners.

A few countries have begun to assimilate these programs into statutory health insurance. The Dutch solution is to use AWBZ, designed to finance programs serving social as well as medical needs. During the 1980s, the mosaic of local community mental health services for adults, children, and pensioners has been combined under fifty-nine Regional Institutes for Ambulatory Mental Health Care (RIAGGs) owned and managed by nonprofit associations unaffiliated with churches. Payments to the RIAGGs are capped more strictly than the payments to doctors and hospitals, where COTG decides the unit prices but patients and providers decide total utilization. Each year, the Ministry of Welfare decides the total amount of AWBZ money that should go to all the RIAGGs. Each RIAGG negotiates with its local sickness fund a global budget estimating utilization, morbidities, staffing, other resources, and money needed next year. COTG then decides the distribution of the total national global budget among all the RIAGGs. COTG tries to use formulas estimating each region's different level of need for mental health services, an elusive task. But COTG must also ensure minimum resources for all RIAGGs, so it gives less money to the biggest— and most troubled—cities than the formulas would provide.[10]

France, like Holland, has long been an innovator in developing community mental health services designed to support the mentally ill at home, keep them out of asylums, and prevent deterioration. In community mental health care at present, the right mix of services is uncertain, a great variety is spread across every country, and financing is confused. Such variety seemed appropriate to Holland in the decades of religious operation of social services (*verzuiling*), weak national government, and responsibility by local government. But it contradicted French customs of central direction, top-down financing, and standardization. During the 1950s and 1960s, France decentralized its mental health care; instead of large centralized asylums, each *département* would establish whatever mental hospitals and community mental health services were appropriate to its needs, priorities, and resources. Gradually the local programs were shifted from government budgets to statutory health insurance. The short-stay and extended-stay public and private mental hospitals were then financed by the daily charge and, at present, by global budgets coming from the sickness funds. The beginnings of insurance coverage for the ambulatory community mental health services were grants from many regional *caisses*—that is, the *action sanitaire et sociale* of the CRAMs, used also to subsidize the long-term care programs described in Chapter Fifteen.[11] The national government finally decided to transfer the community programs completely to statutory health insurance during the 1980s. The transition was suspended in 1987 because of the priority given to stopping the growth in the health insurance accounts. Thus, the precise mechanism of insurance reimbursement of community health services was not settled.

Psychiatry requires prolonged continuity of care between inpatient and outpatient programs. Traditionally, public mental hospitals have been poorly integrated with community services; private clinics with outpatient services and the same medical staffs are better coordinated. Statutory health insurance may be a barrier to coordination if it covers only shorter inpatient stays and leaves community services to government budgets. German statutory health insurance covers both hospital stays and ambulatory visits but prevents continuity of care by refusing to pay the same doctor in both modes. Because ambulatory-care doctors in all fields monopolize office care and refuse membership in the *Kassenärztliche Vereinigungen* to all the salaried members of nonprofit and government hospital staffs, the psychiatrists in those hospitals may not treat and bill for patients after discharge but must refer them to office doctors. Likewise, the office psychiatrists may not treat their patients in nonprofit and government hospitals, but only in private clinics.

The goals of continuity of care were important reasons for the French decisions to phase out the centralized asylums, create networks of inpatient and outpatient programs in each community ("sectorization"), and cover all these programs under the same social insurance financing. The doctors would be paid a single salary for work in all these programs.

Patient Cost Sharing

There are several reasons for any higher-than-usual cost sharing under statutory health insurance. All apply to mental health benefits:

☐ Recently added benefits usually have higher cost sharing than those originally covered by statutory health insurance. The new benefits (such as ambulatory mental care) were previously completely out-of-pocket, so partial reimbursement by the sickness funds is considered a concession. The sickness funds can continue to concentrate their money on acute care. (This is a principal reason for dental cost sharing too.)

☐ Some benefits may be used unnecessarily and wasted merely because insurance covers them. If the patient invests his own money, purchase is more serious. (This "moral hazard" is a principal reason for pharmaceutical cost sharing too.)

☐ Care can be prolonged unnecessarily for the patient's comfort and the provider's profit. This is a particularly important motive for cost sharing in mental care, because the patients are dependent and psychiatry lacks clear-cut criteria of therapeutic success and failure.

☐ Benefits include housing, sustenance, and social support, as well as medical care. If the patient were not institutionalized, he and his family would have to cover these costs at home. Payment-in-full would provide a perverse incentive for institutionalization. (This is a principal reason for cost sharing in long-term care too.)

Ambulatory, Community, and Clinic Care. Psychiatric cost sharing under statutory health insurance usually is coinsurance or copayment rather than unlimited extra-billing at the discretion of the provider. As in acute care, regulators or negotiators decide a per diem hospital rate for each establishment or a standard fee for all psychiatrists. The sickness fund pays a standard percentage or a fixed amount, and the patient pays the rest. The mental hospital and psychiatrist may not extra-bill. In psychiatry as in acute care, statutory health insurance protects its citizen-taxpayers against unpredictability and profiteering.

If a mental health service is paid by global budget, the patient cannot be charged coinsurance for each service. Rather, he is charged a fixed copayment. In Holland, for example, psychotherapy in community programs (through the RIAGGs) and in physicians' offices is the principal source of cost sharing by patients in the normally paid-in-full social insurance. The regulatory agency (COTG) fixes the global budgets for each RIAGG. The national associations of medical specialists and the sickness funds negotiate a schedule of copayments for all psychiatric services throughout the country in RIAGGs and in psychiatrists' offices, COTG approves, and the patient charges are calculated as revenue in each RIAGG's global budget. The difference between copayment revenue and each RIAGG's global budget is billed to the sickness fund. The office-based psychiatrist bills the sickness fund for the difference between the official fee and the patient's copayment.

Private psychiatric insurance differs. The carrier usually pays an indemnity per episode; the patient has discretion in patronizing unregulated and very expensive providers and in paying the difference. This method is used by sickness funds only in a few places where psychiatry is just being adopted by social insurance and social insurance still resembles private health insurance—that is, in certain cantons of Switzerland. In its acute-care benefits, Switzerland allows coinsurance but not extra-billing.

Hospitalization. Most countries lack cost sharing for social insurance of inpatient acute hospitalization, and they do not impose it for psychiatric hospitalization. Cost sharing is avoided on the humanitarian grounds that psychiatric illness is particularly impoverishing for patients and their families. The patient has been disabled for a long time, usually has a poor work history, and—although now eligible for a disability pension—may never have worked long and effectively enough to be entitled to adequate disability benefits.

Statutory health insurance may treat the psychiatric inpatient even more generously than the acute-care inpatient on the grounds that he is particularly impoverished and doomed to a longer stay. For example, France has long required cost sharing of all its acute-care inpatients: coinsurance during the period of per diems, copayments under current global budgeting, and higher rates of cost sharing for longer stays. French patients suffering from certain severe illnesses— including mental illness—are exempt. Therefore, the psychiatric patient pays nothing from the first day.

The structure of cost sharing creates a disincentive to deinstitutionalize mental patients. Although cost sharing is not required by the hospital, it is obligatory in nursing homes, community mental health services, and home care. The financially straitened family must be unusually solicitous of the patient and unusually critical of mental hospitals to assume the burden. In trying to substitute community programs and social insurance for the traditional methods of institutionalization and full public financing, French policymakers search for methods of overcoming the countervailing effects of the cost-sharing rules.

Drugs. Ambulatory mental care depends heavily on prescription drugs. Reimbursement is administered in the usual fashion. The psychiatrist in his office or in the community mental health program writes the prescription, the sickness fund pays the pharmacist, and the patient pays the pharmacist the usual cost-sharing fee for drugs.

Utilization Control

Mental health care is thought unusually vulnerable to moral hazard—excessive and wasteful use merely because insurance is available to pay. Patients may cling to the doctor or community clinic. It is never clear which treatments are effective or when the patient is cured. Feeling underpaid by social insurance, the psychiatrist can easily fill gaps in his schedule by ordering unnecessary visits.

Cost sharing is designed to discourage unnecessary visits by the patient. But mental patients may be unusually dependent, convinced that care is necessary, and not deterred by out-of-pockets. If a patient is very poor, government social welfare programs—which once covered all mental health care—are still available to pay the cost sharing.

Thus, other controls apply to mental health benefits under statutory health insurance. A common method is prior approval by the control doctor of the patient's sickness fund:

☐ Advance authorization of psychiatric hospitalization is common. In several countries (such as France), prior approval of acute hospitalization is required in theory but is not enforced. The control doctor gives *pro forma* approval retrospectively to the attending physician's decision. But prior approval is enforced for psychiatry.

☐ Referral to a psychiatrist for ambulatory care requires both referral by the general practitioner and, often, explicit agreement by the control doctor. For example, in Holland, the psychiatrist must file a proposed treatment plan with the control doctor giving the patient's diagnosis, the procedures, and the necessary number of sessions.

☐ If a patient goes to a community mental health program under statutory health insurance, he must bring a referral slip from his physician and an authorization from the control doctor of his sickness fund. (An example is France.) Then the sickness fund can monitor the appropriateness, length, and outcome of the treatment.

If a country's mental health financing stays close to the ambulatory medical model, which lacks prior authorization for visits, the patient can go directly to a psychiatrist or can go with only his GP's referral. An example is Germany.

Another common control is to limit the length of psychiatric services: either the number of visits or the number of days. One can, for example, set limits on the number of visits to a psychiatrist under statutory health insurance. If the patient wants more, he can continue privately. Holland limits the number of visits in a patient's lifetime to ninety—on the grounds that psychiatric care should succeed by then and continued dependence is life support not provided appropriately by the expensive medically qualified psychiatrist. When coverage by statutory acute-care insurance (ZFW) ends, the patient must apply to a RI-AGG, which provides social supports and is financed by long-term insurance (AWBZ).

Or one can set limits on the number of days spent in the psychiatric service of an acute hospital or in the psychiatric extended-care hospital. The control doctors review lengths of stay for psychiatry as well as for acute care, although the thresholds are higher for psychiatry. The control doctor needs to move patients from the more expensive general hospital into the less expensive extended-care hospital—both under per diem methods of payment (as in Germany and Holland) and under global budgets (as in France). Now that the less expensive and more humane community health services are being developed in France, the control doctors of French sickness funds try to substitute community and home care for prolonged inpatient stays. Several statutory health insurance systems—as in Holland and certain Swiss cantons—have specific limits on numbers of days in the psychiatric hospital. After that limit, the patient must be paid for by a program for the chronically disabled.

Mental patients in the past were often left in institutions for very long times. Control doctors in France are now being encouraged to monitor the quality of mental services and the appropriateness of assignments. If a patient has stayed in a community program or in a hospital for a very long time, the control doctor is expected to evaluate whether reassignment would be better. But control doctors in France and elsewhere are too overloaded to assume the immense task of thorough surveillance of mental services.

Private Mental Health Insurance

Europe. Statutory health insurance adds new benefits cautiously—not only are the outcomes unpredictable and possibly expensive, but revocation of a major set of benefits would be fought by the newly entitled patients and providers. Mental health was added slowly to statutory health insurance partly for these reasons and partly because public policymakers and medical associations considered the illnesses, diagnoses, therapies, and cures unclear. Europe until recently lacked a large mental health lobby of patients, doctors, and community activists to press legislatures.

The European private insurance companies have hesitated about including mental health benefits. Their policies cover conventional acute care, pharmaceutical drugs, and dentistry. Because they have sold policies to large markets not covered by statutory health insurance—and since social insurance covers mental health—the Dutch companies (before 1990) and German companies today must offer some mental health benefits too. These are cash allowances, not guarantees to pay full fees of ambulatory and inpatient psychiatric care. The psychiatrists must rely on private payments from the market for much of their income—that is, large fees they set freely themselves, with the patients recovering lower (or no) indemnity payments from their carriers. Since they are dedicated to the welfare of their members, several French *mutuelles* provide mental health services. These are direct services and not payments to private providers, so the *mutuelles* can regulate admissions, length of treatment, and payments.

Even when a niche appears, private carriers hesitate to enter. Great Britain for centuries had mental hospitals and community mental care programs run by government for the poor. The National Health Service took them over. Because of the blue-collar ambiance and inconvenient location of those facilities, one might expect the middle and upper classes to seek private care and to be willing to pay. Since the managers of British private hospitals and British private insurance had heard that mental health was an important part of American for-profit health services, they investigated private financing of mental health ambulatory visits and hospitalization.[12] But they decided it was too risky. Sales would invite adverse selection, coverage would invite moral hazard, and any case could turn into expensive chronic care. British private insurance focuses on small finite risks. The principal carrier (BUPA) offers no mental health benefits. A few of its competitors (particularly PPP) try to attract business away by offering mental health options in their basic family policies, but the annual limits are strict and additional premiums are substantial.

The United States. Experience in America has differed from that of European social and private insurance—because of the private and competitive structure of its health insurance, because of its large number of psychotherapists and mental health programs, and because of the anxieties of its population. Many Americans have long been concerned about personal relations with their families, work settings, and communities. Business managers—the principal purchasers of health insurance—have long feared that productivity was harmed by alcoholism, tensions, and family troubles in all ranks. The competitive structure of American insurance leads to the introduction of new benefits by carriers trying to take business from the established ones. Therefore, the United States has witnessed a rapid spread in insured mental health benefits for hospitals, psychiatrists, offices, and special community programs. But since American insurance is cost-conscious as well as private, it has also witnessed periods when much coverage was revoked or reduced.

As in other countries, mental hospitalization in America once was confined to public asylums financed by state government budgets and by private clinics paid for by patients out-of-pocket. After World War II, many acute-care general hospitals added short-stay psychiatric wards. Blue Cross had contracts to pay all-inclusive per diems or charges for acute care in these hospitals. During the 1950s, many Plans agreed to add psychiatric inpatient care to their coverage. Blue Shield then covered technical procedures, such as neurological surgery or electroshock,[13] but did not pay for inpatient or outpatient psychiatry. When they entered the group market during the 1960s, commercial insurers offered better coverage than Blue Cross and Blue Shield: their "major medical policies" included both inpatient and outpatient psychotherapy anywhere in the United States. To cover the costs of more generous benefits and to quote lower premiums to employers, the commercial insurers—in psychiatric as well as in acute-care benefits—required deductibles and coinsurance, while the Blues required little or no cost sharing. By the 1970s, the Blues had to match the commercial carriers' psychiatric benefits in order to keep their group and individual markets.

America's only statutory health insurance—Medicare, enacted in 1965 during this evolution—provided generous psychiatric benefits that became a benchmark for the private policies:

☐   Psychiatric services in general hospitals were covered. (Coverage was identical to the acute-care conditions under Part A of Medicare.)

☐ Hospitalization in a psychiatric hospital was limited to 190 days in a lifetime. (This too was paid for under Part A of Medicare.)

☐ Psychiatrists' treatments under Part B of Medicare were limited to 50 percent of charges or $250 per year, whichever was less. In subsequent years, the coinsurance rate per visit and per charge was reduced to the 20 percent rate used for all physicians' charges. But the $250 annual limit remained until 1988 and 1989, when it was increased to $1,100 in two stages.

The scope of mental health benefits has resulted from an interaction among three interest groups:

☐ Persons interested in the cure of the mentally disturbed—particularly the beneficiaries of insurance (such as employees) and their employers.

☐ The providers—particularly the associations of psychiatrists and the managers of community mental health programs. The American Psychiatric Association—whose members are physicians specializing in psychiatry—has vigorously pressed for parity between psychiatry and all other medical specialties by such measures as covering mental care exactly like all somatic care in health insurance.

☐ Organized purchasers of insurance, such as employers and government. Employers encounter a conflict of interest: they favor cure of personnel problems manifested in absenteeism, alcoholism, addictions, and tension; but they also fear commitment to uncontrollable benefits in their insurance contracts.

After the initial decision to include mental health benefits in Medicare, these interest groups deadlocked. Medicare's mental health benefits were expanded only once (while the rest of Medicare was altered more often), but no cutbacks were imposed. Private health insurance coverage of mental health has been more volatile.[14]

Besides Medicare, a benchmark for private employer group coverage during the 1960s was the national government's own health insurance for civil servants: the Federal Employee Health Benefits Program (FEHBP). The program offered "high-option plans" that included generous mental health coverage and "low-option plans." The subscriber and the government contributed higher premiums to high-option plans. During successive expansions, FEHBP went farther than normal acute-care health insurance in the United States and abroad by paying for the services of clinical psychologists, psychiatric social workers, and psychiatric nurses. The program experienced adverse selection: many subscribers and families needing acute and mental care picked the high-option plans; subscribers needing fewer acute and mental services picked the cheaper low-option plans. Utilization and costs of the outpatient mental health benefits increased, FEHBP experienced a general financial crisis during the 1980s, and the much-publicized events contributed to a widespread backlash against the insurance of mental health.[15]

While both private employers and even FEHBP during the late 1970s and 1980s were cutting back mental health benefits, the mental health interest groups found another lever for expansion. Under American insurance law, it is the state governments that regulate. Thus, the interest groups pressed state legislatures to require inclusion of psychiatric inpatient and outpatient benefits, alcoholism treatment, and drug rehabilitation in every group and individual health insurance policy. Once such laws were enacted, the interest groups could block repeal or reduction of benefits. By 1988, such mandated benefits had been enacted in:[16]

☐   Psychiatry and mental health (28 states)
☐   Alcoholism rehabilitation (39 states)
☐   Drug rehabilitation (18 states)
☐   Psychologists' services (36 states)

The states vary in definition of minimum benefits. Carriers can offer more, but not less.

Mandating these and other benefits under insurance laws proved counterproductive. They have been principal reasons why many employers have substituted self-financed employee benefits for insurance contracts. (Self-financing is exempt from state insurance mandates.) The remaining insurance contracts with employers and individual policies must bear the full costs of mental health coverage; to cover actual and unexpected costs, all carriers must raise their premiums. Unable to self-finance and unwilling to pay high premiums, many small businessmen refuse to purchase health insurance for their workers.

By the late 1980s, private mental health insurance was diminishing slightly from its earlier high point—both in numbers of beneficiaries and in generosity of benefits. Employers could cut back substantially if they self-financed or were located in states without statutory mandates. In states with mandates, employers and carriers could cut back to the statutory minimum. But reductions were limited because of the continuing influence of providers and the widespread demand in the population. In nearly all self-financed and insured arrangements, the mental health components are less generous than the acute-care components, and they vary more widely. Here are some common patterns:[17]

☐   Nearly all group and individual coverage includes mental conditions. Even when ambulatory services and psychotherapy are not covered, technical interventions close to acute-care benefits are covered in both inpatient and ambulatory settings. Inpatient psychiatric assignment to general hospitals is also covered.
☐   Inpatient mental hospitalization is often (not always) severely limited in number of days (perhaps thirty per year), but acute inpatient hospitalization under major medical or comprehensive policies usually has no limit.
☐   Inpatient mental hospitalization has higher daily coinsurance than acute hospitalization.

☐ Ambulatory visits to psychiatrists and mental health centers are severely limited in number, but acute-care visits are not.

☐ Coinsurance is much higher for each ambulatory mental care visit than for each acute-care visit. For example, a policy might require 50 percent for the former and only 20 percent for the latter.

☐ An increasing number of medical insurance policies have stop-loss limitations: after considerable out-of-pockets, the carrier pays the patient's remaining obligations. Stop-loss applies to acute care but not to mental care, where the patient's obligations are unlimited.

☐ Major medical coverage often has an obligation to pay no more than a lifetime maximum for each patient. The lifetime maximum is lower for mental care than for acute care.

☐ The methods developed for utilization review in acute care—statistical profiles and peer review committees—once were thought inappropriate for mental care. Limits on number of benefits and substantial cost sharing by patients were the standard methods of utilization control in mental coverage. But to keep offering mental care in a period of cost containment and skepticism about mental services, some insurers and private mental clinics now are offering managed-care screening of inpatient admissions.[18]

Nearly all the bills for enacting statutory health insurance during the 1970s and 1980s have required inpatient psychiatric hospitalization and ambulatory mental health services. The bills allow limits on numbers of days in the hospital, and they allow coinsurance, but their benefits are more generous than the principal patterns in the current private market. These expansions are major reasons for the resistance to statutory health insurance by large employers, by small businessmen, and by political conservatives.

The persons most at risk of mental deterioration—the elderly—are not covered by private mental health insurance. The private policies are for employed groups, whose beneficiaries are younger. The new private long-term-care insurance policies exclude psychiatric problems as principal diagnoses. The principal statutory insurance program—Medicare—limits mental care benefits. The mentally disabled elderly in the United States—as in other countries in the past—ultimately must depend on public welfare. In America, this takes the form of institutionalization in nursing homes under Medicaid.

Effects on Utilization and Health

Since World War II, fewer persons in Europe and North America have been consigned to custodial hospitals for the mentally disabled; more have been treated therapeutically to bring about recovery in special services of acute-care general hospitals and in ambulatory settings.[19] Statutory health insurance has been the financial medium—raising more money than was possible under past custodial-oriented public budgets, defining mental disease as a treatable condition like any other, and reimbursing the providers in the typical acute-care forms.

But one cannot say more than that. The European research reports about historical trends in services and mental health include nothing about simultaneous trends in mental health financing. Since the research reports about services in various countries today include almost nothing about their different financing methods, one cannot compare outcomes as a consequence of financing arrangements. Every country's aggregate outcome—the usual information in national reports—results from several internal programs, but research rarely compares them within countries.

Even in the United States—the principal source of health services research—one cannot draw firm conclusions about the consequences of different mental health insurance arrangements for utilization, clinical outcomes, and costs. Each arrangement that has been studied is unique in important respects. Each research project focuses on one program and rarely compares different ones. Nor can one compare the programs and infer consequences by secondary analysis across all the data, since each set of facts was designed for each program and each research project.[20] Even when several studies have been done on the same topic in mental health insurance design, the results are inconclusive. For example, one cannot judge the effects of cost sharing by patients on the use of mental services: despite the importance of the issue and the ready availability of examples in every mental health insurance policy, very little research has been done and the few studies are contradictory.[21]

All American health insurance arrangements respond to competitive pressures by offering certain mental health benefits. But delivery and reimbursement are less standardized than for acute-care benefits. Mental health benefits range widely among HMOs in service organization, utilization, and costs.[22] Between HMOs and conventional health insurance is an even larger difference that may amount to a division of labor. An HMO must deliver services within its panel of doctors, often (not always) within its health center, and within strictly predictable costs. It specializes in the limited and conventional mental health problems of a good-risk population enrolled primarily in an acute-care program; its psychiatry is primary care that can be integrated into comprehensive medicine. Compared to conventional mental health insurance, the HMO hospitalizes patients less often and allows the patient's primary physician (rather than a specialized psychiatrist) to give more of the psychiatric care.[23]

The self-employed American office practitioners of psychiatry argue that the result is a different and inferior clinical product. They say that HMO psychiatry is oriented toward short-term symptomatic relief and stabilization, heavily reliant on psychotropic drugs, so that an outcome is achieved within the cost limits. But, they claim, only the office psychiatrist under fee-for-service and without a fixed length of care can treat causes and produce true cures. The advocates of HMOs respond that—by combining acute care and mental services in the same group and in the same site—they can treat the patient comprehensively, but the fragmentation of traditional office practice and traditional fee-for-service insurance prevent this. Therefore, the advocates of HMOs say, comprehensive care produces better treatment of conventional mental problems and reduces unnecessary utilization of acute medical services.[24] Because other countries with statutory health insurance do not have different forms of service delivery tied to insurance, one does not hear such claims that rival insurance schemes produce these differences in utilization and outcomes.

Although broad generalizations are elusive, some evidence about the specific effects of mental insurance coverage might be found. Adding certain mainstream tests and treatments on a large scale (as in American state mandates) increases utilization for some of them. The specialists in tasks benefiting from the mandates (such as clinical psychologists) increase in income and number.[25] But merely adding an unusual therapy does not automatically increase its utilization—for example, patients' demand for intensive psychotherapy (such as psychoanalysis) does not greatly increase.[26]

Much more than in somatic medicine, the clinical situation revolves around the personal relation between therapist and patient; other persons play carefully defined roles or are excluded altogether. The introduction of health insurance may alter the methods and results of therapy. The relationship between therapist and patient is no longer exclusively bilateral and confidential. Patients no longer demonstrate their independence, seriousness, and responsibility for themselves by paying with their own scarce resources. Instead they call upon an organization that pays and can wield power over the psychiatrist.[27]

Implications for the United States

A cursory overview of mental health insurance in Europe reveals no salient problems, solutions, or innovations that some American program has not already experienced. Indeed, the United States at present is passing through so much ferment in psychiatric practice and financing that it may provide some ideas for emulation in Europe. For many years, American psychiatry confronted the same doubts from policymakers and insurers as its European counterparts did: mental illness was not an insurable risk; health insurance could not be designed economically for mental illness; and coverage would lead to abuse and waste. The criticisms were (and still are):

☐ Adverse selection is more common in mental health than in acute-care insurance. Given an option—particularly one subsidized by employers—the vulnerable are more likely to choose generous (and expensive) mental benefits coverage.

☐ Moral hazard is more common in mental health than an acute-care insurance. Since need for care is ambiguous and defined by the patient, the beneficiary is eager to use his full entitlement.

☐ Utilization is prolonged unnecessarily until benefits are exhausted. The criteria for cure are unclear and defined by the patient. Unlike acute care, mental therapy does not interfere with continuation of employment and family life. Extended care becomes part of one's lifestyle and is painless personally and financially.

☐ Provider-induced demand is more common in mental health than in acute-care insurance, since treatments can be repeated. Ambulatory mental health providers schedule their work long in advance and can stabilize their incomes by fixing the beginning and end of prolonged patient regimes.

☐ Only substantial cost sharing and strict limits on entitlements can control utilization.

The American Psychiatric Association, state associations, the national government's own National Institute of Mental Health (NIMH), and foundations responded to these criticisms by sponsoring study commissions and empirical research that uniformly argued for full parity between mental health and somatic benefits under health insurance.[28] Some research conceded that mental health insurance is particularly vulnerable to adverse selection, moral hazard, and unnecessarily prolonged utilization, and the authors searched for insurance designs that could avoid the pitfalls.[29]

At the same time, serious work was being done by task forces of the American Psychiatric Association and by others to improve mental health care and, incidentally, to make it a more insurable risk under insurance:

☐ Diagnostic nomenclature was improved in the light of clinical experience and research findings. The new nomenclature has several uses in health insurance—such as providing the basis for diagnosis-related groups in inpatient hospitalization and practice guidelines in utilization review.[30]

☐ When the reliability of the new system of diagnosis was tested, it surpassed that of past methods.[31]

☐ Research about the outcomes and cost-effectiveness of specific services began under the Carter administration, was shelved under the Reagan administration, and became a high priority during the late 1980s as part of the larger thrust in outcomes research in health.[32] Presumably only safe and effective therapies would be paid for under public and private health insurance.

☐ Clinical research into the somatic causes and physical treatment of mental illness continued. Without anyone intending it, the clinical basis of psychiatry was moving the field closer to the medical model that had been the original assumption of health insurance design.

While these long-term foundations were being improved, private American mental health insurance was being swamped by the contagions of emotional disorder and substance abuse that afflicted employees and their families during the 1970s and 1980s. Despite the limits in employer group contracts on length of inpatient hospital stays, on lifetime mental health costs, on numbers of outpatient visits, and on the employer's own contribution to per diems, to hospital charges, and to fees, mental health costs were thought to rise faster than acute-care costs. Because of the paucity and biases in research about mental health insurance, the employers and their managed-care consultants had little knowledge of the facts and few insights into the reasons. The standard reactions were more cutbacks—but they would be resisted by the beneficiaries, might increase the bad health that employee benefits were supposed to reduce, and would not solve the causes. During the late 1980s, managed care was being touted as the salvation of employment-based health insurance. But it did not seem to fit mental health.[33]

A perennial problem in American mental health insurance has been the identity of the provider to be reimbursed. Since health insurance automatically paid physicians, it therefore paid psychiatrists and non-psychiatrically-trained physicians, even when the latter gave psychiatric treatments. Mental health services could also be delivered by psychologists, nurses, and social workers who, under many circumstances, might be clinically superior and less expensive. For years, the psychiatrists and clinical psychologists argued over the right of the latter to prescribe, to file claims, and to receive high fees. The specialist psychiatrists also challenged the right of other physicians to treat and bill for psychiatric care—a particular example of the jurisdictional issues arising in every country's clinical medicine and health insurance.[34]

The clinical and financial jurisdictions of physicians and other professionals are problematic in long-term care as well as in psychiatry. Both fields involve prolonged comforting, life support, teaching, and rehabilitation. A physician is well suited to some tasks but is neither skilled nor interested in others. To maintain his power, he may try to be the case manager and employer, though another professional may be better suited. In both psychiatric care of the young and long-term care of the aged, the issues of comparative reimbursement, authority, and roles are not so sensitive in the hospital and in community health centers, where all the professionals are salaried employees of organizations. But the complications arise in ambulatory mental health insurance, since such financing follows the model of acute medical care. A task in the design of insurance for both mental health and long-term care is coverage not for a physician alone but for an entire team of collaborators—including a case manager who may be a nonphysician and has authority to shift the patient back and forth among various medical and nonmedical services.

The analogy to long-term care can be extended to an important American innovation: the Social HMO for long-term care of the elderly (described in the next chapter). Instead of fitting all mental health care into the conventional model of acute-care insurance—billing by physicians alone, fee-for-service, and inpatient hospitalization paid for by per diems, charges, or DRGs—comprehensive Mental Health HMOs might be created. They would operate community health services and day hospitals, they would offer menus of mental health services, they would involve teams of professionals (psychiatrists and others), and they would use case managers.[35] They might share facilities and staffs with Social HMOs. The Mental Health HMOs, Social HMOs, and statutory acute-care health insurance would be linked but not fully merged. As noted elsewhere in this book, conventional HMOs might not be able to survive under statutory health insurance except as multispecialty groups—because of legislative prohibitions of patient lock-ins and closed physician panels—but HMOs dedicated to special purposes outside acute care might exist and even prosper.

Notes

1. Past and present mental health services in Europe are described in Steen P. Mangen (ed.), *Mental Health Care in the European Community* (London: Croom Helm, 1985); Chris Breemer ter Stege and Martin Gittelman, "The Direction of Change in Western European Mental Health Care," *International Journal of Mental Health*, vol. 16, nos. 1–2 (1987), pp. 6–20 plus the articles about individual countries in the same issue; and Hugh L. Freeman and others, *Mental Health Services in Europe* (Copenhagen: World Health Organization Regional Office for Europe, 1985).

2. The development of payment of short-stay and long-stay psychiatric hospital care under French health insurance is described in Christine Gaston, *L'hospitalisation des malades présentant des troubles mentaux dans les établissements psychiatriques et à l'hôpital général* (Paris: Centre de Recherche pour l'Etude et l'Observation des Conditions de Vie, 1983). Much information about French psychiatric hospital services is scattered throughout Norbert Paquel and others, *Le coût de l'hospitalisation* (Paris: Centre d'Etude des Revenus et des Coûts, 1977–1984).

3. See Norbert Paquel and Pierre Giraud, *Le coût de l'hospitalisation—Les établissements de soins privés—Descriptions et analyse d'ensemble,* Documents du CERC no. 54 (Paris: Centre d'Etude des Revenus et des Coûts, 1980), pp. 33, 35. The substantial numbers of admissions and patient-days are cited on p. 130. Smaller proportions of the for-profit beds are devoted to mental health in countries with fewer psychiatrists. For example, 14 percent of Germany's private clinic beds (not including the establishments at spas) are devoted to psychiatry and neurology; see Bundesministerium für Jugend, Familie, und Gesundheit, *Daten des Gesundheitswesens—Ausgabe 1989* (Stuttgart: Verlag W. Kohlhammer, 1989), p. 265.

4. Methods of paying for inpatient care under German statutory health insurance are described in Steen P. Mangen, "Germany: The Psychiatric Enquête and Its Aftermath," in Mangen, *Mental Health Care in the European Community* (see note 1, above), chap. 5; see also Meinolf Nowak and others, *Modellprogramm psychiatrie: Finanzierung psychiatrischer Versorgung* (Cologne: PROGNOS AG, 1983), pp. 158–184.

5. *Kosten en financiering ZFW en AWBZ* (Amstelveen: Ziekenfondsraad, 1986), p. 22. For a discussion of the complete pattern of management and financing of the Dutch mental hospitals and special institutions for the mentally hand-

icapped, see *Financieel overzicht zorg 1990* (The Hague: Ministerie van Welzijn, Volksgezondheid, en Cultuur, 1989), pp. 51-79. For overviews of Holland's several intramural and extramural programs see S. Rose and N. Steffens, *De geestelijke gezondheidszorg in Nederland* (Amersfoort: ACCO, 1987); Tom E. D. van der Grinten, "Mental Health Care in the Netherlands," in Mangen, *Mental Health Care in the European Community* (see note 1, above), chap. 10; and R. Giel, "The Jigsaw Puzzle of Dutch Mental Health Care," *International Journal of Mental Health*, vol. 16, nos. 1-2 (1987), pp. 152-163.

6. Pierre Chanoit (ed.), *La psychiatrie: aujourd'hui ... demain* (Paris: Mutuelle Générale de l'Education Nationale, 1979); and Inspection Générale des Affaires Sociales, *Les formes complémentaires de la protection sociale* (Paris: Ministère de la Santé et Ministère du Travail, 1975), pp. 236-239.

7. See, for example, the effects of the highly technical and itemized German fee schedule described in Mangen, "Germany: The Psychiatric Enquête and Its Aftermath" (see note 4, above), pp. 83-86.

8. The prolonged (and still only partially successful) struggle of psychiatrists within the medical associations and insurance systems is described in Glaser, *Paying the Doctor* (Baltimore: Johns Hopkins Press, 1970), pp. 158-159, 295; and Pierre Gallois and Alain Taib, *De l'organisation du système de soins* (Paris: La Documentation Française, 1981), vol. 1, pp. 44-47, 181-186.

9. *Le secteur libéral des professions de santé en 1985*, Carnets Statistiques no. 28 (Paris: CNAMTS, 1986), p. 30. Of all French statutory insurance spending for psychiatry, less than 5 percent goes for physicians' fees and 87 percent is spent on hospital care (including the salaries of the medical staffs). The rest (8.3 percent) pays for pharmaceuticals. See Christian Rampht and Christine Meyer, *Evaluation du chiffre d'affaires de la psychiatrie en 1984*, Cahiers de la Division des Etudes no. 9 (Paris: CNAMTS, 1986), p. 25.

10. The RIAGGs and other ambulatory mental health services are described in J. M. Boot and M.H.J.M. Knapen, *De Nederlandse Gezondheidszorg* (Utrecht: AULA, 1983), pp. 99-109; and in *Regional Institutes for Out-Patient Mental Health Care in The Netherlands* (Utrecht: Nederlandse Vereniging voor Ambulante Geestelijke Gezondheidszorg, 1985). Their financing by AWBZ is summarized in Tom E. D. van der Grinten, "Organisatie, beleid en financiering in de ambulante geestelijke gezondheidszorg," *Tijdschrift voor sociale geneeskunde*, vol. 60, no. 16 (Aug. 18, 1982), pp. 418-424; and *Advies inzake verstrekking hulp door of vanwege een Regionale Instelling voor Ambulante Geestelijke Gezondheidszorg* (Amstelveen: Ziekenfondsraad, 1981).

11. Monika Steffen, *L'alternative a l'hospitalisation en psychiatrie* (Saint Martin d'Hères: CERAT, I.E.P. de Grenoble, 1987); and Steen P. Mangen and Françoise Castel, "France: The 'Psychiatrie de secteur'" in Mangen, *Mental Health Care in the European Community* (see note 1, above), chap. 6.

12. William Laing, *Private Health Care* (London: Office of Health Economics, 1985), chap. 5.

13. The mental care procedures that resemble acute care and fit the tradi-

tional insurance model are described in Jeffrey A. Buck, "Should Mental Health Services Be Structured Like Medical Care?", *Inquiry*, vol. 19 (Fall 1982), pp. 211-221.

14. The history of mental health benefits in private health insurance in the United States appears in Louis S. Reed and others, *Health Insurance and Psychiatric Care: Utilization and Cost* (Washington: American Psychiatric Association, 1972); and Steven S. Sharfstein and others, *Health Insurance and Psychiatric Care: Update and Appraisal* (Washington: American Psychiatric Press, 1984). For short summaries of mental health financing (including the ebb and flow of insurance) and mental health services see Thomas G. McGuire, *Financing Psychotherapy* (Cambridge, Mass.: Ballinger, 1981), chap. 2.

15. McGuire, *Financing Psychotherapy* (see note 14, above), pp. 44-51; see also James A. Schuttinga and others, "Health Plan Selection in the Federal Employees Health Benefits Program," *Journal of Health Politics, Policy and Law*, vol. 10, no. 1 (Spring 1985), pp. 127-136; and Edwin Hustead and others, "Reductions in Coverage for Mental and Nervous Illness in the Federal Employees Health Benefits Program, 1980-1984," *American Journal of Psychiatry*, vol. 142, no. 2 (Feb. 1985), pp. 181-186.

16. Greg Scandlen and Brenda Larsen, *State Mandated Health Care Coverage Laws* (Washington: Office of Government Relations, State Services Department, Blue Cross and Blue Shield Association, 1988). For summaries and criticisms of the entire policy of state mandates see Greg Scandlen, "The Changing Environment of Mandated Benefits," *Employee Benefit Notes*, June 1987, pp. 6-9; and Carolyn Peterson, "Mandated Health Benefits: Time to Evaluate," *The State Factor* (of the American Legislative Exchange Council), vol. 12, no. 4 (May 1986), pp. 1-10.

17. For overviews of the present heterogeneous state of private health insurance coverage—by the Blues, commercial carriers, HMOs, and self-insured plans—see Sharfstein and others, *Health Insurance and Psychiatric Care* (see note 14, above); Sam Muszynski and others, *Coverage for Mental and Nervous Disorders: Summaries of 300 Private Sector Health Insurance Plans* (Washington: American Psychiatric Press, 1983); and Allan P. Blostin, "Mental Health Benefits Financed by Employers," *Monthly Labor Review*, vol. 110, no. 7 (July 1987), pp. 23-27.

18. "New Directions in Mental Health Care," *Federation of American Health Systems Review*, vol. 21, no. 3 (May-June 1988), pp. 18-26 passim. The peer review methods previously developed by the American Psychiatric Association and used by some carriers are described in Sharfstein and others, *Health Insurance and Psychiatric Care* (see note 14, above), pp. 40-43 and sources cited.

19. The time series are given in Freeman and others, *Mental Health Services in Europe* (see note 1, above).

20. Richard G. Frank and Thomas G. McGuire, "A Review of Studies of the Impact of Insurance on the Demand and Utilization of Specialty Mental

Health Services," *Health Services Research,* vol. 21, no. 2, pt. 2 (June 1986), pp. 241–265.

21. See Sharfstein and others, *Health Insurance and Psychiatric Care* (see note 14, above), pp. 24–27; and Constance M. Horgan, "The Demand for Ambulatory Mental Health Services from Specialty Providers," *Health Services Research,* vol. 21, no. 2, pt. 2 (June 1986), pp. 291–320.

22. See Bruce Levin and Jay H. Glasser, "A National Survey of Prepaid Mental Health Services," *Hospital and Community Psychiatry,* vol. 35, no. 4 (April 1984), pp. 350–355; and William Goldman and others, special issue about mental health services in HMOs, *Administration in Mental Health,* vol. 15, no. 4 (Summer 1988), pp. 187–261.

23. Daniel Y. Patterson and others, "Health and Mental Health Care of the 1980's," *Journal of the National Association of Private Psychiatric Hospitals,* vol. 10 (1979), pp. 12–18. For a summary of empirical research comparing the services in HMOs and in conventionally insured office practice see Jon B. Christianson, "Capitation of Mental Health Care in Public Programs," in Richard M. Scheffler and Louis F. Rossiter (eds.), *Advances in Health Economics and Health Services Research* (Greenwich, Conn.: JAI Press, 1989), vol. 10, pp. 284–285 and sources cited.

24. The complaints of the office psychiatrists are summarized in David Upton, *Mental Health Care and National Health Insurance* (New York: Plenum Press, 1983), pp. 4–5, 58–59. The offsetting savings in acute care within HMOs are summarized in Upton's book, p. 186 and sources cited, and in Gary R. VandenBos and Patrick H. DeLeon, "The Use of Psychotherapy to Improve Physical Health," *Psychotherapy,* vol. 25, no. 3 (Fall 1988), pp. 335–343 and sources cited.

25. Some tests and treatments increase more than others, according to Richard G. Frank, "Regulatory Policy and Information Deficiencies in the Market for Mental Health Services," *Journal of Health Politics, Policy and Law,* vol. 14, no. 3 (Fall 1989), pp. 494–497.

26. Steven S. Sharfstein and Howard L. Magnas, "Insuring Intensive Psychotherapy," *American Journal of Psychiatry,* vol. 132, no. 12 (Dec. 1975), pp. 1252–1256.

27. Paul Chodoff, "Psychiatry and the Fiscal Third Party," *American Journal of Psychiatry,* vol. 135, no. 10 (Oct. 1978), pp. 1141–1147.

28. Upton, *Mental Health Care and National Health Insurance* (see note 24, above); Sharfstein and others, *Health Insurance and Psychiatric Care* (see note 14, above); and several others. For a summary of the literature arguing that mental disease genuinely exists and is an insurable risk, see Martin Roth and Jerome Kroll, *The Reality of Mental Illness* (Cambridge: Cambridge University Press, 1986).

29. McGuire, *Financing Psychotherapy* (see note 14, above); and Steven S. Sharfstein and Carl A. Taube, "Reductions in Insurance for Mental Disorders: Adverse Selection, Moral Hazard, and Consumer Demand," *American Journal of Psychiatry,* vol. 139, no. 11 (Nov. 1982), pp. 1425–1430.

30. *Diagnostic and Statistical Manual of Mental Disorders,* 3rd rev. ed. (DSM-III-R) (Washington: American Psychiatric Association, 1987). A completely new DSM-IV will appear in 1992. The use of DSM-III in creating psychiatric DRGs is discussed in Donald Scherl and others (eds.), *Prospective Payment and Psychiatric Care* (Washington: American Psychiatric Association, 1988), especially chaps. 2-4.

31. Robert L. Spitzer and others, "DSM-III Field Trials," *American Journal of Psychiatry,* vol. 136, no. 6 (June 1979), pp. 815-820. Diagnostic reliability is said to be no better in somatic medicine; see Roth and Kroll, *The Reality of Mental Illness* (see note 28, above), pp. 94-97.

32. The efforts during the Carter administration—once thought stillborn but now considered essential groundwork—are described in Gary R. VandenBos (ed.), *Psychotherapy: Practice, Research, Policy* (Beverly Hills: Sage, 1980), and in the symposium "Psychology in the Public Forum," *American Psychologist,* vol. 38, no. 8 (Aug. 1983), pp. 907-955.

33. The flux in demand, treatment modalities, utilization, costs, and management is summarized in "New Directions in Mental Health Care," *Federation of American Health Systems Review,* vol. 21, no. 3 (May-June 1988), pp. 10-43. For a summary of recent problems of managed care in mental health insurance and in employer self-financed employee assistance plans, see Lloyd I. Sederer and R. Lawrence St. Clair, "Managed Health Care and the Massachusetts Experience," *American Journal of Psychiatry,* vol. 146, no. 9 (Sept. 1989), pp. 1142-1148; see also Sari Staver, "Employers Turning to Managed Mental Health Care," *American Medical News* (of the American Medical Association), May 26, 1989, pp. 1, 13-14.

34. For the psychiatrists' case for primacy and some rebuttals see Upton, *Mental Health Care and National Health Insurance* (see note 24, above), pp. 33-112, 232-233; Paul Chodoff, "Effects of the New Economic Climate on Psychotherapeutic Practice," *American Journal of Psychiatry,* vol. 144, no. 10 (Oct. 1987), pp. 1293-1297; and the debate between a clinical psychologist and Chodoff in *American Journal of Psychiatry,* vol. 145, no. 8 (Aug. 1988), p. 1049.

35. The whole concept is suggested by Steven S. Sharfstein, "Medicaid Cutbacks and Block Grants: Crisis or Opportunity for Community Health?", *American Journal of Psychiatry,* vol. 139, no. 4 (April 1982), pp. 468-470. Sharfstein was inspired by the need to provide better public financing and community service for Medicaid beneficiaries, but the method could be redesigned for the entire insured population. The effective integration of mental health into conventional acute-care HMOs is explained in John T. Boaz, *Delivering Mental Healthcare: A Guide for HMOs* (Chicago: Pluribus Press, 1988).

CHAPTER 15

Long-Term Care

─────────────────────── **Summary** ───────────────────────

Long-term care requires supplying, combining, and financing nonmedical and acute-care services. Countries vary in their understanding of the mix and in their supply of social and personal services. Need rapidly grows because of the aging of all populations and because of policies to keep the chronically disabled out of acute hospital beds.

The elderly and disabled of every country are now fully covered by statutory health insurance for all their acute-care needs. In the past they had to pay for long-term housing, maintenance, and personal services out-of-pocket, with the help of their pensions and families. The poor without enough money and family support had to rely on public charity.

All countries now search for ways to organize and finance the nonacute long-term-care institutions and benefits. There is no standard model that all might emulate. Governments and health insurance carriers are reluctant to add long-term care to traditional statutory insurance, since new providers would be involved, the need for long-term care is not as clear-cut and as insurable as in the well-established decisions in acute care, utilization can be prolonged and expensive, and utilization control may be difficult. The costs of acute-care insurance have only recently been contained, and governments fear any new measures that might destabilize their systems.

Holland alone has enacted special long-term-care insurance as part of social security. Financed by payroll taxes, it covers nursing home stays, the personal services in home care, and prolonged institutionalization. It has enabled Holland to develop very comfortable nursing homes. The Dutch government has recently won a prolonged struggle to control its costs.

Since both the pension and the health insurance sectors of social security protect the elderly and disabled, both sectors may collaborate in creating the long-term benefits that are beyond the competence of each alone. In France, the two pool money to construct sheltered housing, provide social services, and add medical facilities to old-age homes. They pool money to enable individual beneficiaries to pay for home aids. In Switzerland, the pension system subsidizes a national network of case managers and home-care agencies. Moreover, the pension system helps the poor elderly and disabled pay their acute-care health insurance premiums. Unless such community services are created and unless the pension system pays, the disabled fill up acute-care hospital beds at the expense of the health insurance system, as Germany's experience demonstrates.

Since much of long-term care consists of the housing, personal aids, and food that are part of daily living, all arrangements use means tests and require cost sharing by the user. The indigent alone are subsidized in full. Otherwise, social security will pay for everyone and the heirs of the affluent will enjoy a financial windfall.

Private health insurance carriers are cautiously introducing long-term-care policies. They begin with nursing home benefits, which are insurable risks. Cash benefits for home care and special housing are being added cautiously. A serious problem is how to market these policies to a young population. Age-of-entry lifelong premiums may persuade farsighted buyers and may build up the reserves essential to cover high costs late in life.

The United States debates many of the options heard abroad. In addition, the Americans have experimented with several innovations (such as Social HMOs) that deserve attention abroad. But while Europe eventually makes decisions and will create some sort of system, America continues to debate inconclusively. In lieu of a solution using social insurance, the Americans rely on public welfare for long-term care (that is, Medicaid) while other countries reduce it.

Dilemmas

Health insurance is obligated to add new acute benefits. Doctors and patients demand them; health insurance exists in order to find the money. But the cost containment crisis has led every insurance program to avoid adding new nonacute benefits—unless they clearly work to the advantage of the carrier by attracting new subscribers. Unfortunately for the sickness funds, this is the moment when everyone realizes that more is needed for the growing numbers of elderly members: nursing care at home and in long-stay establishments; physiotherapy; meals; home helps; and more. The elderly have chronic as well as acute conditions, and long-term care may be permanent.

The philosophy of social solidarity has always guaranteed that the pensioners receive full acute-care benefits despite paying low premiums or none at all. The same philosophy now presses for long-term-care benefits. But every country for the moment is uncertain about the content of the benefit package, the source of the money, and the method of administration.[1] The issues are:

☐ What benefits should be provided?
☐ Who should decide the patient's need for benefits?
☐ What are the roles of acute-care health insurance and any other social insurance in paying providers?
☐ How do insurance payments relate to any other financing?

Sources of Money

In the past, the long-term-care needs of the elderly were financed from several sources:

☐ Statutory health insurance covers some benefits. Whether they are in the doctor's office, their own homes, hospitals, or special institutions for the elderly, the aged members of sickness funds continue to get full entitlement to all acute-care benefits. During the 1960s and 1970s, nearly all pensioners were added, even if they had not been members while they (or their husbands) had been working. Often during the 1960s and 1970s they were charged no premiums; later, as sickness funds ran deficits, they were charged low premiums. In a few countries, they benefited from lower cost sharing than the young were obliged to pay.
☐ Out-of-pocket payments were the usual method for home help services, prolonged stays in nursing homes, and permanent stays in old-age homes.
☐ Pension funds under social security provided cash to the retired person. The pensions were based on prior earnings history and not on current need for long-term care. The funds provided pensions and did not pay for health or personal services. These pensions provided much of the cash for the out-of-pocket payments.
☐ Social welfare programs of municipalities became principal sources to pay for home services and nursing home care for the elderly with no or low pensions, with little personal income, with few assets. In every country, the poor elderly constituted a large fraction of the beneficiaries.
☐ Social welfare programs of private religious associations had been the principal source of help for the poor elderly during earlier centuries. During the twentieth century in many countries, they continued to play important roles as owners and managers of nursing homes and home-care services. But they recently experienced declining charitable contributions, declining numbers of nuns, and demands by their employees for normal hours and wages—at a time when the numbers of dependent elderly have been greatly increasing.

The problem is how to expand some of these channels (or combine them) in order to finance and deliver long-term care.

Expanding Statutory Acute-Care Health Insurance

One solution is to add benefits to the existing health insurance that already covers the elderly. This has been done in two forms: extended-care hospitals and home visits by nurses and physiotherapists.

At one time, the chronically ill were mixed together with the acutely ill in general hospitals, a practice that resulted in long average stays. This remains true in much of Germany. But France has attempted a division of labor: a new hospital building is constructed for acute care; the old building is retained for chronic care; the same managers and medical staff service both; the chronic patient is referred back to the acute hospital from time to time as needed. The French hospital receives lower reimbursement from the sickness fund for the extended-care days than for the acute-care days, since the extended-care division has lower operating costs. The control doctor from the French sickness fund reviews the patient's file periodically and must approve extension of the stay. But the extended-stay hospital is a medical and not a residential facility, and the patient eventually must transfer elsewhere. Since the patient receives room and board from the extended-care hospital as well as a pension (either for old age or for disability), he must pay a significant fraction of the cost.[2]

Home visits by nurses and physiotherapists have long been benefits of statutory health insurance in France, Belgium, and French-speaking Switzerland, where district nurses and physiotherapists are self-employed. The prescribing doctor must prescribe the number of visits, and the nurse and physiotherapist bill the sickness fund. The nurses and physiotherapists are paid according to a fee schedule negotiated between their professional associations and the sickness funds in the same manner as in the reimbursement of physicians.

These benefits do not satisfy the needs of long-term care—like all services under statutory health insurance, they are acute-care benefits given under the supervision of physicians. The extended-care hospital is medicalized. The visiting nurse's and the physiotherapist's fee schedules list treatments prescribed by doctors.

These home health services arouse policymakers' anxieties over utilization review and cost containment. During recent years the agency monitoring Belgian health insurance (the *Institut National d'Assurance Maladie-Invalidité*, or IN-AMI) has been trying to identify the cases of unnecessary prescriptions by doctors for courses of treatment by nurses and physiotherapists, unnecessary prolongation of courses of treatment, and false billing. Because the excessive number of doctors in Belgium causes competition and hence the need to please patients, prescriptions and renewals are generous. Because home visits are not easily monitored, unnecessary care and fraudulent billing occur.

A few acute-care insurance systems are now cautiously experimenting with the addition of true long-term-care benefits. In Germany, for example, private health insurance companies are ever eager to demonstrate inventiveness in recognizing and satisfying new needs. The association of private health insurers designed a policy for cash benefits to the family when the subscriber needs long-term care. For higher premiums in the table, the subscriber gets higher benefit payments. For a later age of entry, the subscriber must select from a higher premium table, thereby protecting the insurer from adverse selection. For a rating of greater need—made jointly by the doctors retained by the patient and by the insurance company—the family gets more cash. The family can spend the money for any health, social, and personal needs, thereby relieving the company of the difficulty of specifying benefits. By giving the family cash and freedom to shop, the company avoids having to name acceptable providers and negotiate rates. Since benefits are a fixed cash schedule related to premiums, costs of the program are controlled. Companies compete over the premium tables and the benefits. The policies were offered for the first time in 1986.

In Switzerland, too, Zurich canton in 1986 added home care by salaried visiting nurses and by home health aides to the standard acute-care protection by the insurance companies. As I explain later, such home care at present is widely available to Swiss self-payers and (with the help of subsidies from the pension system) to the poor elderly. Home visits by nurses for acute-care treatments are an insurance benefit in the French-speaking cantons. Swiss insurance companies offered supplementary policies to cover home nursing costs (like those now beginning in Germany), but not enough Swiss bought them; Zurich officials wanted to tap the larger financial base from the main insurance policies. Zurich wanted to add to all insurance offered in the canton long-term care as it is really delivered—by salaried employees of community agencies providing on each visit whatever personal services the home visitor deemed necessary. To the Zurich officials, these were progressive steps to improve the quality of life and to reduce costs by keeping the elderly out of the hospital. To the insurance companies, they were a Pandora's box of unnecessary visits, unreported services, and an add-on to the costs of hospital care. The insurance companies refused to bear the risks, and the canton has had to pay nearly all the costs in subsidies to the sickness funds. To prevent abuse, courses of care are limited, need is recertified periodically by the patient's doctor, and the patient shares some of the cost.

Statutory Long-Term-Care Insurance

The idea of including long-term care in the social security package has been discussed in several countries—for example, as "Part C" of American Medicare—but has been enacted only in the Netherlands. The Dutch government in 1967 passed the General Law for Exceptional Medical Expenses (*Algemene Wet Bijzondere Ziektekosten*, or AWBZ).

At first, the problem was thought to be simply a matter of filling omissions in acute-care health insurance. The first aim was to pool risks and resources for catastrophic conditions that happened rarely but were beyond the financial capacities of the family: the hospitalized patient who exceeded the number of days covered by acute-care statutory insurance; the family with a mentally handicapped child requiring lifelong institutionalization. Until 1967, as in other countries, these Dutch patients depended on religious charities and public welfare. Instead of merely extending public welfare and its means tests, Holland made the benefits an entitlement of every citizen. Statutory health insurance until the 1990s was compulsory only for the 70 percent of the population under an income ceiling, but AWBZ was always universal, covering every person and financed by a payroll tax on every employer. Individuals do not pay premiums; the elderly and the institutionalized pay nothing, and no payroll taxes are paid on their behalf. Since employers alone cannot bear the cost of this very expensive program, the national government pays a large annual subsidy to the AWBZ account.

From the start, AWBZ covered extended-care hospitals (after the patient exhausted his insured days) and nonprofit nursing homes giving skilled care. Their prospective budgets are screened by the regulatory agency that monitors all hospitals (COZ, now called COTG). Allowable costs include staffing, equipment, living expenses, and amortization of the debt incurred to build the facilities. As a result, Holland has new and well-provided nursing homes, patients' costs are covered in full, and a higher proportion of the elderly are institutionalized in nursing homes in Holland—at least 6 percent of those over sixty-five—than in any other country.[3]

Likewise, many special establishments for handicapped children and adults were created in Holland because of AWBZ financing. All are nonprofit, and most are operated by charitable associations, often sectarian. Medical, living, and nursing costs are covered fully by AWBZ. Only educational costs are charged to other budgets.

AWBZ precipitated a familiar dilemma: it had great success in caring for the chronically disabled, placing them in modern and pleasant environments, providing attentive care-givers, and relieving the families. But by the late 1970s, once thrifty Holland had unexpectedly attained one of the highest levels of health and social spending in the world. The government could not reduce benefits. In fact, it kept expanding AWBZ by charging to it new programs—such as preventive examinations and immunizations—that it did not wish to charge to the deficit-ridden general budget of government. During the desperate search for methods of cost control, the government sought alternatives to the excessive institutionalization of the elderly.

One solution was to add home care to AWBZ's benefits in 1980 and to reorganize the home-care system.[4] For over a century, separate Catholic, Protestant, and nonsectarian "Cross Associations" in each locality had provided home care to young mothers, to the disabled, and to the infirm elderly from each religious group.[5] Each local Cross Association had pieced its budget together from annual membership dues from families with incomes, subsidies from public welfare offices and other government agencies, and patient charges. The reorganization of the late 1970s made home care more efficient and more generously financed. All the Cross Associations merged in each locality. Home care became a benefit of AWBZ that covered nearly all the costs of the elderly as well as chronically disabled adults; and home care became a benefit of statutory acute-care health insurance with coverage of nearly all the costs of expectant and newly delivered mothers. If the patient pays the Cross Association an annual subscription fee, he is not billed any charges for services.

The homebound person, as before, is visited by his GP under statutory acute-care health insurance. Home-care benefits under AWBZ cover the employees and services of the Cross Association: the district nurse, home health aide, nutritionist, and physiotherapist. The patient receives home care initially on the the order of the GP or hospital discharge nurse, but he can also ask his Cross Association himself. Thereafter, it is the district nurse who decides to continue or terminate care. The nurse is the case manager and orders all services. Daily rates are negotiated between the Cross Associations and special sickness funds that administer the AWBZ money; the rates are determined by the Cross Association's level of staffing. The special carriers send the Cross Association a steady flow of cash to cover their case load.

As in the case of AWBZ financing of nursing homes, the home-care benefits have been welcomed by the patients and the employees of the Cross Association. Holland has become a model of home services beyond the acute care delivered by doctors. The case manager is a specialist in nonmedical long-term care. But home care in Holland is expensive, and nursing home utilization has not been reduced substantially.

The financial burden on beneficiaries is minimal, but it must be borne by employers and general taxpayers. Although public welfare for the poor is no longer involved in long-term care, a burden remains, and it has been shifted to the social security system.

Cooperation Between the Pension and Health Insurance Systems

The social security pension funds traditionally have only provided cash between retirement and death. It was left to the pensioner and his family to use the cash for his housing and personal services. If their needs were higher than the pensions, they had to seek extra money from charitable associations and municipal welfare offices.

France. Involving the pension system in long-term-care services requires a broader definition of its mission. A precedent long existed in France: the guilds and mutual aid societies provided a range of services to their members, including cash for temporary invalidity, cash upon retirement, and home visits by doctors and other employees. This mixture continued when the *mutualités* were revived during the nineteenth century. An organized and ideologically articulate national movement of the numerous *mutualités* asserted that members could use these agencies of solidarity to meet all their needs for social protection. These mutual aid societies were the carriers for the first statutory pension and health insurance laws. Besides the payment of pensions and the reimbursement of health care providers, they continued to deliver medical and home help services of many kinds.

After World War II, the principal tasks were transferred to three hierarchies of governmental carriers for pensions, health insurance, and family allowances. The law creating the new public pension carriers (CNAV, CNAVTS, and its regional offices) authorized use of their resources for tasks benefiting the pensioners (*action sanitaire et sociale*). A fraction of the revenue from payroll taxes, from earnings from the reserves, and from a few other reserves is earmarked for these expenditures. The spending is administered on behalf of the pension funds by the regional agencies of the health insurance system.

The grants by the pension system are of two kinds:[6]

☐ *Collective.* These grants help construct sheltered housing and community services for the elderly. During the first decades of these grants, most money was used to construct nursing homes, old-age homes, and special housing. Nursing homes and old-age homes are no longer subsidized, since excessive institutionalization is now contrary to public policy. Grants are now provided to build up medical facilities within old-age homes in order to eliminate the need for hospitalization.

☐ *Individual.* These grants pay for services needed for particular pensioners. The purpose is to help the infirm elderly live at home and avoid institutionalization. Most of the grants today are used for these purposes:
  • Home aids of all sorts: wages of helpers, meals, and supplies.
  • Refurnishing homes so the elderly can continue to live there.
The pensioner is expected to pay for part of the individual services according to a scale based on his pension and total income.

The sickness funds have their own *action sanitaire et sociale* for the benefit of all patients, including the elderly:

☐ *Collective.* These are grants and loans to hospitals—including extended-care hospitals—for new construction and renovation.

☐ *Individual.* These are grants helping poor patients—including many elderly—to pay for the cost sharing required by the health insurance law.

The combined efforts of the pension system and sickness funds produce two main thrusts in home care for the same clients:

☐ Medical care by doctors, nurses, and other medical personnel, paid for largely by the sickness funds (*hospitalisation à domicile*)

☐ Personal supports by nurses, housekeepers, nutritionists, and others paid for by *action sanitaire et sociale* with some contributions by municipal welfare departments (*soins infirmiers à domicile pour personnes âgées* and *l'aide ménagère*)[7]

When a program matures in France, it becomes standardized throughout the country by regulations, reimbursement methods, and cost reporting. But long-term care in France is still far from such stability:[8]

☐ One purchaser does not yet dominate the market. The pension fund (CNAV) is important now and its role will grow in the future, but it does not yet set the pattern. Cost containment limits its money for long-term care. Many chronically disabled still must depend on ad hoc help from municipal welfare offices.

☐ Defining the components of long-term care in various settings—in the extended-care hospital, in the mental hospital, in the partially medicalized residential institutions, in home care—is not yet settled. The policy literature has grown recently, but no consensus exists.

☐ Units of payment and rates of cost sharing by patients vary by type of institution. The French have only recently begun to investigate methods of rating patients by the need for long-term care and methods of varying services and third-party reimbursement by need.[9]

☐ Priorities can be reversed quickly. For example, as in other countries, funds once were used primarily to build institutions for the aged, but recent policy has switched completely in favor of home care.

☐ Even if funds were available, the growth of long-term care would be blocked by a shortage of home-care agencies.

☐ Management of benefits has been delegated to the regional and local sickness funds. CNAV issues guidelines that are specific on only some matters. Considerable local variations exist in the roles of case managers—often but not always doctors—in authorizing and renewing home care.

☐ Coordination at the grass roots is not established. Methods of managing the several payers and service providers have not yet been disseminated and standardized throughout the country. The agencies in each locality do not share the same goals and organizational styles.

☐ Planning is not yet possible in each locality, since the separate agencies do not meet together regularly, share the same goals, or contribute to a common pool of information.[10]

Germany: Separation of the Health and Social Sectors. The French method of mixing health and pension insurance in the medical and social sectors might become an ideal model for any country. In contrast, Germany is an example of problems resulting from complete separation of the health and social sectors. There the health insurance accounts under social security may be used only if a physician certifies that the patient is sick. Then the patient is treated by a doctor and placed in an acute-care hospital. If the elderly person is merely disabled but not "sick" in the acute-care sense, he cannot draw upon any third-party social insurance to pay for services.[11]

One result is the complete separation between residences for the elderly and the acute-care hospitals. Germany has few nursing homes, and they lack the medical staffs and medical facilities now being added in other countries. The patient must pay nursing home charges completely out-of-pocket, assisted either by the social welfare offices (for the poor) or the new private insurance policies (for the rich).

Another result of the separation is the use of acute-care hospitals for long stays that, in other countries, would be transferred to nursing homes. Germany therefore has more hospital beds and longer stays than other developed countries. Once they are admitted to a hospital under statutory health insurance, patients are allowed to stay on by hospital doctors and hospital directors, since the providers are guaranteed per diem health insurance payments. The sickness funds' control doctors are supposed to disallow unnecessary days but hesitate to force patients out because medicalized nursing home substitutes do not exist.[12]

Another result of the German financing arrangements is the high involvement of the German family. Reformers in other countries fear that long-term insurance and public financing will result in excessive institutionalization or (if the patients are paid for home care) pecuniary windfalls for the family. But these outcomes are not possible in Germany.

By the 1980s, the German Ministry of Health sought fundamental changes. The acute hospital sector could not be reduced when so many of its beds were being filled by custodial cases. The elderly's needs were not being identified, and appropriate services were not being created. Possible reforms were discussed for several years.[13] The first practical step was the addition of home care to statutory health insurance benefits. Eligibility was limited to the severe cases who otherwise would have filled hospital beds. Respite care for the family was included. Monthly contributions by the sickness funds were limited. Since the benefit was targeted on the severely ill, a long-term-care program still remained to be designed.

Switzerland. Germany illustrates the underdevelopment of long-term care when health insurance concentrates on acute care and pension insurance plays no role. Switzerland demonstrates the value (as in France) of active protection of the total lives of the elderly by the pension program. Swiss health insurance focuses on acute care; the social sector alone organizes and finances long-term care.

Swiss social programs have always been crafted to combine adequate mixed financing, flexible administration, local responsibility, and voluntary participation. Centralized, bureaucratized, and collective organization is avoided. The result is social solidarity with an individualistic spirit.[14]

Home care is delivered by agencies in each community. They train, employ, pay, and supply home aides. In larger cities, executives may be salaried; in smaller ones, many executives are volunteers motivated to protect their neighbors, a role being replaced by functionaries in other countries but still potent in Switzerland. The network of home-care agencies has small cantonal and national offices to deal with governments and financial donors.[15]

Fundraising at the top and case management at the grass roots are done by another network: *Pro Senectute,* an association of volunteers and a few paid executives that protects the interests of the elderly. The national office receives an annual grant from the Swiss statutory pension insurance fund to pay all the administrative and salary costs of all the national, cantonal, and communal offices of *Pro Senectute.* The national office also receives from the pension fund the money to subsidize pensioners with high needs and low incomes (the *Erganzungleistungen* described in Chapter Eight). Cantonal offices raise money from cantonal governments for home care of the low-income elderly who cannot pay out-of-pocket. Communal offices raise similar public grants in the more affluent cities.

The communal staffs of *Pro Senectute* investigate the incomes and living costs of the poor pensioners and distribute the *Erganzungleistungen* money. Persons needing home care come to the attention of the communal staff by the elderly person's application, by a health or social worker, or by the office's own case finding. The case manager arranges for a visiting schedule by the home health agency, determines the family's contributions in work and money, decides the size of the client's out-of-pocket contribution, pays the rest from the communal *Pro Senectute* budget, and monitors the outcomes. The operating money therefore combines contributions by the national pension system, the cantonal and communal social welfare budgets, private donations, and the patients' own out-of-pockets. The patient is not stigmatized, since *Pro Senectute* is a respected organization. Most of its home-care clients are self-payers (some with the help of the *Erganzungleistungen*), the public welfare money merges into a *Pro Senectute* pool, and no client is identified openly as a welfare recipient.

A Private System: The United States

The United States has enacted acute-care statutory health insurance for the aged and chronically disabled who receive pensions from the Social Security system— that is, Medicare. As in all other countries before public intervention, the long-term-care needs of the elderly and disabled were left to families and the person's own financial resources—and they still are today.[16]

Most care is given by family members. Usually there is no financial assistance from insurance and public programs and no help from community services. Families—particularly the adult female care-givers—are burdened emotionally and financially, especially after the patient's condition has deteriorated and is prolonged.[17] A substantial number of the elderly have no family help: the children have moved far away, they are uncooperative, or the person was childless.[18] These problems are probably more common in the United States—with its fragmented and mobile social structure—than in Europe. Unlike Switzerland and several other European countries, America has few community institutions to fill such gaps.

Public Programs. The Social Security pensions for the retired (enacted in 1935) and for the chronically disabled (enacted in 1956) provided cash according to the beneficiary's prior earnings history. But the dependent elderly and disabled still needed the family and neighbors to provide services and most financial support. Some indigent elderly lived in old-age homes, nursing homes, and mental hospitals operated by state governments and private charities. Because the law barred Social Security pension payments to residents of public institutions, a private nursing home industry sprang up.

The "medically indigent" were covered by heterogeneous state and municipal public welfare programs; some paid the costs of nursing home confinement. The national government agreed to share the costs of the state programs beginning in 1960 (the Kerr-Mills Act) and expanded and made permanent in 1965 (Medicaid). Nursing homes multiplied, and the institutionalization of the indigent elderly increased. Medicaid unexpectedly became the largest funder of long-term care. Half of all American nursing home costs are now covered by these public grants, and the other half is paid by patients out-of-pocket—often a stage before they become indigent and are added to the Medicaid rolls. All state Medicaid programs eventually added home-care benefits, but their largest long-term-care share remains nursing homes.[19] Although Medicaid's long-term-care arrangements have been limited in cost, they have never changed in structure. There have been many state experiments in acute-care benefits but little debate and few innovative proposals about the long-term-care benefits.[20]

Medicare was enacted in 1965 to give pensioners the type of acute-care services that Blue Cross and Blue Shield provided the employed groups but that were no longer available to the retired. Long-term care was not included. Medicare's original nursing home benefits and its subsequent home-care benefits were intended for short-term convalescence after discharge from the hospital. Because of this limitation, nursing home benefits were not used much. The home-care benefits in practice were often used for long-term-care needs after the patient had recovered from the acute-care condition—in violation of the regulations.[21] The addition of long-term care—a Medicare Part C, much like the addition of Holland's AWBZ to its acute-care statutory health insurance—has often been proposed but never enacted.[22] The executive branch and Congress have been preoccupied with controlling Medicare costs and shrink from adding a new and unpredictable benefit. Congress eliminated the prior hospitalization requirement in 1988, thereby opening up the use of nursing homes under Medicare. But it repealed the reform and reinstated the requirement a year later when the public protested the higher taxes to pay for this and other new benefits.

As possible harbingers of the future, several social insurance schemes were introduced in Congress during the late 1980s. "Lifecare" covered nursing homes and home care in full for up to six months. The revenue would come from the

Medicare payroll taxes, but not by increasing the rates. Rather, the earnings ceiling would be abolished and the extra revenue would be earmarked for Lifecare. Nursing home care would continue after six months, paid partly by the Lifecare trust fund and partly by a fund created from insurance premiums paid earlier by beneficiaries.[23]

Private Insurance. During the 1980s, Americans discussed at great length the problems of the aged, their need for long-term care, and the deficits in services. But the Reagan administration wanted to reduce the role of government, not extend it into a new field. Long-term care became a new niche for the private commercial health insurance industry. Devotees of free competitive markets argued that the need for long-term care was an insurable risk and that appropriate group and individual insurance policies could be designed and marketed.[24] The United States became a laboratory for demonstrating whether an entire population could be covered by private voluntary long-term-care insurance.

Insurance companies offered policies and, by the early 1990s, had found over a million subscribers. Because the carriers feared adverse selection, excessive costs, and excessive utilization, they hewed close to traditional indemnity insurance for acute care:[25]

☐ The policies are sold almost entirely to individuals and their spouses. Even when the policies are marketed to employed groups, the subscriber (and payer of premiums) is the individual worker and not the employer.

☐ The benefits at first were paid only when a subscriber was institutionalized in a nursing home under doctor's orders. Like Medicare, some private policies require prior acute hospitalization. To avoid the costs of nursing homes, most policies are beginning to cover the alternative use of home care for the convalescent or chronically disabled.

☐ The benefits are cash indemnity payments and not full reimbursement of provider charges. Coinsurance rates need not be calculated. Since the cash payments are lower than provider charges, the patient must add considerable out-of-pocket. A subscriber can choose policies with higher premiums and higher indemnities.

☐ Premiums are lifelong age-of-entry rates—a departure from America's age-graded acute-care rates. Low premiums at young ages of entry are intended to attract and keep young subscribers, who normally are not interested in prepaying for long-term care and mistakenly believe Medicare will protect them in old age. High premiums at older ages of entry protect the carrier from adverse selection on the eve of need, the principal hazard of long-term-care insurance.

☐ A deductible ("elimination period") specifies the number of days that must be spent in the nursing home or in home care before payments begin. It satisfies the carriers' fears of overutilization, moral hazard, and excessive costs from uncontrollable numbers of patient-days.

☐   Some policies vary premiums, coverage, or both after medical underwriting of applicants, particularly the elderly on the eve of need. Since policies are guaranteed renewable, carriers deny coverage to some persons with serious prior conditions, such as mental illness.

Marketing long-term-care insurance encounters several serious barriers:[26]

☐   The American health care system and health insurance are so complicated that most people once thought they would be fully covered for long-term care by Medicare. Only slowly are people learning they are not protected at all.
☐   Insurance requires a pool of good and bad risks. But many young persons think they will never need long-term care and start worrying only late. While sales have been growing, they fall short of the entire population and many eligible persons never hear of long-term-care policies, particularly among workers.[27] The lifelong age-of-entry premiums are unfamiliar to Americans and may not impress the young, who imagine they will never need the benefits.
☐   Americans are accustomed to getting health insurance "free" and resist paying premiums. In the market for individual policies, lapses and changes of carrier are frequent. Americans may object to the rules of a long-term-care insurance market with age-of-entry premiums—rules requiring renewals after a lapse at a higher premium or back-payment of all the unpaid premiums.
☐   Employers are trying to reduce the costs of acute care—not increase the financial costs and administrative effort by adding long-term coverage. But incorporating the young workers and their families into the long-term-care financing system may be essential for a complete societal financial pool: without extensive employer group coverage, social insurance might be the only alternative. (During the late 1980s, a few employers bought group insurance to cover an unexpected problem: workers who were absent to care for elderly parents. The policies enabled the workers to hire care-givers.)

Even if long-term-care insurance can be designed successfully and marketed widely, there are great difficulties in implementing it:

☐   Home nursing care, social supports, personal care, meal services, and the like might be overused and wasted. Methods of rating patient needs (such as the "Activities of Daily Living" scales) are being tested in their early stages and may not be reliable and strict enough for insurers. Identifying improvement in the patient's needs is still not highly reliable. Utilization review in an institutional setting (like a nursing home) is difficult enough, and it is much more difficult in the elderly persons' dispersed homes.
☐   The providers in long-term care are unorganized and cannot yet participate collectively in reimbursement negotiations, quality assessment, and utiliza-

tion review. Each provider is autonomous, and nearly all are for-profit small businessmen.

☐ The United States has few providers in long-term care, let alone providers of high quality.

Some insurance carriers have begun to offer a long-term-care option in life insurance policies. Under traditional arrangements, a substantial amount of money from a paid-up policy goes entirely to the heirs but the insured himself has been ruined by long-term-care costs. Under the option, the insured can reclaim some of the cash to pay for long-term care (and the beneficiaries receive less). Life insurance therefore becomes a form of prepayment for care. Whether state insurance commissioners will allow a mixture of traditionally separate accounts remains to be seen. But the scheme has received an important impetus from the national government, which is now offering an option in the life insurance it gives its own civil servants. An advantage of the method is collection of premiums at a younger age than the usual time when people start buying long-term-care insurance.

Comprehensive Care and Appropriate Financing. Proposals and products in long-term-care insurance in the United States and some other countries have followed a sequence like that in traditional acute-care insurance. Certain services (like hospitals and nursing homes) become widely used, potentially expensive, and underdeveloped because of underfunding. Some persons lack access because they lack money. Social and private insurance are devised to cover these benefits. Other needs are deemed less urgent or less insurable and are excluded. Utilization is thought to be clear-cut and finite.

But long-term care does not fit this image of specialized individual services, clear-cut need, and full recovery by the patient. The long-term-care patient has multiple conditions and needs several services. Most services are not medical; they must be created and coordinated; and the system needs case managers who are not physicians. Patients' needs must be rated according to their competence in daily living and according to the presence and skills of family care-givers. Patients' needs for particular services vary from time to time, and they must be transferred back and forth. Therefore, a range of services must be coordinated— and the financial arrangements must cover their appropriate use at the right time. The services needed are:

☐ Acute care by physicians.
☐ Housing appropriate for the dependent and disabled. If existing housing is used, it must be adapted.
☐ Acute-care hospitalization.
☐ Nursing homes.
☐ Acute-care nursing care and equipment.

- ☐ Personal care and homemaker services not provided by the family. Respite care when the family is not available.
- ☐ Teaching the family care-givers.
- ☐ Meals.
- ☐ Transportation.
- ☐ Case management.
- ☐ Communication between patient and case manager.

Therefore, something broader than the traditional health insurance model is needed. In response, several American arrangements organize these many services and use insurance-like financing:

- ☐ *Continuing care retirement communities (CCRCs).* They provide full special housing and all the foregoing long-term-care services. The person must pay a large entry fee to cover the housing and contribute to the contingency reserves; usually the subscriber brings enough money from sale of his home. Thereafter, the subscriber pays a monthly subscription fee to contribute to the operating costs of the long-term-care services; he has enough cash from his pensions and other assets. He has some out-of-pocket payments for coinsurance (particularly for nursing home care) and for special services (such as extra cafeteria meals and some recreational programs). Usually the doctors and hospitals are in the surrounding community; the subscriber can pay them by the usual methods with Medicare and Medigap. The managers screen out the bad medical and financial risks but welcome subscribers who sign up early in life. The subscription premium is usually a lifelong age-of-entry rate.[28]
- ☐ *Social health maintenance organizations (S/HMOs).* The enterprise includes a prepaid multispecialty medical group (organized either as an HMO or IPA) with full admitting privileges to a hospital. Medicare and Medigap cover the capitation payment. The S/HMO also provides all necessary long-term-care services for an annual subscription paid either by the person out-of-pocket or by Medicaid. The rates cover the S/HMO's current costs. Since the patient remains in his home, the S/HMO need not levy a large entrance fee and maintenance charge for housing. Communication and transportation links must be installed between the case manager's office and the patient's home. In contrast to the many CCRCs, there are only a few S/HMOs.[29]
- ☐ *Life care at home (LCAH).* The program offers all necessary long-term-care services. Since the patient remains in his home, the LCAH needs no large entrance fee or maintenance charge for housing. Subscribers are encouraged to join and prepay while young by means of lifelong age-of-entry premiums. The accumulated reserve guarantees coverage of each subscriber's lifetime costs, particularly the high and less predictable nursing home costs. The patient continues to use his private physicians and their affiliated hospitals

under the customary reimbursement methods of Medicare and Medigap. The LCAH has been proposed but not yet implemented.[30]

These comprehensive service and financing arrangements have encountered several difficulties:[31]

☐ The costs of constructing and maintaining housing often exceed expectation, and the entry fees and age-of-entry premiums for many CCRCs have not been high enough. Bankruptcies leave the residents with low real estate resale values and without long-term-care protection.

☐ Nursing home costs often exceed expectations, both in daily operations and in lengths of stay. Home-care services cannot be substituted well enough to reduce nursing home admissions and stays. To balance the enterprise's budget and avoid abrupt increases in premiums, the program may limit the number of nursing home days—reducing the program's appeal over conventional long-term-care insurance and damaging the marketing image of lifetime protection.

☐ So many elderly have been getting Medicare and Medicaid benefits "free" that they refuse to pay actuarial premiums for long-term care and even resist reduced premiums subsidized by government and employers. They refuse to share their pensions.

☐ The poor do not—and may not be able to—pay the large entry fees for the CCRCs. Therefore, the subscribers are the rich and society is left with the problem of covering most of the population. Since the assets and incomes of the rich are tied up in CCRCs and these programs cannot be folded into social insurance, prospects of redistributive social insurance for long-term care diminish.

☐ Few people have the foresight to start subscribing while young.

☐ Benefits are not portable. The subscriber must stay in the locality.

☐ As in the case of the acute-care HMO lock-in, applicants are put off by the need to give up their regular physicians.

☐ An established acute-care HMO with its own loyal doctors and hospital (like Kaiser) can add long-term-care services. But an S/HMO that starts as a nursing home or home-care agency has difficulty enlisting enough doctors to form a multispecialty panel and has trouble persuading a nearby hospital to give all the doctors admitting privileges.

☐ As in all private long-term-care insurance, marketing and administrative costs are high.

Effects on Utilization and Health

Every country is aware of the need to organize and finance new programs for the elderly. The options are specified with considerable sophistication. But no country has clearly resolved all the dilemmas, and none has produced a successful final model. Because of the variety of financing methods, the changes, and the short-ages of services, one cannot clearly trace the clinical consequences of each third-party financing system.

Development of Services. A well-planned financial method with wide cov-erage can place the disabled elderly in appropriate settings with staffs skilled in long-term care. The elderly and their families need not worry about impoverish-ment. Nursing homes have an attractive rather than miserable atmosphere; home care is delivered by experienced persons with adequate equipment.

A comparison of two neighbors—Belgium and Holland—demonstrates the difficulties in creating satisfactory long-term-care services in the absence of long-term-care insurance. Holland has AWBZ, but Belgium has nothing like it. The disabled elderly have long filled the extended-care wards of Belgium's acute-care hospitals, where they have been fully covered by statutory health insurance. Compared to Holland, Belgium has had more hospital beds per capita, longer lengths of stay in acute-care hospitals, more patient-days in the hospitals, and no advanced nursing homes at all.[32] Most Belgian old-age homes (*maisons de repos*) lack health services on the premises. A few tried to add nursing care and treat-ments during the 1970s and 1980s, but these efforts were underfunded and under-developed. Families had financial incentives to keep the patient in the hospital, not move him to a private *maison de repos*.

During the 1980s, the Belgian government was determined to limit hos-pital costs—in large part by eliminating convalescent occupancy. But its dilemma arose from the general budget deficit (preventing creation of a new nursing home system from general revenue) and from the policy of limiting social insurance (not adding new benefits). Changes had to be made as controls over hospital budgets reduced stays and increased discharges, but the sectors receiving the re-ferrals have expanded only grudgingly. Several dozen old-age homes have added medical services and became *maisons de repos et de soins* (MRS). A patient can be admitted for a prolonged stay—usually after a hospital discharge—by the control doctor of the patient's sickness fund. A special fund of the Ministry of Social Affairs pays a daily grant to the MRS (950 FB in 1984, the first year of the program), and the patient pays the rest of the bill. If the family cannot pay, it must turn to the communal government's welfare office. If the family can pay, the cost-sharing requirements still are an incentive to keep the patient in the hospital. Nevertheless, some patients have moved from hospitals to MRSs. The MRS does not earn enough revenue to attain the levels of staffing and comfort found in Dutch nursing homes.[33]

Also in contrast to Holland, Belgium lacks the universal insurance financ-ing essential to the generous provision and widespread utilization of home-care services. Some Belgian paramedicals are paid fees under statutory health insur-ance—resulting in a possibly excessive number of home visits by nurses and physiotherapists. But other home-care services are underdeveloped and are unequally distributed, since they require completely private out-of-pocket payment or welfare subsidies.[34]

Without widespread home-care services and universal insurance financing, nearly all of Belgium's disabled elderly are cared for at home by their families. The country's tight family bonds have always performed this function. But no one has yet compared underfinanced Belgium and overfinanced Holland in terms of clinical health and patient morale. A surprising number of transfers to nursing homes from home care have occurred in Holland; apparently families are willing to move their parents out of their households if the nursing homes are satisfactory. This expensive trend in Holland has been stopped only by halting the construction of new nursing homes; the result is long waiting lists. New policy proposals in long-term care in Belgium are careful to stress methods of assisting the family in home care without replacing it.[35]

Using the Appropriate Service. When one examines the effects of an insurance reimbursement on acute-care utilization, it is clear which service is being utilized. But long-term care differs: it is a set of roughly substitutable services. The problem is whether an insurance arrangement promotes or deters access to each service and the appropriate level of work for each type of patient. As the patient's condition changes, the financing methods should support appropriate transfers.

Long-term-care financing has developed as a series of separate ad hoc coverages of specific services. Means tests and cost sharing are customary in each, since the patient and his family should still pay for the patient's maintenance and social supports. But the different cost-sharing rates have perverse incentives: comprehensive third-party coverage is introduced to eliminate financial barriers against using any service; but the patient and family prefer services that are clinically less appropriate than those with higher cost sharing. French experience shows how the patient suffers clinically and the long-term-care accounts suffer financially.[36]

The only counterweight to such biases by the family is a case manager. The physician cannot be the case manager: he is biased in favor of acute-care services, he is rarely interested in convalescent and social services, and he has little time and interest for the patient's total life. The only counterweight to fragmented financing and the uneven provision of services unrelated to need is a coordinated method of financing and delivery—as in Social HMOs being tried in America.

Implications for the United States

The Need for a Comprehensive Policy. Acute-care services and acute-care financing developed in an unplanned and narrowly focused manner in all countries. But clearly progress in long-term care cannot be achieved without large-scale management and long-range thinking. Long-term care requires creating and coordinating many services, activating and combining several sources of money, and serving persons with diverse needs.

America's long-term-care policy cannot simply evolve spontaneously out of its past and current long-term-care practices. The public component of care for the chronically disabled, young and old, has always been welfare for the indigent. If one has money, he pays for himself among private providers. One becomes eligible for the statutory program by spending down into indigence. Medicaid has merely expanded welfare financing for acute care and long-term care. Europe, by way of contrast, tries to build on a long history of social services run by municipalities and religious associations: it tries to implement social protection in purpose and social solidarity in financing. Europe uses means tests in long-term care, but usually only to decide the amount of cost sharing and to choose the third-party payment channel, not to determine eligibility for the statutory program.

The United States needs to break away from its custom of trying to solve problems by extending established programs and filling gaps with new categorical programs. Its public long-term-care financing is limited to the indigent, creates new indigence, and stigmatizes the beneficiaries. Long-term care should be humanitarian in goals and in implementation.

Mixed Financing. America might achieve adequate financing and universal coverage by private voluntary long-term-care insurance, but that is unlikely. After all, the country has not achieved universal coverage and adequate redistributive financing by voluntary private insurance to cover the more widely appreciated acute-care services. The greater the coverage by private long-term-care insurance, the greater the problem in covering the entire population: the premiums of private health insurance cover only the subscribers to that risk pool; they are not socially redistributive; and American private subscribers then resist paying additional money to help the poor and the bad risks. In order to sell policies to an apathetic public in a price-cutting competitive market, private long-term-care insurance may always be underfunded in benefits for its own subscribers.

Private long-term-care insurance may never cover the sector because its benefits may always be limited and, in its excessive marketing claims, it may mislead its subscribers. Insurance companies cover insurable risks like posthospital nursing home confinement—which occurs infrequently, is distributed randomly in the population, has predictable costs, and invites little moral hazard. Insurance companies fear the less predictable, less observable, and more manipulable sectors that are at the heart of long-term care, such as the social supports in home care.[37]

An element of obligatory public insurance—other than welfare coverage from general revenue—seems unavoidable. But such statutory insurance need not require the high taxes and high premiums for lavish services. Nor need it displace private participation. A trend in all countries is universal two-tier financing of pensions, and some countries are discussing universal two-tier health insurance.

America might preserve its voluntary private health insurance as a second tier. Statutory insurance for the entire population would cover most acute-care and basic long-term care. But since long-term care includes many amenities and services constituting one's standard of living, private participation related to one's own income is necessary. Private health insurance—purchased voluntarily by anyone—would cover some acute-care services and many long-term-care services. Statutory insurance (perhaps supplemented by Treasury subsidies saved from the terminated Medicaid) would cover basic long-term-care services for all. A person could buy more generous and better-quality services out-of-pocket or by private insurance. Private long-term-care insurance policies could be crafted with a great variety of benefits, reimbursement levels, and premiums.

Long-term-care financing includes both the logic of insurance and the logic of prepayment:

☐ *Insurance.* The degrees of dependency requiring nursing home confinement and advanced home care occur unexpectedly for the individual but in expected frequencies in society. Probability rises with age, but it is never certain for the individual. Social and private long-term-care insurance can be designed accordingly.

☐ *Prepayment.* One form is a supplement to an insurance policy. When events create a need for long-term care, the insured person can collect benefits. Besides the basic services covered by the standard policy, the patient and his family prefer certain forms of delivery and better amenities. The private insurance package can be designed to cover the costs of such discretionary services, triggered by the collection of basic nursing home or basic home-care insurance benefits.

A second form of prepayment is a special savings account accumulated over the years to cover benefits collected by the patient or family whenever they wish. Cumulative over the years, the account would cover costs that become more probable with age but can occur at inconvenient moments and at burdensome costs. The account could cover optional benefits that depend on individual lifestyle and family structure but are not insurable risks in large populations—benefits such as respite help for the family.

Such a mix in financing methods will not arise spontaneously from the recent American policy style of endless discussion, research reports, demonstration projects, and catalogues of policy options. Designing and enacting a new system require leadership and political will.

Case Management. Acute care long begged questions of case management by allowing the doctor and patient to decide everything. Payers recently have made doctors more careful by introducing prospective questions and retrospective review, but the doctors are still in charge.

Long-term care requires new forms of case management.[38] Doctors are not interested or qualified. Patients are uncertain about their true needs; they and their families are interested in excessive provision of certain services. Many providers exist, their quality varies, and someone must choose and oversee them on behalf of both patient and payers. Individual plans of care must be designed and revised as the patient's needs change.

A common American method—unusual in Europe—is to delegate public functions to private for-profit contractors. Competitive bids, detailed regulations, and bureaucratic monitoring are supposed to ensure job performance. Nevertheless, overcharging, underservicing, and fraud occur—often in programs intended to deliver acute care and long-term care to the poor. Neither the government nor (in too many cases) the contractor himself knows about the qualifications and the performance of the contractor's employees.[39] Government then requires elaborate and burdensome written reports. But there is no substitute for well-motivated civil servants. Case management for long-term care should not be handed over to private management firms.

Social HMOs are case managers with reliable services. They are one of America's more important innovations. But they may not be able to attract enough enrollments—thereby leaving most of the elderly in need of a different form of long-term-care case management. One solution could be a national voluntary association devoted to protection of the elderly, an entity like Switzerland's *Pro Senectute*. It would unite local volunteers and staffs earning modest salaries. It would manage the money from several public funds and insurance programs. It would select providers and oversee performance. It would require Americans to think and act like Swiss, no small change. Perhaps the American Association of Retired Persons might add such a network, but it should be independent of AARP's advocacy functions.

Services. It is not enough to enact a law that lists benefits. Americans often legislate in this narrow fashion without visualizing the consequences and spelling out implementation. Therefore, the public and private sectors must collaborate—not only in designing long-term-care financing but also in creating the right number, quality, and mix of services in all communities, arrangements that will mesh with family members and with volunteers.[40] This effort is much more difficult (and less glamorous politically) than merely passing a financing law.

America has already seen in long-term care the failure to plan services when financing was enacted. Medicaid in 1965 suddenly expanded demand for nursing homes. Americans assumed that the free market would respond to the incentives and would automatically generate the supply. Indeed it did. Many disreputable operators quickly created nursing homes.[41] Long-term-care services financed by Medicaid have been stigmatized ever since and have required government machinery to detect and penalize fraud and underservicing.

America would have to develop a program in housing, as well, not merely one for long-term-care services. The care of the aged depends not only on the presence of family care-givers but also on the elderly's housing. Scandinavia demonstrates how long-term-care programs must be coordinated with appropriate forms of housing for the aged. America entered the 1990s without any public policies in long-term care or housing—except for wishful thinking that "free markets" and "pluralism" would automatically yield solutions.

Goals. One lesson from abroad is that publc policy in long-term care should pursue the positive aims of compassion, not merely avoid incurring costs. During the late 1980s, the United States procrastinated in making any decisions about long-term care lest Medicare and government be saddled with new costs. In 1989, it even repealed the limited expansion in its Medicare Catastrophic Coverage Act. Another country that had long struggled to control costs—the Netherlands—at the same time decided that an important protection for the disabled elderly was lacking. In 1989, Holland added nonmedical home-help benefits to AWBZ.[42]

Notes

1. People's needs for long-term care and the services generally required are summarized in Rosalie A. Kane and Robert L. Kane, *Long-Term Care* (New York: Springer, 1987), pt. 1. Options in financing, organizing, and delivering long-term care generally are summarized in Alice M. Rivlin and Joshua M. Wiener, *Caring for the Disabled Elderly* (Washington: Brookings Institution, 1988), especially chap. 1; and Günter Buttler and others, *Wege aus dem Pflegenotstand* (Baden-Baden: Nomos Verlagsgesellschaft, 1985). Descriptions of the still unsystematic arrangements in several countries appear in Klaus Grossjohann and Detlev Zöllner, *Soziale Sicherung bei Pflegebedürftigkeit in europäischen Nachbarländern* (Bonn: Gesellschaft für Sozialen Fortschrift, 1984); Teresa Schwab (ed.), *Caring for an Aging World* (New York: McGraw-Hill, 1989); and Pamela Doty, *Long-Term Care for the Elderly Provided Within the Framework of Health Care Schemes* (Geneva: Permanent Committee on Medical Care and Sickness Insurance, International Social Security Association, 1986).

2. France's institutional services and their financing are described in Pamela Doty and Andrée Mizrahi, "Long-Term Care for the Elderly in France," in Schwab, *Caring for an Aging World* (see note 1, above), pp. 58–62, 66–68, 73–75; and Andrée Mizrahi and Arié Mizrahi, *Financement des soins et des séjours des personnes âgées en institutions* (Paris: CREDES, 1988), chap. 1.

3. Doty, *Long-Term Care for the Elderly* (see note 1, above), p. 24. Over 21 percent of the Dutch above seventy-five years are in nursing homes and special retirement institutions according to Anton Amann and others, *Open Care for the Elderly in Seven European Countries* (Oxford: Pergamon Press, 1980), p. 19. In addition, some Dutch elderly are in nonmedicalized old-age homes not covered by AWBZ.

4. *Opneming werk van kruisinstellingen in de Algemene Wet Bijzondere Ziektekosten* (Amstelveen: Ziekenfondsraad, 1978). At first, policymakers favored

home care for its own sake. Not until later was it justified as a cheaper substitute for institutionalization in nursing homes.

5. These programs have always provided social services as well as health care. See J.M.P. Scholten, "The Development of Home Help Services in the Netherlands," in *Home Help Services Around the World* (Washington: International Federation on Aging, 1975).

6. The early decades of the program are described in Jacques Doublet, *Sécurité sociale*, 5th ed. (Paris: Presses Universitaires de France, 1972), pp. 302–321. The current details are in *Notice sur l'action sanitaire et sociale de la Caisse Nationale d'Assurance Vieillesse des Travailleurs Salariés en faveur des personnes âgées* (Paris: CNAV, 1985); and Elie Alfandari, *Action et aide sociales*, 3rd ed. (Paris: Dalloz, 1987), passim, especially pp. 196–202, 407–443.

7. Monika Steffen, "Entre le social et le médical, quelles alternatives?", *Prévenir*, no. 14 (2nd Trimester 1987), pp. 11–21. The several financing channels also converge to support indigent elderly in intramural long-term care. Mizrahi and Mizrahi, *Financement des soins et des séjours des personnes âgées en institutions* (see note 2, above), chap. 1.

8. The needs, services, and financing are all in flux according to Martine Bungener and others, *Le bilan économique et financier du secteur médico-social* (Paris: Laboratoire d'Economie et de Gestion des Organisations de Santé, Université de Paris XI Dauphine, 1985), pp. 77–97.

9. Claudine Padieu and Lucien Mironer, "Les bénéficiares de l'aide ménagère: Test d'une grille d'analyse des dépendances," *Solidarité-santé: Etudes statistiques*, July–Aug. 1986, no. 4.

10. For case study of financing and service delivery in one area see Marie-Eve Joel and others, *L'action médico-sociale dans le département de la Sarthe* (Paris: Laboratoire d'Economie et de Gestion des Organisations de Santé, Université de Paris XI Dauphine, 1987).

11. The German system and its consequences are summarized in Arbeitsgruppe Fachbericht über Probleme des Alterns, *Alterwerden in der Bundesrepublik Deutschland: Geschichte-Situationen-Perspectiven* (Berlin: Deutsches Zentrum für Altersfragen, 1982), vol. 2, chap. 12; and Margret Dieck, "Long-Term Care for the Elderly in Germany," in Schwab, *Caring for an Aging World* (see note 1, above), chap. 3.

12. Compared to those in other European countries, the acute-care hospital sector in Germany has more beds, higher occupancy, and longer stays: Brian Abel-Smith and others, *Eurocare* (Basle: Health-Econ, 1984), pp. 92–99. Because so many inpatients are receiving custodial rather than acute-care services, German hospitals work with fewer employees and at lower daily costs than those of other countries: William Glaser, *Paying the Hospital* (San Francisco: Jossey-Bass, 1987), p. 403.

13. Several "think pieces" are *Bericht der Bund-Länder-Arbeitsgruppe "Aufbau und Finanzierung ambulanter und stationärer Pflegedienste"* (Bonn: Bundesministerium für Jugend, Familie, und Gesundheit, 1982); and *Bericht der*

Bundesregierung zu Fragen der Pflegebedürftigkeit (Bonn: Deutscher Bundestag, 10. Wahlperiode, Drucksache 10/1943, 1984). Basic facts about the needs of the disabled elderly had to be collected for the first time; see, for example, Werner Bróg and others, *Anzahl und Situation zu Hause lebender Pflegebedürftiger,* Schriftenreihe des Bundesministers für Jugend, Familie, und Gesundheit, vol. 80 (Stuttgart: W. Kohlhammer Verlag, 1980). Nursing homes with medical services had to be designed; see, for example, Ursula Mybes and others, *Zur Organisation pflegerischer Dienste in Altenpflege/Altenkrankenheimen,* Schriftenreihe des Bundesministers für Jugend, Familie, und Gesundheit, vol. 82 (Stuttgart: W. Kohlhammer Verlag, 1983).

14. See Ralph Segalman, *The Swiss Way of Welfare* (New York: Praeger, 1986); and Walter Ruegg, "Social Rights or Social Responsibilities: The Case of Switzerland," in S. N. Eisenstadt and Ora Ahimeir (eds.), *The Welfare State and Its Aftermath* (London: Croom Helm, 1985), pp. 182-199.

15. Services for the elderly are summarized in *Die Altersfragen in der Schweiz* (Bern: Eidgenössischen Drucksachen- und Materialzentrale, 1979), chaps. 7 and 8. Home care in one canton is described in Lilia Ramel and others, *Soins à domicile* (Lausanne: Réalité Sociale, 1982).

16. America had not only few public programs for the poor and dependent elderly, but also few private charitable programs. See W. Andrew Achenbaum, *Old Age in the New Land* (Baltimore: Johns Hopkins Press, 1978), pp. 75-86.

17. Kane and Kane, *Long-Term Care* (see note 1, above), especially chap. 2; and Marjorie H. Cantor, "Strain Among Caregivers: A Study of Experience in the United States," *Gerontologist,* vol. 23, no. 6 (Dec. 1983), pp. 597-604.

18. Judith D. Kasper, *Aging Alone* (New York: Commonwealth Fund Commission on Elderly People Living Alone, 1988), chap. 4.

19. For a summary of the initial coverage of nursing home care for the elderly and the sudden increases in utilization and costs, see Robert Stevens and Rosemary Stevens, *Welfare Medicine in America: A Case Study of Medicaid* (New York: Free Press, 1974), chaps. 1, 3, 5. Recent trends are summarized in Congressional Research Service, *Medicaid Source Book: Background Data and Analysis* (prepared for the Subcommittee on Health and the Environment, Committee on Energy and Commerce, U.S. House of Representatives, 100th Congress, 2nd Session, Committee Print 100-AA, 1988), especially app. C.

20. The most thoughtful book about options for long-term-care financing merely examines an expanded but still means-tested Medicaid: Rivlin and Wiener, *Caring for the Disabled Elderly* (see note 1, above), chap. 15. No American even suggests study of a universal Treasury-financed long-term-care program, such as that found in Canada and described in Robert L. Kane and Rosalie A. Kane, *A Will and a Way: What the United States Can Learn from Canada About Caring for the Elderly* (New York: Columbia University Press, 1985).

21. Judith Feder and William Scanlon, "The Underused Benefit: Medicare's Coverage of Nursing Home Care," *Milbank Memorial Fund Quarterly/*

Health and Society, vol. 60, no. 4 (Fall 1982), pp. 604–632; and Mary O'Neil Mundinger, *Home Care Controversy* (Rockville, Md.: Aspen Systems, 1983).

22. The idea was proposed by the House Select Committee on Aging and voted down by the House in July 1987. The addition of long-term care has been proposed in various forms by several policy research centers and individual authors: Cynthia J. Polich and others, *InterStudy's Long-Term-Care Expansion Program* (Excelsior, Minn.: InterStudy, 1988), 2 vols.; Christine Bishop, "A Compulsory National Long-Term-Care Insurance Program," in James J. Callahan and Stanley S. Wallack (eds.), *Reforming the Long-Term-Care System* (Lexington, Mass.: Lexington Books, 1981), chap. 4; Rivlin and Wiener, *Caring for the Disabled Elderly* (see note 1, above), pp. 210–236, 244–246; and Anne R. Somers, "Insurance for Long-Term Care," *New England Journal of Medicine,* vol. 317, no. 1 (July 2, 1987), pp. 23–29.

23. Jerry Geisel, "Kennedy Asks Employers to Fund Long-Term Care," *Business Insurance,* vol. 22, no. 13 (March 28, 1988), pp. 1, 4.

24. See, for example, Mark R. Meiners, "The Case for Long-Term Care Insurance," *Health Affairs,* vol. 2, no. 2 (Summer 1983), pp. 55–79; Mark R. Meiners and Gordon Trapnell, "Long-Term Care Insurance: Premium Estimates for Prototype Policies," *Medical Care,* vol. 22, no. 10 (Oct. 1984), pp. 901–911; *The Cost of Caring for the Chronically Ill: The Case for Insurance* (Washington: Special Committee on Aging, U.S. Senate, Senate Hearing 98-1224, 1984); and Morris Snow, "The Role of Insurance in Longterm Healthcare," *Generational Journal,* vol. 2, no. 1 (April 30, 1989), pp. 45–51.

25. See Susan van Gelder and Diane Johnson, *Long-Term Care Insurance: Market Trends* (Washington: Health Insurance Association of America, 1989); and Joshua M. Wiener and others, "Private Long-Term Care Insurance: Cost, Coverage, and Restrictions," *Gerontologist,* vol. 27, no. 4 (1987), pp. 487–493. For advice to the designers of policies see Max E. Lemberger: "Getting Better at Long-Term Care," *Best's Review—Life/Health Insurance Edition,* vol. 87, no. 10 (Feb. 1987), pp. 84–87; and Lemberger, "A New Deal for Long-Term Care," *Best's Review—Life/Health Insurance Edition,* vol. 88, no. 6 (Oct. 1987), pp. 50–54.

26. Rivlin and Wiener, *Caring for the Disabled Elderly* (see note 1, above), chap. 4.

27. The insurance industry has commissioned several marketing surveys of the population. Confronted by interviewers who focus on long-term care, respondents claim to be interested and willing to buy insurance policies. See, for example, Mark R. Meiners, *Public Attitudes on Long-Term Care* (Washington: Health Insurance Association of America, 1989). Once the interviewers leave, the respondents forget the subject. Asked about alternative financing, the American public would prefer "the government" to pay for its long-term-care costs: Stephen McConnell, "Who Cares About Long-Term Care?", *Generations,* vol. 14, no. 2 (Spring 1990), pp. 15–18.

28. Ian A. Morrison and others, *Continuing Care Retirement Communities* (New York: Haworth Press, 1986); and Howard E. Winklevoss and Alwyn V.

Powell, *Continuing Care Retirement Communities* (Homewood, Ill.: Richard D. Irwin, 1984).

29. Robert Newcomer and others, "Social Health Maintenance Organizations: Assessing Their Initial Experience," *Health Services Research*, vol. 25, no. 3 (Aug. 1990), pp. 425–454.

30. Eileen J. Tell and others, "Life Care at Home: A New Model for Financing and Delivering Long-Term Care," *Inquiry*, vol. 24, no. 3 (Fall 1987), pp. 245–252.

31. Rivlin and Wiener, *Caring for the Disabled Elderly* (see note 1, above), chaps. 5–6.

32. J. P. Heesters and J. Kesenne, "Financiering en Kosten van gezondheidszorg in Nederland en België," *Gezondheid & Samenleving*, vol. 6, no. 4 (Dec. 1985), pp. 314–320.

33. A van den Bussche and M. Bacten, "De l'hôpital à la maison de repos et de soins," *Dossier* (of the Alliance Nationale des Mutualités Chrétiennes), vol. 2, no. 5 (1984); and B. Hankenne and others, *Structure d'aide aux personnes âgées malades* (Louvain-la-Neuve: Ecole de Santé Publique, Université Catholique de Louvain, 1977), pp. 88–95.

34. Hilde Spinnewijn and Jozef Pacolet, *Kostprijs van de thuisgezondheidszorg* (Leuven: Hoger Instituut voor de Arbeid, 1985). The role of public welfare in home care is described in *C.P.A.S.: L'aide sociale, vous y avez droite* (Brussels: Fondation Roi Baudouin, 1986), pp. 34–54. The home visits by physiotherapists, their reimbursement, and the problems of utilization control are described in Denise Deliège and others, *Kinésithérapie et physiothérapie en Belgique* and *L'exercice de la Kinésithérapie* (Louvain-la-Neuve: Service d'Etudes Socio-Economiques de la Santé, Ecole de Santé Publique, Université Catholique de Louvain, 1982 and 1985).

35. As in Commission "Personnes âgées," "Quelle politique médico-sociale pour les personnes âgées?", *Dossier*, vol. 1, no. 2 (1983), especially chap. 4.

36. Jean-Claude Henrard and Anne-Marie Brocas, "Les obstacles tarifaires à une politique de soins pour les personnes âgées," *Revue française des affaires sociales*, vol. 40, no. 3 (July–Sept. 1986), pp. 59–73.

37. The limitations of private long-term-care insurance are summarized in Rivlin and Wiener, *Caring for the Disabled Elderly* (see note 1, above), chap. 4; in chap. 17 they offer strategy for mixed financing.

38. Numerous American methods are described in *Case Management for Long-Term Care* (Excelsior, Minn.: InterStudy, 1989).

39. The privatized and competitive Arizona Medicaid program broke down in large part because of the performance of the contracted case management. See Diane G. Hillman and Jon B. Christianson, "Competitive Bidding as a Cost-Containment Strategy for Indigent Medical Care: The Implementation Experience in Arizona," *Journal of Health Politics, Policy and Law*, vol. 9, no. 3 (Fall 1984), pp. 427–451 and sources cited; and Bradford Kirkman-Liff and others,

"The Evolution of Arizona's Indigent Care System," *Health Affairs,* vol. 6, no. 4 (Winter 1987), pp. 46–58 and sources cited.

40. Valuable ideas are presented in Kane and Kane, *Long-Term Care* (see note 1, above), chap. 12.

41. See Bruce Vladeck, *Unloving Care: The Nursing Home Tragedy* (New York: Basic Books, 1980), chaps. 3–5; and Mary Adelaide Mendelson, *Tender Loving Greed* (New York: Knopf, 1974).

42. *National Reports: Eighth International Congress* (Bern: International Council of Homehelp Services, 1989), p. 33.

CHAPTER 16

Adding New
Acute-Care Benefits

——————————— Summary ———————————

Selecting medical treatments is considered the prerogative of the medical profession. Coverage of new procedures by statutory health insurance has long been decided by the standing joint committees of doctors from the medical associations and the sickness funds who write the fee schedules. They add new procedures and eliminate obsolete ones.

The recent growth of complex, expensive, possibly ineffective, and potentially dangerous procedures leads to more elaborate screening machinery. Lest expensive but untested methods be installed in hospitals prematurely and proliferate, expensive equipment in countries with statutory health insurance requires grants from public funds, approvals by planning agencies, and approvals by the regulators who screen operating budgets. The hospital and its medical staff cannot install the new methods and cannot operate them by their own decisions. Rather, a consensus must be worked out with lay finance officers and facilities planners. Innovations usually go through an experimental period in academic medical centers. Then the medical faculties and a special monitoring agency in the Ministry of Health agree on wider use. A few specialized centers are given the grants to install the expensive new programs and are authorized to include their operating costs in the budgets covered by health insurance. Some countries have a considerable staff to evaluate innovations and authorize their widespread adoption.

America's private health insurance system has lacked machinery to evaluate and phase in expensive innovations. The country's ideology has always encouraged entrepreneurs to invent and quickly adopt new methods; its competitive style has led to the rapid and widespread use of innovations. Health services planning has never been seriously attempted. But there are drawbacks in this approach: risks to patient welfare and excessive costs to the system. Some payers— particularly Blue Cross and Blue Shield—have attempted to delay coverage of technically advanced benefits until their efficiency is established and have discouraged overutilization of the approved methods. But the hospitals and office doctors can still purchase advanced equipment, and the carriers hesitate to contradict the doctors' judgments about its use.

Covering Acute-Care Benefits

The purpose of statutory health insurance is to pay for the generally recognized treatments that will restore subscribers to health and to work. Until recently, the carriers deferred to the medical profession's judgment about the appropriate treatments (and they still do for the simpler and less risky procedures). These treatments are listed in the fee schedule used by each country's insurance system in the payment of doctors, described in Chapter Ten.

During the early years of health insurance in the nineteenth century, medical practice was simple and fee schedules were brief. The general practitioner's list consisted of the home visit, the office visit, dispensing of drugs (in Holland and in a few other countries), and a few other items. The visit was a global act encompassing most procedures. In addition, the surgeon billed for several types of operation, rated by complexity.

As medical practice became more complex, items were added to the fee schedules. Some lists were issued by medical associations, but they were guides to practice outside statutory health insurance, since the sickness funds refused to accept unilateral documents from medical associations. A fee schedule might be enacted by government as an appendix to the health insurance law and a guide to the payment of doctors—as in the case of Germany's PREUGO—but the drawback was rigidity in the face of clinical progress.

Decisions by the Negotiating System. In most countries, the updating of the fee schedule became part of the standing negotiating machinery between sickness funds and medical associations, as Chapter Ten explained. A permanent joint committee is created: it issues a new fee schedule from time to time, it adds new benefits as specific new items in the list, it interprets the list in response to questions and disputes from around the country, and it decides whether proposed procedures can be paid under existing lines rather than meriting new ones. All members are doctors, including the representatives of the sickness funds. The meetings between carriers and medical associations over money occur only about once a year, but the committee for the fee schedule meets every one or two months.

New clinical methods are reported in the world medical journals, tested in the teaching hospitals, and discussed in the scientific committees of the medical association. Eventually the specialty's representatives on the medical association's tariff committee propose that the new test or treatment be added to the fee schedule. The medical association's representatives in the joint payer/provider committee propose the addition, and the negotiating committee's secretariat checks that the professional literature poses no objections.

The joint negotiating committee eliminates old benefits as well as adding new ones. Treatments that are obsolete or manifestly ineffective (according to the professional grapevine) are dropped from the fee schedule during general revisions and at times individually. Since the fee schedule is an instrument for paying for services and controlling costs, items are reduced in price if they have become simpler.[1]

These methods were sufficient for endorsing new tests and treatments so long as the procedures were cheap for the insurance system and apparently safe for the patients. For a long time, doctors could do no more than simple procedures in their office and home visits, and hospitals too did simple work. But the evolution of expensive and risky methods—performed in nonprofit hospitals, in public hospitals, and in the doctors' own private clinics—led government to screen procedures for safety and led insurance carriers to challenge their need.

Installation in Hospitals. Safer and less expensive new technology can still proliferate through the country's hospitals at the discretion of the hospital chiefs of service and are covered by statutory health insurance in hospitals' operating budgets. But limits now exist in all developed countries.

In Europe, the new procedures usually originate in the few academic medical centers with financing by the educational and research budgets of the Ministry of Education. Drug and equipment companies may donate the materials and contribute cash to the professor's research budget. When a risky program is ready for wider use, each installation requires a license. Most European governments grant the money to a few special centers for the equipment and renovation of the building. The health insurance system then covers the full operating costs of patient care.[2]

Once the treatment is included among the insured benefits, the doctor can prescribe it for any patient. Waiting lists can result in hospital centers, but if care is urgent, something must be done by the sickness funds to fulfill their obligations to members. After open-heart surgery was added to the benefits of Dutch health insurance in the late 1970s, there was at first only one major center and later only a few hospitals with the equipment and staff. During the next years, the carriers cleared the waiting lists by flying patients to Switzerland and to Houston and paying for all costs. The government's hospital planners and rate regulators allowed more academic medical centers to add the equipment and staff for open-heart surgery; by 1986, all patients could be treated in Holland.

Permissive Reimbursement. If a country's statutory insurance system lacks a fee schedule, it cannot specify which tests are covered. America's Medicare is an example. Part B reimburses the doctor for any procedure he considers "reasonable and necessary for the diagnosis or treatment of illness or injury." The

Health Care Financing Administration could standardize practices if it administered its own program, but it does not. HCFA delegates all claims processing and all contacts with doctors to local insurance companies under contract. Forty-five different carriers run the program in over two hundred different administrative areas.

Doctors have performed whatever tests and treatments they used in their regular practice, and the carriers paid under the CPR calculating rules. If carriers reimbursed certain procedures in their non-Medicare business, they continued to do so for Medicare. The claims forms and the carriers' reports to HCFA until recently have carried no standard procedure codes and therefore yielded little detailed information about clinical practice, so HCFA long lacked data to detect problems and set policy.

Doctors have not needed to buy expensive equipment for their own office practices, since the reimbursement system has financed such purchases by hospitals. America's open medical staff structure means that hospitals allow private office practitioners to treat their own patients in hospitals. Nearly every doctor has privileges in his community's hospitals, and the average doctor has more than two affiliations. If a doctor requests that a hospital install new equipment for a new procedure, the hospital must do so lest the doctors refer their patients elsewhere and ruin it. Competition among hospitals for productive doctors results in the early purchase and wide spread of expensive new methods. Hospitals welcome innovation because it increases their revenues and because the reimbursement system covers acquisition costs. Blue Cross and Medicare long paid the full cost of hospital care as the hospital defined it. Allowable costs have included depreciation and interest on any debt incurred to acquire expensive equipment and rebuild the plant. Wages of the many new technicians have been fully covered.[3]

Approval Machinery

For many years, in countries with statutory health insurance, new treatments were almost automatically added to fee schedules and hospital budgets if the medical associations endorsed them. The wording of health insurance laws has always been almost open-ended. But during the last decade, new methods have grown in number and cost: transplants, artificial organs, dialysis, imaging equipment, and so on. Doctors are eager to try out every new method in their specialties, patients want everything that might save their lives, and medical associations argue that sickness funds are obligated to pay for everything that doctors prescribe in their professional judgment.

Every country has groped for a system for investigating the clinical merits of expensive and risky new procedures, estimating the costs, deciding the rules of coverage, and fixing reimbursement rates. Countries with statutory health insurance must eventually develop clear-cut machinery. To design a system, for example, Holland's *Ziekenfondsraad* created a special Subcommittee on Limits of the Insurance Benefits during the early 1980s. Because the United States has many separate payers and an indecisive government, it can lead the world in research about technology assessment but cannot coordinate all the separate efforts and apply them to reimbursement decisions.[4]

Europe. All countries now have government agencies that screen and license expensive and risky technologies after the initial development abroad or in their own academic medical centers. In countries with statutory health insurance, expensive new investments in nonprofit and municipal hospitals depend on government grants. Such grants follow governmental plans for the entire hospital sector, and the screening and licensing machinery are parts of the planning system. A few governments—such as Great Britain and Sweden—maintain careful control by owning and managing, as well as financing, all the hospitals. In order to guide decisions, their Ministries of Health are among Europe's principal grantors and clients for research in technology assessment.[5]

Holland's system for technology implementation differs. It has a special need to screen the installation of very expensive programs. In the past, government in the Netherlands has been very limited; hospitals, doctors, and health insurance carriers were private and autonomous. Almost alone in Europe, Dutch hospitals have been allowed to continue raising their own capital by borrowing in the private market. The amortization costs of new equipment and buildings have been included in the prospective budgets and have been fully paid off in the per diems approved by the rate regulation agency (COTG). The system led to the headlong modernization and cost explosion in Dutch hospital care during the 1970s. New expensive programs might have been installed prematurely, could have proved ineffective, might have soon been replaced by better versions. Competition among hospitals might have resulted in the proliferation of expensive programs, unnecessary and wasteful in a small country.[6]

Screening machinery evolved. First, an innovation (such as organ transplants) is developed abroad and in Dutch academic medical centers. It is not yet covered by statutory health insurance, so the treatment costs of the first patients are covered by AWBZ, which has become a catchall third party. When the method seems promising for wider installation and inclusion under the mainstream statutory health insurance, it is assessed by a joint project conducted by the Department of Physical Health Care of the *Ziekenfondsraad* and by the *Gezondheidsraad* (the Health Council of the national government). The study is led by a committee representing the academic centers that are sites of the project, the association of private health insurers, and the Ministry of Health. The chairman is the General Secretary of the *Ziekenfondsraad*. The report covers both the clinical effectiveness and the costs of the innovation. It presents the arguments for and against including the benefit under statutory health insurance. The final decision is made by the Ministry, which alone can balance the costs, the clinical benefits, and the political pressures from the patients.

Installation of the equipment and staffs follows a plan. The Dutch hospital planning law of 1971 (the *Wet Ziekenhuisvoorzieningen*) was intended to screen plans for new buildings. When advanced technology began to proliferate in the late 1970s and hospital costs grew rapidly, the Minister of Health used one clause (Article 18) as authority to approve or disapprove great changes in the clinical functions of hospitals—as authority, that is, to grant licenses for expensive new programs. The hospital planning agency (the *College voor Ziekenhuisvoorzieningen*) develops a plan for their siting and provisioning around the country. About ten such programs are under license and control at any time.[7]

The license authorizes that hospital to borrow the funds from the private capital market, install the program, obtain a reimbursement rate from the national government's rate-setting agency (COTG), and bill the sickness funds. During its first years, the new program is not mixed into the hospital's prospective operating budget, but COTG fixes a special case payment pursuant to the College's estimate of allowable costs. After a few years, the procedure's clinical value and costs are fully understood: it no longer requires a special license and a special case payment, and its operating costs become part of the hospital's operating budget. But COTG can restrain excessive proliferation after delicensing—by questioning new entries in the operating budgets of hospitals that were not one of the original licensed sites. Every hospital now must receive COTG's approval for purchase of any equipment costing at least f. 75,000.

During the late 1980s, the Dutch government became one of Europe's principal sponsors of research on the costs and benefits of new technology.[8] The ultimate goal was to add an economic dimension to the clinical criteria for approving and reimbursing advanced programs.

Since politicians ultimately have the final say, politics can hasten the widespread adoption of a therapy. For example, associations representing heart patients, kidney patients, and others in a few countries (such as Holland) have pressed government to add the new therapies to hospital budgets, to capital grants, and to insurance fee schedules. If the Minister of Health represents a parliamentary district containing a major manufacturer—as in the case of the spread of CT scanners in France in 1981—he may allow more widespread installation in hospital budgets and more widespread reimbursement under insurance. To stimulate the economy and compete in the world's medical equipment markets heretofore dominated by Americans, the French government increased the purchase of advanced technology by public hospitals during the early 1980s.[9]

But politicians must reduce budgetary deficits as well as distribute largesse. Therefore, recently they have had to enact cost containment measures. They usually delegate this unpopular chore to civil servants, such as the assessment and licensing staffs.

United States. America's permissive reimbursement schemes—particularly Blue Cross/Blue Shield and Medicare—financed an explosion in technology. During the early 1970s, state insurance rate regulators and employer groups began to resist rate increases and insisted that the Blues control provider costs, not merely pass them on to the payers. All the Blues' benefit contracts were supposed to pay only for services that were "medically necessary."

Blue Cross and Blue Shield. The national association headquarters created a Medical Necessity Program to identify wasteful claims and advise member Plans about remedies. Plans were advised not to pay for routine batteries of tests upon admission, for example, but only to pay for tests specifically ordered by the attending physician; someone need not be admitted as an inpatient merely for testing. New procedures of unproved value need not automatically be covered— and obsolete procedures need not be retained—unless the attending doctor can justify his choice. Lists of doubtful and redundant methods have been prepared by the Professional Affairs Committee of the Association with the help of staff reports and advice of medical specialty societies. Screening originally was intended to exclude ineffective and redundant methods and to postpone coverage of unproved methods, rather than approve and price effective new methods.[10] More recently, the Medical Necessity Program has added guidelines of good and reimbursable medical practice in several fields, such as cardiac surgery.[11] Final decisions about coverage and specific payments to doctors and hospitals have always been left to the member Plans. At first the Plans' coverage decisions for a procedure vary, but eventually they agree.[12]

By the 1980s, advanced and expensive technology was spreading and beginning to threaten the Blues' financial viability. It was not merely enough to advise Plans to exclude ineffective, obsolete, or redundant procedures. The problem was to find out which procedures were most effective and to pay fair prices with optimum incentives. The national association since 1986 has conducted the Technology Evaluation and Coverage Program to evaluate advanced procedures. With the aid of the literature and expert consultants, the staff establishes that each procedure has been approved by government regulators where appropriate, that it has been evaluated scientifically, that it improves health, and that it is equally or more effective than other methods. For many methods, the staff suggests reasonable prices in light of their operating costs and the prices of comparable procedures. The goal is to inform member Plans in negotiating prospective prices with hospitals and doctors, instead of merely processing expensive claims initiated by the providers. The association headquarters sends to the member Plans approximately thirty reports each year evaluating individual technologies and advising how to decide complex coverage issues. Typical reports deal with organ transplants, in vitro fertilization, extracorporeal shock-wave lithotripsy, and like topics.

Medicare. Blue Cross/Blue Shield is a private business; it can decide its benefits unilaterally or in negotiations with providers. But Medicare's hands are tied by the generous wording of the original law and by the government's deference to the professional judgment of hospitals and doctors. Providers are always paid by the carriers for established procedures by the customary reimbursement rules.

If the carrier encounters a new and untried procedure, it may pay the providers and HCFA never hears of the episode. In several dozen cases a year, the carriers refer uncertain techniques to the regional and thence to the national office of HCFA. Headquarters investigates the technique in the scientific literature, asks clinical agencies elsewhere in the government for advice, consults its own Physicians Panel, and debates the issue in one of the bimonthly meetings of the Coverage/Payment Technical Advisory Group. This group, which consists of medical directors and executives of many of the HCFA carriers, discusses general policy as well as specific procedures. HCFA then notifies all carriers about covering the procedure. If payment is denied, the provider is not supposed to bill the patient—since it is the provider who failed to check coverage in advance and assumed the financial risk.[13]

For twenty-five years, Medicare denied coverage only on grounds that a procedure was unsafe and clinically ineffective. During the 1990s, HCFA added the criterion of cost-effectiveness: if two procedures are available for a patient's needs and are comparable in results, the carrier pays the provider only the fee for the cheaper one. The economic evaluation and comparison of technologies will be constantly under investigation by HCFA's research office and other agencies of the national government.[14] Whether this policy is technically feasible and politically defensible remains to be seen.

Medicaid. During the 1980s, Washington gave state governments considerable discretion in managing the special programs for the poor. Because budgets were limited, the states needed some methodology for rationing and for setting priorities. At first, the common method was to limit the number of beneficiaries—thereby leaving many uninsured without coverage and leaving the hospitals with bad debts.

The state of Oregon in 1987 decided to use the voluminous cost-benefit literature to prioritize procedures. It identified several procedures that yielded few benefits in return for high costs, such as organ transplants. Moreover, it cited other procedures with more attractive cost/benefit ratios, such as preventive medicine. Therefore, the Oregon Health Services stressed preventive and primary care and avoided transplants and other expensive procedures.[15]

Effects on Utilization and Health

Since medicine is international, the list of insured benefits is nearly the same in all developed countries. The only variations are breadth of participation: whether all doctors or only specialists can bill the sickness funds for a procedure; whether many hospitals or only a few can install and amortize a complex new treatment.

National Peculiarities. A few differences exist in the boundaries of acute care: some treatments are recognized in a few countries, are covered by health insurance, but are not covered elsewhere. They require prescriptions from the patient's primary physician or from a specialist. For example:

☐ *Physiotherapy.* In a few countries, paramedicals can make home visits, are covered by their fee schedules, and can bill the sickness fund directly. The patient cannot retain them on his initiative but needs a doctor's referral form. An example is the large and prosperous occupation of physiotherapists (*kinésithérapeutes*) who have been giving office care and home care in Belgium for many decades.

☐ *Thermal treatments in spas.* Germany, Switzerland, and France include them as benefits under health insurance. They are widely used in Germany, and a large and politically powerful industry depends on insurance coverage and the patients' additional payments. To have coverage of a trip to the spa, the patient must obtain a referral card from his doctor and must be treated in an installation managed by a physician.

Doctors, governments, and sickness funds complain about the large amount of money wasted in excessive use of these benefits. If spending were cut, the insurance systems' deficit would be noticeably reduced. About 4 percent of all Belgian health insurance payments went to physiotherapists in 1982, for example, and the proportion may be higher today.[16] About 5 percent of German health care costs is spent on thermal cures; the sickness funds bear much of this, and the employers must continue to pay the absent worker's salary.[17]

But the sickness funds cannot revoke these benefits, since they have been popular with members for many years and are heavily used by all social groups. One reason they are rapidly increasing in utilization and costs is competition among sickness funds; the carriers keep their present members and seek new ones by offering these benefits more generously. On the other hand, in a few countries, such as Switzerland, all the sickness funds try to reduce their wasteful expenditure by increasing the cost sharing for thermal cures.

Results of Permissive or Strict Reimbursement. If a country's insurance system reimburses hospitals for depreciation and interest, allows hospitals to borrow in the private capital market, and has little regulatory screening of these purchases, then hospitals throughout the country purchase the newest technologies, can operate them with full staffs, and can pay off the debts with high utilization. These tendencies are reinforced if the insurance system pays hospital doctors directly by fee-for-service, instead of paying them indirectly as salaried members of hospital staffs.

These reimbursement arrangements exist in the United States but are much less prevalent in the statutory health insurance or national health services of Europe and Canada. As a result, the United States has had the largest amounts of cash and the strongest incentives for the early adoption of new equipment. It has had the highest per capita frequencies of imaging equipment, cardiac surgical units, organ transplant units, and nearly everything else. In 1980, American firms had between 40 and 65 percent of the world's total sales in medical electronics, medical-surgical equipment, dental equipment, nuclear medicine, cardiac monitors, respiratory monitors, biological analyzers, and cardiac pacemakers.[18]

Americans not only install more advanced medical technology than any other country, but they also use it. The incentives of an activist medical culture and those of health insurance converge. Compared to other developed countries—with clinically comparable populations—American doctors and hospitals perform more organ transplants, heart surgery, kidney dialysis, cataract surgery, radiodiagnostic tests, pacemaker implants, hysterectomies, cesarean deliveries, and other active procedures.[19] Although comparative data about these invasive procedures are not reported by age, the reimbursement methods of Medicare probably result in much more surgery on the elderly in the United States than elsewhere.

The level of utilization of an advanced procedure depends on the insurance reimbursement for both the physicians and the hospitals. One party may encourage early and frequent utilization while the other discourages it. Before 1983, for example, Medicare paid hospitals for all the operating and capital costs of care—including full coverage of the acquisition and use of new methods. The physicians were paid generous fees that rose every year, and they could extra-bill patients at their own discretion. After 1983, Medicare continued to pay hospitals their acquisition costs for all capital (less 10 or 15 percent) but changed to standardized fixed-price DRGs for all operating costs. The system was intended to make hospitals cautious in buying expensive equipment and hiring high-salaried technicians. As a result, the operating costs of many new improved techniques exceeded the allowances of the DRGs for those diagnoses. Many hospitals could not keep up with innovation in as many fields as heretofore. The once affluent and growing equipment manufacturers found that some expensive innovations (such as cochlear implants, hip implants, penile prostheses, and implantable defibrillators) were poor risks for further research and development.[20]

The DRG payment technique therefore succeeded in its intention—to reverse traditional incentives, make all hospitals cost-conscious, and restrain the proliferation of expensive programs and staffs. But unlike European methods of health facilities planning and targeting public capital grants upon centers of excellence, the American DRG method had no instrument for selecting the most meritorious clinical innovations and placing them in the best-qualified hospitals. The free market was supposed to decide. The restraint on Medicare *hospital* reimbursement contradicted the continued high-technology incentives of Medicare *physician* reimbursement.

Some structures of insurance reimbursement can determine the sites where the new benefits are provided. German statutory health insurance, for example, has always paid mainstream hospitals very little for capital and has limited annual increases in operating costs. Depreciation and interest are small items in a hospital's prospective budget. The national and provincial governments were supposed to give generous capital grants to all the nonteaching hospitals during the 1970s, but the governments' budget deficits caused cutbacks. The few academic medical centers receive large capital and operating budgets from the provincial governments; they are the sites for developing new technologies and providing such care long afterward.

But the German insurance system pays office doctors by fee-for-service and the fee schedules are oriented toward expensive invasive procedures. The hospitals are forbidden to compete with the office doctors by treating ambulatory patients, and the office doctors may buy whatever equipment they deem clinically advantageous and financially profitable. From their earnings, German office doctors install advanced technology and high-salaried technicians in their offices, in cooperative laboratories, and in private clinics. Sharing their doctors' fees, German private clinics can attract patients by depicting themselves as more up-to-date than their municipal and nonprofit competitors. [21]

Implications for the United States

Technology assessment and outcome research are not fields where one must preach the value of lessons from abroad. The Americans are already heeding them. Advanced clinical medicine has always been an international field, the equipment and drug companies sell in world markets, and policymakers have commissioned evaluation studies everywhere. America's lavish research spending is well invested in this area and attracts an international audience. When American assessment studies are replicated abroad, Americans can profit from learning whether their findings remain true in other patient populations and other delivery systems. Some international-minded authors offer propositions that synthesize findings from both Europe and the United States. [22]

One lesson that Americans might heed from abroad is the need to make decisions. American officials shrink from making hard political decisions in health care finance. Instead they spend vast amounts on prolonged research projects and naively hope that the final reports will yield popular and simple solutions. But the organized financing systems of Europe and Canada cannot afford drift. They spend less time, money, and manpower on research; they decide about adding benefits and about everything else by deadlines. They realize that prolonged dispute and uncertainty are serious costs. As the expenditures on technology assessment and research on patient outcomes escalate during the 1990s, Americans must realize that creation of an efficient and politically harmonious decision-making system is at least as important as establishing facts about individual benefits.

European statutory health insurance stresses the need for clarity and universal understanding in order to minimize conflicts and frustration—in order, that is, to make the system work. Even when processes are unavoidably complex, they must be understood. An important feature may be unsettled for a while—such as a technically advanced new benefit—but its status at every step of the decision sequence is known widely. Americans pay a high price for the lack of clarity regarding benefits and reimbursement in health insurance, as the recent tightening of "medical necessity" under Medicare demonstrates.

During the late 1980s, HCFA instructed fiscal intermediaries not to pay physicians' claims for procedures that were not "medically necessary," and the carriers complied with varying degrees of strictness. Assigned claims could be handled simply: the carrier refused to pay the doctor for a test or treatment it deemed unnecessary; the doctor was angered; the carrier's denial was private. But if the procedure was included in one of the many unassigned claims, there was trouble: the patient had already paid the doctor; Medicare refused to reimburse the patient, told the patient that his doctor gave him care that it deemed not "medically necessary," and advised the patient to get a refund from the doctor. No one had been forewarned, and everyone was embittered at the end of each episode.[23] If Medicare had simply mandated universal assignment, if the mysterious and confusing assigned/unassigned option did not exist, if the benefit coverage rules were clear and universal by means of a fee schedule, none of this trouble would have occurred.

Notes

1. See the many examples throughout Glaser, *Health Insurance Bargaining* (New York: Gardner Press and John Wiley, 1978).

2. See the examples in Glaser, *Paying the Hospital* (San Francisco: Jossey-Bass, 1987), chap. 9; and in the many national case studies in *International Journal of Technology Assessment in Health Care.*

3. Glaser, *Paying the Hospital* (see note 2, above), pp. 236–241; John H. Goddeeris, "Economic Forces and Hospital Technology: Lessons from the United States Experience," *International Journal of Technology Assessment in Health Care,* vol. 3, no. 2 (1987), pp. 225–228; and Mary Wagner, "Promoting Hospitals' High-Tech Equipment," *Modern Healthcare,* vol. 19, no. 46 (Nov. 17, 1989), pp. 39–50.

4. American methods and the voluminous literature are codified in Institute of Medicine, *Assessing Medical Technologies* (Washington: National Academy Press, 1985). For America's inability to coordinate efforts see Frederick Mosteller and Elisabeth Burdick, "Current Issues in Health Care Technology Assessment," *International Journal of Technology Assessment in Health Care,* vol. 5, no. 1 (1989), pp. 123–136.

5. For basic facts about the numbers, locations, costs, insurance coverage, and other details about the principal new technologies in several European countries, see Veli Müller, "Survey on New, Costly Medical Methods and Technology in Member Countries of the Association," a report prepared for the Sixteenth General Assembly (Geneva: Association Internationale de la Mutualité, 1987).

6. Glaser, *Paying the Hospital* (see note 2, above), pp. 246–251.

7. Frank de Charro and H. David Banta, "Transplant Policy in the Netherlands," *International Journal of Technology Assessment in Health Care,* vol. 2,

no. 3 (1986), pp. 533–545; and Frans Rutten and H. David Banta, "Health Care Technologies in the Netherlands," *International Journal of Technology Assessment in Health Care,* vol. 4, no. 2 (1988), pp. 229–238.

8. Stuurgroep Toekomstscenario's Gezondheidszorg, *Anticipating and Assessing Health Care Technology* (Dordrecht: Martinus Nijhoff, 1987–), 8 vols.

9. Jean-François Lacronique, "Technology in France," *International Journal of Technology Assessment in Health Care,* vol. 4, no. 3 (1988), pp. 385–394.

10. Johanna Sonnenfeld, "The Blue Cross and Blue Shield Associations' Medical Necessity Program," *Voluntary Effort Quarterly,* vol. 3, no. 2 (June 1981), pp. 5–8.

11. *Medical Necessity Program Manual* (Chicago: Blue Cross and Blue Shield Association, constantly updated).

12. Roger W. Evans, "Coverage and Reimbursement for Heart Transplantation," *International Journal of Technology Assessment in Health Care,* vol. 2, no. 3 (1986), pp. 425–449. The intuitive decision making in one Plan is described in Stan N. Finkelstein and others, "The Process of Evaluating Medical Technologies for Third-Party Coverage," *Journal of Health Care Technology,* vol. 1, no. 2 (Fall 1984), pp. 89–102.

13. Described in "Medicare Program: Criteria and Procedures for Making Medical Services Coverage Decisions That Relate to Health Care Technology," *Federal Register,* vol. 54, no. 18 (Jan. 30, 1989), pp. 4302–4308. See also David A. Kessler and others, "The Federal Regulation of Medical Devices," *New England Journal of Medicine,* vol. 317, no. 6 (Aug. 6, 1987), pp. 361, 363–364. Screening and decision making in practice both in Washington and in the fiscal intermediary are described in Finkelstein and others, "The Process of Evaluating Medical Technologies for Third-Party Coverage" (see note 12, above); see also Linda K. Demlo and others, "Decision Making by Medicare Contractors for Coverage of Medical Technologies," in *Medical Technology and Costs of the Medicare Program* (Washington: Office of Technology Assessment, 1984), pp. 191–205.

14. Refer to "Medicare Program" (see note 13, above), pp. 4308–4310; and Alexander Leaf, "Cost Effectiveness as a Criterion for Medicare Coverage," *New England Journal of Medicine,* vol. 321, no. 13 (Sept. 28, 1989), pp. 898–900.

15. Peter Reich, "Health Care Tickets for the Uninsured," *New England Journal of Medicine,* vol. 321, no. 18 (Nov. 2, 1989), pp. 1262–1263; and Charles J. Dougherty and David C. Hadorn, "Setting Health Care Priorities," *Hastings Center Report,* vol. 21, no. 3 (May–June 1991) supplement.

16. Denise Deliège and Paul Minne, *Kinésithérapie et physiothérapie en Belgique* (Louvain-la-Neuve: Service d'études socioéconomiques de la santé, Ecole de Santé Publique, Université de Louvain, 1982), p. 27.

17. These are my inferences from several sources, such as Bundesministerium für Jugend, Familie, und Gesundheit, *Daten des Gesundheitswesens—Ausgabe 1989* (Stuttgart: Verlag W. Kohlhammer, 1989), p. 318.

18. Jean-Georges Moreau and Patrice Bimont, "L'industrie du matériel

biomédical," *Revue française des affaires sociales,* vol. 34, no. 4 (Oct.–Dec. 1980), pp. 191–204.

19. Institute of Medicine, *Assessing Medical Technologies* (see note 4, above), pp. 232–234; R.J.C. Pearson and others, "Hospital Caseloads in Liverpool, New England and Uppsala," *Lancet,* no. 7 (Sept. 7, 1968), pp. 559–566; John P. Bunker, "Surgical Manpower: A Comparison of Operations and Surgeons in the United States and in England and Wales," *New England Journal of Medicine,* vol. 282, no. 2 (Jan. 15, 1970), pp. 135–144; Frances C. Notzon and others, "Comparisons of National Cesarean-Section Rates," *New England Journal of Medicine,* vol. 316, no. 7 (Feb. 12, 1987), pp. 386–389; William A. Knaus and others, "A Comparison of Intensive Care in the U.S.A. and in France," *Lancet,* no. 9 (Sept. 18, 1982), pp. 642–646; G. N. Marsh and others, "Anglo-American Contrasts in General Practice," *British Medical Journal,* May 29, 1976, pp. 1321–1325; Eugene Vayda and others, "A Decade of Surgery in Canada, England and Wales, and the United States," *Archives of Surgery,* vol. 117 (June 1982), pp. 846–853; and many other comparative studies.

20. Nancy Kane and Paul Manoukian, "The Effect of the Medicare Prospective Payment System on the Adoption of New Technology," *New England Journal of Medicine,* vol. 321, no. 20 (Nov. 16, 1989), pp. 1378–1383.

21. The low capital and operating reimbursement of German public and nonprofit hospitals is explained in Glaser, *Paying the Hospital* (see note 2, above), pp. 90, 216–225. Much more is spent on hospital care than on physicians' reimbursement in other countries, but the two accounts under German statutory health insurance are closer. Until the hospitals received more money under the financial reforms of the 1970s, German health insurance always spent more on physicians' fees than on the capital and operating costs of the hospitals. Time series for provider spending appear in Bundesministerium, *Daten des Gesundheitswesens—Ausgabe 1989* (see note 17, above), pp. 228–229.

22. See, for example, the Stuurgroep Toekomstscenario's Gezondheidszorg (the Netherlands) cited in note 8; the Copenhagen Collaborating Center for the Study of Regional Variations in Health Care; and many contributors to the *International Journal of Technology Assessment in Health Care.*

23. Sharon McIlrath, "Medicare May Use Costs as Part of Coverage Criteria," *American Medical News,* Feb. 17, 1989, pp. 1, 46–47.

PART FOUR

Reforming
the Health Insurance
System

Statutory and private insurance are strained in every country because of steady increases in utilization, service intensity, operating costs, and capital costs. In every country, health insurance must operate within the fiscal capacity of the society. Chapter Seventeen describes the many methods of deciding and implementing expenditure targets while preserving society's commitment to its sick and aged.

Statutory health insurance has achieved much for the populations of Europe as well as other countries. One hears proposals to make fundamental changes, particularly by devotees of competitive markets. But it is easier to theorize about great changes than to bring them about—especially if the changes jeopardize achievements. Chapter Eighteen summarizes the debates and their outcomes.

The only country that has not enacted universal (or nearly universal) statutory health insurance is the United States. As noted here in chapter after chapter, America's private system cannot meet the country's health financing needs. Chapter Nineteen, the final chapter, describes a statutory health insurance system for the United States that is based on the experiences of other developed countries.

CHAPTER 17

Cost Containment

──────────────── Summary ────────────────

Every country experiences increases in health care costs that strain its payroll taxes, government budgets, and premiums. The causes are universal and very difficult to control: the general level of inflation in prices and wages; extra price increases charged by health providers; larger demand due to the growth and aging of populations; greater utilization per capita; and the greater intensity of services per contact. Countries grope for the best ways to eliminate waste and contain costs without depriving their populations of care.

The problem is to contain costs for the entire system, not merely for one payer. Shifting claims from one payer to another insurance program or to the patient often introduces disputes and higher costs. Almost all countries—but not the United States—have all-payer systems governed by collective negotiations or rate regulation, so that providers' costs are fully covered, costs are no longer shifted, and each payer's liability is predictable.

Regulation of capital investment and provider rates has steadily been tightened in Europe and is one of the instruments that has reduced the once rapid increase in costs. But government rate regulation does not fit all situations: the medical association insists on negotiations. Without any of these instruments, the United States experiences larger annual increases in spending.

In the negotiations with doctors and in rate regulation, payers have tried to limit the annual increases in total costs by reducing the annual increases in physicians' fees and hospital charges. But price control alone has had only partial success, since utilization of doctors and hospitals can rise, more expensive treatments replace the less expensive, and payers are obligated to cover the hospitals' costs. One of America's few cost containment efforts has been the adoption of

DRGs for hospital care under Medicare. This policy has slowed the annual increase in inpatient claims by persuading hospitals to transfer many cases to the outpatient department, thereby accelerating the increase in extramural costs. A few countries now try to link unit prices and total volume of physician's services: if utilization approaches expenditure targets, fees are reduced for all or for the busiest doctors.

Health insurance carriers try to reduce unnecessary spending by reviewing utilization. But this measure requires challenges to their subscribers' visits and to doctors' clinical decisions, when health insurance was intended to assist use. Hospital admissions are screened, excessive stays are questioned, the doctor's tests and treatments are compared with peer group averages. But doctors resent interference by health insurance carriers and government, and the carriers are legally obligated to pay. In Europe, these methods may discourage manifestly unnecessary care, but they cannot substantially reduce national norms of generous servicing. Small "managed-care" efforts in the United States try to reduce utilization, but their total administrative costs offset part of any savings and there is no national system. American payers are now developing "practice guidelines" that will recommend to doctors a sequence of decisions of high clinical quality and high economic efficiency.

A widespread American belief is that market incentives—such as substantial point-of-service cost sharing by the patient—will motivate him to avoid unnecessary visits and shop for the most efficient provider. But social insurance was intended to encourage use, not interject obstacles. The substantial cost sharing that would make a difference in utilization is never imposed in statutory health insurance, except for minor benefits. In practice, cost sharing is so small that patients become accustomed to it. Deterrent effects further disappear if the patient can buy supplementary health insurance. However, cost sharing may discourage waste in some sectors, such as pharmaceutical drugs.

Americans try to use differential cost sharing to persuade subscribers to choose a preferred panel of more cost-conscious doctors instead of providers without special contracts. Some savings may result, but many subscribers do not forgo their regular family doctors in favor of the slightly cheaper "preferred provider" option. Managing care on such a small scale in individual cases is (on the aggregate) complicated and expensive.

Because the numerous methods of regulation, negotiation, and financial incentives have had mixed results, have elicited protests from providers, and have required constant administration, some payers and governments have resorted to the most direct form of cost containment—that is, requiring providers to give all necessary service within an expenditure cap set in advance. Global budgets are a common method of paying hospitals in countries with full public financing. Applying the method to statutory health insurance is possible but more difficult, since that system has multiple payers, autonomous providers, and legislative guarantees of full services on demand. Physician reimbursement in German health insurance has long used fixed annual caps, and some countries attempt to introduce fixed budgeting into other health markets. Negotiation with providers must be combined with financial guidelines from government. Several countries have introduced and then steadily tightened the less fixed expenditure "targets."

The effects of any cost containment effort depend on how it is administered: the same method may be generous at one time and restrictive at another. The long-term trend in countries with statutory health insurance and national health services is toward tighter limits—forcing health care to function within the country's fiscal capacity. Even countries with several cost containment methods for different sectors can follow guidelines, coordinate the methods, and limit the annual growth of the total. The hospital sector was the first to be constrained, but controls are now being tightened on physicians' services and pharmaceuticals. If a country has no leadership and no system—as in the United States—it cannot limit the growth in costs as well.

Cost Increases and Their Causes

The costs of health care and, therefore, the expenditures of health insurance rise in all developed countries. The growth seems inevitable,[1] but the task of public policy is to decide whether spending on health should exceed the allocation of society's resources for other purposes. Without any monitoring or restraint, health care spending can grow very rapidly, and society's priorities are reshuffled unintentionally.

Policymakers must identify the causes of year-to-year spending increases, decide whether these increases can be restrained, craft appropriate instruments for each, and specify expenditure targets. Several causes of rises in spending may be distinguished:[2]

☐ Higher prices and wages in the general economy from one year to the next. Health services must pay employees and must buy supplies, fuel, electric power, and food from outside markets.

☐ Higher prices charged for each service by doctors, hospitals, and other providers—beyond the rise in general prices.

☐ Greater demand due to a larger population.

☐ More inpatient admissions, ambulatory visits, and home-care services per capita ("utilization").

☐ More tests and treatments per inpatient admission, ambulatory visit, or home visit ("service intensity").

Prices and Wages. In a labor-intensive industry such as health, trends in the rest of the economy are the key component of health care spending increases. Until the 1960s, health services insulated themselves from outside labor costs by employing many religious, paying low wages to lay workers, paying them in part in room and board, and requiring long working hours. The health cost explosion of the 1970s was due in large part to a wage catch-up with the rest of the economy: the religious declined in numbers and were replaced by lay nurses; workers (including the nurses) joined unions and obtained normal wages and normal hours; many more workers had to be hired, because of shorter hours and greater service intensity.[3]

The health care cost explosion of the 1970s was due in large part to the high inflation that afflicted all countries. Health expenditures inevitably rise because of this general force. As all countries fought to bring down the general inflation rate during the 1980s, health spending increases declined. Once the wage catch-up occurred in health, this source of health spending increases stabilized.

Any economies in labor and in purchases must come not from paying lower prices but from hiring fewer workers and buying fewer supplies. This is difficult to do in most countries, because they used the growth in third-party coverage to improve their once parlous staffing and cannot easily cut back services. Perhaps the United States has some scope for saving in labor costs, since it staffs organizations more lavishly than other countries.[4] But America's health cost policy is in disarray with respect to the definition of problems and application of remedies: of all developed countries, it is the last to bring down annual spending growth in health close to the annual levels of growth in wages and prices in the general economy.[5]

Price Increases Above the General Market. Health care providers have taken advantage of the great increases in third-party funding—particularly during the permissive periods of statutory and private health insurance—to increase their prices faster than prices in other sectors in the economy. The incomes of health care managers and physicians rose substantially in all countries.

Fees rose faster in some medical specialties than in others. In all countries, doctors in primary and cognitive fields once received modest incomes comparable to those of other executives and professionals. But as they became more influential within medical associations, they received higher fees and more patients from the sickness funds and began to approach the income levels of the surgical specialties. Since the health sector can influence the charges of providers, these prices are a leading target of cost containment.

Size and Composition of the Population. Health services must adapt to total demand. Size changes only slowly. If government has a population policy—usually aimed at reducing fertility in a developing country—it has motives other than health cost containment.

Aging is one of the principal sources of increase in health care spending. Since it is a trend that cannot be halted, the problem is how to manage its implications. In developed countries, the elderly have higher rates of morbidity and chronic disability. In every developed country, persons over sixty-five incur a large share of the country's health services utilization and health insurance costs—at least one-third of statutory health insurance spending in every country. Since the proportion in each population older than sixty-five—and in the vulnerable level over seventy-five—steadily grows, this powerful stimulant of costs relentlessly increases everywhere.[6]

Utilization. Visits to providers inevitably increase as the population grows and ages. The policy problems are to determine whether utilization rises even more than population trends, whether it can be justified on clinical grounds, and whether the benefits justify the costs. Utilization is one important cause that health care providers can influence (usually upward) and that policymakers try to limit. Overutilization of a particular service must be detected and limited. Patients who need care must be directed from the less to the more cost-effective services.

Service Intensity. This is another important cause of cost increases that the health sector itself has created and policymakers now try to control. Throughout the world, technology and pharmaceuticals steadily grow in number, complexity, and utilization. Testing and treatments per patient, per admission, and per visit steadily increase in number—even when the methods do not become more technically advanced—particularly in the countries with invasive clinical styles. In addition, much of the new technology and drugs is more elaborate and often far more expensive than the methods they replace, both in acquisition costs and in operating costs.[7]

Cost Containment Versus Cost Shifting

Shifting Costs to Other Carriers. The policy problem is how to limit spending for the system as a whole, not merely to limit it for one payer. Each sickness fund everywhere would be happy to limit its own spending and shift providers' bills to other sickness funds or to government. For this reason, carriers in most countries have welcomed assumption of hospital investment costs by government. Particularly where sickness funds compete for members by offering lower premiums or higher benefits—as in Belgium, Germany, and Switzerland—each would be delighted to reduce its own costs and increase the others' burdens.

But shifting operating costs of providers among sickness funds is not possible in Europe. In the payment of hospitals in France, Belgium, Holland, and Switzerland—as noted in Chapter Eleven—government regulators fix the identical hospital unit rates for all payers. In the payment of hospitals in Germany, all sickness funds form a joint negotiating committee and fix a standard daily rate for each hospital. In the payment of doctors in every country with statutory health insurance—as noted in Chapter Ten—all the sickness funds form joint negotiating committees and agree on standard fees for all doctors. (In the only European exception, German *Ersatzkassen* voluntarily pay the doctors more and not less.)

The only exception among developed countries is the United States, which

has no statutory health insurance, many competing carriers, no collective negotiations by payers with providers, and (in most states) no rate regulation of hospitals. Each carrier tries to pay hospitals—and, if possible, doctors—as little as
possible, and each invites the providers to make it up from other payers. Each
payer restricts the definition of allowable costs if its contract with hospitals
pledges the reimbursement of the subscribers' clinical costs. Other restrictive
payers limit their per diems, charges, fees, or case payments. Cost shifting becomes a tactic in the competition among American insurance companies for
business: the restrictive carriers offer lower premiums to employed groups and
individual subscribers, while the victims of cost shifting must quote higher premiums.[8] Instead of creating order, the United States government is a principal
cause of cost shifting: for twenty-five years, the national government has tried to
limit its Medicare spending and has encouraged hospitals and doctors to shift
costs to other payers.[9]

Shifting Costs to the User. Cost shifting to patients can be found occasionally in Europe: if the sickness funds cannot afford to pay all bills, they expect
their subscribers to pay a part—but they do not expect that the divided arrangements will somehow reduce total utilization and spending. An example is Switzerland. For physicians' care, the patient is expected to pay 10 percent of every
bill; he is supposed to pay a deductible (*franchise*) each quarter, with a certain
minimum and maximum, which is often met by the accumulation of 10 percent
of every bill. Whenever the sickness funds run chronic deficits, the national Cabinet raises the deductible: after the national electorate in 1974 voted down a law
to impose payroll taxes on employers, the deductible was increased the next year;
after the national government reduced its subsidies during the early 1980s, the
deductible was raised again in 1986. In service-benefit arrangements in Switzerland, the sickness funds pay providers in full and then bill the patient for the
coinsurance, for the deductible (if the accumulated coinsurance has not satisfied
it), and for the quarterly premiums.

Increases in cost shifting to patients have been common in the United
States. Nearly all private health insurance policies have required deductibles and
coinsurance; even statutory health insurance for pensioners (that is, Medicare) has
followed this pattern; and the United States has long had higher out-of-pocket
payments than any other country.[10] To demonstrate to potential subscribers that
it offers better benefits than its competitors, a carrier may at times require little
or no cost sharing by patients at the point of service. For long periods, Blue Cross
and many HMOs offered "first-dollar coverage."

But when the commercial insurance companies—with their customary
requirements of deductibles and coinsurance—quoted lower premiums and won
larger market share from employers, some Blue Cross Plans and HMOs during
the 1980s were forced to abandon their pledge to offer Americans the equivalent
of paid-in-full social insurance. Annual deductibles and point-of-service coinsurance in commercial insurers' major medical group policies steadily increased.[11]

(The growing financial burden on subscribers was limited by "stop-loss" clauses: beyond a very high out-of-pocket total each year, the carrier or employer pays the rest. Since few patients reach the limits, the aggregate trend is toward more cost sharing by patients.)

Methods of Cost Containment

Total health care costs can be contained by any of the following methods:

☐ Limiting the total volume of resources by either:
  • Government regulation of health care providers.
  • Collective contract between all providers and all payers.
☐ Limiting prices by either:
  • Regulation of rates by government or by an independent commission.
  • Collective contract between all payers and each provider (or between all payers and all providers).
☐ Limiting the utilization of services by:
  • Prior authorizations from payers or regulators.
  • Machinery to monitor utilization statistically (managed either by the payers or by governments). Excessive billing by certain providers is investigated and dealt with.
  • Patient incentives to minimize visits to providers and minimize consumption of materials.
☐ Limiting the total amount of money available. All payers unite under a ceiling.

Recent cost containment efforts have reversed traditional policy. Once very little was spent on health care. But public policy for over a century in every country has steadily increased spending for several purposes: to increase coverage so that everyone has access to mainstream services; to subsidize clinical progress and spread the new technology throughout the society; to increase the number of health care workers and give them normal wages and hours.

Costs could easily be contained by reducing coverage and benefits. Among developed countries, this is possible only in the United States, since it alone has no national health insurance law—in fact, the Americans attempted to contain total health costs during the 1980s by precisely this method.[12] As noted in Chapters Three and Four, American employers have tried to limit their labor costs by eliminating employee health coverage completely, by eliminating employee dependent coverage, and by reducing benefits. But these methods do not seem to have contained America's total health care costs: they save money for individual employers, but spending for the entire system grows as before.

Cutting coverage, slowing access, reducing benefits, and diminishing services are impossible in any other developed country, since they would require amendments to laws that have become sacrosanct. Again, the United States has been the only exception. When the U.S. Congress repealed the Medicare Catastrophic Coverage Act one year after its initial passage in 1988, it eliminated expanded nursing home benefits (already in effect in 1989) and eliminated the new ambulatory pharmaceutical benefits (to be phased in during the 1990s). The United States thereby became the first country to repeal a significant part of its statutory health insurance. Unable and unwilling to repeal its social security laws, every European country is wrestling with the more difficult task of controlling costs of services that are central institutions of society.[13] The aging of the population and the improvements in technology relentlessly increase costs; the problem, therefore, is how to spend money well.

Limiting the Total Volume of Resources

Direct Ownership by Payers. If an insurance carrier owns a hospital or health center, it can avoid deficits and premium increases by efficient management. It can avoid purchasing unnecessary equipment and materials, and it can avoid hiring too many employees. But direct control is rare in mainstream health insurance: in universal statutory systems, only the sickness funds of Belgium retain from the past a significant number of hospitals;[14] in America's private health insurance system, HMOs own health centers and a few hospitals. Otherwise, as noted in Chapters Ten and Eleven, hospitals and doctors have insisted that statutory health insurance recognize their private and autonomous status and that insurance carriers be restricted to the payment of claims.

If government owns and manages hospitals and ambulatory-care polyclinics, it can reduce total costs by supplying these installations sparingly. But the effects on system-wide costs would be small, since national and provincial governments own few hospitals and almost no health centers in countries with national health insurance. In practice, public installations are usually more expensive than the private ones, since political pressures from community groups, politicians, doctors, and civil service unions result in more modern equipment, more staffing, higher salaries, permissive management, and higher budgets.

Regulation and Grants in Europe. National and provincial governments use their granting and regulatory powers over private and municipal hospitals to prevent excessive operating costs that the insurance system will have to pay—since ultimately it is government that has to raise payroll taxes or increase subsidies. In the countries with statutory health insurance and with government grants or government loans to hospitals—such as France, Germany, and Switzerland—government restricts new buildings and advanced equipment to major regional centers. Dutch hospitals may self-finance but now must obtain government approval of expensive projects. Capital projects both large and small must conform to plans.[15]

Government regulators decide the rates that the sickness funds must pay to hospitals in France, Holland, Switzerland, and Belgium. Since rapidly increasing hospital operating costs were the principal strain on the health insurance systems during the 1970s, the regulators have become much stricter. They examine the hospitals' prospective budgets and cut back any unusual increases in number of personnel and other lines. For a long time, the carriers played no role in hospital rate regulation, but—as part of the attempt to detect waste of resources—now they do. In France and Holland, the hospital's prospective budget and retrospective cost report are sent to the local office of the sickness fund, which advises the regulator of any evidence of financial waste and underservicing. The local office has closer insights into the individual hospital than the overloaded government rate regulator does.[16]

If government exercises these powers strictly, hospital costs can be contained. During the 1980s—as explained later in this chapter—nearly every country with statutory health insurance reduced the annual rate increase almost to the general rate of inflation. As a proportion of GNP, therefore, hospital spending became more nearly constant.

While these controls can be exercised over hospitals—the private clinics as well as the municipal and nonprofit hospitals—they cannot be used in all health sectors. Sickness funds and government regulators cannot investigate office doctors and order cuts in their equipment and staffing, since the reimbursement of doctors is not based on strict coverage of allowable costs and since doctors do not buy their capital with public grants. Doctors everywhere oppose any invasion of their professional practice by laymen. They refuse to report their styles and costs of practice; they refuse to accept site visits.

The United States. Since America lacks direct controls over both the capital and operating costs of hospitals, its hospital costs continue to rise considerably faster than the general rate of inflation. Public capital grants have been only a temporary method of quickly expanding facilities, not a permanent system for locating services where needed. Although the country has had national health planning laws, they were administered permissively and were repealed during the 1980s—at precisely the time when Europe was strengthening its own enforcement.[17]

The national government once debated—but has never enacted—machinery for regulating the budgets and reimbursement rates of hospitals. Only a few state governments have enacted comprehensive regulation of hospital rates: a few retain it (New York, New Jersey, Massachusetts, and Maryland), while others have repealed it (Washington). The states with regulation have slower annual increases in operating costs than the majority of states.[18] America's rate regulation in these few markets is much less effective than Europe's in promoting the most efficient use of resources: American regulation often is merely an annual update of total spending by a formula, rather than a detailed screening of individual signs of waste in each hospital's prospective budget; political influence forces concessions; regulators have limited information; and so on. Unable and unwilling to enact detailed controls over lines in hospitals' budgets, the Americans search for reimbursement formulas yielding prices that will give hospitals incentives to become efficient voluntarily.[19]

Limiting Prices

Doctors. Controlling prices was the principal method of limiting the cost of physicians' services under statutory health insurance in the past. By itself, it was not successful for several reasons:

☐ Sickness funds did not begin to bargain strictly with office doctors until the 1950s and 1960s. By then, the medical profession had become the best-paid occupation throughout Europe. The sickness funds could not propose any lower starting point for calculations.

☐ Medical associations have been well led and very militant. The laymen from the sickness funds have always been cautious in arguing with them. The doctors have dominated the crucial committee that monitors and modernizes the fee schedule. Sickness funds have feared strikes by the medical association lest they—and not the doctors—be blamed by politicians and the public for any interruption of services.

☐ The sickness fund could not apply fixed ceilings as the criterion for granting annual increases in fees:
  • Rarely has any country used a total figure as the limit for all payments to doctors. (Recent attempts are cited later in this chapter.)
  • For many years, the negotiators set the annual increase in fees as no less than the expected increase in the country's rate of inflation or rate of wage increases. When inflation exploded during the 1970s, annual awards to doctors tended to overshoot these rates.

☐ Certain factions in the medical profession—especially the GPs—constantly pressed for fee increases to narrow the gap between their incomes and those of the specialists. This pressure greatly increased the average fees and average incomes of all doctors.

☐ Fee schedules set higher prices for the more complex procedures. With technological progress, service intensity and cost per office visit and per hospital stay have grown. Diagnostic testing grew rapidly as well, and patients have been reclassified into new intensive-care programs.[20]

☐ Utilization grew per subscriber, thereby increasing the incomes for each doctor and for the entire medical profession.[21]

☐ The number of doctors greatly increased. Since all can bill in full under the fee schedule, total costs for physicians' services grew substantially.[22]

During the 1970s and early 1980s, statutory health insurance systems experienced crises. Governments warned they could not automatically increase payroll taxes and subsidies, and they urged the sickness funds to bargain more strictly with providers. The sickness funds then began informally the calculations to fall within expenditure targets next year: the total spending for office care should be no more than last year's total plus inflation; if utilization were rising rapidly, the bargainers would offer providers only a very small increase in the unit fees. If the target were exceeded, no money would be recaptured—but the sickness funds would be even stricter bargainers next year.

Relating fees to expenditure targets in this flexible fashion differs from fixed expenditure caps of the type practiced from time to time in the payment of German doctors. As described in Chapter Ten and later in this chapter, a cap requires downward prorating of all fees in the current year if utilization during the current year exceeds predictions. Although insurance carriers and government would like to impose expenditure caps, providers (particularly physicians) resist adamantly. Thus, the payers press for stricter implementation of targets. The medical association must agree, and all practicing doctors must be willing to cooperate. A later section in this chapter will describe the failure of the Dutch government and the Dutch sickness funds to impose caps and degressive fees on specialists. The Dutch compromise is to negotiate fees under guidelines designed to fulfill expenditure targets.

Hospitals. Rate regulation of hospitals under European statutory health insurance does not focus on the allowable annual increase in the daily charge. Rather, as noted in Chapter Eleven, the starting point for European hospital regulation and negotiation is the resource use recorded in statistical reports and requested in the prospective budget of each hospital. The daily charge is the arithmetic outcome for each hospital when the approved prospective budget is divided by expected patient-days. If hospital utilization is greater than predicted, the resulting costs cannot be controlled in the short run. Decisions about admissions and length of stay are made by the doctors, and greater revenue from the sickness funds is welcomed by the hospital administrators. Direct utilization controls, as we shall see, must be added.

The United States, as usual, differs. Medicare avoids any negotiations between HCFA and each hospital over the latter's prospective budget. Because of ideological suspicion of government regulation—as well as the administrative difficulty of investigating so many accounts in depth every year—the country lacks regulatory machinery to screen and revise each hospital's prospective budget and retrospective costs. America's DRG payment system tries to calculate a fair price for each type of case and then to offer it to all hospitals throughout the country. In contrast to the hospital-specific cost reimbursement that results from negotiation or regulatory arbitration in Europe, the American government performs all the calculations. Some hospitals can earn profits; others risk losses. The method is supposed to provide incentives for more efficiency: if a hospital loses money on a case, the manager reduces personnel, tests, or days in the ward. By themselves, DRGs do not control costs for the entire hospital sector: as in any reimbursement scheme, it depends on how they are administered. The payer can be generous or stingy, depending on the financial level for all DRGs—that is, the "standardized amount" that is set each year and multiplied against the unique weight for each DRG.[23]

The use of DRGs has been accompanied by a variety of cost-saving, cost-increasing, and cost-shifting responses. Some results were expected, some not. At the time of the Medicare reform, the country excitedly predicted unforeseen cost squeezes and operating difficulties for hospitals; hospital managers adopted new methods of financial administration; and hospitals stopped expanding employment.[24] Administrative overhead rose while other operating costs grew less rapidly than before. During the first years of DRGs, hospitals saved more money than they needed to and net profits rose. Since then, the government has increased average rates (the "update factor") more generously in some years than others, and operating margins fluctuate. Although hospital costs for both Medicare and non-Medicare business have steadily grown, payroll tax revenue for the Hospital Insurance Trust Fund has risen faster than Medicare's DRG payments—so a threatened Social Security deficit was averted. But hospital costs as a whole were not strictly controlled because of loopholes and the long phase-in: for example, capital costs incurred by hospitals at their discretion are not limited by DRGs but continue to be reimbursed separately by Medicare nearly in full.[25]

DRGs did not limit costs for the entire American health care sector because of the unusual fragmented structure of American health insurance—including the national government's own Medicare. DRGs were adopted only for inpatient care paid for the HI Trust Fund (Medicare Part A). The costs of hospital outpatient care continued to be reimbursed in full by the separately financed SMI Trust Fund (Medicare Part B). Therefore, hospitals treated many cases in outpatient surgery—thereby shifting costs from the Part A trust fund to the Part B trust fund. The cases shifted were those with low DRG inpatient rates, such as surgery on the eye.[26] The apparent reduction in inpatient admissions and patient-days was offset by an increase in outpatient hospital services and same-day surgery. The costs of inpatient housing and personal care were saved, but little else. The Part A trust fund saved money and increased its revenues; the Part B trust fund incurred a growing deficit and had to increase its subscriber premiums and Treasury subsidies. The system did not permit financial transfers from one fund to the other.[27]

Limiting Utilization

Doctors. Direct controls over patients' and doctors' utilization are difficult to design and implement. The reason for creating universal and statutory health insurance was access for everyone. Every subscriber has unlimited entitlement to visit a doctor and receive all the services he needs for recovery. It is the doctors—not the laymen running sickness funds—who decide the treatments needed by the patient and the length of these treatments. The professional responsibility and freedom of the doctors are specified in every country's medical practice laws and often in the health insurance laws. Chapter Ten described utilization review methods set up by health insurance carriers in cooperation with medical associations. This section points out possible consequences for health care costs.

Some health insurance rules limit the patient's ability to shop at the expense of the system. Every Dutch subscriber, for example, must enroll with a general practitioner who is paid by capitation fees. If the subscriber sees a second GP, the latter cannot collect a fee from the sickness fund: the patient must pay him privately or petition for a permanent change in primary physician. In neighboring Belgium, the patient is free to shop and the health insurance funds pay all fees (less the usual coinsurance). The greater opportunities for self-referral to doctors in Belgium may lead to more frequent patient/physician contacts, greater pressure on doctors to please the patient by writing prescriptions, higher ambulatory-care costs, and higher pharmaceutical costs.[28]

Under the Dutch insurance rules, the patient cannot see a specialist without a referral form from his GP. The Belgian patient may self-refer whenever he wishes. Again, the result may be more patient/specialist contacts and higher costs in Belgium.[29] But the data may not be broken down well enough for reliable comparisons, and many other influences (such as the larger number of doctors) may account for Belgium's high utilization. The Dutch method does not automatically minimize referrals and costs: some observers believe that reimbursement by capitation fees rather than fee-for-service gives Dutch GPs an incentive to minimize difficult work and refer to specialists too often. Since one of the few fees available to Dutch general practitioners is that for obstetrical delivery, this exception to the system may discourage rather than encourage cost-saving referrals to midwives.

Quarterly assignments may also limit the patient's ability to shop. For many decades, a German patient obtained an authorization form from the sickness fund (a *Krankenschein*), took it to any doctor, and had to stay with that doctor and case manager throughout the quarter. (He could change when the *Krankenschein* expired.) It was long thought to be an effective restraint on shopping and costs. But as sickness funds are pressed by competition to offer more discretion to subscribers, this method has declined in use. The subscriber now can obtain several *Krankenscheine* from the sickness fund at the start of the year and can use them at his discretion. A doctor can make referrals to specialists in ambulatory care but—since all are paid according to the same fee schedule— usually tries to do everything himself and not lose patients to his competitors. Each German doctor therefore tries to develop well-equipped, well-staffed, and expensive offices either by himself or in partnership with other doctors, each performing a range of specialized procedures. This is one reason why hospital care seems less expensive in Germany than in other countries, while ambulatory care is more expensive.

Before attacking unnecessary and wasteful utilization, the sickness funds must detect it. A common technique in both Europe and the United States is the statistical profiles described in Chapter Ten: all bills are read into a computer system, frequency counts for each procedure are made for each specialty in each region, and individual doctors are singled out if they greatly exceed the average.[30] "Control doctors" employed by the sickness funds demand explanations from the offenders and advise restraint.[31] Until now, this method has had little effect on overutilization:

☐ It calculates the norm from actual practice. If the entire medical profession overutilizes, the method has no standard for criticizing the trend. Diagnostic tests have proliferated in all countries, for example, but the profile system must accept the expensive increases as the baseline.

☐ The system cannot be managed and enforced in Europe without cooperation between the medical association and the sickness funds. The doctors oppose it as an invasion of professional judgment by statisticians who do not understand medicine and by finance officers who think money is more important than human life. Medical associations delayed the development and enforcement of the profile in France for over a decade, and they block its use in Belgium today. Utilization control has worked strictly only in countries (such as Germany) where the medical association itself manages it and deals with offenders.

   One of the few countries where insurers administer utilization control unilaterally over the entire community of office doctors is the United States. The country has no standing negotiating machinery, and medical associations avoid assuming any responsibility for health insurance. Medicare's orders to reduce certain "medically unnecessary" procedures have not been widely heeded by practitioners.[32] Blue Cross/Blue Shield Plans calculate and evaluate statistical profiles, but their control doctors approach the clinicians gingerly. They punish only the few cases of fraud. More often, they counsel the outliers and try to persuade them to practice more like the average doctor.

☐ Many European control doctors are former GPs, from small communities, with limited professional attainment. They are very cautious about criticizing urban specialists.

☐ In practice, many outliers in the statistical profiles are very hard workers. They are models for economists' preachings that medicine should cease to be a primitive cottage industry and should become more productive. Some of these doctors practice a style of medicine that is unusual but legitimate— many short contacts instead of infrequent long ones, for example, but each contact recorded as a separate act in billing.

☐ Some apparent overbilling is due to statistical errors—for example, often all the billing by a group of doctors in radiology or pathology has gone out in the name of the manager.

   Since Americans shrink from punitive regulation and believe in the efficacy of financial motivation, they search for automatic pecuniary incentives that will reward doctors for saving money. But the dominant model of individual practice seems to defy this goal: the patient comes to the doctor with a problem;

the doctor is expected to use his time and full resources to diagnose and treat the problem; the doctor's professional commitments require him to work and not to risk neglect. The doctor earns his living from performing work, not by collecting small rewards for refusing work.

The Americans try to combine such financial incentives with expenditure caps for collective networks. The Independent Practice Association (IPA) contracts with insurers and self-insured employers to deliver physicians' care within a fixed annual amount. Doctors earn fees for their work. If the total fund is not spent, the collective savings are distributed among all the doctors. The first evaluation of IPAs shows that performance over the long run does not differ from that of conventional office practice. The incentives do not reduce utilization—and thereby save money—for several reasons:[33]

☐ Each IPA covers only a small part of the doctor's total work. He cannot change his practice style for his IPA business alone.

☐ If the doctor has affiliations with several IPAs, he is subject to different utilization rules and financial rewards. He may not understand all the nuances. He cannot apply the different rules to the flow of patients each day. He thinks about patients and clinical needs, not about IPA rules and minutely different incentives.

☐ He is rewarded financially by clinical work in individual cases. The small rewards he must share with the rest of the IPA network seem trifling.

Hospitals. Utilization of hospital care can be controlled by the methods described in Chapter Eleven. But these measures are difficult to implement under European statutory health insurance.

One strategy might be to reduce admissions. But this decision is the prerogative of doctor and patient, and both oppose any interference by the sickness funds or by government. Patients' entitlement for hospital care is unlimited under the law. In theory, the control doctors of the sickness funds in some countries (such as France) are supposed to approve hospitalization in advance. But in practice the attending doctor sends the patient to the hospital on short notice, and the control doctor gives pro forma approval later.

American hospitals now try to conserve money in the face of limited reimbursement by substituting day surgery and home care for inpatient admissions. Day surgery is only now starting in Europe. German statutory health insurance pays doctors only for care in private office and private clinics. Since it pays hospitals only for inpatient care, nonprofit and municipal hospitals lack outpatient departments. Hospital-based home care does not yet exist in Europe, and home care usually is not reimbursed under statutory health insurance.

Another strategy might be to reduce the length of stay. But sickness funds and government regulators have no direct sanctions over length of stay. At most, they can force the hospital to reduce its prospective budget, which would require it to treat the same number of patients with fewer personnel in a shorter time.

Sickness funds and rate regulators exhort hospitals with excessive stays to reduce them. (Compared to the United States, Europe has always had more hospital beds and longer stays.) But per diem payment units are incentives to maintain and not reduce existing stays. Nevertheless, the spreading norms of medical practice are steadily reducing stays in every European country, although they still exceed America's.[34]

American private health insurance and Medicare for many years deferred to doctors and hospital managers on the appropriateness of initial admission, length of stay, discharge, and readmission. Blue Cross was pledged to cooperate with hospitals; commercial insurers for a long time had few hospitalization policies and relied on cost sharing by patients to deter unnecessary admissions; the politically driven Medicare assumed that doctors and hospitals (like all good citizens) would not waste taxpayers' money. But as Chapter Eleven reported, Blue Cross Plans and commercial insurers have developed several techniques to prevent unnecessary utilization of the inpatient hospital services:

☐ Preadmission screening—requiring the attending physician to justify non-emergency hospitalization
☐ Second surgical opinions—to confirm the need for elective surgery
☐ Ambulatory testing before admission—and a stipulation that surgery and other treatments must begin upon admission
☐ Specifying a maximum length of stay for each diagnosis
☐ Concurrent review during the stay—to ensure that treatments are not prolonged
☐ Discharge planning—so that the patient is willing to leave promptly (and the family, home-care agencies, or nursing home are ready)

America's health policy literature has depicted the widespread achievements of "managed care." Insurance companies claim they have saved employer groups and individual subscribers much money with their "managed-care packages"; management consulting firms and third-party administrators have proliferated to help insurance companies and self-insured employers deal with hospitals and doctors; conferences and workshops have taught the methods. America was said to have created a "new managed-care environment" superseding the bad old system.

Managed care—plus the structure of Medicare DRGs described earlier—has probably been the cause of the decline in inpatient hospital admissions and inpatient days, the cause of the shift to ambulatory care in hospital outpatient departments, in free-standing centers, and in physicians' offices. From 1976 to 1989 among all Blue Cross Plans, for example, inpatient admissions per subscriber dropped 28.3 percent and outpatient visits nearly doubled. The cost per inpatient day in 1989 was over three times the cost per outpatient visit—but the outpatient unit costs rose faster each year, and the total number of outpatient visits produced a rapid increase in total spending for them.[35]

Yet impartial researchers and indignant employers noted that total spending for all of health—the hospital sector in particular—continued to grow.[36] There were several reasons:

☐ "Managed care" was a series of small autonomous activities within a larger environment that was unmanaged. But cost containment requires a single policy and comprehensive implementation for an entire sector. Since the typical hospital must deal with many managed-care firms (insurance companies, TPAs, and others) with different policies and procedures, the hospital cannot develop the single methodology that contains costs and protects quality. Many large hospitals had to add administrative employees to process the unique questionnaires and authorizations from so many payers.[37]

☐ Cost shifting is common:

- Hospitals responded to controls by shifting work to high-priced outpatient departments. Managed-care programs have few instruments of utilization control in outpatient departments and other ambulatory settings. If a payer covers the hospital but not ambulatory care—for example, a Blue Cross Plan that has a group contract for inpatient care while commercial insurance covers the rest—the inpatient payer encourages the hospital's cost shifting.

- Insurance for ambulatory care both inside and outside the hospital usually requires deductibles and coinsurance. To conserve their own payments, self-insured employers and insurance companies have been increasing cost sharing by patients. The final result does not reduce costs but spreads them.

☐ Insurance companies may claim to provide managed care but fail to enforce it. To win subscribers and keep them in a highly competitive market, a carrier must offer satisfactory coverage. To the individual patient and doctor, full coverage and satisfactory care are more important than saving money for the purchaser—that is, the employer. Denials irritate patients and doctors.

☐ Hospitals and doctors may refuse to cooperate with the payer's rules. Even if the doctor cooperates, his hospital may not. And the managed-care firm cannot force him to hospitalize the patient in an establishment where he lacks admitting privileges. The hospital may be too important in the community for the managed-care firm to antagonize it.

☐ Managed care requires a great volume of expensive investigations, reports, and communications.[38]

☐ In a competitive private market, managed-care firms must compete with each other for contracts with self-insured employers and insurance companies. This means they must advertise and send out salesmen. If they are creating a preferred provider panel, they must advertise and visit the doctors and hospitals. All this adds to their own operating costs.[39]

☐ The executives of managed-care firms pay themselves high salaries and perquisites, maintain expensive office suites, and have many employees. Despite their ostensible mission to contain costs, they follow the lavish style of American management.[40]

Probably America's "managed-care" activity has reduced total health costs below what they might have been otherwise.[41] Even so, the total rose substantially. Some programs were probably more successful than others. But no one could tell: not only was each program's experience a secret between the insurer and the employer, but the carriers and managed-care firms exaggerated their public claims in order to win business. If the entire system were managed—as in European statutory health insurance—American costs would be controlled more strictly.

Forcing Patients to Share Costs

Americal medical economists have long attempted to calculate the precise effects on utilization, system efficiency, and aggregate savings from finely tuned variations in cost sharing by patients.[42] But designing cost-sharing methods that implement theoretical goals proves very difficult:[43]

☐ Market theory claims that consumer prices will signal buyers that some providers are more cost-effective than others—and thus inspire consumers to choose those with lower charges. But buyer-seller relations in a competitive market imply many different prices and many different patient cost-sharing requirements. Such a complex and flexible set of transactions cannot be administered in social insurance or in large-scale private insurance.

☐ Flat-rate coinsurance or copayment can be legislated, administered, and understood easily. But flat rates are not targeted individually to motivate consumer choice and provider efficiency. The standard rate has different meanings and effects among all providers and patients.

Social Insurance. Cost sharing has existed for some time in European health insurance to discourage waste:

☐ Drugs, prostheses, and other supplies that might be ordered unnecessarily often have considerable cost sharing, even in countries with full insurance coverage of doctors and hospitals. Few countries have full third-party payment of drugs.

☐ Cost sharing of ambulatory visits to doctors exists in a few countries where office doctors are paid by fee-for-service—for example, France, Belgium, and Switzerland. The intention is partly to discourage patients from making unnecessary visits (*les cas bagatelles*).

☐ Few countries expect cost sharing of hospital stays. Where it exists, it is waived for the poor and the seriously ill. If these patients were expected to pay, they and the hospital would have to appeal to public welfare. But as noted earlier, governments are reducing welfare programs and are trying to route financing through the health insurance system.

Cost sharing has not been effective in bringing about large reductions in utilization and costs for several reasons:

☐ It is usually insignificant. A large amount would clearly reduce utilization and system costs—euphemistically called a "high deductible" by American advocates—but that contradicts the very purpose of statutory health insurance. The programs were designed to encourage, not discourage, use. Some recent additions of cost sharing—such as Germany's charge of 5 DM per day of hospitalization during the 1980s—cost more to collect than they bring in and increase hospitals' administrative burden. (Even when the copayment was doubled in 1991, the affluent German population could easily bear it.) After struggling to limit the costs of specialists' care for decades, Holland in 1987 reluctantly adopted a copayment for the first time. But it is probably too small to make a difference: it is f. 25 per visit, and the patient is liable for no more than six copayments a year.

☐ Long-term effects must be distinguished from short-term results. During the first year after introduction of cost sharing for an important procedure, utilization of that procedure drops; thereafter it resumes at its previous rate. This sequence has occurred in French radiology in 1959, in Saskatchewan office practice in the late 1960s, in German pharmaceuticals in the 1970s and again in 1983, and elsewhere.[44]

☐ If significant cost sharing exists and government does not forbid it, insurance carriers sell supplementary policies to cover the cost sharing. Therefore, the financial deterrent disappears and a windfall in business results for the carriers. Examples are France and American Medicare. Indeed, selling coverage of the cost sharing has enabled France's mutual aid societies to survive. Several attempts by conservative French governments to forbid such supplementary insurance by the *mutuelles* have been politically suicidal.[45]

If the government, sickness funds, and medical association agree that a procedure is medically useless, is overused, and provides undeserved financial windfalls, they may agree to substantial cost sharing. For example, physiotherapy was widely used in Belgium, utilization grew, and it became a significant proportion of all health insurance costs. Physiotherapists made home visits and billed the sickness funds according to a fee schedule.[46] Then, in 1982, INAMI and the government increased coinsurance on every bill from 25 to 40 percent. Thereafter, during the first years, utilization rose less rapidly. Reductions were not as great as hoped (and might even disappear in the long run) since many physiotherapists in this overstaffed and competitive field tried to keep business by waiving the cost sharing.[47]

Another example is thermal cures at spas. They have long been benefits of German statutory health insurance. Sickness funds and medical associations cannot eliminate them, since the benefits are popular. Sickness funds competed for members and were permissive in covering the mounting costs. Removal of the benefit from the law would have aroused the many communities depending on the thermal services, the housing, and the related tourist facilities. The general insurance reform of the 1970s transferred much of the burden to the patient's employer by forcing him and not the sickness fund to pay the worker's salary during all leaves—presumably the employer would discourage unnecessary and prolonged absences at spas. During the mid-1980s, the patient was required to pay 10 DM per day for the thermal medical bills as well as all nonmedical expenses—and utilization leveled off.

If a population is determined to use health services, cost sharing makes a greater difference for those who can least afford it. The statistics are rarely analyzed to identify the contrasting reactions of patients by disease and by class. One of the few such studies—in Saskatchewan during the late 1960s and early 1970s—showed that the short-run reduction in hospital admissions was concentrated primarily among the poor and elderly.[48] But these are precisely the people whom statutory health insurance and national health services are designed to protect.

A policy of exempting vulnerable patients from cost sharing must be delicately crafted according to the facts and the ideology of the policymakers. For example, French hospital patients have long been expected to pay a share of their costs. Patients suffering from very serious illnesses were exempt. The law listed twenty-five specific diagnoses and also allowed exemptions for any other "long and expensive" illness not on the list (*la 26ᵉ maladie*). When the French government and sickness funds tried to contain the costs of hospitals during the early 1980s, they discovered that a considerable proportion of all exemptions from cost sharing fell under the ambiguous "26th illness." A hospital doctor could specify any "long and expensive" diagnosis, the law courts would back up such exemptions, and the sickness funds had become permissive. One part of the new conservative government's cost containment policy (the *Plan Séguin*) was the elimination of the "26th illness." The measure was believed to be a principal reason for the success of health cost containment in France.

When the Socialists regained power in 1988, they faced a familiar dilemma of the Left: how to protect the poor and vulnerable while avoiding a new explosion of costs. The new government preserved its predecessor's cost containment policy by avoiding restoration of a catchall "26th illness." But it added additional specific diagnoses relieved from cost sharing and created a new exempt category of multiple illnesses, applied in practice to the elderly. The conservative government had increased pharmaceutical cost sharing for the severely and chronically ill, and the socialist government restored their exemption.

Cost sharing is based on the economists' assumption that all people wish to maximize cash savings. But it may have the reverse effect of attracting some customers to the more expensive providers. Medical care is a field where customers want "the best," and the most expensive may be interpreted as "the best," while cheap or free services and products may be thought ineffective. When Belgium's national health insurance adopted variable copayments for drugs to deter purchase of proprietaries and motivate acceptance of generics, the immediate result was the opposite: patients opted for the more expensive proprietary drugs with the higher copayments.[49]

Rebates. Indirect incentives such as cost sharing have limited effects on important procedures: people use health care because they and their doctors think they need it, and the risk of damage outweighs small out-of-pocket payments. Direct rewards are more effective. Several private health insurance companies in Germany offer rebates on premiums if the subscriber does not use insurance that year (*Kostenerstattung*). If the carriers offer high enough rebates, subscribers do not merely refrain from submitting claims—utilization itself is lower, and everyone saves.[50]

The German social insurance system experimented with such rebates in 1970 (the *Krankenscheinprämie*). If a subscriber did not go to the doctor in a quarter and therefore did not submit a quarterly bill (the *Krankenschein*), the sickness fund sent him 10 DM. He could "earn" up to 30 DM a year. The bonus caused a rescheduling of services but not a reduction: to collect a bonus during a quarter, the patient scheduled all his visits in the previous or subsequent quarter. Total medical costs did not diminish. Moreover, the financial situation of the sickness funds declined instead of improved: the many subscribers who would not have gone to doctors anyway received bonuses; the administration of the records was a new expense. And the attempt to reduce utilization contradicted another law designed to increase it: in 1971 the German government and sickness funds added preventive examinations to the fee schedules; patients were expected to visit the doctor regularly, even when they did not feel sick. The *Krankenscheinprämie* was phased out in 1972 and repealed from the law in 1974.[51]

United States. Because of its history, American health insurance has always required considerable cost sharing. While European health insurance was created by the labor movement to protect the poor by redistributive financing, American health insurance was first created by elites for their own protection and designed on common principles of insurance. Point-of-service cost sharing by patients was intended not only to reduce premiums for all subscribers and for employers but to discourage the inevitable temptations for moral hazard. Other insurance had deductibles, and so did American health insurance. Many Blue Cross Plans tried to emulate European social insurance by avoiding cost sharing, but Blue Shield never did. The indemnity methods of commercial health insurance left considerable cost sharing and balance-billing. But the carriers thought them necessary to make the patient vigilant, since the carriers had no contacts with providers and no utilization review. As employers contained their own health benefit costs during the 1980s, cost sharing by patients increased.

During the 1970s, health policy analysis in the United States was captured by neoclassical welfare economists. The advocates of social solidarity, redistributive finance, and generous insurance were eclipsed. To the new economists, the problem was to make the health care sector more efficient and to assign it an appropriate place in society's priorities. This could be achieved by a competitive market in which a well-informed and self-interested consumer made rational choices among providers, drove hard bargains, and maximized his savings. When health care suffered from market failure, the culprit was overinsurance among employed groups and in Medicare. People could not be rational consumers: they patronized wasteful providers and overutilized services because they did not buy their own insurance and did not use enough of their own cash in paying providers.[52]

The new economists recommended that all employees and their dependents become purchasers of health insurance by changes in the tax laws—in this way, all group insurance premiums could be counted under wage income. Many persons might then self-insure or might select policies with point-of-service cash liability. The leading medical economist recommended restricting all health insurance to catastrophic coverage.[53] Having captured the grant-making machinery of the national government, these economists created a major demonstration project devoted in large part to identifying the effects of different cost-sharing rates on patient utilization, provider performance, health, and service delivery generally.[54]

Despite all the talk about the beneficial or adverse effects of cost sharing—and despite its widespread use in the United States—the country has only rudimentary knowledge about its volume, the type of people who must pay what amounts for what services, how much of the out-of-pockets is subsequently reimbursed by insurers, and the effects on patients and providers.[55] Empirical generalizations are impossible: millions of people are subject to different cost-sharing rules in their various coverages, their cost-sharing varies by benefit, cost-sharing rules in each policy may change from year to year, and the individual encounters different extra-billing demands by different doctors. Often the cost sharing cannot influence the patient's market behavior since it is not known in advance; it is the subsequently unreimbursed part of the total fee that the patient has paid the doctor at the time of the visit. Even when an insured carrier thinks it has a consistent cost-sharing policy, a substantial number of doctors fail to collect it—either to attract patients from their competitors or to ease the burden on their own longtime patients.[56] In sum, then, the effect on the average patient is not rational market choice but confusion and complaint.[57]

Instead of taking advantage of their large and diverse natural laboratory of cost sharing, American researchers have studied the issue only in controlled and atypical insurance arrangements. Some of their findings have been the following:[58]

☐   Point-of-service cost sharing reduces adults' visits to office doctors.
☐   Point-of-service cost sharing reduces children's visits to office doctors, but not to the same extent as adults' visits.

☐ Cost sharing reduces the rate of admission to hospitals but does not reduce the consumption of services after admission.

☐ The visits forgone are not those for urgent care. Therefore, cost sharing is not associated with lower health.

☐ Cost sharing reduces all services uniformly. Patients are not motivated to reduce "inappropriate" or "unnecessary" services selectively.

☐ Cost sharing reduces visits for preventive care.

☐ Cost sharing might raise the costs of the health care system if it discourages ambulatory visits to office doctors and patients instead visit the better-insured hospital outpatient department.

☐ Cost sharing reduces utilization among the poor more than the rich.

☐ Since the richer have better insurance coverage, better health, and lower utilization, they have lower out-of-pocket spending in proportion to income.

☐ Some persons—particularly the poor and elderly—have very high and often disastrous bills.

In the few research studies of typical health insurance over long periods, the long-term effects are much like those in the European data—for example, the introduction of cost sharing briefly reduces utilization, but then the historic trends resume.[59]

Preferred Provider Organizations. The Americans attempt to use the economic incentives from differential cost sharing to persuade the insured to cooperate with managed care voluntarily. While policymakers have preferred HMOs to conventional office practice covered by traditional insurance, the public has refused to accept the lock-in. Closed panels violate the conservative American belief in free markets governed by prices. The PPO is designed to combine several distinctively American desiderata: the most cost-effective providers are offered to the subscriber; the patient is free to visit any doctor or hospital either inside or outside the preferred panel; the PPO pays the in-plan doctor and hospital directly (with minimum or no cost sharing by the patient); the patient is reimbursed by the PPO at less than the full charges of out-of-plan providers. The financial savings are supposed to motivate users to choose the in-plan doctors and hospitals who obey fee schedules and utilization controls. Economic incentives therefore result in lower costs. The more efficient its doctors and hospitals, the greater the cash savings the insurer can pass on to its subscribers, the more attractive its doctors, the greater its sales.

PPOs were intended to enlist subscribers who opposed the lock-in of HMOs and otherwise would have remained in conventional insurance. PPOs have become a common method whereby mainstream insurance companies constrain costs while preserving good relations with all doctors and hospitals. Blue Cross/Blue Shield, for example, is committed to participation by any licensed doctor and hospital willing to accept its contract. Since it promises free choice to subscribers, it cannot create closed-panel HMOs or IPAs, and the PPO arrangement is its ideal solution. Because the United States has no laws (except for Medicare) fixing provider reimbursement and cost sharing by patients, private insurance companies and self-financing employer benefit plans can offer such "discounts" to patients who select doctors on the preferred list. In return for more patients—presumably attracted away from the higher-priced community doctors—the doctors who join are willing to conform to a fee schedule and not extra-bill. The in-plan providers contain costs not only by following fee schedules but also by restraining hospitalization and utilization in other ways.

The PPO option arrived at an opportune moment during the late 1980s. Employee benefit managers needed to control costs, and closed-panel HMOs seemed the only solution. But the workers and their unions would have been outraged by restrictions on their free choices and the elimination of coverage of their family doctors. The PPO option enabled the benefit managers to pass the risks and choices on to the insurers, the provider panels, and the patients. Unable to expand enrollments and fearing the loss of subscribers to PPOs, some HMOs have added the PPO option (called "open-ended HMOs" or "point of service managed care") as Chapter Ten and Appendix A report.

By the 1990s, many group policies covering millions of persons included PPO options.[60] During these first years, this form of health insurance may have restrained costs below those of unmanaged conventional financing. But PPOs also encountered several growing pains:[61]

☐ Clinical costs have been higher than expected. The additional cost sharing is not sufficient to deter many patients from selecting out-of-plan doctors either regularly or occasionally. In order to obtain services and not antag-onize the subscribers, the carrier often must pay the out-of-plan provider more than the in-plan provider.

☐ Selection is adverse—contrary to the pecuniary incentives at the heart of PPOs. The lower utilizers are more willing to select in-plan providers. The higher utilizers, despite the financial incentive to switch, are reluctant to abandon their regular doctors in the community.

☐ The fees paid to in-plan doctors and hospitals—as in the case of all IPAs—have often been raised faster than expected to ensure enough participants in that PPO.

☐ Since utilization of out-of-plan providers is hard to predict, setting premi-ums is very difficult. Meanwhile, employers are forcing competing insurers to underbid against each other in order to win contracts.

☐ The health care system as a whole becomes increasingly complex. The same doctors may have agreements with several PPOs and IPAs, each with differ-ent fees and rules. The fees and rules change from year to year.

☐ Doctors join and quit PPOs unpredictably. They quit if they believe the PPO rules are burdensome and if business from that source does not increase to offset conformity to its fees.

☐ In-plan doctors make referrals to physicians who seem most appropriate clinically. They rarely think about whether the physicians are on the preferred list.

☐ The PPO management cannot easily monitor the doctors and enforce the rules. If it finds the doctor has charged the patient directly (*tiers garant*) and has extra-billed over the agreed fees, it cannot be sure whether the doctor has dropped out, deliberately violated the agreement, or committed a clerical error. There follows the sort of administrative inquiries that irritate doctors.

☐ HMOs and IPAs have often made guarantees of minimum business, capital costs, and operating costs to their doctors. Until they became "open-ended," all their insurance was dedicated to covering the guarantees. Adding the PPO option enables the patient to redirect the plan's revenue outside, and the plan faces deficits from the continued guarantees. If open-ended options spread, staff-model and group-model HMOs—with their expensive health centers—may no longer be viable.

☐ While the rules about differential reimbursement procedures and differential cost sharing for in-plan and out-of-plan providers are self-evident to PPO designers and employee benefits managers, the patients often do not understand them. Complaints about extra-billing—some justified and others not—contribute to America's general dissatisfaction about health care finance.

☐ PPOs have high administrative costs.

Limiting the Total Amount of Money Available

Many partial and indirect methods have proved contentious, or ineffective, or both. The most effective method is simple and direct: provide a predictable sum of money, retain full entitlement for all subscribers, and expect doctors and hospitals to provide all necessary care within that limit. The official financing system—as in statutory health insurance—therefore can suffer no cost overruns. If they dislike the consequences, health care providers and patients have an escape hatch in the form of outside private practice, financed by either cash or private commercial insurance.

An "expenditure cap" is usually associated with the centralized financing and strong management of a national health service. An "expenditure target" is usually associated with the decentralization and flexibility of health insurance. If targets cannot contain health costs, the problem is to achieve caplike control and predictability without the governmentalization that statutory health insurance is supposed to avoid. Every developed country except the United States now uses either caps or targets for several health sectors.

Definitions. An expenditure cap (sometimes called "global budget") is a fixed amount of money within which health care providers must serve patients during the next year. Expenditure caps may be applied in three different ways:

☐ They may apply to all health care. However, such comprehensive limits—controlling all private as well as public spending—are unusual. Although

93 percent of all British health expenditure passes through the National Health Service and is constrained by government, the remainder is left to an uncontrolled and decentralized private market. Canadian provinces control about 74 percent of all Canadian health spending, either by expenditure caps or by strict expenditure targets, leaving the rest to the private market.

☐   They may apply to only that part of health care covered by the third parties. For example, the British National Health Service covers hospitals, doctors, drugs, dentistry, mental care, and certain other benefits. Canadian public expenditure covers hospitals and nursing homes (by expenditure caps) and covers doctors (by strict expenditure targets that are evolving into caps in some provinces).

☐   They may apply to a single clinical sector such as physicians' services, hospitals, pharmaceuticals, or laboratory tests. At various times, all German doctors providing care in offices and in private clinics have had to operate under a cap. No such cap applied to other sectors under German statutory health insurance.

A cap may be either nationwide or regional. Britain's National Health Service begins each year with an amount listed in the general budget of the national government. The Ministry of Health then divides it into 14 regional amounts and then into 192 district amounts. Each district must provide all specified services under its cap. Each Canadian province has its own health budget, but it is then subdivided into sectors (such as hospitals and physicians' payments) rather than into geographical districts.

A cap may be subdivided among certain providers in advance. It is very common to give each hospital a global budget for the next year.[62] The method is used under government financing in Britain, Canada, and Sweden; it is used under statutory health insurance financing in France and the Netherlands. If the method is used in ambulatory medical care, as in Germany from time to time, it is a cap for the entire medical profession's billings. Individual doctors and individual medical groups are not given fixed budgets in advance under which they must perform all their services.

In contrast, an expenditure target is a voluntary agreement among payers, providers, and government to try to hold health care spending at a specified level for a specified time. A target may refer to all health care, health care traditionally covered by third parties, or a specific health care service (such as physicians, hospitals, pharmaceuticals, or laboratory tests). Expenditure targets may be calculated in two ways: either as the total annual amount of spending or as a percentage increase over the previous year's total expenditure. In the latter case, this may be either a real or a nominal increase—that is, corrected or not corrected for expected price inflation. To ensure that the projected total is realistic, the agreement usually includes unit prices and utilization guidelines. In practice, providers are paid more (or occasionally less) than the totals. The time period for an expenditure target may be next year or several years together.

With expenditure targets, there is no fixed amount of money under which providers must give all services. There need not be a single payer or a small cohesive group of payers. All-payer cooperation for a common target is possible, or (more rarely) the principal payers might have slightly different targets. Usually the providers continue to collect full fees even if utilization exceeds expectations and defies controls. If costs exceed revenue during the current year, the provider (such as a hospital) may receive a rate increase during the current year. If it does not, it is allowed to borrow, receive a supplement to its rates next year, and pay off the debt. Therefore, targets often are exceeded in practice without sanctions. But if government and the insurance carriers must contain their costs and limit their payments to the targets—and the targets are being exceeded substantially— government and the insurance carriers in subsequent years may reduce fees or limit utilization. Deficits then no longer are carried over and retrieved next year.

An expenditure target system is adopted instead of an expenditure cap in countries where governments traditionally have had limited power over health care. The target method is adopted because health care spending must be restrained but government is not accustomed to controlling the health sector. (Examples today are the Netherlands and most of the health sectors in Germany.) Expenditure targets are also used in countries where the payers are too numerous and too competitive to agree on a fixed collective payment. And targets are adopted in countries where, if the payers run deficits, government is committed to subsidizing them but lacks the power to impose caps.

Sometimes, an expenditure target system is tightened to become an expenditure cap because the target is persistently exceeded. The change requires amendments to health insurance and related laws, magnifying the power of government. Such changes in payment to hospitals occurred during the 1980s in France and Holland and may be evolving now in Belgium.

Expenditure Caps in Practice. Until the 1980s, there was only one example of an expenditure cap under social insurance. To settle a series of disputes during the first decades of the twentieth century—as Chapter Ten reported—German sickness funds turned over lump sums (the *Kopfpauschalen*) for all ambulatory care to associations of their doctors. The method spread to all sickness funds in each province, and doctors in insurance practice created province-wide associations (the *Kassenärztliche Vereinigungen*, or KVs). The KVs negotiated lump sums from the sickness funds and then distributed the money among their members according to services performed, priced by a fee schedule. Since the total was set by annual negotiations between the sickness funds and the KV, higher utilization during the year led to lower unit prices before the year ended. This method was abandoned amidst the economic prosperity and utopian hopes of the 1960s: each doctor was now guaranteed payment of his bills in full according to a fee schedule negotiated between all the sickness funds and the KVs, and the *Kopfpauschale* was dropped.[63] A cost explosion then followed, the economic recession of the 1970s created financial problems for the sickness funds, and the funds tried to negotiate annual increases in fees so that expected total costs would rise no higher than expected increases in their revenue—a typical form of expenditure targeting.

Meanwhile, other countries became discouraged with their fragmented and contentious methods of cost control and adopted global budgets and fixed limits (*enveloppes*) in various sectors:

☐ *Hospitals.* Several countries were inspired by the methods of public financing as in Britain and Canada. Public subsidies require fixed appropriations without provider-initiated cost overruns: Britain and Canada practiced such predictable global budgets for the entire hospital sector and for every individual hospital. France, the Netherlands, and several Swiss cantons (particularly Vaud during the 1980s) have emulated the method under insurance: at the start of the year, goals for the country's aggregate hospital spending are set by a government agency; a regulator or commission approves each hospital's share of the total and screens its budget in advance; shares of the hospital's budget are distributed among sickness funds by various formulas; if the hospital overspends, it has to make compensating economies.[64]

☐ *Pharmaceuticals.* Beset by critical cost-control problems, Belgium imposed *enveloppes* on several sectors. A cap was set in 1985 on all spending for drugs by all the sickness funds. If consumption rises above predictions, unit prices paid to drug companies automatically are reduced by a regulatory commission.

☐ *Diagnostic testing by CT, NMR, and other imaging methods.* In 1986, a scheme was proposed in Belgium allowing each installation a maximum amount of tests. If the installation wished new equipment, it had to discard old units. Such a general policy was blocked in INAMI; the medical associations feared this would be the first of many caps over medical practice. Instead, each teaching hospital was given an annual global budget for all its NMR amortization and operating costs, including the radiologists' fees.

☐ *Ambulatory care by doctors.* The German sickness funds and KVs in 1986 agreed to reestablish the *Kopfpauschale.* At the beginning of each year, the sickness funds and the *Kassenärztliche Vereinigung* negotiate a lump sum sufficient to cover all expected costs. The unit rate for the fee schedule (the "conversion factor") is calculated by the KV for the year. Doctors are paid at those rates during the first quarter. If total costs exceed the first quarter's target, the conversion factor is reduced during the second quarter. Similar adjustments are made during the third and fourth quarters, so the KV breaks even at the end of the year.

☐ *Clinical laboratory tests.* In Germany, the rapidly growing clinical laboratory tests were placed under their own *Kopfpauschale* in 1984, and their conversion factor has been reduced faster than the unit price for clinical specialties. To make sure they do not absorb too large a share of ambulatory health care money in the future, laboratory tests may always be kept under a *Kopfpauschale,* even if the cap is again abandoned for the rest of medical practice.

Each of the foregoing caps refers to one sector; each motivates the providers to reduce unnecessary services that they deliver. Statutory health insurance systems usually lack clinical budgets that apply to all sectors and are governed by the doctor's own pecuniary self-interest. An experiment in Bavaria in the late 1970s replaced the provincial *Kopfpauschale* with a larger sum that covered physicians' ambulatory services, referrals to hospitals, work disability certificates, and drug prescriptions. If doctors made fewer expensive referrals, the conversion factor governing their own fees would increase. One might expect underreferral and underservicing—a common fear when this method is used in American HMOs. But the Bavarian doctors did not respond. Some referred less; some unexpectedly increased their own service intensity; and others continued their normal practice styles. Professional customs were stronger than new pecuniary incentives. Some doctors understood the goals and methods of the arrangement, while many others did not. The experiment saved little money and was abandoned.[65]

The voluminous research on American HMOs finds some cases where doctors' referrals and testing are affected by their own pecuniary share in the savings.[66] But these doctors have a self-interest in joining such arrangements; all understand the rules and pursue their personal gains. In contrast, the Bavarian experiment demonstrated the reactions of the entire medical profession.

At first sight, one might think the new Dutch dental rules are an expenditure cap. As noted in Chapter Thirteen, coverage of crowns and dentures was added for adults during the 1980s when Dutch health insurance was trying to control its deficit. To prevent deficits in the new dental benefits, adult patients' cost sharing rises if the carriers' dental spending seems to be exceeding the annual plan. This unusual method is an automatic shifting of costs from the sickness funds to the patients—not a firm lid over the insured dental sector.

An expenditure cap does not mean that the payers give the providers lump sums and allow them to use the money at their complete discretion. Under expenditure caps, the payers and governments impose permanent rules about the use of the money, usually impose (by regulation or negotiation) some kind of prospective budget in advance, and always require an annual retrospective accounting.

Barriers to Expenditure Caps. The virtues of controllable and predictable budgeting may seem self-evident to finance officers and policy analysts. But it can rarely be adopted in health. No important policy in health can be enacted without the cooperation of the medical profession, which opposes "arbitrary" limits on its resources, work, and earnings. If statutory health insurance is strained financially, the medical profession will accept expenditure targets provided their creation and implementation are negotiated.

Dutch experience demonstrates the inability of governments to dictate caps and the need for caution by medical associations. During the years when the Dutch health insurance accounts were being strained (the late 1970s and early 1980s), the Secretary of State for Health and the mass media denounced specialists' excessive incomes—a sin in a country long devoted to economic restraint and charitable services. The medical association feared that a few high earners would prevent other specialists from earning adequate incomes. Thus, during the early 1980s, the sickness funds and medical association agreed to recapture some money paid to very high earners. If a radiologist performed more than 10,000 tests a year under statutory health insurance, for example, he would be asked to refund part of his fees for each test above the 10,000. If a pathologist earned more than f. 200,000 per year, he would be asked to repay one-third of his revenue between f. 200,000 and 225,000 and two-thirds of his revenue over f. 225,000. High earners in several surgical fields would also be asked to refund portions.

As part of its general effort to control costs, the Dutch government in 1986 asked for an increase in the refunds in the short run and proposed a phase-in of a fixed cap, like the German method. The Dutch specialists responded with an unprecedented one-day protest strike. Eventually, the medical association and the association of health insurance carriers agreed to generalize the foregoing degressive method for all specialists: the physician would collect full fees for his first f. 200,000 of billing under statutory health insurance; he would refund one-third of the next f. 50,000; and he would refund two-thirds of all billings over f. 250,000. A special office jointly directed by the medical association and the sickness funds (the *Centraal Bureau voor de Administratie der Specialistenhonorering*) would administer the method.[67]

The agreements were never implemented because the practicing doctors refused to cooperate and the medical association's leadership had to side with its members. All calculations by the *Centraal Bureau* depended on data from the practicing doctors, who refused to send it. Most high earners refused to send refunds. The national government tried to make the arrangement official and enforceable—not merely a bilateral agreement negotiated between sickness funds and the medical association—by instructing the official rate-setting agency (COTG) to issue regulations. Substituting government action for negotiated agreements is anathema to all doctors. The procedural dispute was exacerbated by substance: the Ministry and COTG issued a new guideline reducing specialists' fees on the grounds their practice costs were covered by the sickness funds' reimbursement of the hospitals. The medical association disengaged from its agreement and filed lawsuits against the Ministry and COTG. Groups of specialists around the country called brief wildcat strikes from hospital work. Many specialists imposed administrative strikes by billing patients directly instead of sending the bills to the sickness funds—that is, substituting *tiers garant* for the traditional *tiers payant*.

The sickness funds and medical association then resumed negotiations; a distinguished citizen served as chairman and mediator. The Five-Party Agreement of December 1989 adopted the principle of an annual expenditure target (*macrobudget*) for 1989 through 1992. Whether total spending for doctors exceeds the target for that year will be reported by the national government's statistical office (the *Centraal Bureau voor de Statistiek*). If the target is exceeded, data on billings must be reported for each medical specialty by the associations of sickness funds and of private health insurance companies (VNZ and KLOZ). The standing negotiating body from the payers and medical association will then judge whether the excess over targets is due to unusually rapid increases in spending for certain specialties, so that their share of the total relative to other specialties rises. If so, that specialty's fees for next year will be restrained or even cut. All payments in that specialty are cut at the same rate, not those of high earners alone. The degressive arrangements of the 1980s (whereby impending cost over-runs trigger reductions in current fees) are canceled; any doctors who were not paid in full will be reimbursed. The high-earning specialties that were the first objects of degressive reimbursement (such as radiology and cardiac-thoracic surgery) receive across-the-board cuts in the conversion factor during the early 1990s, while certain cognitive specialties receive extra increases. The Dutch agreement makes formal and permanent a method that has long been used informally and unsystematically in negotiation over physicians' fees: if the incomes of certain specialties rise very fast, the negotiators restrain their relative weights or their conversion factors.

The French government and sickness funds—like the Dutch—might have liked to extend their achievements in hospital global budgeting into physicians' services during the 1980s. Unlike the Dutch, the French did not try and fail. They knew they could never impose expenditure caps on their notoriously militant doctors: none of the three medical associations would have signed any such agreement. After prolonged and passionate wrangling, the French negotiators achieved an outcome much like Holland's: an annual expenditure target for all physicians' services and a commitment to set the next year's conversion factor in the light of this year's experience. The 1990 contract set an expenditure target for physicians' services 106.4 percent over the current year. A timetable for increases in the conversion factor was set as well. If current total spending exceeds 106.4 percent, the Minister approves the next scheduled increase in the conversion factor, less a reduction that will reduce total spending. Fees are not reduced during the current year to ensure no more than the 106.4 percent increase. A negotiated agreement that created expenditure targets and tied fees to them was an important turning point for the French medical associations and sickness funds. A trend was crystallizing in European statutory health insurance.

Setting the Amount. Government can announce and enforce levels of costs where its general budget pays all providers—as in Great Britain, Sweden, and Canada. But it cannot dictate total spending so easily in countries with statutory health insurance—since the carriers are autonomous, the providers are private, every subscriber is guaranteed access to all benefits without waiting, and doctors have complete authority to decide patients' needs. Therefore, payers and providers have evolved machinery to set and implement expenditure levels for both caps and targets. Procedures differ among these countries, but all have multicentered negotiations.

In Holland, Belgium, France, and many Swiss cantons, the guidelines are negotiated among the Ministries of Social Affairs, Health, Budget, and Finance. Each Ministry is influenced by various interest groups in the population and by different factions in the governing coalition. Social Affairs (which usually directs the social security system) speaks for the trade unions, the health insurance carriers, and the left wings of the political parties in the governing coalition. Health speaks for providers (particularly hospitals), the workers in health, and patients. Budget must balance the demands from all Ministries, from all existing government programs, and from the governing coalition's new proposals; Budget must also minimize public subsidies to health insurance. Finance tries to avoid raising payroll and other taxes; in practice, finance represents business interests in expenditure and social policies. Each Ministry develops its case for higher or lower health spending with the help of its own statisticians. In the past, viewpoints diverged and Prime Ministers often had to mediate. But now everyone agrees that increases in payroll taxes and public subsidies should be avoided; all the Ministries agree on basic facts (particularly the expected yield of the payroll taxes next year); and all the Ministries agree on this expenditure level.

In Germany, a standing forum represents all the interest groups: the associations for doctors, hospitals, dentists, and pharmaceuticals; the business associations; the trade unions; the health insurance carriers; and others. It meets at least once a year and is called the *Konzertierte Aktion im Gesundheitswesen*. A staff from the Ministry of Labor provides data, particularly about the expected yield of payroll taxes. A committee of neutral experts—chiefly university professors—prepares option papers and special reports. The forum negotiates annual expenditure targets in all health sectors, usually within the expected fiscal capacity of the payroll taxes. If the bilateral negotiators from the sickness funds and providers (such as doctors and hospitals) deadlock over the amounts of money for next year, the case goes to arbitration and the arbitrator usually selects a figure within the *Konzertierte Aktion*'s target. Thus, the negotiators usually settle on the target.[68]

When laws and regulations creating the system of expenditure caps are first announced, the government regulators and payers promise to keep pace with inflation. The expectation is that expenditure caps can be adjusted to match the inflation rate. The providers will not suffer reductions in their incomes or facilities and can accept the new approach. Guaranteeing increases against inflation is important for nonprofit providers, such as hospitals, that are expected to cover their costs.

In practice, however, the fiscal capacity of the payers soon overrides initial promises to protect the providers against inflation. Caps are first proposed because the payers need protection against rapid increases in health care spending; the payers soon claim they still face deficits. The caps may be frozen or increased less than the inflation rate. Such has been the history of the payment of hospitals and doctors in Canada and the payment of hospitals in France.

Effects on Costs, Utilization, and Health

Does one method of cost containment reduce waste and improve efficiency better than another? How much money does each method save? These questions are much discussed but cannot easily be answered for several reasons:

☐ Since countries cannot be compared by cost containment system, one national arrangement cannot be judged more "effective" than another.

- One reason is that no developed country subjects the entire health sector to financial constraint. As noted in a previous paragraph, for example, not all health spending in Britain and Canada is governed by expenditure caps—and the uncontrolled sectors in other countries are larger.
- Many countries have a complex mixture of methods. For example, hospital spending may be governed by rate regulation and physicians' pay by negotiations; the controls over physicians may impose holdbacks and degressive payments in some countries and carryovers in others. Countries differ in the full configuration.
- Aggregate national data about health spending are published and often compared. But they are not reliable enough for sweeping conclusions that one set of methods is x percent better than another.[69] Rather, the data are legitimate only for rough comparisons.

☐ Since the expenditure problems, administrative organization, and cost containment methods differ among sectors within health, countries can be compared one sector at a time. In *Paying the Hospital*, for example, I compared methods of cost containment in the hospital sectors of seven countries. The methods of cost containment in each country can be described thoroughly as they are in the present book. But the effects on costs and utilization cannot be pinpointed with great accuracy because of limitations in the data: information is available from all countries only for a few sectors, such as hospitals and physicians' services; the data are not collected and reported in identical fashion across all countries; and there are other weaknesses described elsewhere.[70]

National Styles. Earlier this chapter described the effects of cost containment methods within individual countries. The following pages compare the effects of nationwide controls on the entire level of costs. In Table 17.1, countries are grouped by their configurations of cost containment method. Some characteristic configurations are the following:

☐ *Expenditure caps ("global budgets").* The entire hospital sector, nearly all physicians' services, and certain other sectors must perform their work within annual government appropriations. A few sectors in the total figures may be private and uncontrolled.

Table 17.1. Effects of Predominant Cost Containment Methods on Nationwide Costs.

Predominant method	Proportion of GDP spent on all health care in 1987 (%)	Expenditure per capita in 1987 (converted to $US)	Average annual increase in total health care spending (1980–1987)	Average annual increase relative to rise in GDP price deflator (1980–1987)
Expenditure caps				
United Kingdom (NHS)	6.1	721	9.4	1.7
Sweden	9.0	1,275	9.1	1.2
Expenditure caps and strict expenditure targets				
Canada	8.6	1,517	11.3	2.1
Different methods for different sectors (each centralized or highly coordinated)				
West Germany	8.2	1,071	4.8	1.8
France	8.6	1,087	11.8	1.6
Netherlands	8.5	1,037	4.2	2.0
Belgium	7.2	876	7.6	1.7
Heterogeneous and decentralized				
Switzerland	7.7	1,248	7.1	2.2
Uncontrolled				
United States	11.2	2,061	10.6	2.4

Note: Gross domestic product (GDP) = GNP + (income in domestic market accruing to foreigners abroad) – (income accruing to domestic residents arising from investment abroad). Purchasing power parities against the United States dollar (1.00 in 1987) were British pound = 0.60, Canadian dollar = 1.23, Swedish krona = 8.65, German mark = 2.47, French franc = 7.45, Dutch guilder = 2.41, Belgian franc = 44.7, Swiss franc = 2.42.

Sources: My calculations from Jean-Pierre Poullier, "Health Care Expenditure and Other Data," *Health Care Financing Review*, annual supplement, 1989, tables 1, 3, 5; and *OECD Main Economic Indicators*, table 32.

☐ *Mixed.* Different sectors have different cost containment methods—in France, for example, rate regulation and global budgeting in hospitals, rate negotiation with some expenditure targets for physicians' services, other methods in other sectors. Swiss hospitals are subject to a mixture of grants and rate regulation by provincial governments. Certain sectors, such as physicians' services in Holland and Germany, have a substantial share under private health insurance that relies on consumer choice guided by patients' cost sharing; most remaining physicians' services are governed by the negotiations between social insurance carriers and medical associations. Countries do not have perfectly comparable configurations.

☐ *The essentially uncontrolled American market.* A few payers (such as Medicare Part A and most Medicaid programs) use more or less strict expenditure targets. Some HMOs approach true expenditure caps. Blue Cross and hospitals in half the states negotiate rates. Miscellaneous hospital admission rules and forms of patient cost sharing abound.

The data in Table 17.1 come from the 1980s, when countries with statutory health insurance reformed and tightened their methods of cost containment, American payers sought new methods, and the countries with expenditure caps continued their methods. The goal of current cost containment policy in every country is to maintain a steady relationship between growth in the health sector and growth in the economy's ability to support it. The proportion of gross domestic product (GDP) devoted to health services should be nearly constant. Nominal spending should rise nearly at the same rate as inflation.

Before the recent preoccupation with cost containment, costs at times rose rapidly in accordance with public policy. As noted earlier in this chapter, nearly every developed country during the 1960s and early 1970s increased wages, shortened hours, and expanded staffing. All modernized their hospital buildings, hospital technology, and physicians' offices. Governments and health insurance carriers now prevent new cost explosions. But some increases over the general inflation rate seem inevitable: populations age, need more care, and become more expensive; new medical techniques multiply and become more expensive. Cost containment policies are not yet clear enough—and cost containment methods are not yet subtle enough—to relate health spending to the general economy stably over long periods.

The time series summarized in the third column of Table 17.1 shows fluctuations in each country during the decade: nominal increases are larger in some years than in others. Fluctuations in general inflation could account for some increases, but they average out in the time series summarized by the numbers in the fourth column. The fourth column shows the average annual increase in health spending as a multiple of inflation: the larger the number, the greater the increases due to utilization, service intensity, and extra price increases within the health sector.

A combination of expenditure caps and government management of services can restrain costs strictly and stabilize spending from year to year. Examples might be Sweden and Great Britain. But it all depends on how expenditure caps—and all other reimbursement methods—are administered. The Treasury in a democratic country can be generous as well as austere. During the 1960s and 1970s, for example, the Swedish national and county governments poured money into the popular health services (particularly the hospitals); but recent financial crises have forced the country to restrain spending. Great Britain has had to budget strictly; but at times—in response to public protests—it has substantially increased appropriations for the National Health Service, contrary to foreigners' stereotypes about chronic British underfunding.

Canada illustrates the effects of private management of services on governmentally imposed expenditure caps. The national and provincial governments have been able to impose and enforce global budgets on the hospitals but never on the medical profession. Instead, physicians' reimbursement is negotiated with provincial governments under expenditure targets that all provinces set and some enforce strictly. At times, the caps and targets are tight. But the hospitals and doctors complain they are falling behind the spendthrift Americans, the mass media protest, and the provincial legislature appropriates more money. The result is a recurrent cycle of squeeze and catch-up.[71]

During the 1970s, European statutory health insurance had severe problems in balancing its accounts: costs had risen steadily, but the slowdown in national economies made them more difficult to bear.[72] Each country developed its own distinctive mixture of restraints. By the 1980s—the annual growth had slowed. Even when a potpourri of regulation, negotiation, operating targets, and supply constraints is used, and even when the providers are privately owned, Table 17.1 shows that determined governments and payers can bring about the same constraints as centralized and fixed expenditure caps.

While the numbers in the fourth column of Table 17.1 are low, they do not consistently reach 1.0. It seems impossible to limit health spending increases only to the growth of GDP and inflation. For reasons mentioned at the start of this chapter, health spending grows somewhat faster. If a country has a low rate of general inflation, health care spending increases—although modest—are significantly larger than inflation and slowly absorb more of GDP. Examples are Germany, Holland, and Switzerland.

A decentralized and less coordinated reimbursement system—as in Switzerland—can result in higher increases. The Swiss national government has responded by limiting its subsidies to the sickness funds and allowing higher cost sharing by patients. But otherwise Switzerland lacks national machinery for setting and implementing expenditure targets. The health insurance carriers are competitors—free to set their own rates, to offer extra benefits, and to offer services. Each provincial government is free to set its own subsidies and guidelines. Hospitals and doctors improve their services to attract both the Swiss (including some from other cantons) and a lucrative foreign clientele.

The United States differs. According to Table 17.1, it spends more of its

GDP on health than any other country does (in column one) and its annual increases relative to inflation are higher (in column four). But this was not always so. Once the United States spent no more than other developed countries.[73] Both European and American spending grew during the 1970s, the American at a faster rate, and gradually the United States became the leading spender.[74] The difference widened during the 1980s—as Table 17.1 shows—since the other countries instituted effective cost controls of various types while the United States did not.

Hospitals. Cost containment methods are specific to each sector. The best way to evaluate each method is to compare it with others across the same sector. Since hospital costs constitute such a large fraction of all health care spending and were the principal source of the general cost explosion of the 1970s, they were the first costs subjected to firm and nationwide containment machinery.

In *Paying the Hospital,* I described the effects of the various cost containment methods during the 1970s as they were first being perfected and implemented.[75] Every method had to pass on to payers higher costs due to the inflation of wages and prices; every method had to concede increases due to the population's utilization and medicine's technical progress. The precise outcomes from year to year depended on how each system was administered. Global budgeting provided the payer motivation and administrative instruments for strict control, but the funds for hospitals were sometimes increased intentionally. Rate regulation and rate negotiations kept annual spending increases close to the rate of inflation in some years but conceded larger increases in others. The decentralized forms of cost containment in the United States and Switzerland produced uneven results. By the early 1980s, the countries with global budgeting, rate regulation, and rate negotiation had lowered the annual increases.

Table 17.2 shows the results during the 1980s when governments and health insurance carriers were determined to limit their spending on hospitals. While the regulators, negotiators, and grantors tried to be strict, they had to pass through costs of national labor contracts and supplies that the individual hospital could not control. The regulators, negotiators, and grantors occasionally had to mollify the complaints of the hospital industry. Therefore, the average figures in the fourth column were revised by extra one-time increases given to many hospitals: in Belgium in 1987, in Holland and in Canada in 1986, in Germany in 1985.

If a strict new reimbursement method is introduced, the entire hospital industry can respond in collective shock and save more money than anyone expected. In Holland, for example, strict guidelines about hospital spending were phased in during the early 1980s and hospital managers were warned that caps would apply by the mid-1980s. The managers made adjustments at once in anticipation: during 1984 admissions were suddenly reduced, stays were shortened, economies were made, and real total insurance spending on acute-care hospitals dropped 5.5 percent. The declines continued thereafter.[76] Since hospital spending

Table 17.2. Effects of Predominant Method of Hospital Rate Control on Hospital Operating Costs.

System	Proportion of GDP spent on all hospitals in 1987 (%)	Expenditure on all hospitals per capita in 1987 (converted to $US)	Average annual increase in total hospital spending (1980–1987) (%)	Average annual increase relative to rise in GDP price deflator (1980–1987)
Global budgeting				
United Kingdom (NHS)	3.0	353	7.2	1.3
Canada	4.4	754	10.4	1.9
Sweden	6.3	874	9.3	1.3
Rate regulation				
France	3.9	500	10.9	1.4
Netherlands	4.8	592	3.6	1.6
Negotiations				
West Germany	4.8	422	5.2	1.9
Mixed				
Switzerland	3.6	736	7.5	2.2
Belgium	2.4	296	8.1	1.7
United States	5.3	969	9.9	2.2

Note: Swiss data are calculated for 1980–1986, when different accounting methods were introduced. Therefore, Swiss data in the first two columns were derived in 1986.
Sources: See Table 17.1.

constituted such a large proportion of all statutory health insurance spending, the payroll taxes could be reduced.

The same sudden shock from a new restrictive payment method resulted in America when Medicare adopted DRGs. They were phased in slowly from a generous cost base in 1984. America's hospital managers made immediate economies in anticipation of much tighter rules in the late 1980s. Outpatient care was substituted for less remunerative inpatient care, length of stay was reduced, the number of beds diminished, fewer workers were employed, and fewer supplies were bought.[77] The savings were not passed on in lower payroll taxes, however, but were divided between the Hospital Insurance Trust Fund and the hospitals themselves.

A cost containment system makes permanent the short-run reductions, as in Holland. Larger-than-normal increases are given occasionally, but they are controlled and intended. Uninhibited by an all-payer structure, American hospitals resumed and even surpassed their previous high annual increases during the late 1980s, regularly approaching three times the annual inflation rates.[78]

Physicians. During the 1980s, governments and payers expanded cost containment to the services of doctors so that annual spending would stay within targets. The doctors proved more resistant than the hospitals: there were too many to investigate and rate individually; government avoided applying to them the intrusive regulation that it used upon the hospitals; payers could not obtain from the doctors the detailed reports of costs and profits that were routine in hospital reimbursement.

Table 17.3 shows the outcomes. The negotiators granted only small annual increases in unit fees—that is, the "conversion factors" applied to relative value scales. It proved difficult for mere negotiation schemes to control total costs, since total expenditures are also governed by higher utilization and service intensity. If an expenditure cap applies to the entire sector, it does not automatically lower total spending, as Germany's experience demonstrates. The German negotiators decide that higher utilization and service intensity are legitimate, are popular with the public, and can be afforded by the health insurance system. German sickness funds have long squeezed the hospitals in order to leave plenty of money for ambulatory care. An organized and comprehensive reimbursement system can set priorities among sectors.

Any of the organized negotiation arrangements can contain physicians' costs better than a market with many small-scale and permissive arrangements. In column four of Table 17.3, annual increases are higher in the United States than in other countries. Despite increased American rhetoric during the late 1980s about the need to contain costs, the annual increases accelerated to nearly five times the rate of inflation.

Utilization and Health. So far, cost containment under statutory health insurance has improved efficiency and reduced waste. It has not reduced or de-

Table 17.3. Effects of Predominant Method of Determining Physician Rates on Costs of Physician and Related Services.

System	Proportion of GDP spent on all ambulatory care in 1987 (%)	Expenditure on ambulatory care per capita in 1987 (converted to $US)	Average annual increase in total ambulatory care spending (1980–1987) (%)	Average annual increase relative to rise in GDP price deflator (1980–1987)
National negotiations with expenditure caps				
West Germany	2.3	305	4.9	2.0
National negotiations				
France	2.3	300	13.1	1.9
Netherlands	2.2	268	3.5	1.7
Belgium	3.0	359	8.6	1.9
Province-by-province negotiations				
Switzerland	3.4	708	6.9	2.0
Uncontrolled				
United States	3.5	646	12.7	3.0

Note: Sources of data, their definitions, and their limitation are summarized in Jean-Pierre Poullier, *Measuring Health Care 1960–1983* (Paris: Organisation for Economic Co-Operation and Development, 1985), pp. 19–25. The data include physicians' reimbursement by fee-for-service and capitation fees in offices, hospital outpatient departments, and inpatient wards. They do not include the salaried reimbursement that is part of inpatient hospital accounts. The data probably omit patients' out-of-pocket payments and private insurance payments. Some countries may include NHI fee-for-service payments to dentists and home nurses. Other definitions and sources are those used in Table 17.2. Swiss data in columns 1 and 2 refer to 1986; Swiss time series in columns 3 and 4 refer to 1980 through 1986.

layed access because it cannot do so: the wording of the law and the political monitoring in democracies guarantee that all bad health risks must be accepted by carriers, that every insured person can use health care, that doctors decide the appropriate services, and that carriers pay in full according to the reimbursement rules. If patients have any unmet needs or are underserviced, the causes are not cost constraints but other reasons:

☐ The services and benefits are not covered by statutory health insurance. Persons who need them must find private cash or private insurance. Examples are long-term-care services.

☐ The benefit is new and not enough providers have become adequately trained and supplied. An example is dentistry. (A common problem in statutory health insurance is overprovision rather than underprovision—that is, too many hospital beds, doctors, and drugs—and cost containment is directed at overservicing.)

☐ Although the benefit is covered by statutory health insurance, there are no definitive proofs and professional consensus about the most effective services. An example is mental health.

If cost containment reduces patients' access and providers' services, this happens not in countries with statutory health insurance but in countries with national health services and with expenditure caps made strict by deficits in government budgets. But even there, many accusations about underservicing are spawned by political controversy and are exaggerated.[79]

Implications for the United States

During the 1990s, every developed country—even one as decentralized as Switzerland—implemented various methods and limited its annual increase in health care costs. In the United States, costs continued to rise more rapidly. After a decade claiming that they had developed original methods of "managed care" that would soon restrain costs, improve efficiency, and raise quality, Americans had to admit that savings were modest, that the principal achievement was in preventing even worse overruns, and that techniques still needed improvement.[80]

The central problem is that the United States has many small-scale "managed-care" ventures, but the system as a whole is unmanaged. The national government is preoccupied with Medicare and Medicaid alone; no one inside or outside government formulates policy for the entire health care sector. A number of the favorite nostrums of American health policy analysts and health executives actually raise costs rather than containing them.

Competition. One set of proposals makes a virtue of necessity. Since the United States lacks a coherently unified system of financing and service provision, its payers and providers are autonomous and compete against each other for advantage. American health financing policy has for decades been dominated by free-market enthusiasts who believe that excessive costs are due to provider collusion, excessive third-party money, and misconceived government interference. They contend that costs would be reduced if all health care markets became more competitive.[81]

The many competitive situations in American health care at present do lower costs of the total system in some ways:

☐ Business firms compete with each other in their fields. Each tries to reduce its labor costs, including employee benefits. Periodically a firm calls for competitive bids by insurance companies for its health contract, and the result is lower premiums. Some save insurance company loadings by self-insuring.

☐ Several limits on providers—such as preadmission screening before hospitalization, concurrent review of hospitalization, concurrent review of length of stay, restraint on fees, and prior authorization of expensive procedures—are adopted by some insurers so that their total costs lie within the limits of their contracts with employers. The less expensive the groups' experience and the more effective these controls, the lower the premiums asked of employer groups and the larger the insurance carrier's market share.

☐ Some HMOs deliver satisfactory care with minimum cost sharing by patients, so they gain a substantial share of the local market. To remain attractive to employers and individual beneficiaries, other carriers and other HMOs must lower their costs, premiums, and cost sharing too.

☐ Bad medical risks may be unable to buy an individual policy; or they may be accepted and prior conditions excluded. These people receive less care than if they were fully insured.

But competition also increases the costs of the entire health sector in several ways:

☐ Each insurance carrier must maintain a marketing staff. Extra marketing and actuarial costs are incurred during the renegotiation of group contracts.[82]

☐ Each employer must maintain an employee benefit staff.

☐ In the market for individual policies, many persons are persuaded to buy more insurance than they need.

☐ Hospitals compete for market share by wooing the physicians who bring patients. Lest doctors affiliate elsewhere, each hospital tries to install the equipment and staff desired by the doctors. Considerable duplication in expensive programs results among hospitals. To amortize the debt incurred to pay for the new equipment and construction, the hospital presses all the doctors to utilize the new service and bill the carriers. To attract and retain affiliated doctors, hospitals compete in offers of professional office space, bonuses, administrative fees, and income guarantees.[83]

☐ The large number of managed-care enterprises adds to administrative and marketing costs.

☐ Disputes are handled not by standing negotiating machinery nor by government mediation but by lawsuits in civil courts of general jurisdiction, sometimes before juries of laymen. Patients can sue managed-care agencies and payers for liability if they think they were underserved and damaged by cost containment.[84] The lawyers' fees and court costs add to the total costs of the system. Doctors and hospitals perform many tests and generate many documents to protect themselves in case of future lawsuits.

Competition produces some benefits, such as the creation and rapid proliferation of clinical and administrative innovation. But it also yields disadvantages for the delivery of services:[85]

☐ Since consumers are at risk, some are priced out of the market. Patients with poor health and little cash are unable to buy health insurance. Public welfare programs (such as Medicaid and municipal hospitals) cannot cover all of them and cannot deliver mainstream services.

☐ Since providers are at risk, some attract few purchasers and go bankrupt. Some American hospitals close because they have too few paying patients and too many bad debts. To protect themselves from expensive nonpayers, many close their emergency rooms. Doctors gravitate to the affluent neighborhoods of cities. Rural communities and urban ghettoes lack sufficient services.

☐ If a hospital or the management company that owns it incurred too much debt during periods of expansion and modernization, it cuts staff, services, and quality in order to retain cash for debt service.

☐ Hospitals strongly resist trade union organization of their employees.

☐ The system has hardly any guardians of quality, since all discussions revolve around money. The principal purchasers of coverage—employee benefit managers—try to minimize their expenditures, usually regardless of clinical consequences. In theory, patients deal with poor quality by changing providers. But in practice they cannot understand quality, they cannot comparison shop, and it is their doctors (not they) who select the hospitals.

Organizing a System. If the United States—or any other country—is to contain its health care costs, it must install the following elements:

☐ *Effective evaluation.* There must be methods of evaluating the clinical practices, technology, and pharmaceuticals that are effective and accomplish their purpose economically. Statutory health insurance is supposed to promote and not restrict clinical care; therefore, cost containment should foster efficiency and not denials. As noted in Chapters Ten and Sixteen, Americans are conducting much valuable research. But they abandoned their health planning machinery during the 1980s and will have to recreate it in order to translate research findings into decisions.

☐ *An all-payer system.* Restricting payments by one insurance carrier or third-party program will cause providers to refuse services to subscribers or to shift costs and income aspirations to other payers. For example, strict Medicaid payments cause doctors to refuse Medicaid patients and cause hospitals to shift costs elsewhere; strict Medicare payments cause doctors to extra-bill patients and cause hospitals to shift costs to other carriers; and the costs of the entire system are not constrained. Cost shifting leads to concealment and dispute—costs no less serious than money. Because of standardization of procedure and centralization in administration, an all-payer system has lower administrative costs.

☐ *Expenditure targets.* A research staff drawn from government and from the health insurers must develop guidelines about the probable fiscal capacity of the system. Negotiating machinery must be created whereby government Ministries, the principal carriers, the provider associations, and other interest groups debate their initial claims and converge. The targets should be simple and comprehensible. Such negotiating machinery is now spreading in Europe. As the recent adoption of expenditure targets in the once polarized sector of French medical services shows, limits can be created and implemented for an all-payer system determining the medical profession's entire income, but only by open negotiations. America's initial adoption of the principle of expenditure targets—adopted shortly after the French agreement—is much less promising: after a year of confusing controversy, Congress in late 1989 enacted formulas to limit the growth of Medicare Part B costs—formulas full of compromises, differentials applying to different classes of doctors, regional differentials, and opportunities for exemption. Despite its overload from so many other tasks, each year Congress will try to enact amendments to the formulas and the annual financial update.[86]

☐ *A variety of instruments to implement the targets.* As this chapter has shown, countries with statutory health insurance and private providers cannot simply apply one across-the-board technique such as centralized public financing. The right mix of methods can constrain costs while protecting services. Government regulation cannot be avoided. If American interest groups and health policy analysts continue to oppose government regulation, costs cannot be controlled at the rates of other developed countries. Regulation should be implemented with political will and without the legislative log-rolling that has weakened American hospital rate regulation.[87] One instrument that should be restricted to appropriate situations is that American cure-all, the "financial incentive." Normally, monetary rewards are earned for performing work and thereby increasing costs, not for avoiding work and reducing costs.

☐ *Improvements in the organization and management of providers:*

- *A coordinated system of provider delivery.* Expensive, technically advanced facilities should not be allowed to proliferate too widely with full financing by all payers. Concentration with high utilization at each site will save money and raise quality.
- *Simpler organization within hospitals.* The present style of many small departments built around individual technologies and numerous layers of management results in overstaffing, inefficient communication, and excessive costs.[88]

Notes

1. Jean-Pierre Poullier, "Les dépenses de santé: une croissance inéluctable?", *Revue française de finances publiques,* no. 18 (1987), pp. 55–78; and Odin W. Anderson and Duncan Neuhauser, "Rising Costs Are Inherent in Modern Health Care Systems," *Hospitals,* vol. 43 (Feb. 16, 1969), pp. 50–52.

2. Explained in Mark S. Freeland and Carol Ellen Schendler, "National Health Expenditures: Short-Term Outlook and Long-Term Projections," *Health Care Financing Review,* vol. 2, no. 3 (Winter 1981), pp. 100–104. The reasoning is applied to time series from several developed countries in Poullier, "Les dépenses de santé" (see note 1, above), pp. 60–68.

3. William A. Glaser, *Paying the Hospital* (San Francisco: Jossey-Bass, 1987), chap. 10 and sources cited.

4. Ibid., p. 403.

5. George J. Schieber and Jean-Pierre Poullier, "International Health Care Expenditure Trends: 1987," *Health Affairs,* vol. 8, no. 3 (Fall 1989), pp. 169–177. As a multiple of general inflation, American health care costs have increased: C. Wayne Higgins, "Competitive Reform and Nonprice Competition: Implications for the Hospital Industry," *Health Care Management Review,* vol. 14, no. 4 (1989), pp. 57–58.

6. Working Party on Social Policy, *The Implications of Aging Populations for Social Policy and Expenditure* (Paris: Organisation for Economic Co-Operation and Development, 1984), especially the special paper "The Implication of Aging Populations for Health Care Policy and Expenditure." Every country has produced statistical breakdowns showing that small fractions of the population (between 5 and 10 percent) incur large fractions (50 percent or more) of all the health insurance costs. American time series suggest that the concentration of all spending among the aged is intensifying: Marc L. Berk and others, "How the U.S. Spent Its Health Care Dollars: 1929–1980," *Health Affairs,* vol. 7, no. 3 (Fall 1988), pp. 50–54. In all countries, a steadily larger share of all welfare state expenditure goes to the elderly in pensions and other benefits: John Myles, *Old Age in the Welfare State* (Boston: Little, Brown, 1984).

7. Christa Altenstetter (ed.), *Innovation in Health Policy and Service Delivery* (Königstein/Ts.: Verlag Anton Hain, 1981), pp. 60–64, 90–99; Louise B. Russell, *Technology in Hospitals: Medical Advances and Their Diffusion* (Wash-

ington: Brookings Institution, 1979), chaps. 3–5; and Jonathan Showstack and others, "Changes in the Use of Medical Technologies, 1972–1977," *New England Journal of Medicine,* vol. 306, no. 12 (March 25, 1982), pp. 706–712.

8. The typical hospital's cost shifting among the entire range of payers is complex because each carrier has different practices. See Bruce R. Neuman and others, *Financial Management* (Owings Mills, Md.: National Health Publishing, 1984), pp. 329–332. European and American practices are compared in William Glaser, "Juggling Multiple Payers: American Problems and Foreign Solutions," *Inquiry,* vol. 21, no. 2 (Summer 1984), pp. 178–188.

9. The accounting and billing techniques necessitated by Medicare are described in Donald F. Beck, *Principles of Reimbursement in Health Care* (Rockville, Md.: Aspen Systems, 1984).

10. Since the precise numbers are uncertain in the United States, exact cross-national comparisons are impossible. But insured Americans may pay over 25 percent of the acute-care claims that are covered in Europe with much less cost sharing. Some comparative estimates appear in Robert J. Maxwell, *Health and Wealth* (Lexington, Mass.: Lexington Books, 1981), pp. 61, 65. Total American figures—both insured and uninsured persons and for both insured and uninsured benefits—are in Suzanne W. Letsch and others, "National Health Expenditures, 1987," *Health Care Financing Review,* vol. 10, no. 2 (Winter 1988), p. 116.

11. Regina E. Herzlinger and Jeffrey Schwartz, "How Companies Tackle Health Care Costs," *Harvard Business Review,* vol. 63, nos. 4–5, and vol. 64, no. 1 (July–Aug. 1985, Sept.–Oct. 1985, and Jan.–Feb. 1986); Judith Feder and others, "Falling Through the Cracks: Poverty, Insurance Coverage, and Hospital Care for the Poor, 1980 and 1982," *Milbank Memorial Fund Quarterly,* vol. 62 (Fall 1984), pp. 544–566; *Health Benefits: Loss Due to Unemployment—Staff Report Prepared for the Subcommittee on Health and Environment of the Committee on Energy and Commerce, U.S. House of Representatives* (Washington: Government Printing Office, 1983); and Joyce Jensen and Ned Miklovic, "High Medical Costs Forcing Patients to Postpone Seeking Medical Care," *Modern Healthcare,* vol. 15, no. 14 (July 5, 1985), pp. 209–210.

12. For overviews of recent events see Jean-Pierre Dumont, *L'impact de la crise économique sur les systèmes de protection sociale* (Geneva: International Labour Office, 1986), chap. 5; and Brian Abel-Smith, *Cost Containment in Health Care: A Study of Twelve European Countries 1977–83* (London: Bedford Square Press, 1984). For a compendium of the quite different—and less successful—American methods, see Karen Davis and others, *Health Care Cost Containment* (Baltimore: Johns Hopkins University Press, 1990).

13. The trends in group policies are described in Pamela Farley Short, "Trends in Employee Health Benefits," *Health Affairs,* vol. 7, no. 3 (Summer 1988), pp. 186–196; and Stacy Adler, "Health Plan Deductibles Climb: Survey," *Business Insurance,* July 11, 1988, pp. 1, 32.

14. Thus, the Belgian *mutualités* have had an incentive to squeeze the hospitals they did not own. They might then reserve more of their revenue to

develop their own hospitals. See J. Petit, *Rapport sur la situation de la réforme de l'assurance maladie* (Brussels: Ministère de la Prévoyance Sociale, 1980), pp. 11–12.

15. Described briefly in Chapter Eleven and at greater length in Glaser, *Paying the Hospital* (see note 3, above), chap. 9.

16. Described briefly in Chapter Eleven and at greater length in Glaser, *Paying the Hospital* (see note 3, above), chap. 7.

17. Bonnie Lefkowitz, *Health Planning: Lessons for the Future* (Rockville, Md.: Aspen Systems, 1983); and Glaser, *Paying the Hospital* (see note 3, above), pp. 211–213, 241–245.

18. Carl J. Schramm and others, "Controlling Hospital Cost Inflation: New Perspectives on State Rate Setting," *Health Affairs*, vol. 5, no. 3 (Fall 1986), pp. 22–33 and sources cited.

19. William A. Glaser, "Hospital Rate Regulation: American and Foreign Comparisons," *Journal of Health Politics, Policy and Law*, vol. 8, no. 4 (Winter 1984), pp. 702–721; and Glaser, *Paying the Hospital* (see note 3, above), pp. 146–157, 349.

20. See, for example, Theo de Vries, *Het klinisch-chemisch laboratorium in economisch perspectief* (Leiden: H. E. Stenfert Kroese, 1974); *Having a Baby in Europe* (Copenhagen: World Health Organization Regional Office for Europe, 1985), pp. 77–78, 85, 89–90, 102–103; and Theo Siebeck, *Zur Kostenentwicklung in der Krankenversicherung* (Bonn: Verlag der Ortskrankenkassen, 1976), pp. 87–89.

21. Jean-Pierre Poullier, *Measuring Health Care 1960–1983* (Paris: Organisation for Economic Co-Operation and Development, 1985), pp. 82, 85, 104–107. For the joint effects from both steadily greater utilization per capita and steadily greater service intensity per encounter, see George Schieber, *Financing and Delivering Health Care* (Paris: Organisation for Economic Co-Operation and Development, 1987), pp. 58–59.

22. Poullier, *Measuring Health Care* (see note 21, above), pp. 31, 33, 90.

23. The intricate calculations are summarized in Paul L. Grimaldi and Julie A. Micheletti, *Prospective Payment: The Definitive Guide to Reimbursement* (Chicago: Pluribus Press, 1985). The cost containment intentions are described in Stuart Guterman and Allen Dobson, "Impact of the Medicare Prospective Payment System for Hospitals," *Health Care Financing Review*, vol. 7, no. 3 (Spring 1986), pp. 97–114. The effects on hospital operations and costs are summarized in Stuart Guterman and others, "The First Three Years of Medicare Prospective Payment: An Overview," *Health Care Financing Review*, vol. 9, no. 3 (Spring 1988), pp. 67–77; and Louise Russell, *Medicare's New Hospital Payment System* (Washington: Brookings Institution, 1989).

24. How hospital managers actually responded to the introduction of DRGs is described in Sanford L. Weiner and others, "Economic Incentives and Organizational Realities: Managing Hospitals under DRG's," *Milbank Quarterly*, vol. 65, no. 4 (1987), pp. 463–487.

25. Some expected short-term effects did not occur—for example, hospitals did not suddenly and universally become more efficient. See Jerry Cromwell and Gregory C. Pope, "Trends in Hospital Labor and Total Factor Productivity, 1981–1986," *Health Care Financing Review*, vol. 10, no. 4 (Summer 1989), pp. 39–50. Perhaps the intended results might appear in the long run, but Americans are uninterested in research about permanent effects and unwilling to leave a reimbursement system in place without tinkering.

26. *Medicare Prospective Payment and the American Health Care System: Report to the Congress, June 1989* (Washington: Prospective Payment Assessment Commission, 1989), p. 50. The decrease in Medicare inpatient admissions for certain types of surgery and the steady increase in Medicare outpatient treatment are described in Shelah Leader and Marilyn Moon, "Medicare Trends in Ambulatory Surgery," *Health Affairs*, vol. 8, no. 1 (Spring 1989), pp. 158–170. For all payers during the 1980s, the shift is documented in Carolyn S. Donham and Anne E. T. Vanek, "Community Hospital Statistics," *Health Care Financing Review*, vol. 10, no. 3 (Spring 1989), pp. 125–126. The site is changed for the simpler surgical cases; inpatient admissions remain the same for the more complex procedures. The new capacity for ambulatory surgery results in a much higher total surgical volume.

27. Expenditure by the Medicare Part B trust fund had long increased rapidly each year (between 8 and 10 percent with some exceptions). During the years just after the introduction of inpatient DRGs, inpatient-days suddenly dropped, outpatient visits suddenly increased, and the annual increase in Part B trust fund spending suddenly increased (between 11.9 and 12.5 percent in 1985, 1986, and 1987). Thereafter, annual outpatient spending increases from the new service delivery style and from the new higher expenditure base resumed at the "normal" 8 to 10 percent rate. See Louise B. Russell and Carrie Lynn Manning, "The Effect of Prospective Payment on Medicare Expenditures," *New England Journal of Medicine*, vol. 320, no. 7 (Feb. 16, 1989), pp. 441–442.

28. J. Heesters and J. Kesenne, "Le financement des soins de santé en Belgique et aux Pays-Bas," *Dossier*, vol. 3, no. 11 (1985), pp. 38–39, 49.

29. Ibid.

30. Robert Soete, "Survey on Medical Profiles," reports presented at the triennial General Assembly (Geneva: Association Internationale de la Mutualité, 1981, 1984, and 1987).

31. A Dutch control doctor's work schedule is described in Arnold M.F.B. Crousen, *Analyse van het werk een controlerend geneeskundige voor de ziektewet* (Assen: Van Gorcum, 1968). For a textbook on the control doctor's duties in Holland see Jan A. van der Hoeven, *De controlerend geneesheer* (Leiden: Uitgeverij L. Stafleu, 1960).

32. John A. Nyman and others, "Changing Physician Behavior: Does Medical Review of Part B Medicare Claims Make a Difference?", *Inquiry*, vol. 27, no. 2 (Summer 1990), pp. 127–137.

33. Laura D. Gates and Nancy T. Lukitsh, "Salvaging Managed Care,"

Best's Review: Life/Health Insurance Edition, vol. 90, no. 6 (Oct. 1989), pp. 38–41, 127–128.

34. Glaser, *Paying the Hospital* (see note 3, above), chap. 13, passim, especially pp. 350–353.

35. Unpublished information from the Blue Cross and Blue Shield Association.

36. *Environmental Analysis 1989* (Chicago: Blue Cross and Blue Shield Association, 1989), pp. 3–17; Alison Kittrell, "Unfulfilled Expectation: Benefit Managers Report Little Savings from HMO's or PPO's," *Business Insurance,* Dec. 1987, pp. 6, 8; survey by A. Foster Higgins & Co., summarized in "Survey: Businesses Believe HMO's Don't Save Money," *American Medical News,* Dec. 1, 1989, pp. 13–14; and Stanley B. Jones, "Multiple Choice Health Insurance: The Lessons and Challenge to Private Insurance," *Inquiry,* vol. 27, no. 2 (Summer 1990), pp. 161–166.

37. Bradford H. Gray and Marilyn J. Field (eds.), *Controlling Costs and Changing Patient Care? The Role of Utilization Management* (Washington: Institute of Medicine Committee on Utilization Management by Third Parties, National Academy Press, 1989), pp. 107, 154.

38. Paul Tarini, "Managed Care's 'Hidden Costs' May Erode Containment Efforts," *American Medical News,* Aug. 18, 1989, pp. 13, 17.

39. For a description of how competition for subscribers and preferred providers adds to HMO costs, see Catherine G. McLaughlin, "Market Responses to HMO's: Price Competition or Rivalry?", *Inquiry,* vol. 25, no. 2 (Summer 1988), pp. 213–214.

40. Patrick Mullen, "Managed-Care Executives Fare Well on Pay Incentives," *Managed HealthCare,* Sept. 11, 1989, pp. 1, 5.

41. Paul J. Feldstein and others, "Private Cost Containment: The Effects of Utilization Review Programs on Health Care Use and Expenditures," *New England Journal of Medicine,* vol. 318, no. 20 (May 19, 1988), pp. 1310–1314.

42. The American literature is summarized and evaluated skeptically by three leading Canadian economists in Morris L. Barer, Robert G. Evans, and Glen L. Stoddart, *Controlling Health Care Costs by Direct Charges to Patients: Snare or Delusion?* (Toronto: Ontario Economic Council, 1979).

43. Ibid., pp. 16–27.

44. Simone Sandier, "L'influence des facteurs économiques sur la consommation médicale," *Consommation,* vol. 13, no. 2 (April–June 1966), pp. 85–87; R. Glen Beck and John M. Horne, *An Analytical Overview of the Saskatchewan Copayment Experiment in the Hospital and Ambulatory Settings* (Toronto: Ontario Council of Health, 1978); and *Bilanz der Kostendämpfungspolitik im Gesundheitswesen 1977–1984* (Bonn: Wissenschaftliches Institut der Ortskrankenkassen, 1986), pp. 36–38.

45. Because of exemptions, only one-third of French hospital patients are actually liable for coinsurance. Coinsurance for over half of this group is fully covered by *mutuelles.* Therefore, only 15.4 percent of French hospital patients

actually paid the out-of-pockets that theoretically apply to everyone. See Lola Jean Kozak and others, *Hospital Use in France and the United States,* Comparative International Vital and Health Statistics Reports, series 5, no. 4 (Washington: National Center for Health Statistics, 1989), pp. 39–41, 65.

46. Denise Deliège and Paul Minne, *Kinésithérapie et physiothérapie en Belgique* (Brussels: Service d'Etudes Socio-Economiques de la Santé, Université de Louvain, 1982); and Andrée Sacrez, "Pour une véritable politique de la Kinésithérapie," *M Informations* (of the Alliance Nationale des Mutualités Chrétiennes), no. 103 (Feb. 28, 1982), p. 1.

47. *Rapport Général: Service des Soins de Santé—Partie Statistique 1984* (Brussels: Institut National d'Assurance Maladie-Invalidité, 1988), pt. 4B, pp. 57, 159–160, 163–164.

48. Beck and Horne, *Overview of the Saskatchewan Copayment Experiment* (see note 44, above); and John M. Horne, "Copayment and Utilization of Publicly Insured Hospital Services in Saskatchewan: An Empirical Analysis" (Ph.D. dissertation, Carleton University, Ottawa, 1978).

49. Theodore E. Chester, "The Effects of Copayments and Charges on the Utilisation of Health Care" (Manchester: Department of Social Administration, University of Manchester, 1973), p. 26.

50. Peter Zweifel, "Premium Rebates for No Claims," in H. E. Frech (ed.), *Health Care in America* (San Francisco: Pacific Institute for Public Policy, 1988), pp. 323–352; and Peter Zweifel, "Bonus Systems in Health Insurance: A Microeconomic Analysis," *Health Policy,* vol. 7 (1987), pp. 281–287.

51. Bundesminister für Arbeit und Sozialordunung, *Bericht der Bundesregierung an den Bundesrat über Erfahrungen mit dem neugefassten §188 der Reichsversicherungsordnung (Zahlung einer Prämie für nicht in Anspruch genommene ärtzliche Behandlung und Krankenhauspflege—Krankenscheinprämie)* (Bonn: Bundesrat, Drucksache 98/72, March 16, 1972), pp. 5–29.

52. See Mark V. Pauly (ed.), *National Health Insurance: What Now, What Later, What Never?* (Washington: American Enterprise Institute for Public Policy Research, 1980), pt. 3; and many other publications.

53. Martin Feldstein, *Hospital Costs and Health Insurance* (Cambridge: Harvard University Press, 1981), chap. 9.

54. Joseph Newhouse and others, "The Rand Health Insurance Study," *Inquiry,* vol. 11, no. 1 (March 1974), entire issue; and Kathleen N. Lohr and others, "Use of Medical Care in the Rand Health Insurance Experiment: Diagnosis- and Service-Specific Analyses in a Randomized Controlled Trial," *Medical Care,* vol. 24, no. 9, supplement (Sept. 1986), entire issue.

55. Louis F. Rossiter and Gail R. Wilensky, "Out-of-Pocket Expenses for Personal Health Services," National Health Care Expenditure Study Data Preview 13 (Washington: National Center for Health Services Research, 1982); and Charles Wilder, "Personal Out-of-Pocket Health Expenses," Vital and Health Statistics, series 10, no. 122 (Washington: National Center for Health Statistics, 1978).

56. Mark S. Lachs and others, "The Forgiveness of Coinsurance: Charity or Cheating?", *New England Journal of Medicine,* vol. 322, no. 22 (May 31, 1990), pp. 1599-1602.

57. M. Susan Marquis, "Consumers' Knowledge About Their Health Insurance Coverage," *Health Care Financing Review,* vol. 5, no. 1 (Fall 1983), pp. 69-72. If a policy is simple, standardized, and well publicized, subscribers' understanding of their liability improves; ibid., pp. 74-78. Under present circumstances, Americans do not even understand the size of their contributory premiums and the benefits their policies cover: Daniel C. Walden and others, *Consumer Knowledge of Health Insurance Coverage* (Washington: National Center for Health Services Research, 1982).

58. Summarized in Barer, Evans, and Stoddart, *Controlling Health Care Costs by Direct Charges to Patients* (see note 42, above), pp. 36-46; and "The Rand Health Insurance Study: A Spanner in the Works?", *Lancet,* May 3, 1986, pp. 1012-1013.

59. See, for example, Pamela C. Roddy and others, "Cost-Sharing and Use of Health Services: The United Mine Workers of America Health Plan," *Medical Care,* vol. 24, no. 9 (Sept. 1986), pp. 873-876.

60. The precise numbers of plans and beneficiaries are unknown, since a PPO is an option in what otherwise is conventional insurance. The Health Insurance Association of America conducts periodic surveys of large employers and estimates that 11 percent of the workers were enrolled in PPOs in 1987 and 16 percent were in HMOs. See John Gabel and others, "The Changing World of Group Health Insurance," *Health Affairs,* vol. 7, no. 3 (Summer 1988), pp. 48-65. The numbers should be higher during the 1990s.

61. See Paula Diehr and others, "Use of a Preferred Provider by Employees of the Preferred Provider," *Health Services Research,* vol. 23, no. 4 (Oct. 1988), pp. 537-554; James A. Hester and others, "Evaluation of a Preferred Provider Organization," *Milbank Quarterly,* vol. 65, no. 4 (1987), pp. 575-613; and many news articles in the business magazines and newsletters in health.

62. Glaser, *Paying the Hospital* (see note 3, above), chap. 8.

63. I have described the system after abandonment of the *Kopfpauschale* in Glaser, *Paying the Doctor* (Baltimore: Johns Hopkins Press, 1970), pp. 29-34, 121-123.

64. Glaser, *Paying the Hospital* (see note 3, above), chap. 8. For a description of how Holland decided to adopt expenditure caps for hospitals and how it implements them, see J.A.M. Maarse, "Hospital Budgeting in Holland: Aspects, Trends and Effects," *Health Policy,* vol. 11 (1989), pp. 257-276.

65. Detlef Schwefel and others (eds.), *Der Bayern-Vertrag—Evaluation einer Kostendämpfungspolitik im Gesundheitswesen* (Berlin: Springer Verlag, 1986).

66. See, for example, Alan L. Hillman and others, "How Do Financial Incentives Affect Physicians' Clinical Decisions and the Financial Performance

of Health Maintenance Organizations?", *New England Journal of Medicine,* vol. 321, no. 1 (July 13, 1989), pp. 86–92.

67. *Financieel Overzicht Zorg 1989* (Rijswijk: Ministerie van Welzijn, Volksgezondheid en Cultuur, Tweede Kamer de Staten-General, vergaderjaar 1988–1989), pp. 39–40. The Dutch did not realize it, but degressive fees for the high earners had been used for some time in Quebec, where they effectively constrained the once rapid increase in the costs of general practitioners' services. See Morris L. Barer and others, "Fee Controls as Cost Controls: Tales from the Frozen North," *Milbank Quarterly,* vol. 66, no. 1 (1988), pp. 24–31.

68. For a description of how the *Konzertierte Aktion* works in practice see *Bericht der Bundesregierung nach Artikel 2§6 des Krankenversicherungs-Kostendämpfungsgesetzes* (Bonn: Bundestag, Drucksache 9/1300, Feb. 2, 1982); see also Helmut Wiessenthal, *Die Konzertierte Aktion im Gesundheitswesen* (Frankfurt: Campus Verlag, 1982); and Harald Bogs and others, *Gesundheitspolitik zwischen Staat und Selbstverwaltung* (Cologne: Deutscher Arzte-Verlag, 1982), chap. 8.

69. I have discussed the pitfalls in comparisons of aggregate national financial statistics in Glaser, *Paying the Hospital* (see note 3, above), pp. 3, 341–343, 413–414. In particular, note the experience of the leading specialist in collecting and presenting cross-national time series: Jean-Pierre Poullier, "OECD Experiences with the Initiation and Coordination of Health Indicator Systems . . . ," in Detlef Schwefel (ed.), *Indicators and Trends in Health and Health Care* (Berlin: Springer-Verlag, 1987), pp. 23–36.

70. See, for example, the hospital data described in Glaser, *Paying the Hospital,* pp. 3, 341–343, 413–414.

71. The cycle has long been true. See A. J. Culyer, *Health Care Expenditures in Canada: Myth and Reality; Past and Future* (Toronto: Canadian Tax Foundation, 1988), pp. 57–59. But costs are more predictable and controllable and conflicts are lower in Canada than in the neighboring unorganized and uncontrolled United States. See Robert G. Evans and others, "Controlling Health Expenditures—The Canadian Reality," *New England Journal of Medicine,* vol. 320, no. 9 (March 2, 1989), pp. 571–577.

72. The statistics for the 1960s and 1970s are reported and explained in Brian Abel-Smith and Alan Maynard, *The Organization, Financing and Cost of Health Care in the European Community* (Brussels: Commission of the European Committees, 1979), pp. 107–124.

73. *The Cost of Medical Care* (Geneva: International Labour Office, 1959), p. 76; Brian Abel-Smith, *An International Study of Health Expenditure* (Geneva: World Health Organization, 1967), p. 41.

74. *Public Expenditure on Health* (Paris: Organisation for Economic Co-Operation and Development, 1977), p. 10.

75. Glaser, *Paying the Hospital* (see note 3, above), pp. 344–350.

76. *Financieel Jaarverslag* (Amstelveen: Ziekenfondsraad, 1984), table

2.6.3; and Maarse, "Hospital Budgeting in Holland" (see note 64, above), pp. 264-270.

77. Stuart Guterman and Allen Dobson, "Impact of the Medicare Prospective Payment System for Hospitals," *Health Care Financing Review*, vol. 7, no. 3 (Spring 1986), pp. 102-113; and Stuart Guterman and others, "The First Three Years of Medicare Prospective Payment, An Overview," *Health Care Financing Review*, vol. 9, no. 3 (Spring 1988), pp. 67-77.

78. They increased employment in numbers, skill mix, and, therefore, in costliness. Carolyn S. Donham and others, "Health Care Indicators," *Health Care Financing Review*, vol. 12, no. 2 (Winter 1990), pp. 139-158. Employment grew in health while it was declining in the rest of the economy, according to Cathy A. Cowan and others, "Health Care Indicators," *Health Care Financing Review*, vol. 12, no. 3 (Spring 1991), pp. 121-127.

79. I have compared fact and fancy over hospital waiting lists and over denials in national health services in Glaser, *Paying the Hospital* (see note 3, above), pp. 364-368.

80. Cathy Tokarski, "1980's Prove Uncertainty of Instant Cures: Cost Containment, Competition Fail to Cap Rising Prices," *Modern Healthcare*, vol. 20, no. 1 (Jan. 8, 1990), pp. 51-52, 58; Carl J. Schramm, "The Sorry State of Cost Containment," *Best's Review: Life/Health Insurance Edition*, vol. 90, no. 6 (Oct. 1989), pp. 43-44, 125-126; and Gray and Field, *Controlling Costs and Changing Patient Care?* (see note 37, above).

81. See, for example, Clark C. Havighurst, "The Role of Competition in Cost Containment," in Warren Greenberg (ed.), *Competition in the Health Care Sector* (Washington: Bureau of Economics, Federal Trade Commission, 1978), pp. 359-406; Paul Ginsburg, *Containing Medical Care Costs Through Market Forces* (Washington: Congressional Budget Office, 1982); and Stuart Butler and Edmund Haislmaier (eds.), *A National Health System for America* (Washington: Heritage Foundation, 1989).

82. The high administrative costs due to this and other sources in the decentralized and unstandardized American financing system are estimated in David U. Himmelstein and Steffie Woolhandler, "Socialized Medicine: A Solution to the Cost Crisis in Health Care in the United States," *International Journal of Health Services*, vol. 16, no. 3 (1986), pp. 340-346; and "The Administrative Burden of Health Insurance on Physicians," *SMS Report* (of the American Medical Association), vol. 5, no. 2 (March 1989), pp. 2-4. Single-payer publicly financed systems—such as Canada's and Great Britain's—have the simplest and cheapest financial administration. Comparisons appear in Steffie Woolhandler and David Himmelstein, "The Deteriorating Administrative Efficiency of the U.S. Health Care System," *New England Journal of Medicine*, vol. 324, no. 18 (May 2, 1991), pp. 1253-1258.

83. Glaser, *Paying the Hospital* (see note 3, above), pp. 236-245, 299-301, 327-329, 374; Harold Luft and others, "The Role of Specialized Clinical Services in Competition Among Hospitals," *Inquiry*, vol. 23 (Spring 1986), pp. 83-94; and

David Burda, "Healthcare's Hidden Costs," *Modern Healthcare,* vol. 20, no. 2 (Jan. 15, 1990), pp. 22-30.

84. William A. Helvestine, "Legal Implications of Utilization Review," in Gray and Field, *Controlling Costs and Changing Patient Care?* (see note 37, above), pp. 169-204. If a carrier denies reimbursement to a subscriber on the grounds that the services were not medically necessary, a civil jury might find for the subscriber and order payment. See *Taylor* v. *Prudential Insurance Company of America,* 775 F. 2nd 1457 (1985).

85. Full details appear in the business magazines and newsletters in health, particularly *Modern Healthcare* and *Managed HealthCare.*

86. "Medicare Program: Physician Performance Standard Rate of Increase for Fiscal Year 1990," *Federal Register,* vol. 54, no. 249 (Dec. 29, 1989), pp. 53818-53821; and *Annual Report to Congress* (Washington: Physician Payment Review Commission, 1990), chaps. 2, 11-14.

87. See Glaser, "Hospital Rate Regulation" (see note 19, above); and Stuart H. Altman and Marc A. Rodwin, "Halfway Competitive Markets and Ineffective Regulation: The American Health Care System," *Journal of Health Politics, Policy and Law,* vol. 13, no. 2 (Summer 1988), pp. 323-339.

88. David Burda, "Untangling Management Structures," *Modern Healthcare,* vol. 20, no. 17 (April 30, 1990), pp. 20-25, 28.

CHAPTER 18

Achievements and Reforms

──────────────────── **Summary** ────────────────────

Statutory health insurance has steadily expanded in coverage and financing. It has enabled entire populations to receive mainstream health care in place of the class-based differentials of the private market. It has developed redistributive methods of financing in place of variations by subscribers' own incomes. "Good" and "bad" health risks are fully covered by the same financing principles. A generous and steady flow of money increases the facilities and incomes of providers. The newest licensed clinical methods and drugs are available. Because of full entitlements to subscribers and the generous facilities, access is prompt under statutory health insurance. There are no denials and waiting lists.

If many carriers are retained under statutory insurance, administration can be complicated. An advantage is their competition to please subscribers. Competition adds benefits rather than reduces premiums. Where several carriers exist, each can seek the better risks but cannot reject the less healthy risks. Some deteriorate financially if they have an aging membership and cannot recruit new young subscribers. A considerable machinery of subsidies, interfund transfers, and mergers protects the system and the subscribers.

Statutory health insurance protects the full entitlements of aging populations and covers increasingly expensive clinical methods. It must also operate within society's fiscal capacity—within the yield of the payroll taxes and public subsidies. Every developed country—except for the unorganized United States— has developed methods for setting expenditure targets and controlling health care costs.

Statutory health insurance can prove unworkable. One reason is the inability of health services to provide the care guaranteed by the law. Another reason is the inability to spread and expand financing by means of autonomous sickness funds and payroll taxes. Government then steps in and creates national health services: now government owns, manages, and expands hospitals; it pays all providers from general revenue; it guarantees full coverage for all citizens.

One hears proposals for reform. One must distinguish the types of system that are being discussed: many proposals are designed to reorganize and energize national health services; they do not apply to national health insurance, which already allows considerable discretion by providers and subscribers, and which preserves the private character of providers and carriers. The only opportunity for major structural changes in statutory health insurance occurs when large numbers of uninsured are added—and this has occurred recently only in the Netherlands. After a prolonged period of stabilized costs, governments shrink from major changes that will make the NHI systems unstable and unpredictable. Some proposals would introduce "market incentives" and "competition" into statutory health insurance. But providers and subscribers avoid reintroducing financial and personal risks after countries have developed systems designed to be protective and stable.

Effects of Statutory Health Insurance

Health insurance has existed for hundreds of years. Statutory health insurance was created a century ago. That particular model of acute-care benefits survives and has spread. Coverage was expanded to more groups in each developed country. Financing has been improved to cover greater utilization and more expensive treatments. In place of the limited panels of providers that once delivered care, all doctors and hospitals now participate.

What difference does it make? What are the accomplishments and weaknesses of statutory health insurance—in contrast to the former situation and in contrast to modern alternatives such as national health services and America's predominantly private system? Each chapter has concluded with generalizations about the effects on utilization and services from specific forms of insurance structure and financing. Detailed evidence appears in the text and in the citations.

Following are highlights about the effects of the alternative systems: what difference does it make if the predominant system is statutory health insurance in contrast to a national health service or a private market?

☐   Statutory health insurance has expanded coverage and access to all vulnerable groups: all occupations, dependents, the elderly, the unemployed, and the disabled. If anyone is omitted from the main scheme, it is the elites—and they buy private coverage for the same or more generous benefits.

☐   Universal and prompt access by the subscriber is guaranteed for all recognized therapies by all licensed providers. The patient and his primary physician decide need—subject only to an occasional second opinion by the carriers' control doctors or by a utilization review managed by the carrier and the medical association. Under statutory health insurance, access is the same for all subscribers from all carriers. It is the doctor, not the system, who decides whether he has the time and resources to see a patient. Waiting lists—caused by constraints in resources and slowdowns in work—occur more often in national health services. In a completely private system, patients lacking coverage may be unable to find providers and may hesitate to search.

☐ Statutory health insurance places all beneficiaries on the same footing. Social class differences in services survive only in limited form for the privately insured. Social class differences remain in the rest of the economy.

☐ Because income is inverse to subscribers' costs, redistributive financing machinery exists. The rich and healthy pay more than their actuarial costs. The health insurance system is integrated in some fashion—either by unification of carriers, by interfund transfers, or by subsidies derived from general taxation. The financing system is more complex than the use of general revenue alone in national health services.

☐ The organization of health insurance can be complex. One reason is that all the established carriers—representing different occupations, ideologies, or regions—survive and grow. Another reason is that some politically influential groups—such as small businessmen, miners, and farmers—obtain special regimes with slightly different benefits and tax rates. But the organization can become streamlined if the carriers voluntarily merge or cooperate. A national health service is less complex and less expensive to administer. America's private health insurance system is more complex and more expensive.

☐ Adverse selection by subscribers and preferred-risk selection by carriers are still possible where enrollment is not automatic. But their effects are limited by the large membership in carriers and by financial transfers. No one may be denied coverage by the system. Adverse selection and preferred-risk selection do not arise in national health services, which automatically cover every inhabitant. They are common in America's private system, resulting in elaborate maneuvers between carriers and subscribers.

☐ Where free choices by subscribers and by carriers exist, carriers compete for members. They compete in offers of extra benefits, in image, and in client services. If some experience adverse selection, aging of members, and high costs, these carriers deteriorate but are saved from bankruptcy by mergers and subsidies. America's private carriers are very competitive and unstable.

☐ In organized financing systems, there are tradeoffs between coverage and costs. Under statutory health insurance, coverage is universal, benefits are generous, and providers are paid well. Payroll taxes are high and policymakers fear that industry is overstrained. Therefore, government must develop elaborate machinery that contains costs without violating the decentralized and private character of service provision. National health services can control costs directly by limiting access and amenities. A disorganized private insurance system may have considerably lower utilization because of incomplete coverage, but it has no control over costs.

☐ Higher utilization and early referral result from universal coverage, generous benefits, and the development of services. As a result, the health of the populations—particularly among the poor and elderly—has improved. Any residual variations in clinical methods and their results are due to practice styles and not to the financing system. National health services can accomplish the same clinical results but private insurance systems cannot.

☐ Statutory health insurance enables providers greatly to improve their resources and incomes. After an initial stage of modernization, national health services limit their resources and income more strictly. Private insurance systems with weak cost controls and much competition unintentionally increase providers' resources and incomes even more than statutory health insurance does.

☐ Statutory health insurance has few instruments to reorganize service delivery and redistribute resources around the country. Doctors and the managers of organizations are private and autonomous. National health services control expenditure, employ the managers and many of the clinicians, and can implement plans. Private health insurance systems cannot produce their own plans, and government in such countries lacks the authority to implement policies of its own, except in its few public programs.

☐ By providing an assured market for new methods, statutory health insurance fosters a steady flow of new techniques. It is more cautious about unorthodox new methods. Because of cost constraints and the power of a single set of decision makers, national health services are slower to approve and invest in expensive new programs.

Such are the achievements of statutory health insurance. Then it survives and grows. But it can also encounter crises beyond its capacity.

When Services Fail

Under what conditions does statutory health insurance succeed? Under what conditions does it fail? It can finance the care of entire populations, as current European experience demonstrates. But it can break down. One reason is the failure of service delivery.

Statutory health insurance was supposed to preserve the private character of health services. Hospitals, doctors, and sickness funds remained autonomous. Government's role was limited. All European countries had mutual aid funds and health care providers at the beginning of the century. Most converted them into statutory insurance programs for health, disability, pensions, and work accidents.[1] The model assumed that service providers were sufficient in number and in competence to expand and cope with the work load as coverage, benefits, and financing grew. But if doctors and hospitals are inadequate in resources, numbers, and locations, a mere increase in payroll taxes for the sickness funds is not enough to assure adequate health care delivery. The obligation to serve the insured patient cannot be met. Government may then step in, make service delivery a public responsibility, and take charge of financial administration as well.

Soviet Union. The Soviet Union was the first country where statutory health insurance collapsed in this fashion. Before World War I, cities had private office doctors, hospitals, and mutual aid societies. The mutual aid funds had small memberships in cities and could not cover the country. Several industries (such as mines and metals) were better insured.[2] The national government employed a corps of physicians and medical assistants to treat the immense rural population.

Statutory health insurance for industrial workers and many city-dwellers was enacted in 1912. But it was too late to build up a system modeled after Germany's. World War I and the Civil War destroyed the hospitals, killed many of the doctors, and ruined the sickness funds. The country was overwhelmed by epidemics. The new Soviet government had to create a new system by direct intervention. It established new hospitals, trained medical assistants, and financed everything from general revenue.[3]

United Kingdom. British experience shows how a breakdown in both service delivery and financing leads to substitution of a national health service. It also suggests that once it is abandoned, NHI cannot be restored.

Between 1911 and 1948, Great Britain had a statutory National Health Insurance that covered only general practice for manual workers. Their dependents were not automatically covered but could join voluntarily by paying premiums. Several private insurance and prepayment arrangements also existed. The middle and upper classes bought private insurance for the services of specialist physicians and hospitals. The voluntary hospitals also sold subscriptions to all classes; members of these "contributory schemes" were assured of admission at reasonable rates. Local government supported community health services and some hospitals. The national government did not try to recognize and improve services.

Europe slowly improved statutory health insurance and services before World War II, but Britain remained frozen. Britain's separate financing channels and its total system were underfunded. General practitioners had primitive offices. Hospitals had out-of-date equipment and buildings, and they deteriorated during World War II. The country was underserved, since the hospitals and specialist physicians clustered in the large cities, where the paying patients lived.

One war aim of the coalition government was the modernization of health services. The national government would create a network of agencies to coordinate and expand services. Financing would be increased through general revenue. The National Health Insurance—like other social insurance programs—would be amended but would be retained in some form.[4]

The organization and reform of a national financing system are not simple rational creations of "the government" but result from the orientation of the political parties and interest groups in power at the moment. If the Conservative Party had ruled during the postwar reconstruction, it probably would have tried to emulate European statutory health insurance by preserving and strengthening the insurance carriers (the "Friendly Societies") and by modernizing the non-profit hospitals with public grants. But the Labour Party won the election of 1945. It decided to abolish National Health Insurance in favor of a National Health Service for several reasons:[5]

☐   The hospitals could be satisfactorily modernized only by outright national-
     ization. They would then be financed in full for both capital and operating
     costs by public funds. Their managers and physicians would then cooperate
     with public financing.
☐   Hospital services could spread throughout the country only by public plan-
     ning and public funding. Only then would specialist physicians practice
     throughout the country.
☐   The Ministry of Health and the civil service could administer collections,
     expenditures, and financial control far more efficiently throughout the coun-
     try than the small and inept Friendly Societies could.
☐   A universal NHS would treat everyone alike. Under even an expanded NHI,
     the rich would not be included—and they would create a large private sector
     that would draw money and physicians' loyalties away from the NHI for the
     general population.
☐   Public funding is based on progressive taxation and is preferred by the Left.
     Health insurance uses regressive payroll taxes and premiums and is less
     attractive to the Left.

During subsequent decades, control of government alternated between the Labour Party and the pragmatic wing of the Conservative Party. The National Health Service was left in place and never questioned (except for a few academics devoted to free markets financed by voluntary insurance).[6] When the Conserva-tives won the election of 1979, they were led by the libertarian wing, which favored privatization of government services and the reduction of public expen-ditures. A team of civil servants was assigned to study European statutory health insurance and design a form that could replace the National Health Service's Treasury financing. Advisers close to the Prime Minister were assigned to devise a completely privatized health care sector—government would provide little more than vouchers.[7] The NHS administrative structure would be replaced by giving the District Health Authorities autonomy in the short run and denationalizing the hospitals in the long run. Having missed the opportunity in 1945, the Con-servatives would create an effective health insurance system—either statutory and obligatory in the European form or private with public vouchers. In either case, services would be owned and managed privately.

But the eggs could not be unscrambled. Substituting statutory health insurance and privatization of services could not be designed and would invite a political defeat at the next election.[8] There were too many obstacles:

☐ The administrative basis for a large number of health insurance carriers no longer existed.

☐ Without substantial guarantees that violated the purposes of the transition, the existing private health insurance companies were not willing to insure the entire population for all benefits. They had recently suffered when—in the spirit of the new government-of-the-day—they tried to recruit more subscribers and cover more expensive benefits.

☐ To support the health care market, payroll taxes of a very high and visible level would be necessary. If the payroll taxes were lower and more palatable, government would have to contribute much money in addition—either by subsidizing the carriers or by giving vouchers to most of the population.

☐ In a less controlled health care market, total costs would rise to the European level. But the Thatcher government wanted to reduce—not increase—public spending.

☐ While private investors were willing to buy other nationalized industries, no one wanted to buy hospitals.

☐ Few welcomed the risks of a private market. Providers and the population had become accustomed to stable financing and set procedures. Suspicions that the Thatcher government wanted to dismantle the sacrosanct NHS aroused widespread outrage.[9]

Unable to convert the entire NHS into a statutory or private insurance system, the Thatcher government settled for methods of making it more flexible and more efficient. Each District Health Authority may send its patients to any NHS or private provider in order to save money or clear waiting lists. Hospitals may seek out-of-area business and attract it by quoting lower prices. General practitioners may compete more vigorously for patients; if they refer and prescribe less, they may keep the savings. District Health Authorities and hospitals may contract some services out to private companies. All the money remains public; none uses governmental or private insurance. All these reforms began as mandates for limited privatization and for competition, all have been enacted as options for managers and providers, and the long-term result may be limited.[10]

When Financing Fails

Statutory health insurance now presumes that everyone enjoys equal benefits. The system redistributes money to cover the costs of the higher users who pay in less than their costs. When health insurance was completely private, each carrier tapped the resources only of its own membership and its own industry. The sickness funds with more affluent members had more generous benefits than the others. Social class differences in coverage, benefits, and services offered by providers characterize every private and competitive system and can be maintained (to the advantage of the rich) only if the system remains private.

When statutory health insurance is first enacted, the private arrangement is merely regularized. As the program expands in coverage and benefits, the trade unions and the political Left protest that the poor and the pensioners are being treated unjustly. Payroll taxes and earnings bases are raised so that each carrier can cover the costs of its own poor and elderly members. To cover the beneficiaries in economically weak industries, their sickness funds are merged with carriers in more affluent industries or (if their sickness funds are preserved) their limited revenue is supplemented by government subsidies or interfund transfers. Therefore, the private insurance model of many independent carriers—each operating within its own resources—is abandoned. But if sufficiently redistributive financing is not adopted, statutory health insurance cannot succeed and a national health service is substituted.

Italy. The country had a long history of guilds and mutual aid funds. But they varied in resources and in efficiency. Most occupations and most of the population were not covered.

Italy never enacted a comprehensive health insurance law following the much-copied German model that standardizes benefits from the start, soon leads to all-payer reimbursement, and eventually reduces fiscal inequalities among the carriers. Rather, the Fascist government and the postwar democratic government created many new official funds (*enti mutualistici*), standardized and coordinated all the old and new carriers in many respects, but did not pool all the revenue. Different funds had widely different yields from payroll taxes. One large public corporation was created by merging several occupational funds (the *Istituto Nazionale per l'Assicurazione contro le Malattie,* or INAM); it was decentralized into financially autonomous regions with wide differences in revenue, benefits, and provider reimbursements. Benefits and reimbursement of providers varied across all carriers. Some sickness funds (particularly INAM) operated health centers and employed their own doctors. All carriers were underfunded because payroll taxes on employers were often evaded (as Chapter Six reported). To pay for physicians' services and pharmaceutical drugs, sickness funds paid hospital claims late or never, damaging the services of the hospitals.[11]

For several decades after World War II, trade unions, the political parties of the Left, and social reformers called for change. But they could not invoke any national feelings of social solidarity: Italian society in those years was fragmented among interest groups, ideologies, and regional loyalties. The national government was ruled for decades by Center-Right coalition governments—too weak to enact social reforms and too committed to traditional methods. The system deteriorated because of the regional differences within INAM. The health insurance system seemed beyond redemption, and reformers called for a clean sweep. They were much impressed by the National Health Service of Great Britain as a model to solve Italy's problems of reorganizing service delivery, universalizing coverage, standardizing benefits, and increasing and redistributing finances.

The deadlock was resolved in the 1970s when the Left for the first time unexpectedly joined the Cabinet. Social disorder originated in Italy during the late 1960s and spread to all developed countries. Like many others, Italy installed a new government of national unity. As the price for their cooperation on other issues (such as wage controls), the Socialists, Communists, and trade unions forced the Cabinet and Parliament to enact a National Health Service (the *Servizio Sanitario Nazionale,* or SSN). INAM, the *enti mutualistici,* and the hospitals were nationalized; payroll taxes and general revenue were merged; services were administered by regional councils.[12]

When the all-party Cabinet was replaced by the traditional Center-Right coalition during the late 1970s, the new Cabinet inherited the SSN. It could not repeal the SSN and go back to the previous heterogeneous arrangement; and it had no understanding of the typical European statutory health insurance arrangement. So, it dragged its feet in implementing the SSN. Slowly the new system was put into place.

Spain. The country did not have the long history of crafts, industry, and trade union action that produced guilds and mutual aid societies elsewhere in Europe. A few mutual aid funds existed in the Northeast. Many rural communities prepaid their local doctors. During the 1940s, the Falangist national government tried to emulate European statutory health insurance by organizing governmental insurance, requiring membership, and levying payroll taxes on workers and employers. The principal agency (the *Seguro Obligatorio de Enfermedad,* or SOE) covered barely more than half the population at its peak. Other workers had their own official funds. The rich were not obligated to participate and bought private health insurance. The carriers differed in fiscal capacity, organization, and reimbursement to providers. Official carriers and even private insurance companies had closed panels of doctors. SOE developed for its own subscribers the country's best hospitals.

After Franco died in 1975 and the Falange fell, the new democratic government inherited the problem of improving health care finance and service delivery. The principal carriers were government corporations; they were not private organizations protected by social movements and determined to defend their autonomy. If the conservatives had won the government, they might have created a semiprivate market with many carriers and subscriber choice. But the conservatives were discredited by their cooperation with Franco, and democratic Spain has been ruled by the moderate Left. The Left in every country prefers completely pooled financing over complex and incomplete interfund transfers; revenue from progressive general taxes rather than payroll taxes; equal benefits for all citizens rather than special benefits for each fund's subscribers; and universal access to the best providers over closed panels. Like the reformers in Italy, Spain's policymakers admired Great Britain's National Health Service. Without the struggles that characterize governments with coalition Cabinets, Spain easily enacted such a scheme in stages during the 1980s by creating the governmental *Instituto Nacional de la Salud* (INSALUD), by transferring all the public carriers (such as SOE) and their delivery facilities into it, by extending its coverage to almost the entire population, and by mixing new general revenue and the traditional payroll taxes.[13]

Structural Reforms in Insurance

Insurance systems are abandoned only if they cannot solve crises in service delivery and crises in the structure of financing. When these systems fail, national health services are substituted. But mere cost overruns are not enough to precipitate a fundamental change. In all countries after World War II, costs increased and demands rose on the payers of payroll taxes and on government subsidies. The financial situation deteriorated during the 1970s. Then it looked as if the decentralized and private model would fail, that all statutory health insurance would go bankrupt, and that national governments would have to take over the financing and management of all health services. The threat seemed particularly severe in Belgium and France.

However, during the 1980s, every country with statutory health insurance managed by a variety of instruments to stabilize its spending and financing. Governments now guide the containment of costs but do not take over financing and service delivery. The original structure of payers, providers, benefits, and patient entitlements survives. Everyone sighs with relief. Remarkably few changes have been made during the last decade: policymakers and government financial monitors fear that structural alterations will disturb the delicate financial balance and create deficits; they fear upsetting the delicate political balance in relations with doctors and hospitals. The problem is not addition of new benefits. The problem is financial stabilization in the face of the growing costs of existing benefits because of the aging of every population and the advances in medical technology.

Realistic Reforms. It is easy for academic theorists to spin out idealized utopias that promise more than current humdrum reality. These writings can be widely read and discussed.[14] But they are never seriously proposed by policymakers or by the special commissions that recommend reforms. The authors are left to fume.

In established statutory health insurance systems, the dominant policy goal has been stabilization. That is precisely the problem, complain the principal voices for structural change—conservatives who believe that the Welfare State is too generous, too heavy a burden on national economies. Providers and payers are said to be inefficient and wasteful. The critics are inspired by American medical economics.[15] They favor introducing into European social insurance "competition" and "market incentives" in the following forms:

☐ Subscribers will not be automatically assigned to sickness funds by occupation or region but can choose.

☐ Subscribers can choose among benefit packages offered by the same or by different carriers:

- If the subscriber picks a cheaper-than-average package, he can pocket savings or use them for nonacute protection, such as long-term care.
- If the subscriber picks a more expensive-than-average package, he can purchase it by supplementing the standard social security benefit with his own cash.

☐ Patients (or their insurance carriers) can bargain for special fees with doctors and hospitals. There would no longer be all-payer fees for all doctors established by industry-wide negotiations. There might no longer be all-payer hospital rates.

☐ Payers can selectively contract with the most cost-effective doctors and hospitals.

All countries have experiments and demonstration projects.[16] The number of experiments increased during the 1980s. Some innovations are adopted. But they do not fundamentally alter the systems. Basic structural reform can be enacted only if a health insurance system is being expanded substantially. Then no enrollee or provider loses established benefits, and the new subscribers still gain much. The last country where that could occur was the Netherlands: the expansion of social health insurance into the large competitive private market inspired at the start proposals that the entire social insurance sector become more like the private market, more "competitive," more sensitive to "market incentives." The Dekker Commission in Holland—described earlier in this book— proposed a new universal statutory health insurance system combining features of the old statutory and private sectors.[17]

Barriers to Basic Structural Change. Ambitious and much publicized reforms of established statutory health insurance schemes founder for several reasons:

☐ A national consensus has developed behind all social security programs. By the late 1980s, everyone receives health care and costs are contained successfully. Even many doctors are adjusting. After the prolonged organizational effort to combine generous entitlements with discipline over costs, free-market reforms seem risky, they invite new trouble, and they promise few benefits.[18]

☐ Despite publicity, hardly anyone supports the reform. For example, a few French academicians and their American guests recommended reorganization of the relations between French health insurance and the medical profession so that HMOs would be encouraged.[19] Soon afterward, a powerful national commission investigated social security and its possible reforms.

Appointed by a conservative Prime Minister, the commission searched for methods of introducing more competition into French health insurance. But when the commission called for witnesses and written proposals, hardly anyone advocated HMOs—either as a preferred form of practice or as an option.[20]

☐ Many proposals—such as increased cost sharing by patients—are publicized as "rational" methods to improve consumer awareness and market efficiency. Actually, they are the favorite schemes of conservative political parties and employers with high payroll taxes. These proposals are automatically opposed by the political parties of the Left, the trade unions, and the advocates of social solidarity. Parliaments are deadlocked, coalition Cabinets are threatened with breakup, and the proposals are shelved.[21]

Democratic politics torpedoed the publicized Dekker reforms in Holland. The sponsor and enthusiastic supporter of the commission was a Center-Right coalition government. It enacted a framework law to carry out the scheme for a two-tier insurance system with many competitive features. The coalition broke up during 1989, the electorate strengthened the Socialist Party and reduced the Liberal Party, and a new Center-Left Cabinet took office. Its new *Plan Simons* cut back the shift of benefits from the statutory first tier to the optional second tier, and it reduced other competitive features.

Even if a conservative government-of-the-day converts statutory benefits into consumer options, the Left might invoke guarantees in the national constitution or in international treaties enshrined when it was in power. For example, the advisory constitutional council of Holland gave the new Dutch Center-Left government the ammunition to repeal an essential feature of the law of 1988. The council held that earlier EEC treaties and International Labor Office agreements protected workers by forbidding cutbacks in entitlements once enacted. The council held that the planned transfer of pharmaceutical and dental benefits from the universal and obligatory first tier into the second tier was a violation.[22]

☐ Some privatization proposals undermine the redistributive foundations of social insurance by emulating the private insurance market. For example, citizens might select less coverage; in return, they would pay lower payroll taxes and premiums, or they would receive vouchers to purchase other social services. Persons could opt out of all social security and use their money to buy private income security insurance and private consumption goods. The better health risks would pay less into the system or would withdraw money. The proposals would reverse history, convert social insurance into a welfare program for the poor and disadvantaged, and throw social insurance into deficit.[23]

☐ Some proposals may sound reasonable to their authors but are anathema to the medical profession and violate agreements between the medical associations and governments fundamental to the creation of statutory health insurance. As Chapter Ten reported, every law guarantees that every licensed physician can treat patients under health insurance and any beneficiary may select any doctor; in Germany, doctors have this right under the constitution. Therefore, closed panels and patient lock-ins (as in HMOs)—a favorite idea of reformers influenced by American medical economics—cannot be created under statutory health insurance. No Parliament would consider such a fundamental revision of the law. None would risk a disruptive fight with the entire medical profession.[24]

☐ Financial incentives to subscribers may also be excluded by the standardized rules of statutory health insurance. Even in Switzerland, the country with the most flexible system, the cost-sharing rates for patients are set by the national law fixing conditions for *Bund* grants to the sickness funds. Therefore, the American PPO option—with lower cost sharing if the patient selects the more economical or the better-quality doctor—cannot be emulated by the established sickness funds.

☐ Including HMOs or IPAs as independent sickness funds—even if they are legally and administratively possible—is very risky. Such special carriers have been proposed in Switzerland, and a demonstration project was conducted during the 1990s in Zurich.[25] The reward for subscribers is lower premiums. Their presence endangers the established carriers; as in the American market, their better risks would join the HMOs and IPAs, thereby forcing them to raise their own premiums. Therefore, the Swiss national association of sickness funds does not endorse proposals and demonstration projects—and the national government does not guarantee the subsidies essential to their survival. Joining an HMO or an IPA is risky for the subscriber: if he changes his mind, he would rejoin a conventional carrier at a higher lifelong premium.

☐ Some NHI statutes might allow PPO options—provided the carriers have discretion to offer lower premiums to those patients who accept a permanent lock-in to the preferred doctors. The carrier would contract with the doctors it deems most economical or better in quality. A Swiss sickness fund is trying to implement the arrangement in Bern canton.[26] It encounters two barriers. Appropriate data about physicians' practice costs must be collected in Bern, in the carrier's other markets, and (for comparison) in the rest of Switzerland—and this effort takes years. Even if a scheme can be set up, the medical association threatens a lawsuit.

The amendments to the Dutch health insurance law in 1988 allowed selective contracting. A leading Dutch private insurance carrier (Silver Cross) set up a demonstration project in Utrecht consisting of a health center for a panel of GPs and special contracts with a few specialists in the community. The method depends on the response of the market: it cannot succeed if doctors and subscribers do not sign up. The financing of those carriers' mainstream accounts would be strained if the healthier risks pick the PPO option, as they do in the United States.

If any major structural change is in the offing, it might be the addition of a second voluntary tier in health insurance. New benefits are now added to statutory health insurance only cautiously and are hedged about, as in the example of dentistry in the Netherlands. A niche for private health insurance might be to cover benefits absent from statutory health insurance (such as long-term care) or to expand limited benefits under mainstream insurance (such as mental health, dentistry, and rehabilitation). The second tier of health insurance might cover the nonclinical personal services that acute-care health insurance omits, as is the case in long-term care and mental health occasionally now. This step requires building up private carriers in countries that lack them, such as Belgium. Dutch experience is a warning that the second tier must offer new benefits; important acute-care benefits cannot be transferred from the first to the second tier.

Greater Standardization and Predictability. Despite the publicity surrounding competitive schemes, the only significant structural reforms have been of the opposite form. The public policy problems are to guarantee patients' protection and stabilize the providers. As Chapter Eight explained, Germany after many decades of debate cushioned the flight of healthier risks and more prosperous subscribers to the *Ersatzkassen* by requiring financial transfers to the *Ortskrankenkassen*. Competition is no longer so profitable to the *Ersatzkassen,* and the market shares of the carriers might stabilize.

The grand design for a competitive Dutch health insurance system ended with enactment of universal statutory health insurance of the traditional sort. The first scheme of the Dekker Commission foresaw full participation in health insurance by all sickness funds and private companies. But they could compete in designing and selling a substantial second tier of benefits, they could freely bargain with providers, and their savings in selective contracting with providers would enable them to market better policies at lower premiums. The Center-Right government that sponsored and welcomed this plan was replaced in late 1989 by a Center-Left government. The law that was enacted (the *Plan Simons*) increased the scope of benefits for mainstream universal statutory insurance and reduced the benefits for the second-tier optional insurance. The final result made universal the coverage of the Dutch population under the standard benefits and rules of social insurance.[27] In order to participate in the larger market of social insurance, the private insurance companies became fiscal intermediaries like the sickness funds, no longer completely free enterprises.

Structural Reforms in National Health Services

Policymakers now try to stabilize statutory health insurance systems, not upset them. But proposals for competition, choice, and market incentives attract serious attention in other countries. One must realize that these are proposals to energize government programs and vertical bureaucracies, a very different situation from statutory health insurance.

These proposals do not follow from any recent worldwide triumph of neoclassical health economics. Rather, they are welcomed because of a decades-long interest in decentralizing public administration. The problems are how to perform important and expensive public services throughout a large and demanding society, ensure that the grass-roots providers follow general policy, distribute authority and responsibility from the center to the periphery through levels in a hierarchy, ensure enthusiasm and efficiency at all levels, ensure that service providers and their overseers adapt to the varied localities, contain costs, and obtain accurate reports. Every government in the world has been reforming a few or many national and provincial public services in this manner. The literature proposing, describing, and evaluating these changes has been enormous.[28]

A national health service is always a particularly controversial department of government: the public and the mass media always complain about inadequate health care, Left and Right disagree over policies and levels of spending, the medical profession tries to be independent, and the hospital managers constantly juggle conflicting demands. Thus, established national health services periodically reorganize in order to instill more energy and innovation at the grass roots— to increase local citizens' satisfaction. Great Britain twice during the 1980s adopted reforms that gave authority and discretion to local managers. The Soviet Union's stagnating health services were one of the first sites for Mikhail Gorbachev's *perestroika*.[29] Italy and Spain constructed their new national health services at the same time both governments were being decentralized into strata of regional and local authorities, and, therefore, much attention was given to the assignment of health planning, operations, and monitoring to the appropriate levels.

Policymakers were attracted to the economists' ideas because theory made a virtue of necessity. Doctors and hospital managers wanted maximum independence from the Ministry of Health and its detailed regulations. One could decentralize civil servants, but not health care providers. Thus, according to the economists' reforms, each general practitioner, health center, and hospital would become more autonomous in selecting patients and earning operating revenue. Instead of accepting patients from only one catchment area, doctors and hospitals could compete for business everywhere. Instead of receiving a fixed public budget, doctors and hospitals would obtain more money from more business and would risk losses if they did not attract enough patients.[30] Whether national health services will ever operate in this manner is doubtful: the Thatcher government first wished to mandate these methods for all general practitioners and hospitals—but, after prolonged protests by the British Medical Association, the final legislation made them mere options. In practice, British providers and patients may prefer to continue in the conventional manner. However they may develop in national health services, these innovations do not apply to statutory health insurance (which already can use them but rarely does) because subscribers and providers prefer wide choice, they experience no "inefficiencies," and they prefer stability over risk.

Rethinking the Aims of Health Insurance

By the 1990s, statutory health insurance and national health services had become stable in organization and successful in guaranteeing widespread access to acute care. Were these outcomes good enough? Were some of society's health needs underserved?

Statutory health insurance and the alternative modes of financing and service delivery had been limited to the support of services defined by the medical providers. The accumulation of clinical knowledge and technological innovation had made medical care more somatic and technical in orientation, more insistent in claiming society's resources. The influence (and incomes) of the technical specialties widened over the influence (and resources) of primary care, preventive medicine, mental health, long-term care, and community medicine. But the latter services were used by more people and might be more effective contributors to health.

Study commissions and policy thinkers began to suggest that statutory health insurance had become successful in an unduly narrow manner.[31] The fundamental character of health insurance was now questioned. As a result, during the 1990s, statutory health insurance might be channeled toward more primary-care and preventive goals. As Chapters Fourteen and Fifteen demonstrated, the traditional methods of social insurance would have to be coordinated with greater government intervention in service delivery and with other modes of private and public financing. To follow these new proposals and to learn whether fundamental reforms are possible will require a new research project and a new book.

Notes

1. Described in "Workmen's Insurance and Compensation Systems in Europe," *Twenty-Fourth Annual Report of the Commissioner of Labor 1909* (Washington: Government Printing Office, 1911); and I. M. Rubinow, *The Quest for Security* (New York: Henry Holt, 1934).

2. "Workmen's Insurance and Compensation Systems in Europe" (see note 1, above), pp. 2206–2209, 2235–2255; and I. M. Rubinow, *Social Insurance* (New York: Henry Holt, 1913), chaps. 16 and 17.

3. Christopher Davis, "Economic Problems of the Soviet Health Service: 1917–1930," *Soviet Studies*, vol. 35, no. 3 (July 1983), pp. 343–361; and Mark G. Field, *Soviet Socialized Medicine* (New York: Free Press, 1967), chaps. 2, 4.

4. For the compromise proposal by the wartime government see Ministry of Health, *A National Health Service* (London: His Majesty's Stationery Office, 1944), Cmd. 6502; the retention of "social insurance" appears in chap. 8 and app.

E. The formulation of this White Paper and the subsequent creation of the National Health Service are described in John E. Pater, *The Making of the National Health Service* (London: King Edward's Hospital Fund for London, 1981).

5. Pater, *The Making of the National Health Service*; Brian Abel-Smith, *The Hospitals 1800-1948* (London: Heinemann, 1964), chaps. 19-23; and Rudolf Klein, *The Politics of the National Health Service* (London: Longman, 1983), chap. 1.

6. Arthur Seldon, *After the NHS* (London: Institute of Economic Affairs, 1968); and Arthur Seldon (ed.), *The Litmus Papers* (London: Centre for Policy Studies, 1980).

7. "Thatcher's Think Tank Takes Aim at the Welfare State," *Economist*, Sept. 18, 1982, pp. 57-58.

8. Some of the technical and political barriers are described in Rudolf Klein, "Privatization and the Welfare State," *Lloyds Bank Review*, Jan. 1984, pp. 12-29; and Rudolf Klein, "The Politics of Ideology vs. the Reality of Politics: The National Health Service in the 1980's," *Milbank Memorial Fund Quarterly*, vol. 62, no. 1 (1984), pp. 82-109. The Thatcher government was able to transfer many other public services to private owners and to private operating finance, but the NHS proved resistant: Julian LeGrand and Ray Robinson (eds.), *Privatisation and the Welfare State* (London: Allen & Unwin, 1984).

9. Robert J. Blendon and Karen Donelan, "British Public Opinion on National Health Service Reform," *Health Affairs*, vol. 8, no. 4 (Winter 1989), pp. 55-59.

10. Robert Maxwell (ed.), *Reshaping the National Health Service* (Hermitage, Berks.: Policy Journals, 1988). The watering-down of the reforms is described in John Lister, "Reform of the British National Health Service," *New England Journal of Medicine*, vol. 322, no. 6 (Feb. 8, 1990), pp. 410-412.

11. Arnoldo Cherubini, *Storia della previdenza sociale* (Rome: Editori Riuniti, 1977); Arnoldo Cherubini, "Note sulla assicurazione sociale de malattia nel periodo 1923-1943," *Previdenza sociale*, vol. 29, no. 6 (Nov.-Dec. 1973), pp. 1585-1655; and Aldo Piperno (ed.), *La politica sanitaria in Italia* (Rome: Franco Angeli, 1986), chap. 1.

12. The creation of SSN is described in Antonio Brenna and others, *Il governo della spesa sanitaria* (Rome: Servizio Italiano Pubblicazioni Internazionali, 1984); Lawrence D. Brown, "Health Reform, Italian-Style," *Health Affairs*, vol. 3, no. 3 (Fall 1984), pp. 75-101; and Giovanni Berlinguer and Fiorella de Rosis, "Balance Sheet of Health Organisation Reform in Italy," *Effective Health Care*, vol. 1, no. 3 (Oct. 1983), pp. 143-151.

13. The issues and steps in the reform are described in Pedro Pablo Mansilla Izquierdo and others, *La Sanidad Española 1982-1986* (Madrid: Ministerio de Sanidad y Consumo, 1986); Pedro Pablo Mansilla Izquierdo (ed.), *Reforma Sanitaria en España* (Madrid: Ministerio de Sanidad y Consumo, 1984); and J. I.

Cuervo and Eduard Portella, "Espagne: La réforme du système de santé," *Journal d'économie médicale*, vol. 4, no. 5 (1986), pp. 275–285.

14. For German and French reform proposals from all sources see Hartmut Reiners, *Ordnungspolitik im Gesundheitswesen* (Bonn: Wissenschaftliches Institut der Ortskrankenkassen, 1987); and Robert Launois (ed.), *Des remèdes pour la santé* (Paris: Masson, 1989). In recent years, the principal policy options and their probable consequences were formally presented to the *Konzertierte Aktion* by its steering committee (the *Sachverständigenrat*). The annual reports are published by Nomos Verlagsgesellschaft in Baden-Baden.

15. A few examples are Jörg Finsinger and others, "Some Observations on Greater Competition in the West German Health-Insurance System from a U.S. Perspective," *Managerial and Decision Economics*, vol. 7, no. 3 (Sept. 1986), pp. 151–161; Wissenschaftliche Arbeitsgruppe, "Krankenversicherung," *Vorschlage zur Strukturreform der Gesetzlichen Krankenversicherung* (Gerlingen: Bleicher Verlag, 1988), especially pp. 110–136; Wynand P.M.M. van de Ven, "Studies in Health Insurance and Econometrics" (Ph.D. dissertation, University of Leiden, 1984), especially chap. 3; and J. J. van Dijck and H. A. Tiddens (eds.), *Van koepel naar markt? naar een marktbenadering in de gezondheidszorg* (Lochem: De Tijdstroom, 1987). See also a proposal for competitive reforms by a European economist and rebuttals by other Europeans who argue that established methods now control costs while the competitive reforms will prove illusory or troublesome: Jürg H. Sommer, "Health Care Costs Out of Control: The Experience of Switzerland," *World Health Forum*, vol. 6, no. 1 (1985), pp. 3–9 plus the rebuttals on pp. 9–19.

16. Bradford L. Kirkman-Liff and Wynand P.M.M. van de Ven, "Improving Efficiency in the Dutch Health Care System: Current Innovations and Future Options," *Health Policy*, vol. 13 (1989), pp. 35–53.

17. *Derde Dekker-brief (Nota 'Verandering verzekerd')*, 7 maart 1988 (Rijswijk: Ministerie van Welzijn, Volksgezondheid, en Cultuur, 1988; Tweede Kamer, zitting 1987–1988, 19,945, nos. 27–28), app. A-4; summarized in *Changing Health Care in the Netherlands* (Rijswijk: Ministerie van Welzijn, Volksgezondheid, en Cultuur, 1989), pt. 3.

18. Monika Steffen, "Privatization in French Health Politics: Few Projects and Little Outcome," *International Journal of Health Services*, vol. 19, no. 4 (1989), pp. 651–661.

19. Pierre Giraud and Robert J. Launois, *Les réseaux de soins, médecine de demain* (Paris: Economica, 1985); and "Les R.S.C: Une organisation du système de santé," *Journal d'économie médicale*, vol. 4, nos. 3–4 (May–Aug. 1986), special issue. The French were inspired by exaggerated accounts of the American experience in such sources as *Politiques et management public*, vol. 3, no. 4 (Dec. 1985), pp. 1–16, 39–86, 149–180.

20. *Rapport du Comité des Sages* (Paris: Etats Généraux de la Sécurité Sociale, 1987), pp. 94, 99–100.

21. For a case study of a major structural reform that was pushed by an

unusually powerful government but was blocked nevertheless by opposing interest groups and political parties, see William Safran, *Veto-Group Politics: The Case of Health-Insurance Reform in West Germany* (San Francisco: Chandler, 1967). The West German cycle of promising initiatives, deadlocks in coalition Cabinets, and compromise reforms is described in Douglass Webber and Bernd Rosewitz, *Reformversuche und Reformblockade im deutschen Gesundheitswesen* (Frankfurt: Campus Verlag, 1990). Structural reform of a system as amorphous as Switzerland's has repeatedly been blocked by widespread ideological opposition to expansion of governmental authority and by deadlocks among interest groups and provider groups. See, for example, the events described in Gerhard Kocher, *Verbandseinfluss auf die Gesetzgebung*, 2nd ed. (Bern: Francke Verlag, 1972).

22. "Memorie van toelichting" (The Hague: Raad van Staat, 1990), pp. 28–36.

23. Jef van Langendonck, *Privatisation et Sécurité sociale* (Louvain: Institut européen de Sécurité sociale, 1986), pt. 2, chaps. 2–3; and Alain Euzéby and Jef van Langendonck, "Néo-libéralisme et protection sociale: la question de la privatisation dans les pays de la CEE," *Droit social*, vol. 52, no. 3 (March 1989), pp. 256–265.

24. Therefore, realistic European devotees of competitive markets in health concede that HMOs cannot be incorporated into statutory health insurance. See, for example, Heinz Hauser and J. Mattias Graf von der Schulenburg (eds.), *Health Maintenance Organizations—eine Reformkonzeption für die gesetzliche Krankenversicherung in der Bundesrepublik Deutschland?* (Stuttgart: Bleicher Verlag, 1987).

25. How to design HMOs and IPAs under Swiss statutory insurance is discussed in Heinz Hauser (ed.), *Mehr Wettbewerb in der Krankenversicherung* (Horgen: Schweizerische Gesellschaft für Gesundheitspolitik, 1984). Several schemes are described in Stephan Hill, "Neue Krankenversicherungsmodelle für die Schweiz," *Schweizerische Krankenkassen-Zeitung*, vol. 78, nos. 15/16 and 17 (Aug. 16 and Sept. 1, 1986), pp. 235–237, 249–251; and Jürg Baumberger, *Versicherungsplan Gesundheit/HMO Rohmodell* (Winterthur: Interessengemeinschaft für Alternative Krankenversicherungsmodelle, 1986).

26. Heinz Schmid, "Finanzielle Anreize und fehlender Markt im Gesundheitswesen," *Schweizerische Krankenkassen-Zeitung*, vol. 78, nos. 13 and 14 (July 1 and July 16, 1986), pp. 193–195, 208–211.

27. The original Dekker proposal was Commissie Structuur en Financiering Gezondheidszorg, *Bereidheid tot verandering* (The Hague: Distributiecentrum Overheidspublikaties, 1987). The law enacted in 1988 was explained in the sources cited in note 17. For the *Plan Simons* see *Werken aan zorgvernieuwing* (Rijswijk: Ministerie van Welzijn, Volksgezondheid, en Cultuur, 1990; Tweede Kamer, vergaderjaar 1989–1990, 21,545, no. 1), app.

28. See, for example, "Symposium on Administration Without Bureaucratization," *International Review of Administrative Sciences*, vol. 55, no. 2 (June

1989), pp. 165-181; and L. J. Sharpe (ed.), *Decentralist Trends in Western Democracies* (London: Sage Publications, 1979) and sources cited.

29. The initial plan of action was summarized by Minister of Health Evgenii Chazov, "Zadatchi organov i outchrejdienii zdravookhranienia," *Sovietskoie Zdravookhranienie,* no. 2 (1989), pp. 3-22.

30. These ideas are summarized and applied to Sweden in Richard B. Saltman and Carsten van Otter, *Planned Markets and Public Competition: Strategic Reform in Northern European Health Systems* (London: Open University Press, 1991).

31. The redirection of statutory health insurance is recommended in *Strukturreform der gesetzlichen Krankenversicherung: Endbericht der Enquête-Kommission* (Bonn: Referat Offentlichkeitsarbeit, Deutscher Bundestag, 1990), vol. 1, pp. 54-162, 251-278; and Philippe Lazar, *12 thèses pour le renouveau de la médecine libérale* (Paris: INSERM, 1990). The same proposals are seriously considered in countries with direct public financing, as in *Pour améliorer la santé et le bien-être au Québec: Orientations* (Québec: Ministère de la Santé et des Services sociaux, Gouvernement du Québec, 1989).

CHAPTER 19

Lessons
for the United States

-------------------- Summary --------------------

For income protection, the United States enacted a social security program that
is typical of all developed countries. For health, it substituted a mosaic of employer group contracts and special categorical programs for the retired and the
unemployed.

America's health financing methods have failed. Many persons have no
health insurance coverage, since their employers do not buy it. Government does
not fill the entire gap with special programs. The insured experience many inequalities in benefits and services. There is no mechanism for redistributive financing, but the trend has been increasingly self-centered, whereby the rich and
employed pay only for their own actuarial costs. The system is difficult for patients and providers to understand, and disputes are common. Administrative
costs are high. There is no method for planning and controlling clinical costs.
The present situation is the inevitable real-life *reductio ad absurdum* of a free
market in which everyone pursues his own pecuniary self-interest at everyone
else's expense.

Government officials and policy analysts are baffled about reform. Thinking about the entire health sector and designing comprehensive machinery are
unfashionable. A widespread vogue is to propose mandating employer group
coverage for all workers and supplementing it with special pools, but this will
not remedy the many defects in the present group insurance system. Universal
coverage through mandating employer coverage cannot be enacted by Congress
because of opposition by small business and ideological conservatives. Universal
coverage through full government financing ("the Canadian model") cannot be
enacted because of opposition by business, providers, and insurers.

If Americans are serious about reform, they will do what they once repeatedly debated: add statutory health insurance to Social Security in the form common in Europe. This arrangement will yield universal coverage, standard benefits, standard and comprehensible rules, administrative simplicity, and the instruments for containing costs. Doctors, hospitals, and insurance companies will function much as they do now. Patients will have free choice among providers and even greater choice than they now have among insurers. The poor will have mainstream coverage and a range of choice that they now lack.

But American elites and the American government may be unwilling to enact a genuine health insurance system, since it assumes social solidarity and financial redistribution. Many Americans have become accustomed to thinking of health care as a private consumer product and not as a social sector: they seek the best services for themselves, wish to pay as little as possible, resist contributing to the less disadvantaged, complain about the outcomes, and do not grasp that only a total reform of the system can alleviate the difficulties of its individual members. Another obstacle to reform is the parlous state of policy thinking and leadership in the American national government.

The American Health Financing Model

By the late 1960s, American health insurance financing was supposed to be fulfilled by a set of private and governmental efforts:

☐ *Employer-provided health insurance.* All employees and their dependents—nearly the entire population—were to be covered by groups paid for entirely by employers. Coverage for health and pensions were fringe benefits provided by employers either voluntarily or under contracts with trade unions. The employer would place the group with a health insurance carrier, which would offer standard benefits, administer beneficiaries' claims, and pay providers. The principal carrier was Blue Cross/Blue Shield.

☐ *Medicare.* All retired persons were fully covered by a special program of the national government: Medicare. The benefits and payments to providers were modeled on those for the employment-based insurance of the young. Hospital care of the elderly was paid for under a form of statutory health insurance financed by Social Security payroll taxes on the economically active. All the elderly were covered. Physicians were paid for under a hybrid arrangement not fully integrated into Social Security. Every person over sixty-five could join voluntarily and pay premiums. The Treasury contributed in lieu of payroll taxes on employers. All doctors were expected to cooperate voluntarily.

☐ *Medicaid.* Public welfare survived to cover costs of the chronically disabled and socially handicapped. But they would receive mainstream medicine. The national government contributed half the costs of the state-administered Medicaid programs. Benefits and payments of providers were modeled on

Medicare and therefore on Blue Cross and Blue Shield. All doctors were expected to cooperate voluntarily.

☐ *Private insurance for individuals.* Nonprofit and for-profit insurance companies were free to sell extra cash-benefits health insurance policies. They sold special policies to the elderly (Medigap) to cover the Medicare cost sharing.

☐ *Unemployed.* The foregoing arrangements would cover the population completely. A "war on poverty" and nationwide prosperity would ensure that all able-bodied persons under sixty-five had jobs and coverage.

Since this mixture of private and public programs would cover the entire population with generous benefits, government intrusion by enactment of statutory health insurance was unnecessary.

Failure of the American Model

By the 1990s, this idyll obviously had evaporated.

Employer-Provided Health Insurance. Many workers had no group coverage. It had always been voluntary. Some industrial employers now terminated health coverage in order to cut their labor costs during tighter business conditions. Many workers switched jobs to service industries and to small employers, who offered no fringe benefits. Trade unions, the traditional guarantor of fringe benefits, declined in importance.

Where group coverage existed, often it was no longer paid for completely by employers. Workers were expected to contribute premiums. Many employers economized by reducing benefits. Workers were expected to pay higher shares of the providers' bills. Part-time employment grew, and many part-time workers were not covered. To avoid private fringe benefits, some employers classified a number of their regular jobs as "temporary."

Dependents. Most dependents lost automatic coverage in groups at the employers' expense. They could continue with group membership if they paid premiums. Probably dependent coverage dropped substantially.

Unemployed. Losing a job resulted in immediate loss of coverage. During business recessions, many persons and their families lacked health insurance. If a worker got a new job with group coverage, he might have a waiting period. Persons who changed jobs had intermittent coverage during the year. This was common in industries with high labor turnover. Young workers were often in limbo, since they were no longer dependents in their parents' groups. Many early retirees were in limbo too. They had Social Security pensions at sixty-two years and employer-provided private pensions even earlier. But Medicare did not begin until age sixty-five.

Medicare. As the population aged and life expectancy lengthened, gaps in Medicare coverage—that is, its focus on customary acute-care coverage—became more serious. The very old needed long-term care, prescription drugs, and other benefits that were not provided.

In addition, Medicare proved very contentious. For many years, a permissive method of paying hospitals resulted in rapidly increasing costs, ineffective attempts to control costs through unilateral government action, and constant disputes between the national government and hospitals. Congress and the courts were repeatedly involved. In addition, the method of paying doctors proved permissive and confusing. Costs rose quickly, resulting in large Treasury subsidies. Attempts to control payments and utilization produced repeated disputes between the national government and the medical associations. Individual doctors refused to accept assignment, extra-billed patients, and let the patients deal with the reimbursement system. Patient out-of-pockets exceeded original plans. The national government tried to persuade doctors to cooperate by means of incentives and penalties that made the system more confusing and contentious.

Medicaid. The Medicaid program has proved disappointing for several reasons. It did not succeed in making its subscribers indistinguishable from all other patients by giving them equal access. Fees were limited in order to control costs. As a result of low fees and the aura of welfare medicine, few office doctors have accepted Medicaid patients. For ambulatory care, many beneficiaries have had to rely on the outpatient departments of public and nonprofit hospitals.

Because the program was considered cheap government charity and patients were uninformed, Medicaid attracted providers with penchants for underserving and fraudulent billing. To cut costs, the national and state governments reduced coverage during the early 1980s, even though poverty worsened.

Absence of a System. The several health care financing programs have not reached a consensus in coverage and benefits so that the entire population is treated alike. The differences among the programs have not produced cost-reducing efficiency nor lessons in prudent purchasing by consumers. Despite the widespread lack of coverage and the underinsurance of benefits, American health care is the most expensive in the world. The many different programs, their varying coverage, and their diverse payments for the same services impose confusion and administrative costs on providers.

Therefore, the United States is again faced by the policy agenda of 1960: how to construct a general system of health insurance for the economically active, for the elderly, for the disabled, and for the poor. The country can make wiser decisions now, because of the failure of the fragile and utopian financing arrangements created during the 1960s. Americans now can also profit from the experiences abroad, which proceeded from different decisions and encountered their own difficulties. This chapter describes how statutory health insurance might be designed in the United States in the light of European experiences.

I do not argue that the United States *should* enact statutory health insurance. Rather, I describe the designs implied by European precedents *if* the United States enacts the methods established as least troublesome and most comprehensive in normal practice elsewhere and *if* the United States implements its own legislative proposals of past years.

More Years of Deadlock and Drift?

One possible course of action is inaction. Perhaps no single reform will find support greater in numbers and political energy than the critics who fear its consequences. Every program involving money income and economic autonomy arouses the interest groups who might lose. Every program seems ideologically impure to many. Health care financial reforms always touch off political alarms about high costs and government intervention.

Such impasses have occurred previously in the United States. A considerable number and variety of health insurance schemes were introduced into Congress during the 1970s. Each was criticized for some reason; the free-for-all was not converted into a serious effort to maximize support and minimize opposition around one principal scheme; no President was willing to adopt one scheme on his own—and foreign experience shows that enactment of any major health care financing innovation requires all-out leadership by the head of government.[1]

The failure to enact universal health insurance seemed tolerable during the early 1970s. Policymakers assumed that the population was sufficiently covered by employee groups, Medicare, Medicaid, and privately purchased policies. Researchers underestimated the numbers of people without coverage and the amount of underinsurance in employee groups. Proponents of financing reform were inhibited by distrust of hospitals and doctors; the reformers had no experience in designing cost containment and feared that the providers would exploit any new arrangement. Some policymakers believed it untimely to finance the status quo; they believed that health care delivery and financing were about to be transformed spontaneously by en masse adhesion to health maintenance organizations.

The present impasse may continue for several reasons. Health care finance has become so complicated and troublesome that American politicians cannot understand it and so they avoid it. They fear they will be identified with wrong decisions that will make things worse. Instead of taking responsibility for designing a comprehensive reform, leading policymakers in health confess bafflement and hope that future study commissions and debate will somehow produce a "consensus."[2]

There is a grimmer explanation for delay. As noted in earlier chapters of this book, statutory health insurance—like all social security—requires redistributive financing. The healthy rich pay more than their actuarial costs in order to finance full benefits for the poor. But, more than in other developed countries, the poor in the United States are nonwhite. For two centuries, American whites have refused to subsidize equal social benefits for nonwhites. The present health insurance system is financed primarily by experience-rated premiums for employed groups: insurance carriers are not given extra cash to subsidize the uninsured; Medicaid covers many nonwhite poor, but government budget limitations restrict its coverage and benefits. Americans rarely speak of "social solidarity," because their society is divided. A comprehensive reform of health care financing will require a reform of the public conscience.[3]

Deadlock and drift have become so pervasive in American health care policy that reformers have become dispirited and pessimistic. Once they crusaded optimistically for grand designs. Now many hesitantly suggest a small set of limited categorical improvements that might improve coverage, benefits, and financing. Nothing more can be enacted, they fear.[4] But all the essential problems will remain. Pessimism will guarantee that the problems will only grow.[5]

Mandating Employer Group Coverage

Every country builds on its past structure of health insurance when making it compulsory and extensive. In all other countries, individuals and their dependents belonged to sickness funds and paid their own premiums. The laws made membership obligatory, expanded coverage, standardized the members' premiums, and added payroll taxes on employers.

When the United States enacted no law, private employer group coverage was added to the pattern of individual policies and became the principal vehicle. Americans have become so accustomed to group coverage in its short forty-year history that they assume it is the normal form of health insurance and design their proposed statutes around it. American Social Security follows the universal pattern of social redistribution, pay-as-you-go, and individual entitlements, but the Americans may enact an entirely different arrangement in health insurance.

Since the mid-1970s nearly every serious proposal for extensive health insurance coverage of the American population has required all employers to buy group coverage for their workers and dependents. One might have expected the health insurance crisis of the 1980s to have generated an explosion of original ideas, but all current proposals remain wedded to the model of employer group insurance.

In comparison to the conventional form of statutory health insurance, it will be far more difficult to achieve extensive coverage, satisfactory benefits, and orderly administration through mandated group coverage for the following reasons:

☐   Big business can block enactment of all benefit levels beyond the minimum already offered by the least generous large corporations.
☐   Small business opposes enactment of all such laws. Usually it has enough

leverage in the legislature to emasculate the law: all very small business would be exempt; others have lower obligations than larger employers; small business may be phased into coverage over a longer timetable.

☐ Benefits vary widely. Even if each group contract lists minimum benefits, employers are allowed considerable latitude in negotiating terms with insurers and providers. Some proposed laws may not even specify a benefit list but may merely specify a total financial obligation per worker (as in the Massachusetts Health Security Act of 1988), and the employer is allowed to offer any benefit package priced at that sum. Government and unions may be unable to monitor whether all employers are fulfilling their obligations under the law—a difficulty that does not arise under the present voluntary situation.

☐ The top managers can provide for themselves slightly more generous benefits than they give their workers.

☐ Benefits may fluctuate from year to year if employers have discretion. The result is just as baffling to beneficiaries as the present situation. But it may be more frustrating, because they think they are being cheated of an entitlement under law.

☐ The burden of financing falls on the employers. The American proposals make the workers responsible for one-quarter or less of the premiums, resulting in lower financing than other countries have.

☐ The burden of shopping among insurers, administering the benefits, and monitoring the carriers falls on the employers. But their mission is to perform their own production and services, not administer health benefits. American employers are trying to reduce their roles in health, not increase them.

☐ The many separate employers cannot bargain effectively with carriers and providers. At best, they can threaten to change contracts from year to year, producing an unstable situation. To reduce their own burden in bargaining, employers may have to rely on third-party administrators whose costs may or may not offset savings and whose presence contributes to the instability and complexity of the system.

☐ Employers vary in the claims experience of their labor forces. The individual worker who is a good risk may not enjoy even average (let alone superior) benefits because his group is a poor risk. Employers have an incentive to avoid hiring anyone who might be superior in work but whose family is expensive medically.

☐ The system's premiums are not redistributive if groups are experience-rated. The system lacks intergroup or interindustry financial equalization.

☐ There would still not be a comprehensive financing system stabilized by government. The insurer's reserves would be at risk. Therefore, the underwriting cycle continues for employer groups and individual policyholders with weak bargaining power: the insurers try to raise premiums very high

during certain years in order to restore reserves and expand them in anticipation of future cost squeezes.

☐ Special categorical programs survive for the retired and the unemployed. All
of their weaknesses remain:

- The complexity of rules and wide variation among the states in Medicaid
supplementary coverage of poor Medicare beneficiaries
- Fluctuating coverage and benefits for the poor according to the budgetary
constraints of the states
- Wide variations among the states in programs for the unemployed

☐ Employers have an incentive—greater than under Social Security—to keep
workers completely off the books, or as part-timers, or as nominal tempo-
raries. Small businessmen have an incentive to keep their labor forces below
the threshold where they are obliged to participate.

☐ If every group and insurance carrier sets its own payment arrangements with
hospitals and doctors, the present situation worsens rather than diminishes:
cost shifting by providers among payers; refusal by providers to accept assignment with extra-billing of patients regardless of the group's assurances
to patients; variations in administrative procedure (such as billing by *tiers
payant* or by *tiers garant*) among providers dealing with the same carrier and
the same patient; confusion among patients and doctors; disputes over extra-
billing and suspected underservicing; and high administrative costs. Complaints will rapidly spread that statutory health insurance is a sham because
it cannot be understood, providers are profiteering, and the public is not
getting its money's worth. Washington will respond with its usual cycle of
indignant oversight hearings and involved regulations that make the system
yet more incomprehensible and contentious.

☐ If each employed group is a distinct entity, an extra (and expensive) tier of
administration is placed between the subscriber and the insurance carrier.

☐ Writing and pricing insurance policies for many small and medium-sized
groups is a complex and expensive business.

☐ Since group health arrangements become a variable part of personnel costs,
they become an instrument of competition among firms. Each employer
invites carriers and providers to shift costs to its competitors.

☐ Certain anomalies of current employer group insurance will stay in place
unless a new law clearly eliminates them. For example, employers might still
evade state insurance regulation by declaring that they offer self-financed
employee benefit plans governed by ERISA. The arrangements will continue
to vary and fall short of any public policy supposedly enacted in the national
health insurance law.

Key Principles for a Financing System

Foreign and American events suggest many guidelines for the redesign of health
care financing in the United States during the coming years. Every chapter in this

book has concluded with specific lessons for the United States. This section offers some general and particularly important conclusions.

One must think about designing a national system. At first sight, Americans seem not to think this way. Many idealize free markets, decentralization, competition, and innovation. The struggle of interest groups, the caution by elected politicians, the leverage by each interest group to minimize limitations and maximize advantages—all produce legislation full of special concessions and ambiguities.

Nevertheless, Americans have planned strategically and have enacted coherent national structures in some sectors where such action was preferable to chaos and financial collapse. The Founding Fathers created national systems in postal services, in currency, in the courts. Since then, Congress has enacted—in a field closely connected to health—an unusually standardized and comprehensive Social Security pension system. Using its powers over interstate commerce, taxation, and currency, Congress has created national systems in many areas of banking, labor/management relations, air travel, railroads, and elsewhere.

In federal systems, some variations always occur among provinces. But effective programs involving the welfare of all citizens require considerable uniformity across the country. Some proposals for statutory health insurance during the 1970s authorized each state and its interest groups to design and finance their own programs. Other proposals would have allowed every employee group and insurance carrier to devise its own benefit package and methods of reimbursing providers. No national policy can be framed, understood, and implemented in these ways. Medicare Part B and Medicaid demonstrate the confusion and conflict that ensue if patients, providers, and lawyers are confronted with systems that are unduly variable and incomprehensible.

A national health service—whereby government owns hospitals and employs the doctors—is enacted only if the management of health services has collapsed. If the problems are only insufficient financing and barriers to access, facilities are left with their owners, doctors remain independent, and statutory health insurance is enacted. Since the American problems revolve primarily around financing and access, the real issue is the form of statutory health insurance. Arguments for and against a national health service are diversions.[6] Arguments on behalf of certain "uniquely American" reforms as salvation from the horrors of British and Swedish alternatives are diversions too.[7] The question is whether these American proposals are superior to the normal form of statutory health insurance.

Universal health insurance cannot be enacted and implemented without the cooperation of the medical profession. Government cannot dictate to them, no matter how popular the statute. (Medicare has been an unusual exception—the only important health financing law passed over the opposition of the American Medical Association. But it was drafted in excessively ambiguous and permissive ways so that individual doctors would not be forced to participate and not be forced to accept governmental price controls.) Government enacts a law setting forth the institutional framework and imposing payroll taxes. Permanent decision-making machinery is necessary so that the medical association and the payers can implement and constantly update the details.

The established health insurance carriers will insist on becoming the carriers under the official program. Unless they are bankrupt or decide that health insurance is less attractive than other lines, they will oppose any law replacing them with governmental financial administration. Since they would rather deal with private carriers than with government agencies, the medical associations will defend the private carriers' role. Thus, no law can be enacted in the United States that supersedes the private health insurance carriers with government agencies. Few may wish to stay in the basic scheme. A large number of insurance companies now offering medical expense policies do so reluctantly—in order to prevent competitors' raids on their more lucrative group life and pension business—and they would be relieved to transfer this complex and deficit-ridden field to Social Security.[8] Private carriers could still insure extra benefits as well as manage the basic package as fiscal intermediaries.

Under universal obligatory health insurance, a categorical program for the elderly is no longer necessary. Subscribers can remain in their preretirement sickness funds with no change of benefits. Therefore Medicare—with all its administrative complexities and disputes—can be abolished.

The poor and disabled can also be enrolled in the official carriers with standard benefits. Thus, Medicaid can be abolished—eliminating another political trouble spot. Medicaid's public money can become subsidies to the sickness funds. Distinct "welfare medicine" would disappear.

Because heavy users are underpayers, redistributive features must be included in financing. The payroll taxes must cover the costs of the economically active and their dependents. These subscribers often must pay a surcharge to cover the costs of the elderly and poor members. The pensioners and the poor are expected to pay health insurance premiums. American elderly already do so in Medicare Part B. Additional subsidies from the Treasury or pension funds are unavoidable.

Because health care costs rise and press for even higher payroll taxes and public subsidies, government intervenes to limit health care costs. The United States therefore will need to formulate and apply a general cost containment policy. Up to now, Americans have talked much and acted little, aside from capping Medicare Part A and Medicaid. Medical associations and sickness funds in America may start by assuming that statutory health insurance is essentially private, but they cannot long avoid government guidelines to limit costs.

Statutory health insurance with several carriers uses all-payer rates. All carriers pay the same hospital rates and the same physicians' fees. To arrive at these prices, the sickness funds form a common bargaining committee to face the hospitals and doctors. Except in a few states with hospital rate regulation at present, all-payer arrangements would be a novelty in the United States.

In federal systems of government—as in the United States—statutory health insurance is less centralized and less standardized than it is in unitary systems. Many decisions are made by provincial bargaining committees of payers facing provincial bargaining committees of providers. Many details and rates vary from province to province. Doubtless such decentralization would characterize statutory health insurance in the United States.

A Possible American Design

Coverage and Access. Every other developed country has learned that provision for the poor and vulnerable can be handled satisfactorily only by including them under universal financing—under obligatory health insurance if the country does not have a national health service. In the past, the poor were not covered and local welfare offices had to pay for them. But this very common method had many defects. Paid for by the general budget of government, welfare medicine was limited in the best of times and cut back during economic declines, regardless of patients' needs. Establishing eligibility was laborious and controversial; some persons were added and dropped capriciously; some people were too confused and ashamed to use the program. Deferring care through administrative denials and patients' inhibitions often cost government higher medical costs in the long run. Welfare medicine became a political pawn between Right and Left—starved under the former and expanded under the latter. Health care providers complained about inadequate reimbursement and demanded normal rates. Local welfare programs still survive abroad to support incomes and living standards, but no longer to finance acute health care benefits.

The United States now experiences all the foregoing difficulties in its patchwork approach to coverage and access. To integrate the poor and vulnerable into mainstream medicine, they must be integrated into mainstream financing—as all other developed countries have done. Their health care costs require funding from several sources. The unemployed, the poor, and the disabled abroad are expected to pay premiums to the sickness funds, often a small percentage of their benefits and disability pensions. (America already has a precedent in the Medicare Part B premium paid by persons with Social Security disability pensions.) The rest of the financing is redistributive: the economically active with high payroll taxes are overcharged to cover the extra costs of the poor and disabled who bring in little cash. (American workers and their employers already pay surcharges for the elderly in the Medicare Part A payroll taxes.) American universal insurance—like the financing of some European countries—might require general government subsidies to cover the shortfalls for the poor and disabled. (America already has a precedent in Medicare Part B.)

When countries lack complete obligatory health insurance coverage, the gaps are no longer at the bottom but at the top. The rich—who can clearly protect themselves—are given discretion to join sickness funds voluntarily, buy limited coverage from private companies, or self-insure. Since all buy *some* insurance, the only variation is in type of coverage. As recent Dutch events show, the trend now

is to eliminate these last exceptions in the name of social solidarity. Financing
for the entire population requires contributions by the rich at full payroll tax
rates into the main sickness funds. Their large payments are needed to cover the
expensive underpayers. (America has a precedent in its universal Social Security
pension system.)

Carriers. The established health insurance carriers continue to administer
the money after the enactment of statutory health insurance abroad, and they will
insist on this role in the United States. Such prospects make them a potential
political force in favor of the law. If a bill proposes to replace them with a
government agency—as in the Kennedy-Griffiths and Kennedy-Corman Bills of
the 1970s—it cannot pass any legislature.

In several countries, the subscriber can choose among a few carriers. This
policy would probably hold in the United States too. Instead of one carrier receiving a local monopoly by government—like a fiscal intermediary in Medicare—there would be competition for subscribers. At present in the United States,
many companies offer health insurance of various types, but probably only a few
principal companies would want to do so under statutory health insurance for
the following reasons:

☐   The American law would probably mandate a minimum benefit package as
    in every other country. The law might fix a standard payroll tax; or it might
    give the carrier discretion to set its own premiums, up to a limit. Few carriers
    could count on breaking even under these constraints. If most of an insur-
    ance company's business and home office expertise is not in basic health care,
    it might choose to specialize in other less risky lines.
☐   Enrollment might always be open. Carriers might be forbidden to reject bad
    risks or to charge extra premiums for bad risks.
☐   Since the revenue comes from payroll taxes or premiums set by law, each
    carrier's accounts would be audited and perhaps published annually.
☐   If the carriers were subsidized to cover the costs of the elderly and poor, or
    if they received equalization transfers from other carriers, they might be
    forbidden to earn profits and run up high management costs.
☐   Each carrier must maintain an office in the region to manage subscribers'
    affairs and pay the providers.

In the past, insurance companies would have opposed any health insurance design that relegated them to the mere administration of funds flowing from
government Treasuries to health care providers. They had been trained in underwriting, the assumption of risks, and the setting of rates. These functions
generated their ideology. But during the 1980s, their group business has rapidly
shifted from classic insurance to the work of fiscal intermediaries under Minimum Premium Plans and Administrative-Services-Only contracts for employers.
The insurance business has become riskier as employers recapture profits (under

premium-rebate clauses) and change carriers when the latter try to recover their
deficits by increasing rates. Some employers try to eliminate the insurance
companies completely by self-managing benefits or by using third-party administrators. Thus, insurance companies can accept the fiscal intermediary role—
particularly if they retain a foothold in the group for the rest of their business.

Coordination Among Carriers. In a private financing arrangement like
America's at present, each carrier is self-centered and seeks to maximize its revenue, reputation, and market share to the disadvantage of the others. Each is
secretive and attempts to be innovative. Even the government programs refuse to
cooperate with the private ones; they invite providers to shift costs to the private
payers.

Statutory health insurance standardizes benefits, enrollment rules, and
many other features. Government monitors and audits all the sickness funds
pursuant to standard reporting requirements. Even if they do not cooperate, the
sickness funds become more alike. Even if they compete, they will need to cooperate in some matters. Usually no carrier wishes to pay a provider more than the
others for the same services, and all can drive a harder bargain with providers if
they form a common front. Then they can set the standard rates required in all-
payer systems and screen hospitals' prospective budgets.

If there is more than one significant carrier in an area—particularly, as in
America, if there are many—they can join in a common bargaining committee
with its own secretariat. In every German city, the sickness funds subscribe to an
Arbeitsgemeinschaft der Krankenkassen that screens hospitals' prospective
budgets, works out common positions about hospital rates, and negotiates an all-
payer per diem with every hospital.[9] The provincial associations of sickness funds
meet jointly to face the medical associations on some matters (such as the contract) and meet separately with the doctors on other matters (such as the monetary
conversion factor for fees).[10] American carriers would need to form bargaining
committees on the national, state, and local levels, and probably they would need
something like an *Arbeitsgemeinschaft.*

An American health insurance statute would have to authorize such cooperation among payers so that the providers do not file antitrust suits. However,
all the foregoing arrangements might be completely legal at present. Few persons
realize it, but the insurance industry is largely exempt from antitrust laws.

Negotiations Between Payers and Doctors. Standing negotiation machinery is always created under statutory health insurance, as Chapter Ten explained.
The negotiations decide and oversee the implementation of the basic contractual
agreements, the fee schedule, the financial value of the weights, and utilization
review.

This privatized method of negotiations is less conflictual and less prone
to deadlocks than one that pits government directly against the medical profession. Government always claims the last word, so it cannot negotiate with doctors

as equals. For this reason, the medical profession fights the enactment of health care financing systems where government unilaterally fixes the rules of practice and payment rates and merely consults the medical profession. Democratic legislatures shrink from enacting such systems,[11] and Congress will not pass one in the United States. Governments can dictate the payment of hospitals—as in Medicare Part A—but not the payment and working conditions of doctors.

Because they define Medicare as a government program, Americans have been unable to think of any alternative to acts of Congress and bureaucratic regulations in Medicare Part B. The reforms of the 1990s have merely inserted a government advisory commission with public members—the Physician Payment Review Commission—into the annual decision cycle about reimbursement and rules of practice. The procedure has many disadvantages—all avoided in other countries with statutory health insurance:[12]

☐ Congress is overloaded with investigating and settling the details of physicians' practice and reimbursement. Congress has little time left to think about the American health care system as a whole.

☐ Congress is so constantly involved in listening to rival provider groups and resolving their conflicts that it shrinks from legislating about a larger insurance system.

☐ The management of the national government's budget and cost containment dominate policy on physicians' services for the elderly.

☐ The formulas for paying the doctors are constantly altered to please influential factions within medicine while also appearing to contain costs. The payment system becomes less understandable, more difficult to administer, and more ridden by disputes.

☐ The decision-making cycle involves too many executive and legislative agencies. Each has a different approach, responsibility is diffused, decisions are delayed, and administrative overhead costs increase.

☐ Practicing physicians' hostility toward government and all third-party reimbursement increases.[13]

Medicare limits organized medicine to the roles of petitioner and behind-the-scenes political lobby—instead of giving it responsibility for the success of the program. One of the most serious drawbacks of this experience is to make doctors resist any universal health insurance with an effective structure, lest Congress universalize the Medicare management and reimbursement methods.

These are not the only ways of governing Medicare and health generally. In other complex and contentious fields—some close to health such as environmental protection and occupational safety—Congress and executive agencies have begun to delegate rule making to bargaining sessions among all the interested parties. If their deliberations follow prescribed procedures and the outcome is reasonable, the agency adopts the agreement with legal effect upon the public and all providers. Negotiated rule making ("reg-neg") is designed to relieve all executive agencies of the problems that now beset HCFA and the health sector: overloading the civil servants by the volume and technical complexity of the subjects; arousing providers' hostility against government; orienting the providers, the payers, and their lawyers toward adversarial litigation instead of negotiation and settlement; and overloading the courts.[14] Of course, negotiated rule making should not replace the governmental functions that can best be performed by executives and Congress, such as health facilities planning.

Paying the Hospital. Hospital finance is the most important issue in provider reimbursement under national health insurance, since it involves more than half the money. Usually NHI at first adopts a payment system already widely used in a country. The Americans are adopting DRGs in many third-party programs and might retain them under statutory health insurance. The number and structure of the DRGs and the financial value of the "standardized amount" would have to be made uniform across all payers.

The present attempt to motivate efficiency and contain costs by dictating a standard price across all hospitals is not working well. There is no substitute for scrutinizing and regulating each hospital's budget. The United States will need an agency like Holland's COTG, which monitors quality of care and houses the negotiations between the sickness funds and the medical associations. Once screening machinery for individual hospital budgets is in place, the United States might join the trend toward global budgeting.

Centralization or Decentralization. Statutory health insurance differs in organization according to the type of government:

☐ *Unitary.* It is enacted by the national Parliament and applies uniformly throughout the country. All payroll tax rates, regulations, contracts, and medical fee schedules apply everywhere. Local offices of sickness funds and those of government are subdivisions of national headquarters. Local regulators follow instructions from the center. All payroll taxes pass through a single collection system and a central fund.

☐ *Federal.* Each province has legal authority to regulate and finance statutory health insurance. The national government at most can enact a framework and collect some taxes, but it is the provinces who decide whether to participate. Negotiations between payers and providers are conducted in each province, with varying outcomes across the country. The provinces vary in their pay rates due to their differences in fiscal capacity, health policies, and bargaining outcomes. In some federal countries, the national government encourages provincial participation and uniformity by granting money and imposing program conditions.

The United States is a unique federal system because it can use its constitutional authority over taxes, spending, and interstate commerce to enact universal health insurance and occupy the field completely. Or it can enact a national law and use the states as agencies. Or it can delegate considerable discretion and responsibility to the states. Thus, the United States will need to decide the structure of its statutory health insurance—in contrast to other countries, where constitutional practice allows only one form.

I have spelled out possible American structures elsewhere.[15] The decisions would settle:

☐ *Financial audit and quality review of health insurance carriers.* Screening of prospective hospital budgets. Whether by regional offices of the national government or by agencies of the state governments (as at present).

☐ *Contracts and fee schedules of doctors.* Whether negotiated and updated by national offices of sickness funds and medical associations or negotiated independently within each state by the state-level associations of the carriers and doctors. If negotiated nationally, whether state-level associations must implement them by their own contracts; state-level leeway in revising and supplementing the national frameworks.

☐ *Financing and costs.* Whether payroll taxes or premiums are uniform throughout the country or vary from state to state. Whether practice costs (for both doctors and hospitals) should become similar across the country. Whether doctors' fees are similar (with regional variations that diminish with time). Whether interfund transfers cross the country to redistribute revenue from rich to poor states.

☐ *Determination of hospital costs.* Whether wages for the professional and other staffs are settled locally or determined by nationwide or regional collective bargaining.

☐ *Organization of the medical association.* Power of the state societies relative to the national leadership.

☐ *Subsidies.* Whether there should be grants to health insurance funds from national and state governments.

☐ *Regionalization.* If fifty states is too great a number to organize certain aspects of statutory health insurance, whether interstate consortia can be created.

Whether the organization is centralized or decentralized, Americans must maintain some uniformity in implementation. Even in ostensibly centralized programs, such as Medicare, implementation at present varies widely across the country and invites abuse and waste in some places.[16] One pitfall is the practice of confining civil servants to the mass production of complicated regulations in their headquarters in Washington while implementation is delegated to private management firms with their own profit motives. The Americans usually delegate monitoring and evaluation to other private firms, who then inform headquarters with reports that are always voluminous, often ambiguous, and often late. The experience of other countries shows that statutory health insurance can be administered in a simpler and cheaper manner with civil servants, conscientious carriers, and dedicated providers.

Payroll Taxes or Premiums. One future decision will be whether American statutory health insurance uses payroll taxes or premiums. Medicare has precedents for both: Part A uses payroll taxes with standard percentages applying to all but yielding higher revenue from the better paid; Part B uses premiums with uniform amounts paid by all.

Standard rates result in different financial balances among sickness funds, depending on the incomes and medical costs of their subscribers. One issue is whether the payroll taxes or premiums should be universal or whether each sickness fund should vary them according to its financial balance and the economic strategy of its management. An insurance regulator—if it has such power—would insist on actuarial soundness and would raise the rates of certain companies.

American health economists think that competition for subscribers might reward carriers who quote lower premiums achieved through greater efficiency and tighter control over providers. But lower premiums in health insurance often are achieved by preferred-risk selection, which usually is not possible under statutory health insurance. Often health insurance carriers in Europe—both social and commercial—compete by offering better benefits, not by quoting lower premiums. The other sickness funds then demand that the extra cash be shared on the grounds that windfall profits result from their competitors' more affluent and healthier subscribers—that statutory health insurance should be considered a single integrated system inspired by social solidarity. This is a far cry from current American economic imagery, but health care may be different.

Division of Payroll Taxes. If the United States adds NHI to the rest of Social Security—the normal method abroad—it will expand the usual payroll taxes. The precedent already exists in Medicare Part A. The pension taxes fall equally on employees and employers in the United States, and employers probably will resist a larger share for health. Larger employers will not protest, since they already bear the costs of groups. Opposition will come from smaller employers who now pay nothing for groups—though they do have experience in paying Social Security taxes for pensions. (Employer-paid group coverage for basic benefits would be replaced by NHI payroll taxes. It might survive for optional, extra, and cheaper benefits, as in the case of private pensions in America today.)

An equal NHI tax would be an unwelcome novelty for workers, who now pay only for Social Security pensions. For many years, while employer-paid group coverage seemed viable, the labor movement and the Left proposed American NHI schemes paid completely by employers. No other country has this as a permanent policy.[17] Such financing was opposed by American business and could not be enacted by Congress. Since realistic 50–50 financing was not supported by the American labor movement—the traditional political constituency for NHI in every country—a realistic NHI could not be enacted in the United States.

But the mirage of an employer-paid NHI is now fading. The final proposals by the Carter administration and the mandated benefits bills of the 1980s concede that the worker should pay up to 25 percent. An increasing number of employer group arrangements now require the worker to pay a partial premium for himself and a full premium for his family. The financing of employer groups in America is gradually evolving toward the mix of a jointly financed German *Betriebskrankenkasse*. The American labor movement can no longer hold out against realistic 50–50 financing, because the fallback against contributory legislation is disappearing.

Noncontributory financing developed under union pressures in collective bargaining during the 1950s and 1960s, when the American economy was unusually prosperous and skilled labor was scarce. It was not the original method in employment-based groups. At first, the workers paid all or a large share. Gradually unions and management agreed on a total wage package, and the contract gave some of it in fringe benefits.[18] Thus, financing recently has returned to the earlier form.

Cost Sharing. America has always had cost sharing by patients and probably will retain it out of custom and ideology under statutory health insurance. In many other countries, third parties directly pay providers; cost sharing for physician and hospital services is small—but growing. America characteristically may make its cost-sharing rules complex and expensive to administer. In many of the American NHI bills during the 1970s, the heavy users who would be most deterred—the poor and elderly—are exempt if they satisfy certain criteria.

Cost-sharing rules in America will probably be rendered meaningless for the economically active too. Because of the freedom of the market, insurance companies will be allowed to sell coverage of the cost sharing, as in American Medigap and the French *mutuelles*.

The most troublesome issue in cost sharing is extra-billing by providers over the official fee ("balance-billing" in American terminology). For hospitals and most providers, this is usually illegal under the NHI law and impossible administratively, since the sickness fund pays the provider directly and in full. The problem arises with doctors who were accustomed to charging flexibly before the advent of statutory health insurance, who wish to collect extra money from the rich, and who complain when the negotiated fee schedule does not yield enough. A particular problem arises with the most distinguished and highest-price specialists, who wish to collect their usual high private fees while also treating patients under the official health insurance system.

In every country, sooner or later, a dispute between the medical association and government occurs over whether every doctor wishing to treat insured patients must accept assignment and must forgo extra-billing. (He can always treat patients privately—with the help of the patients' private insurance—and charge what he likes.) The showdown occurs either during passage of the law (if the law mandates assignment and precludes extra-billing) or during its implementation (if the law tried to buy peace and evaded the issue). Citizens protest extra-billing at the discretion of doctors on the grounds they have paid high payroll taxes and do not get their money's worth.

The American government and the medical associations will have to settle this issue. There is no way to evade it. As Chapter Ten reported, assignment has been a source of much of the trouble surrounding Medicare Part B. The participating physician scheme of the 1980s has been a partial and perhaps only temporary compromise. Congress has enacted price controls over the amount of extra-billing (125 percent over the prevailing Medicare CPR and less during the 1990s), and an exhausted medical profession has had to conform. But so many doctors have been willing to waive or reduce extra-billing only because the patients are the impecunious elderly who have patronized them for years. The medical profession and Congress will probably resist even these limited controls over billings under universal health insurance.

Voluntary Private Health Insurance. Many countries have two-tier social security systems: besides a basic obligatory and universal program, each person is free to buy (or not to buy) voluntary pensions or other types of benefit from nonprofit and for-profit companies. Since no law fixes the contributions, benefits, and eligibility, each country has a different arrangement. Some schemes are integrated into social security, some are not.

Earlier, in every country, voluntary private health insurance provided cash benefits (indemnity protection) to the upper classes outside the statutory scheme. But as obligatory coverage became universal, private insurance has specialized in supplementary benefits such as private rooms in hospitals, specialists' private fees, and cash benefits during disability. Second-tier American health insurance benefits might also include dentistry, mental health, and long-term care.

European health insurance companies that did not wish to become carriers under the official scheme (or were excluded) switched to offering the supplementary benefits. Doubtless many commercial health insurance companies—particularly the specialists in individual mail-order policies—will survive in this form if statutory health insurance is enacted in the United States.

HMOs and PPOs. Many Americans hope that a health insurance law will be a lever to reshape the organization of hospitals, ambulatory medical care, and other providers. A favorite goal is to replace traditional office practice by HMOs. Some American NHI bills during the 1970s tried to give HMOs a preferential position and tried to steer patients into them. But that is not done in health insurance statutes abroad: as this book has explained, any licensed provider freely selected by a subscriber is eligible for full reimbursement, and no patient can be locked into one group.

Perhaps a PPO could survive under American statutory health insurance—

if the law requires or allows coinsurance. A physician could attract more patients by offering to waive the cost sharing. But as Belgium's experience suggests, such an option may create new complications: these doctors might encourage more visits and treatments, all "free" to the patient but more expensive to the system.

HMOs and PPOs exist in the United States at present only because there is no national health insurance law and because private insurers are free to create preferential arrangements with certain physicians. They are admired by policy-makers as instruments of cost containment. But a national health insurance system should not become so complex and so anticompetitive as to single out particular providers for special protection. Cost containment would be pursued by other methods.

Multispecialty groups and special panels might flourish if their mission were redefined. Financially, they would conform to the same reimbursement rules as other providers. Statutory health insurance would deal only with financing and would standardize it. Groups and panels could strive to offer the best quality and the best service to patients. Competition among American physician groups is already making these nonpecuniary appeals. Competition for patients among doctors and hospitals cannot reduce costs—as American experience already shows—but it can improve quality and service. This effort will require a system to identify and publicize quality; the groundwork has already begun.

Reinforcing or Reforming the Delivery System. If American NHI bills include extensive reorganization of the delivery system, their partisans will fight each other and nothing will be done about the problems of coverage, access, minimum benefits, and revenue raising. For example, the advocates of rival schemes during the 1970s had incompatible aims about how to restructure a supposedly inefficient delivery system—the Kennedy-Waxman Bill, the Ullman Bill, the Stockman-Gephardt Plan, the Enthoven Plan, and more. They found common ground only in rejecting the Carter administration's National Health Plan because of its modest effects on delivery structures.

In practice abroad, statutory health insurance has limited functions: it guarantees coverage and access to the entire population and guarantees recovery of costs of all acute-care providers. It pays every licensed hospital and doctor and—in the absence of other public policies—reinforces the status quo. To be enacted and implemented, the law requires the cooperation of the hospitals and doctors currently in practice. If the bill includes overt proposals to discriminate among providers or to reorganize all of them, the threatened providers will pro-test and the legislature will back away.

There may be severe weaknesses in the delivery system—an excessive number of beds, the maldistribution of physicians, and so on. These cannot be remedied by the health insurance system but require separate governmental and private efforts targeted on the specific problems. The results must then be coor-dinated with the insurance system: if a hospital plan tries to reduce the number of hospitals, for example, the sickness funds should not continue to pay those being phased out.

If health care needs drastic reorganization and creation of new services, the country should enact a national health service—that is, public ownership and management as well as financing—and not merely national health insurance. For this reason, Great Britain in 1948 and Italy in 1978 abandoned their limited health insurance systems in favor of national health services.

Long-Term Care. Acute-care health insurance accepts the established providers, eliminates financial barriers to access, and guarantees generous incomes. Doctors are accepted as case managers.

But long-term-care financing cannot be built on a traditional image of needs and services. The patient's problems are of several different types—implying a wider range of providers, practice settings, and financing methods. The nature of the problems is only recently being defined in public policy. Appropriate providers are in short supply. Unlike statutory acute-care health insurance, there has been no long history of private long-term-care financing that needs only to be regularized in law and in taxation.

While some have advocated a full-scale statutory program for long-term care—Medicare Part C—it is more likely that the coming years will be a period of reflection on the components of long-term care and a period of experimentation in financing. If enacted prematurely, a generous social insurance program cannot be cut back. At present, a number of private long-term-care insurance schemes are serving as a financing laboratory in the United States, and HCFA and private foundations support many demonstration projects in service delivery. No ready-made foreign precedents are available for a complete long-term-care system.

Simple and Clear Arrangements. Once a program is enacted, all patients, carriers, providers, and civil servants must understand it. This is possible only if the United States government abandons its custom of tinkering with every program every year and sending out an annual stream of voluminous and complex regulations. Public education is essential. It is also essential that Washington heed lessons from abroad such as the following two from France.

In 1988, the new French government-of-the-day amended the cost containment policy of its predecessor (the *Plan Séguin*). It added new conditions for exemption from patient cost sharing and added nuances to the old conditions. In the United States, such changes in Medicare would have made the system more complex and occasioned pages of new regulations in the *Federal Register*. In France, the reformers deliberately avoided making the arrangement more complicated. "Simplification" was a stated goal of the reform. The changes were issued in a few paragraphs in the *Journal Officiel* and in clearly written memoranda from the Ministry of Social Affairs.

During the mid-1980s, France replaced the per diem for hospital reimbursement by the global budget. The Ministry realized that the cooperation of all hospital doctors was essential. All throughout the country received explanatory modules and attended special local seminars explaining the new method. When I told leading American medical policymakers that hospital doctors and employees did not understand the new DRG payment system and were misinforming each other, the patients, and the public, and when I recommended emulation of the French method, the American policymakers saw no need.

New Thinking About Policy

Defining the Problem. The United States has a crisis not only in health financing policy but also in its policy analysis. The generation of economists who designed Social Security examined all the problems of income and living standards in the total society; they then designed appropriate institutions and processes for a national system. Of course, the results had to run the gauntlet of American pressure groups and legislators, but the original schemes and the policy analysts' perspective throughout the events were always societal and institutional.[19]

America now must correct the omission of health benefits from Social Security, but a different generation of economists and policy analysts now dominates. Instead of studying and designing actual institutions, they focus on idealized microeconomic buyer/seller relations. They are interested in technical efficiency in the allocation of resources, not in social justice. They believe that competition will achieve the best results in every way in every health market, and they oppose the machinery of social solidarity and professional organization. They recommend health financing based on the individual's use of his own money for his own self-interest, and they oppose redistributive financing for a social policy. Effort is poured into management consulting firms and research centers to support conferences, reports, and research projects addressed to interesting theoretical topics, but the result is to draw talent and focus away from the essential tasks of designing a system and distributing public resources according to social need.

Proposals. Because the United States lacks leadership to dramatize the urgency of a solution and formulate a single policy, there is a free market in proposals. Many study commissions and individuals now write schemes—each calculated to publicize its author over his competitors, each therefore designed to be unique. Since the country lacks any serious timetable to enact a solution, none of these schemes is scrutinized carefully to evaluate its administrative feasibility or likelihood of enactment and implementation. The endless series of proposals increases rather than reduces the uncertainty of the population and the caution of Congress.

Some proposals for universal health insurance attempt to preserve the American system despite its inherent contradictions. They mandate universal employer coverage. The goal is a private insurance market preserving free choice by patients, competition among insurers and providers, coverage of the population, and adequate financing of all benefits. To avoid the underfinancing, under-enrollment, gaps in benefits, and other weaknesses inherent in the current private group insurance market, the best-known schemes propose legislative and administrative rules of great number and complexity. The result is an ostensibly private market with massive government intervention.[20] Congress is unlikely to comprehend—much less enact—all the rules. If it were enacted, such an arrangement would be difficult for patients and providers to understand, it would be vulnerable to self-interested evasions, it would experience recurrent disputes, and it would require constant fine-tuning by Congress, by the executive branch, and by the courts.

During the late 1980s, a brief vogue commended "the Canadian model" for the United States.[21] Canada was said to have combined universal coverage, advanced clinical care, and stable costs. While very successful, Canada's methods have no chance of adoption in the United States since they use full government financing, not insurance. To prevent deficits in its general budget, government would have to force all organizations (such as hospitals and nursing homes) to operate under expenditure caps and would have to force all doctors to work under strict expenditure targets, as in Canada today. American hospitals and medical associations have heard the Canadian complaints about underfunding for decades and will desperately oppose transplanting them to the United States.

And if government pays the hospitals and doctors directly—as in Canada today—the private insurance industry would play no part (except for minor supplementary services). America's powerful insurance industry would oppose this design. A few proposals to reform American health care financing during the 1970s included such full government payments—for example, the Kennedy-Corman Bill—but none reached the floors of Congress. To avoid their fatal political veto, the Kennedy-Weicker-Waxman Bill of the 1980s preserved the role of the insurance companies as fiscal intermediaries.

Goals and Values. Creating a solution for the United States requires not only political will to enact an appropriate administrative apparatus but, above all, it requires dedication to certain values. Health care in all societies is a social system and not merely a personal service: it is designed to help the unfortunate and not only protect one's own self. Health care in all countries evolved out of religion, not out of commerce. The United States can continue to endorse self-interest in other economic markets. But it cannot resolve its difficulties in health care without institutionalizing social solidarity and compassion.

Americans also need to be reminded of professional norms. Health care is a humanitarian social service once delivered by religions and, in the modern era, by laymen supposedly devoted to the same ideals and governed by professional corporations. Money was supposed to provide the resources and suitable rewards. The goal of work was not supposed to be the maximization of personal incomes; the choices among patients and clinical methods were not supposed to follow differences in fees. Nothing could better demonstrate the bankruptcy of contemporary American health care policy thinking than the fact that it revolves around money. Health financing must be governed by professional ethics and strong professional responsibility, as well as by social justice. The best "incentive" for a health professional is to perform one's duty to society. That is no mere "exogenous factor."

Notes

1. The principal schemes during the 1970s are summarized in Karen Davis, *National Health Insurance: Benefits, Costs, and Consequences* (Washington: Brookings Institution, 1975), chap. 8; Saul Waldman, *National Health Insurance Proposals: Provisions of Bills Introduced in the Congress . . .*, rev. ed. (Washington: Office of Research and Statistics, Social Security Administration, U.S. Department of Health, Education, and Welfare, 1976); *National Health Insurance Working Papers* (Washington: Public Health Service, U.S. Department of Health and Human Services, 1980), 2 vols.; and Judith Feder and others, *Insuring the Nation's Health* (Washington: Urban Institute Press, 1981). Extensive hearings were held; see, for example, *National Health Insurance: Public Hearings Before the Subcommittee on Health of the Committee on Ways and Means, House of Representatives, 94th Congress, 1st Session* (Washington: Government Printing Office, 1975), 3 vols. The political deadlocks are described in Jonas Morris, *Searching for a Cure: National Health Policy Considered* (Washington: Berkeley Morgan, 1985), chaps. 2-3; and Benjamin Heineman and Curtis Hessler, *Memorandum for the President* (New York: Random House, 1980), pp. 266-301.

2. See, for example, Louis W. Sullivan, "Remarks by the Secretary of Health and Human Services to the Atlanta Business Roundtable" (Washington: U.S. Department of Health and Human Services, 1990); and William L. Roper, "Financing Health Care: A View from the White House," *Health Affairs*, vol. 8, no. 4 (Winter 1989), pp. 97-102.

3. During the 1980s, only a few policymakers invoked social solidarity as a guide to health financing reform. Their reports were quickly forgotten. See, for example, *Securing Access to Health Care: The Ethical Implications of Differences in the Availability of Health Services* (Washington: President's Commission for the Study of Ethical Problems in Medicine and Biomedical and Behavioral Research, 1983).

4. See, for example, Rashi Fein, *Medical Care, Medical Costs: The Search for a Health Insurance Policy* (Cambridge: Harvard University Press, 1986), chaps. 10-11.

5. The United States government is baffled not only by health but by all other domestic problems. America's declining ability to govern has become so obvious that it was the cover story of the leading newsmagazine: Stanley W. Cloud, "The Can't Do Government," *Time*, Oct. 23, 1989, pp. 28-32.

6. A few serious designs for an American National Health Service have

been proposed but ignored. See, for example, Leonard S. Rodberg, "Anatomy of a National Health Program: Reconsidering the Dellums Bill After 10 Years," *Health/PAC Bulletin*, vol. 17, no. 6 (Dec. 1987), pp. 12–16.

7. See, for example, Alain Enthoven and Richard Kronick, "A Consumer-Choice Health Plan for the 1990's," *New England Journal of Medicine*, vol. 320, no. 2 (Jan. 12, 1989), p. 94; and Stuart M. Butler and Edmund F. Haislmaier (eds.), *A National Health System for America* (Washington: Heritage Foundation, 1989), pp. 37–47.

8. In the present competitive market, health insurance has become concentrated in a few principal carriers. Historical trends are summarized in Albert Woodward, "The U.S. Health Insurance Industry: An Alternative View," *International Journal of Health Services*, vol. 8, no. 3 (1978), pp. 491–507. During the intense competition of the 1980s, several stopped offering individual (that is, nongroup) policies and some dropped out of health completely.

9. William Glaser, *Paying the Hospital* (San Francisco: Jossey-Bass, 1987), pp. 91–92.

10. William Glaser, *Health Insurance Bargaining* (New York: Gardner Press and John Wiley, 1978), pp. 100–102.

11. Explained in William Glaser, "Lessons from Germany," *Journal of Health Politics, Policy and Law*, vol. 8, no. 1 (Summer 1983), pp. 359–361.

12. William Glaser, "The Politics of Paying Physicians," *Health Affairs*, vol. 8, no. 3 (Fall 1989), pp. 129–146, and vol. 8, no. 4 (Winter 1989), pp. 87–96.

13. The demoralization of the American medical profession because of the administration of reimbursement is so obvious that it became the theme of a series of essays in the country's leading newspaper: "Doctors in Distress," *New York Times*, Feb. 18, 19, and 20, 1990.

14. Philip J. Harter, "Negotiated Regulations: A Cure for Malaise," *Georgetown Law Journal*, vol. 71, no. 1 (Oct. 1982), pp. 1–118; David M. Pritzker (ed.), *Sourcebook on Negotiated Rulemaking* (Washington: Administrative Conference of the United States, 1989); and the speeches by Senators Levin and Grassley upon introduction of the Negotiated Rulemaking Act of 1988, *Congressional Record—Senate*, July 17, 1987, pp. S10209–S10213, and April 12, 1988, pp. S3818, S3822.

15. Possible structures for American statutory health insurance are in Glaser, *Health Insurance Bargaining* (see note 10, above), pp. 197–201. Possible national/state arrangements in other American health programs are described in William Glaser, *Federalism in Canada and West Germany: Foreign Lessons for the United States* (New York: Center for Social Sciences, Columbia University, 1979; distributed by the National Technical Information Service), especially chap. 16.

16. For examples see Timothy Jost, "Administrative Law Issues Involving the Medicare Utilization and Quality-Control Peer Review Organization (PRO) Program," *Ohio State Law Journal*, vol. 50, no. 1 (1989), pp. 5–37, 53–60; *Medicare Carrier Assessment of New Technologies*, OA1-01-88-00010 (Washington:

Office of Inspector General, Department of Health and Human Services, 1989); and many reports in many fields by the General Accounting Office.

17. The unhappy experiences in Italy have been described here in Chapter Six.

18. Raymond Munts, *Bargaining for Health* (Madison: University of Wisconsin Press, 1967), pt. 1.

19. I. M. Rubinow, *The Quest for Security* (New York: Henry Holt, 1934), especially chaps. 35–36, 40, 46; and J. Douglas Brown, *An American Philosophy of Social Security* (Princeton: Princeton University Press, 1972), especially chap. 1.

20. Alain Enthoven and Richard Kronick, "A Consumer-Choice Health Plan for the 1990's," *New England Journal of Medicine*, vol. 320, nos. 1 and 2 (Jan. 5 and 12, 1989), pp. 29–37, 94–101; and Alain Enthoven, "Management of Competition in the FEHBP," *Health Affairs*, vol. 8, no. 3 (Fall 1989), pp. 33–50.

21. David U. Himmelstein and others, "A National Health Program for the United States," *New England Journal of Medicine*, vol. 320, no. 2 (Jan. 12, 1989), pp. 102–108; and David U. Himmelstein and Steffie Woolhandler, "Socialized Medicine: A Solution to the Cost Crisis in Health Care in the United States," *International Journal of Health Services*, vol. 16, no. 3 (1986), pp. 339–354.

APPENDIX A

Principal
Countries Studied

This book has been written analytically and avoids country-by-country descriptions. The reader can find many books and articles describing individual countries at length. The principal sources are listed below.

Table A.1 surveys the separate statutory health insurance programs in the countries in this research. I do not present a compendium of statistics for each, because it can be found elsewhere: Jean-Pierre Poullier, *Health OECD* (Paris: Organization for European Cooperation and Development, 1991). Table A1 gives an overview. The entries are brief. Similar charts with full administrative details about each country exist for attributes of the statutory health insurance systems:

☐ Payroll tax rates by occupation
☐ Eligibility rules by occupation, age, and relation to breadwinner
☐ Special rules for pensioners
☐ Qualifying period before start of eligibility
☐ Commencement and duration of each benefit
☐ Specific benefits: physician's care, hospitals, dentistry, pharmaceutical drugs, prostheses, and so on
☐ Disability benefits: short-term and long-term pensions
☐ Social security generally

These detailed charts can be found in:

> *Comparative Tables of the Social Security Schemes in the Member States of the European Communities: General Scheme* (Luxembourg: Office for Official Publications of the European Communities, periodically updated).

Table A.1. Key Indicators of Insurance Programs Studied.

Indicator	West Germany	France	Netherlands	Belgium	Switzerland	United States
Population, estimated in 000's, midyear 1987	61,077	55,627	14,671	9,868	6,619	243,934
Per capita spending on health in 1987 (in US$ standardized by GDP purchasing power parities)	1,071	1,087	1,037	876	1,248	2,061
Proportion of GDP spent on health in 1987	8.2%	8.6%	8.5%	7.2%	7.7%	11.2%
Year of NHI law	1883	1928	1941	1944	1911 (*Bund* grants to carriers)	1965 (Medicare)
Original basis of sickness funds	Occupational	Occupational	Diverse	Ideological, religious	Mutual insurance companies	Diverse
Number of sickness funds in each area	Several	Very few, one principal	One or a few	Several	Several	Many
General Treasury subsidies to sickness funds	Almost none	Recently began	Yes	Yes	Yes	Only Medicare Part B
Family or individual coverage	Family	Family	Family	Family	Each individual separately	Entire family; insured worker and family separately; or each individual separately
Approximate proportion of population (late 1980s)						
Obligatory coverage	79%	98%	51%	98%	25%	13% (Medicare)
Voluntary membership in social insurance carriers	12%	0	19%	1%	71%	0
Voluntary membership in private insurance companies	7%	1.5%	30%	1%	2%	66%
Not insured	2%	0.5%	0.1%	0	2%	21% (including Medicaid)
Benefit coverage standard for all	Yes (for those covered by NHI)	Yes	Yes (for those covered by NHI)	Yes	Yes	Only for those covered by Medicare
Patient cost sharing in NHI						
Deductibles	No	No	No	No	No	Yes
Coinsurance or copayments	Almost none	Yes	No	Yes	Yes	Yes
Payment of NHI cost sharing by supplementary private insurance	No	Yes	Does not apply	No	No	Yes
Balance-billing under NHI by:						
Hospitals	No	No	No	No	No	No
Doctors	No	A few	No	Yes	No	Yes

Comparative Tables of the Social Security Systems in Council of Europe Member States Not Belonging to the European Communities (Strasbourg: Council of Europe, periodically updated).

Social Security Programs Throughout the World (Washington: Social Security Administration, biennial).

For a detailed comparative chart about hospital reimbursement, see my *Paying the Hospital* (app. A).

The following books are collections of descriptions of health services and health financing in several countries. Chapters cover many of the countries in this research.

Report on the World Health Situation (Geneva: World Health Organization, quadrennial).

Brian Abel-Smith (ed.), *Eurocare* (Basel: Health Service Consultants, 1984).

Marshall W. Raffel (ed.), *Comparative Health Systems* (University Park: Pennsylvania State University Press, 1984).

Richard B. Saltman (ed.), *The International Handbook of Health-Care Systems* (Westport, Conn.: Greenwood Press, 1988).

Markus Schneider and others, *Gesundheitssysteme im internationalen Vergleich* (Bonn: Bundesminister für Arbeit und Sozialordnung, 1990).

Eurohealth Handbook (New York: Robert S. First, periodically updated).

Jack Paul DeSario (ed.), *International Public Policy Sourcebook* (Westport, Conn.: Greenwood Press, 1989), vol. 1.

Odin Anderson, *The Health Services Continuum in Democratic States* (Ann Arbor: Health Administration Press, 1989).

Chapter Four gave an overview of the structure of health insurance. Following are more detailed descriptions of the principal countries.

Germany

Sickness Funds. For centuries, social protection in Europe was organized by guilds and other associations of workers. This structure survives in Germany.[1] To the other functions of their guilds, all masters, journeymen, and apprentices in a particular trade in a medieval German town might have added cash benefits during illness. Examples were the separate guilds for butchers, tanners, bakers, and goldsmiths. These arrangements remain as carriers under modern health insurance: the "crafts sickness funds," or *Innungskrankenkassen.* The small funds in each city have merged, since only larger ones are financially viable, and each carrier now combines all the handicraft employers and workers in the region.[2]

During the Middle Ages and later, mining was organized like other crafts:

the owners and employees worked side by side. Since they were not town-dwellers, they did not organize typical guilds, but miners in many communities formed "brotherhoods" or *Knappschäfte*. Because of the high rates of mortality and disability, each *Knappschaft* provided cash benefits to disabled members, widows, and orphans. During the nineteenth century, they offered medical care by bringing doctors to the mining communities. The Prussian government during the nineteenth century admired the *Knappschäfte*, since nearly all Prussian miners had joined voluntarily and the employers contributed premiums and management help. When the Prussian government enacted workmen's compensation laws beginning in 1838, it allowed the *Knappschaftskassen* to administer the program in the mining industry and encouraged employers to create the same arrangements in all other industries. All these sickness funds eventually became the carriers both for statutory health insurance and for the employers' liability for accidents at work.[3]

The new German national government enacted obligatory health insurance for workers in 1883. Instead of assigning administration to a special agency of the national government—Bismarck's preference for the pension and work accident systems—administration was assigned to the many sickness funds already in existence for craftsmen, miners, sailors, and industry. Many employers created "workplace sickness funds" (*Betriebskrankenkassen*) for their individual work forces. The employers contributed administrative support and part of the premiums. These sickness funds were the most numerous in Germany, but the average size was small.[4]

After World War II, obligatory health insurance was enacted for farmers. Some sickness funds had already existed in rural areas and were superseded by a substantial network of agricultural sickness funds (*Landwirtschaftliche Krankenkassen*) for self-employed farmers and farm workers.[5]

Because the law requires widespread coverage of the population and recognizes all the foregoing occupational sickness funds as primary carriers, the law must create a fallback for those without occupational funds. Therefore, every section of the country has an "area sickness fund" (an *Ortskrankenkasse*) for those without primary affiliations.[6] Some countries permit free choice of basic carriers, but assignment in Germany is automatic under the law:

☐ If someone is a farmer, miner, or sailor, he and his family must join one of those sickness funds. (At present there is one national fund for miners and one for sailors.)

☐ If he works in a craft and an appropriate *Innungskrankenkasse* exists in the area, he and his family must join it.

☐ If his workplace has a *Betriebskrankenkasse*, he and his family are automatically assigned to it.

☐ He and his family are automatically assigned to the local *Ortskrankenkasse* if:

- None of the obligatory funds are available to him.

- The *Betriebskrankenkasse* at his workplace is dissolved and is not absorbed by another *Betriebskrankenkasse*. His original fund can disappear either because it goes bankrupt or because the business firm goes out of existence.
- He changes jobs and the new employer has no *Betriebskrankenkasse*.

Blue-collar workers must join a particular sickness fund according to the foregoing rules. In Germany, as in other countries, white-collar workers and other salaried employees were added at a later time. In most countries from the start or during later legislative reforms, the white-collar and other salaried workers are included in the general regime and are treated like everyone else. In Germany, they have the right to refuse automatic assignment to a *Betriebskrankenkasse* or *Ortskrankenkasse* and instead can join a "substitute fund" (an *Ersatzkasse*). They must join something; they cannot self-insure.

The *Ersatzkassen* were formerly mutual insurance companies for the large number of managers, white-collar employees, and self-employed not yet covered by statutory health insurance. When some managers and white-collar workers were added to the obligatory system, these insurance carriers were given the option of keeping their enrollment under the official scheme or competing for the remaining business in the private market. The *Ersatzkassen* operate completely under statutory health insurance and must conform to its rules: like the other sickness funds, they cannot earn profits, cannot refuse eligible applicants even if bad risks, cannot charge extra premiums of applicants in bad health, cannot advertise or pay salesmen, and must contribute to the equalization funds described in Chapter Nine.[7] The numbers of sickness funds and their shares of total coverage appear in Table A.2.

A social insurance system based on occupation inevitably changes as the economy evolves. Germany once had thousands of *Betriebskrankenkassen*, but

Table A.2. German Sickness Funds in 1989.

Type of fund	Number of sickness funds	Distribution of subscribers
Ortskrankenkasse	269	44.1%
Betriebskrankenkasse	722	11.6
Innungskrankenkasse	155	5.1
Landwirtschaftliche Krankenkasse	19	2.1
Bundesknappschaft	1	2.7
Seekrankenkasse	1	0.1
Ersatzkasse	15	34.3
Totals	1,182	100.0%
Total number of subscribers (not including dependents)	(36,544,069)	

Source: Data extracted from Bundesministerium für Jugend, Familie, und Gesundheit, *Daten des Gesundheitswesens—Ausgabe 1989* (Stuttgart: Verlag W. Kohlhammer, 1989), pp. 225–226.

the number diminishes every year. These funds were created by employers and trade unions in the older smokestack industries with stable and cohesive labor forces. But whenever such an employer goes out of business, its sickness fund is automatically dissolved and all its members are automatically transferred to the local *Ortskrankenkasse*. If the company is absorbed by another with an established *Betriebskrankenkasse*, the latter must take the active workers and the retirees. But if the business firms' merger takes the form of a new national headquarters, standing above many divisions, the more prosperous sickness funds in the network can allow the less prosperous ones to go bankrupt, and the workers and retirees go to the *Ortskrankenkasse*. New companies with younger labor forces and no retirees may create new *Betriebskrankenkassen*, since their experience-rated payroll taxes for those workers are lower than the community-rated payroll taxes for the *Ortskrankenkasse*, where the workers would otherwise belong. But few new *Betriebskrankenkassen* are created: new companies are too small for viable free-standing sickness funds; modern employers do not wish to help administer complicated health carriers; health care costs can quickly exceed predictions; many employers are ideologically opposed to social insurance.

As white-collar employment grows in the German economy, the membership in the *Ersatzkassen* steadily rises. The white-collar and management members of *Betriebskrankenkassen* and *Ortskrankenkassen* alone can choose. Many switch, because the younger and more genteel membership of the *Ersatzkassen* results in lower premiums, higher benefits, greater attentiveness by doctors, and greater social prestige. Self-employed craftsmen once assigned automatically to the *Innungskrankenkassen* sometimes switch to the *Ersatzkassen*. Other low-income self-employed after World War II were added to obligatory health insurance, and many prefer the *Ersatzkassen* to the *Ortskrankenkassen*. The once diffuse occupational structure of German health insurance is being eclipsed by a bipolar distribution between the *Ortskrankenkassen* and the *Ersatzkassen*.

The decline in market share by the *Ortskrankenkassen* and the *Betriebskrankenkassen* was reversed temporarily during the 1990s by the reunification of Germany. West German statutory health insurance and the system of autonomous sickness funds were extended throughout East Germany. Enrollment at first grew most among the *Orts-* and *Betriebskrankenkassen*. Eventually the *Ersatzkassen* will grow there too.

Private Insurance Companies. The only Germans with complete freedom of choice are the salaried employees with high earnings, the self-employed with high incomes, and the higher ranks of the civil service. They may choose among voluntary enrollment in the ordinary sickness funds, voluntary enrollment in the *Ersatzkassen*, self-insurance, or buying a policy from a private insurance company. The earnings threshold for salaried employees and the urban self-employed rises each year; in 1989, it was 54,900 DM. The earnings threshold for self-employed farmers was 60,000 DM.

The number of eligible persons rises or falls annually, depending on whether the earnings ceiling rises more quickly or more slowly than the German population's earnings. Despite the increasing prosperity of the German population, the private companies' market share gradually diminished during the 1960s and 1970s. The earnings ceiling rose rapidly—in order to keep prosperous employees in the statutory health insurance tax base—and the chief gainers were the *Ersatzkassen*. Many of those free to choose now remain in the *Ersatzkassen* or in the social sickness funds where they had been before they surpassed the earnings ceiling. The private companies regained some market share during the 1980s— largely because the civil service grew and because young and healthy salaried employees were attracted by cheap policies with benefits limited to large bills. During the late 1980s, about 20 percent of the German population could choose freely. About 10 percent was left to the private companies, since over 6 percent of the German population were free-choosers who selected the *Ersatzkassen* and nearly 4 percent were free-choosers who picked the social sickness funds.

Staying voluntarily with the *Ersatzkassen* and social sickness funds can be advantageous. They charge high percentage-of-earnings payroll taxes, but they offer full family coverage with complete benefits. Since the family must buy a separate *private* policy for each member, the total can be substantial—particularly if it wants the complete coverage comparable to that of the statutory system. If a person gains free choice late in life, he must join the private company at high lifelong premiums—explained in Chapter Seven—and the *Ersatzkassen* and social sickness funds do not seem so much more expensive.

Once privately insured persons could choose to return to the *Ortskrankenkassen*, which were obligated to accept them. In old age, the subscriber thereby gained more comprehensive and cheaper coverage. The option was advantageous to the insurance companies: after having collected lifelong premiums capitalized to cover the subscriber in old age, the company was free of further costs but was not required to refund past overpayments. The *Ortskrankenkassen* were saddled with additional expensive patients. During the reforms of the late 1980s, the option was eliminated. If a subscriber has been paying a private company for many years, he must keep the policy in old age, and the carrier must provide the benefits purchased. The reform was one of the measures enacted to protect the social insurance sector from the drawbacks of a competitive market.

Forty-two private carriers sold health insurance in Germany in 1989, divided as follows:

Type	Number	Percentage of premium income
Mutual insurance company	26	51%
Stock corporation	15	45
Public corporation	1	4
	42	100%

All companies must specialize in health alone, and all must keep their accounts separate from other lines of business. Some stock companies belong to conglomerates with other lines. Profits go to the shareholders of the stock companies and to the policyholders of the mutual companies, either in dividends to all subscribers or in bonuses to those subscribers who filed no claims. The industry is highly concentrated. Three firms have over one-third of all premium income.

All companies sell supplementary insurance policies to members of the *Ersatzkassen* and social sickness funds, as well as selling full coverage to those free to choose the private market. About 8 percent of the population is covered by statutory health insurance for mainstream protection and also buys supplementary benefits from the private companies.[8]

France

As in other countries during the nineteenth century, the craftsmen and workers of France had many mutual aid funds. They were numerous—over five thousand at times—and small. They provided cash benefits during unemployment, illness, and retirement. Some maintained health centers and employed doctors, but most reimbursed subscribers after visits by independent physicians. During the political compromises permitting enactment of statutory health insurance in 1928, the mutual aid funds were retained as carriers. But they were too small and poorly managed to be efficient. A war aim of the Resistance was creation of expanded and efficient social security in all forms.[9]

Sickness Funds. Writing on a clean slate, the drafters of the new social security system in 1945 at first intended a simple structure of government funds (*caisses*) that would administer all benefits for all covered occupations. But simple streamlined arrangements never emerge from any political process—even in France, the democracy with the strongest tradition of centralized government, pervasive top-down regulation throughout the country, and equal treatment of all affected groups. During the debates of 1945–1948, groups interested in certain sets of benefits (such as family allowances) insisted on separate *caisses* with earmarked payroll taxes to prevent the money going to more expensive programs. Occupations with established pension programs offering benefits better than the ones generally proposed in 1945—civil servants, miners, railwaymen, and others—insisted on retaining these better arrangements, protected by their own pension *caisses*. Other groups depending on financial transfers, public subsidies, and lower patient cost sharing—such as farm workers—pressed for their own *caisses* under their control. The result was a very large number of nominally governmental *caisses* in different fields of social protection—all dominated by their occupational interest groups and by the political parties through election of the governing boards.

After several reorganizations, the many *caisses* for the majority of citizens were placed under a single hierarchy (the *régime générale*). All employed persons are required to join, from the poorest to the richest, with a few exceptions assigned to special regimes. Separate hierarchies of *caisses* deal with health insurance, pensions, and family allowances in this and all other regimes. In the general regime, a *caisse primaire* in health insurance administers the affairs of subscribers and pays money to providers. The local funds report to the regional coordinating offices, which in turn are directed by a *Caisse National de l'Assurance Maladie* (CNAMTS) located in Paris. The national office is regulated and monitored by the national government Ministry responsible for social security (at present the *Ministère des Affaires Sociales et d'Emploi*). All employees of the *caisses* are civil servants paid from tax funds.

Several other occupations pressed Parliament to retain their own regimes outside the general one. Some differences in benefits or taxes result, usually to their advantage. The headquarters and the grass-roots *caisses* in a few occupations (such as railroads) are government agencies staffed by civil servants, supported by tax revenue, and overseen by government Ministries. In most special regimes, such as agriculture and the self-employed, both the headquarters and the *caisses* are legally private entities performing a public service.[10] The *mutualités* and private insurance companies that had been the health and pension carriers for the farmers and self-employed continue under the special regimes. They are empowered to administer public money, they must follow laws and regulations, they are audited by government, but otherwise they fiercely resist government "interference."

Once the political decision was made to preserve the private entities in these special regimes, the injection of much new social security revenue and the expansion of coverage resulted in creation of many new nongovernmental social insurance funds. (In addition, as later paragraphs will explain, the *mutualités* and private insurance companies now flourish as carriers for supplementary benefits in both the general and special regimes.) The result is a bewildering mosaic. France demonstrates that governmentalization is not synonymous with simplification and standardization. The distribution of the French population among the regimes in 1987 appears in Table A.3.

In other countries, sickness funds are forced to merge if some can no longer attract new members and some are overloaded with expensive members. These pressures do not exist in France: the citizen cannot shop among the regimes for his basic care but is assigned automatically to one appropriate to his occupation. *Caisses* with adverse dependency ratios survive because of interfund transfers and public subsidies. Since the interest groups prefer to keep their special regimes, the mélange of *caisses* will survive for a long time.

The Mutuelles. One might have expected the *sociétés mutualités* to disappear after 1945, when mainstream financial administration was given to the new public corporations. Nevertheless, some niches remain in the French health insurance system, and the *mutuelles*—as they were recently renamed—fill them:[11]

☐ *Insurance of cost sharing.* France has more cost sharing by patients than any other statutory health insurance system. If one pays subscription fees to a *mutuelle,* the fund covers his cost sharing in full. This role is the same as the insurance of American Medicare's cost sharing by the Medigap policies of the Blues and commercial carriers.

☐ *Administration of billing.* France has one of the few reimbursement systems of any statutory health insurance systems: the provider bills the patient, the patient pays the provider, the patient is reimbursed by the *caisse primaire.* Since the *mutuelle* member lets the *mutuelle* handle all this, he does not have to lay out any cash or keep track of the documents and rules: his provider mails the bill to his *mutuelle,* the *mutuelle* checks that the bill conforms to the reimbursement rules of statutory health insurance, the *mutuelle* then bills the *caisse primaire,* and the *caisse primaire* reimburses the *mutuelle* the official rates less the patient's cost sharing. The difference is the contribution by the *mutuelle.*

☐ *Services for statutory health insurance.* Many *mutuelles* maintain pharmacies and dental clinics for their own members, either alone or in cooperation with each other. Some manage health centers and hospitals with salaried physicians. The *mutuelle* member may gain in convenience and in cash if he uses these facilities: the *mutuelle* may insist on some cost sharing if he patronizes doctors and pharmacies in the community. Some of the *mutuelle* services—such as the psychiatric day hospitals created by the national educational *mutuelle* (MGEN)—are the best in the country. These prepaid services of the *mutuelles* are the last European vestige of the closed panels that have disappeared under statutory health insurance but have survived across the Atlantic in the American HMO.

☐ *Long-term care.* All countries realize the need for nonacute services for the elderly. As Chapter Fifteen reported, all grope for the best method of orga-

Table A.3. French Sickness Funds in 1987.

Regime	Distribution of entire French population
Employed earners of wages and salaries (*régime générale*)	78.4%
Self-employed	6.0
Farmers and farm workers	9.2
Railroad managers and workers	2.1
Miners	0.9
Nine other special regimes	3.4
	100.0%
Total numbers of subscribers and dependents	(57,862,000)

Source: Statistiques des régimes d'assurance maladie en 1988, Carnets Statistiques no. 52 (Paris: Caisse Nationale de l'Assurance Maladie des Travailleurs Salariés, 1989), pp. 108, 111.

nizing and financing these services. Some French *mutuelles* now offer long-term-care services to their members and (for fees) to the public.

☐ *Ideological movement.* In a society where businessmen, the professions, and farmers were individualistic and self-interested, the *mutuelles* formed a nationwide sodial movement preaching social solidarity and defending the social security system against any cutbacks. Their meetings and publications—led by the national headquarters of their *Fédération Nationale de la Mutualité Française*—have been important reasons for the general commitment to social solidarity in the social services by a population that otherwise thinks and acts very differently. The *mutuelles* have been valuable local cadres for the Socialist Party.

☐ *Extra benefits.* The *mutuelles* always could offer additional health and social benefits not fully covered by statutory health insurance—such as convalescent care, dentistry, long-term care, and death benefits. During the 1980s, the private commercial health insurance carriers invaded the *mutuelles's* niche by selling policies to cover the cost sharing under social security and by offering convalescent care, dentistry, and the like. The *mutuelles* retaliated by obtaining amendments to government regulations allowing them to invade the private companies' turf by offering life insurance, accident insurance, and pensions.

☐ *Special regimes.* During the legislative battles of the mid- and late 1940s, the self-employed businessmen, professionals, farmers, and civil servants obtained separate arrangements like the prewar schemes: a government agency oversees the management and financial accounts of the sector; occupational *mutuelles* administer the money at the grass roots like *caisses primaires* in the general regime. Every citizen in each sector—for example, every self-employed person and his family—must participate, but he has free choice of carrier. In addition, each *mutuelle* can offer insurance to cover the cost sharing and supplementary benefits. These special regimes in France operate like mainstream health insurance in Belgium; their *mutuelles,* like those in Belgium, have become large and prosperous.

Mutuelle membership seemed less valuable after transfer of mainstream functions to the *caisses* in the 1940s. Around 1960, only about one-third of the French population belonged. Unexpectedly, membership since then has steadily increased and approached four-fifths of the population in 1988. An incentive has been the increased out-of-pockets required by statutory health insurance. One's medical bills now are divided between one's *caisse* and *mutuelle.* [12]

Small *mutuelles* for the workers in individual business firms or for special health risks disappear every year. More than 22,000 *mutuelles* existed in 1930, but there are fewer than 6,500 today. Consolidation continues: three-quarters now have fewer than 1,000 members; one-quarter have fewer than 50 adherents; fifty-seven *mutuelles* with more than 100,000 subscribers have more than half the members in France and nearly half the business. [13] The trends are toward nationwide *mutuelles* representing one economic sector (such as education) and toward regional *mutuelles* with members from many similar occupations.

Private Insurance Companies. France has a very large private insurance industry. One hundred companies specialize in life insurance and also offer coverage in work accidents, auto accidents, and short-term disability. Many are affiliated with insurers of property damage. The life insurance companies offer health insurance: full coverage as the carriers for the self-employed and farm proprietors under statutory insurance; supplementary coverage for other employees belonging to CNAMTS and other sickness funds.

If the self-employed subscriber buys full coverage from the private insurance company under statutory health insurance, the carrier—like every *caisse*—pays the hospital directly (*tiers payant*) and reimburses the patient for physicians' claims (*tiers garant*). The list of benefits is the same as in the rest of statutory health insurance. The members of the regime for the self-employed (CANAM) have higher cost-sharing rates—50 percent and not 30 percent—for physicians, dentists, and several other benefits since they pay lower premium rates.

Unlike the *mutuelles'* coverage of exact statutory cost sharing in their supplementary market, the private companies' supplementary policies provide cash upon hospitalization or upon physicians' visits—the amount of cash depends on the premiums of the policy bought. Such sliding scales are common in all private insurance markets. The French patient may use the money to cover the official cost sharing, buy extra amenities and private rooms during hospitalization, or cover the extra-billing allowed for some doctors.

The insurance carriers are diverse: six are nationalized companies legally owned by the French national government; fifty-eight are for-profit stock companies; and sixteen are mutual insurance companies. The nationalized companies are very large and sell half of the country's life insurance.[14] Two-thirds of the insurance companies' life and related business is sold under group contracts between employers and carriers. Instead of organizing a *mutuelle* to administer supplementary health insurance separately, the employer and employees are content to let their life insurance carrier cover the supplementary health benefits as well, just like any *mutuelle*. The employees and not the employer must pay the premiums individually. While a *mutuelle* usually offers full benefits at standard premiums, the private insurance companies offer policies with various combinations of coverage and premiums. Employers with healthy young white-collar workers and managers increasingly have contracts with the insurance companies, since the employees can opt for limited benefits and lower premiums.

It is the employees and not the employers who choose between creating their own *mutuelle* or allowing the life insurance or pension company contracting with the employer to add supplementary health insurance. The law provides for a vote of the workers. If the workers are represented by a militant trade union (such as the *Confédération Générale du Travail* or CGT), they create their own *mutuelle* allied to the union, rather than give business to an insurance company.

(The workers employed by some insurance companies therefore have created their own *mutuelles*.)

The insurance companies energetically sought supplementary health insurance business during the 1970s and 1980s. Their group life and auto insurance contracts gave them access to employers and the salaried employees. By 1988, the private companies had gained a significant foothold: among workers and employees, the companies had about one-fifth of the supplementary market, the *mutuelles* had nearly three-quarters, and other organizations (chiefly pension managers) had the rest; in the special full-service regime for the self-employed (CANAM), the insurance companies covered one-third and *mutuelles* had nearly three-fifths.[15]

The Netherlands

Sickness Funds. Before Holland enacted statutory health insurance during the 1940s, it had hundreds of mutual assistance arrangements and insurance companies. Some—those that appealed to diverse groups in large cities or enlisted members from several regions—were large. Most were small, consisting of prepaid agreements between a general practitioner and a few subscribers in a town, or the workers in a single workplace, or the members of a religious congregation. Their character was diverse: some were sectarian, reflecting the religious basis of much of Dutch social protection; some were associated with the labor movement; some were secular prepayment arrangements organized by doctors.

The enactment of statutory health insurance during the 1940s required order. The law specified standards for recognition as carriers under the system. Many small carriers merged in order to become viable financially and administratively. During the first registration in the late 1940s, some 205 sickness funds qualified. Funds of a similar type created national federations to perform several functions: exchange technical advice; petition the government and the new *Ziekenfondsraad;* enable a subscriber to obtain benefits if he took sick outside his locality; and so on. Persons under a certain earnings ceiling were required to subscribe to statutory health insurance. They could select any sickness fund. The carriers were very competitive, with only one restriction: if the subscriber picked a fund sponsored by one or a few general practitioners, he was locked into them.

Dutch sickness funds steadily merged. By 1958, there were 117 registered funds distributed among the associations listed in Table A.4. By the 1970s, only ninety sickness funds existed throughout the country. By the late 1980s, all sickness funds within nearly every community had merged. Only a few large cities, such as Amsterdam, had two or three. During the late 1970s, all the associations merged into the Union of Dutch Sickness Funds (the *Vereniging van Nederlandse Ziekenfondsen* or VNZ).[16]

Private Insurance Companies. Until the 1990s, about 60 percent of the Dutch population—sometimes less—was required to join statutory health insur-

Table A.4. Dutch Sickness Funds in 1958.

Association	Sponsorship	Number of funds	Distribution of socially insured
Centrale Bond van Onderling Beheerde Ziekenfondsen	Mutual aid funds of secular workers	29	21.5%
Bond van Rooms-Katholieke Ziekenfondsen in Nederland	Catholic trade unions	5	9.6
Stichting Autonome Ziekenfondsen	Catholic mutual aid movement	6	7.3
Het overleg van Ondernemingsziekenfondsen	Employers	21	3.0
Federatie van door Verzekerden en Medewerkers bestuurde Ziekenfondsen	Physicians	50	44.4
Organisatie van Algemene Ziekenfondsen in Nederland	Physicians' associations	4	13.4
Nederlandse Bond van Ziekenfondsen	Commercial life insurance	2	0.8
Totals		117	100.0%
Total number of subscribers		(8,069,000)	

Source: Data extracted from L. V. Ledeboer, "Medical Care in the Netherlands," *Bulletin of the International Social Security Association,* vol. 11, no. 9 (Sept. 1958), pp. 401–402. In addition, two small sickness funds were registered under social security but were not affiliated with any association.

ance. The rest could join the sickness funds voluntarily, buy full benefits from private companies, or self-insure. Thirty percent or more selected private carriers, providing a large market.

During the late 1980s, health insurance was sold by thirty-three stock companies, nineteen mutual insurance companies, and six agencies affiliated with sickness funds (colloquially called *bovenbouw* or "superstructures"). The stock companies and mutual insurance companies were multiline in nonlife as well as life business. At one time, private health insurance was overwhelmingly dominated by a few mutual insurance companies (such as Nationale Nederlanden), and they remain the largest. During the 1970s and early 1980s, several stock companies added health lines, offering policies with lower premiums and higher cost sharing, designed to attract young subscribers away from the mutuals. The market became less concentrated.

A person had to enter the private market as soon as his annual income rose above an annual earnings ceiling (f. 50,150 in 1989). Earlier, during his childhood or employment, he belonged to a sickness fund. Almost two-fifths remained in their sickness funds as voluntary subscribers. The others were attracted to the private carriers by the lower premiums. To keep these subscribers within their orbits, consortia of sickness funds created their own mutual insurance companies (the *bovenbouw*) offering the same private policies—that is, sliding scales with lower premiums for lower coverage.

Almost 40 percent of the private market consisted of group contracts between employers and insurance companies. The employers paid half or more of the group premium and the participating employees contributed the rest. The remainder of the private market consisted of individual policies. In those cases, the employer gave the employee extra cash along with his paycheck, and the employee picked his own carrier. In all group and individual contracts, each person could select either personal or family coverage.

The reforms of the 1990s eliminated the distinction between social insurance and the private market. Statutory health insurance and its payroll taxes now apply to everyone regardless of income. The distinction between sickness funds and private insurance companies was abolished, but all must be nonprofit. The for-profit stock companies wishing to participate in statutory health insurance reorganized as mutual insurance companies. All are entitled to offer both first-tier statutory health insurance coverage and second-tier supplementary policies. The social insurance market again has become competitive.

Belgium

Sickness Funds. As in other European countries, a mosaic of guilds and mutual protection funds existed for centuries. In France and much of Belgium, they were abolished by the anticorporatist governments of the Revolution and then Napoleon, but the social protection groupings (the *mutualités*) revived during the nineteenth century. They were associations of workmen in a locality;

some were drawn from places and tried to expand their base by recruiting workers from different occupations. The Catholic church had managed hospitals and social protection programs for centuries, and they encouraged some *mutualités*, but most were not yet involved in politics and religion.

Industrialization and electoral democracy introduced ideology into working-class politics during the final decades of the nineteenth century. Marxists and other Socialists captured existing *mutualités* and organized new ones. At first, particularly in industrial Wallonia, the Socialist Parties were underorganized and underfinanced. The local *mutualité* became an ideal place to meet, discuss, recruit new followers, and conduct each community's election campaigns.

The Catholic Church matched the Socialists' appeal to the working class. It took over existing *mutualités* and organized new ones, in both Wallonia and Flanders. The Socialist and Catholic movements became large conglomerates of trade unions, political parties, and associations of all sorts, including the sickness funds. Eventually the *mutualités* handled the largest budgets and were called colloquially "the bankers of the political parties." To the present day, the meetings of the Socialist *mutualités* are marked by red flags, calls for fundamental economic change, and the singing of "The Internationale"; the Christian *mutualités* still hear prayers delivered by priests and relate their social insurance functions to the protection of the Christian family.

While most *mutualités* were being politicized by the Socialists and Catholics, some were organized by those preferring Liberal politics—that is, non-Marxist secular ideology and free-market economics. Other *mutualités* were organized by those who wished social insurance to remain entirely free of political and ideological ornaments.

Belgium did not enact obligatory health insurance until 1945.[17] After 1894, it tried to encourage widespread voluntary subscription by means of government subsidies to the *mutualités*. A citizen could join any recognized sickness fund and was free to transfer. The funds therefore competed for members. Each was open to all occupations, emphasized its ideological image, but also tried to enlist dissenters by keeping premiums low and benefits high. When health insurance became obligatory, the *mutualités* continued to be the administrators of revenue and payments, everyone could continue to choose any *mutualité*, and the funds continued to appeal to all occupations.

For a long time, Belgians belonged to five national unions of *mutualités*. They are listed in Table A.5. The distribution of members remained nearly the same among the five sectors for several decades. The local sickness funds have become administrative agencies instead of local clubs of political militants. But ideology survives in the meetings and publications of the union and those of some of their constituent federations as a raison d'être for the survival of distinct unions.

Ideology and the integrated leadership of the union bridge the fundamental cleavage of Belgian life—the tense division between Flanders and Wallonia, between the Flemish-speakers and the French-speakers. Each sickness fund is

Table A.5. Belgian Sickness Funds in 1985.

Union	Political tendency	Distribution of entire Belgian population
Alliance Nationale de Mutualités Chrétiennes	Social Christian (Catholic)	44.9%
Union National des Mutualités Socialistes	Socialist	26.3
Ligue Nationale des Mutualités Libérales	Liberal	6.6
Union Nationale des Mutualités Neutres	Nonpartisan	9.8
Union Nationale des Mutualités Professionnelles	Nonpartisan	11.5
Caisse Auxiliaire d'Assurance Maladie-Invalidité	Nonpolitical	0.9
		100.0%
Total population		(9,578,822)

Note: This table lists the French titles, but each union has an equally valid Flemish title.

Source: Rapport Général: 3ᵉ Partie, Rapport Statistique (Brussels: Institut National d'Assurance Maladie-Invalidité, 1984), pp. 21, 61.

local and belongs to a regional federation. Each federation is exclusively or over-whelmingly either Flemish or francophone, since it is based in that part of the country. The federations join in an ideological union that represents both the Flemish and French, instead of joining in nonideological unions that are exclusively ethnic. The unions of sickness funds are one of the few unifying institutions in Belgium.

Ethnic disruptions can occur if overriding ideology is absent. During the 1980s, the fourth and fifth unions in Table A.5—the *Neutres* and the *Professionnelles*—planned to merge. Unification seemed "rational" according to modern insurance strategy: the unions were not divided by ideology; their members were similar in occupations and economic behavior; a merger would give them larger size and greater political influence; they could share a large and more efficient computing system for financial management; they could eliminate administrative duplication. The *Union Neutre* split along Belgium's fundamental fault line: all but one of its Flemish federations refused to dissolve its union and refused to join the new merger on the grounds they would be "drowned" in a large entity with a francophone majority; all the francophone federations and one Flemish federation seceded and joined the *Union Professionnelle*. The long-stable structure in Table A.5 was partially revised in 1990. A new *Union Nationale des Mutualités Professionnelles et Libres* had about 16 percent of the Belgian population, and the *Union Neutre* was reduced to about 5 percent. Whether the *Union Neutre* could survive financially was uncertain. If it proves inefficient, subscribers can easily give it the *coup de grâce* by switching from its sickness funds to the local offices of the *Union Professionnelle*.

Private Insurance Companies. The commercial carriers specialize in auto accidents and invalidity payments, and they find no niches in mainstream health insurance. They cannot compete with *mutualités*—even in the sectors for the professionals and self-employed—since the registered *mutualités* receive large administrative subsidies from government and the insurance companies cannot. The *mutualités* in all unions offer supplementary policies to their members at low premiums, and the insurance companies cannot compete profitably. Insuring the statutory cost sharing contradicts public policy, it is opposed by the government and the *mutualités*, and (unlike the market niche in France) it cannot be profitable for Belgium's insurance companies.

Switzerland

Like other European countries, Switzerland during the nineteenth century had a wide variety of small mutual aid societies, special workplace funds, private insurance companies, and other arrangements. Many were local. A few insurance companies marketed life, accident, and sickness coverages in wider areas.

The country could not enact German-style health insurance because of businessmen's resistance to payroll taxes, localities' fears of the growth of the national government, and religious associations' distaste for a growing secular role in social protection. Instead, the national government enacted a law (the *Kranken- und Unfallversicherungsgesetz* of 1911, or KUVG) that grants subsidies to carriers meeting certain conditions. A sickness fund is recognized if it accepts any citizen, offers certain minimum benefits, pays providers according to certain rules, is a nonprofit legal entity, and reports its accounts to the national government.[18]

Sickness Funds. The carriers that are recognized and subsidized vary in organizational form and size. Some are large centralized organizations that market all over the country; many others are local. Some are public corporations sponsored by cantonal governments; most are private and nonprofit. Some are confined to workers and their dependents in a particular workplace; most are open to all applicants. Many were once mutual insurance companies; others originated in Socialist or Catholic labor movements. Table A.6 shows the types of sickness funds and their enrollment.

Once there were nearly a thousand sickness funds, and each had a respectable share of the market. The large centralized organizations have steadily grown in membership, since they can market eloquently, manage their accounts efficiently, and protect subscribers at the same premiums upon change of workplace or area of residence. A few companies (such as Helvetia) enlist large proportions of the entire Swiss population. The smaller nonprofit funds and the public funds have steadily lost subscribers to the large nonprofit firms. More than half of all carriers have disappeared or have concentrated on other lines in twenty-five years.

Table A.6. Swiss Sickness Funds in 1988.

Type of fund	Number of funds	Distribution of subscribers
Private nonprofit		
More than 100,000 subscribers	12	71.3%
Fewer than 100,000 subscribers	140	16.7
Public (sponsored by cantonal or communal governments)	140	5.2
Workplace (*Betriebskrankenkasse*)	77	6.8
Totals	369	100.0%
Total number of subscribers		(7,391,482)

Source: Data extracted from *Statistik über die Krankenversicherung vom Bunde anerkannte Versicherungsträger 1988* (Bern: Bundesamt für Sozialversicherung, 1990), p. 12.

Private Insurance Companies. Switzerland's many multiline insurance companies sell property, accident, disability, and life insurance at home and abroad. Five mutual insurance companies and thirty-two stock companies in 1987 sold health insurance policies in Switzerland.

Their market is small and specialized. They cannot compete with the sickness funds for basic and comprehensive acute-care coverage, since they do not receive subsidies from the *Bund*. Instead, they offer supplementary cash benefits when the patient is hospitalized and cash to pay the cost sharing under statutory health insurance. Their supplementary market is small, because the sickness funds also sell policies to cover private rooms and other additional expenses during hospitalization. In 1987, 226,583 Swiss—3.5 percent of the population— had private policies for extra cash during hospitalization; 102,614 had private policies to cover out-of-pocket costs in ambulatory care.[19]

The United States

During the nineteenth and early twentieth centuries, the United States was much like other developed countries. At times it debated enactment of typical European statutory health insurance, which would have imposed some structure and standardization. The United States did not do so and evolved differently, as Chapter Four explained. The result is a complex and unstable mixture.

Private Insurance Companies. The population under the age of sixty-five is covered by a number of nonprofit and for-profit arrangements:[20]

☐ *Blue Cross and Blue Shield.* One or more Plans operate in each state. All are franchised by the national Blue Cross and Blue Shield Association. Legally, each is a private nonprofit organization created by a special law of its state legislature. Some are mutual insurance companies under state insurance law. Each is governed by its state or regional headquarters. The national association sets standards as conditions for the franchises, manages national accounts, manages inter-Plan communications and financial transactions, deals with the national government and public, and performs other tasks. In the late 1980s, there were fifty joint Blue Cross/Blue Shield Plans, thirteen Blue Cross Plans, and fifteen Blue Shield Plans.

☐ *Commercial insurance companies.* All are nationwide firms with headquarters that can be situated anywhere in the country. In order to sell insurance in a state, each must conform to state insurance law. (In the United States, regulation of insurance and chartering of an insurance company are functions of the state and not the national government.) Few have local offices for anything except marketing. In the age of the computer, claims from the entire country are processed centrally. About 1,200 companies sell health and disability insurance, but the market is concentrated: the twenty leading companies in 1988 wrote 53 percent of all the health and accident premiums among all commercial insurers.[21] Turnover is common: some carriers add a small health insurance line so they can negotiate a complete set of products with employers, unions, or individuals; but they drop the health insurance during periodic downturns in profits.

☐ *Self-funded employment-based plans.* Such plans are independent of the Blues and commercial carriers. The share in the total market has grown rapidly and is difficult to estimate: America lacks a comprehensive and regular method of recording health insurance arrangements. Some plans are administered by insurance companies like any third-party-administrator arrangement; some plans are hybrids wherein the carrier insures for large cost overruns; the numbers and forms changed from year to year during the 1980s. A survey of 1,638 plans with large and medium-size employers in 1987 estimated:[22]

- Forty-nine percent were completely self-funded and were administered either by insurance companies ("Administrative-Service-Only" contracts) or by third-party administrators.
- Fifteen percent were hybrids ("Minimum-Premium Plans").
- Twenty-three percent were experience-rated contracts with insurance companies.
- Thirteen percent were conventionally insured.

☐ *Prepaid multispecialty physician groups.* These entities combine insurance and services. Subscribers pay premiums and are guaranteed ambulatory care, hospital care, and certain other services. Some own their own hospitals, but most contract with conventional community hospitals. Most lock in subscribers to physicians and hospitals within their lists. Each is a local entity under state insurance and medical practice laws, but some belong to chains owned by statewide, regional, or nationwide nonprofit or for-profit companies. The types are:[23]

- *Staff-model HMOs.* The doctors are employees of the organization and work in its health center. Fifty-nine existed in early 1990.
- *Group-model HMOs.* The doctors are members of a single medical group, the group has a contract with the organization, and the doctors work in its health center. Sixty-five existed in early 1990.
- *Network-model HMOs.* The doctors are members of several private groups; some are independent office practitioners. They contract with the HMO to treat its patients for the fixed fees, continue to work in their private offices, may use equipment and supplies provided by the HMO, and continue to treat other patients covered by other insurance. Eighty-nine existed in early 1990.
- *Independent practice associations (IPAs).* The doctors are private groups and independent practitioners. They agree to treat the IPA's subscribers within the limits of an expenditure cap and fee schedule, and they continue to treat other patients covered by other insurers. In early 1990, 362 independent IPAs existed. In addition, several Blue Cross/Blue Shield Plans and commercial insurance companies started to organize their own IPAs in large cities.

☐ *Independent plans.* Some are run by trade unions; some are consumer cooperatives. There may be several dozen.

Table A.7 shows the distribution of the American population younger than sixty-five among insurance plans in 1986. The table omits the 31,800,000 of the entire population older than sixty-five and covered by Medicare. It also omits the 17 percent of the population younger than sixty-five without health insurance and without Medicaid. The figures in Table A.7 total more than 100 percent because of much double coverage: many people have Blue Cross for hospital insurance and a private company's major medical for physicians, drugs, and other benefits; some people own several private individual policies. The table omits the many additional individual policies for cash benefits during hospitalization, for loss of wages during disability, for long-term care, and for other purposes. The self-insured employer group plans appear in the "other plans" line if insurance companies play little or no role as managers and insurers; otherwise, they are mixed into the line for private insurance group business or into the line for the Blues.

Medicare. A private health insurance system has no relationship to the statutory Social Security machinery. American private carriers are completely independent of Social Security for their normal business. But Medicare is part of Social Security. Its trust funds (for hospital and physicians' financing) resemble the other Social Security trust funds (for old-age and disability pensions), all the trust funds are managed by the Treasury Department, and all the trustees must report annually to Congress. The only contracts between private carriers and the Social Security system are indirect and derive from their Medicare tasks:

□   The Blues and commercial carriers win contracts as "fiscal intermediaries" that administer claims from hospitals and doctors.

□   The Blues and commercial carriers sell "Medigap" policies to Medicare beneficiaries to cover the statutory cost sharing. The carriers who are fiscal intermediaries have a head start in marketing. The Medigap policies were long supposed to be free and unregulated. But Congress heard that some private companies were misleading the elderly by selling excessive insurance coverage with excessive premiums. Thus, Congress occasionally legislates about the Medigap policies and holds oversight hearings.[24]

Table A.7. Coverage of Americans in 1986.

Carrier	Percentage with hospital insurance	Percentage with major medical	Percentage with comprehensive coverage
Insurance companies			
Group policies	40.3	54.1	
Individual and family policies	4.1	2.3	
Blue Cross/Blue Shield	32.3	18.4	
Other plans (primarily self-insured employee benefit coverage)	23.5	23.0	
Medicare for disabled under 65	1.4	1.3	
Medicaid at any time during year (1986)			9.1
HMOs and IPAs (1988)			
Staff model			2.0
Group model			3.7
Network model			2.6
IPA			6.3

Estimated total population under age of 65: 211,566,000 (in 1986)
214,749,000 (in 1988)

Note: This table gives the number of persons who had some Medicaid coverage for part or all of 1986; as Chapter Three reported, the proportion of persons with Medicaid at the time of a sample survey is less than 8 percent; the number with Medicaid throughout 1986 is even lower.

Source: Source Book of Health Insurance Data—1988 Update (Washington: Health Insurance Association of America, 1988), pp. 4–5; *InterStudy Edge,* Fall 1988, p. 10; *1987 HCFA Statistics* (Washington: Health Care Financing Administration, U.S. Department of Health and Human Services, 1987), pp. 6 and 9.

Notes

1. For good overviews of German statutory health insurance see Donald W. Light and Alexander Schuller (eds.), *Political Values and Health Care: The German Experience* (Cambridge: MIT Press, 1986); Fritz Kastner, *Monograph on*

the Organisation of Medical Care Within the Framework of Social Security: Federal Republic of Germany (Geneva: International Labour Office, 1968); and Romuald Schicke, *Soziale Sicherung und Gesundheitswesen* (Stuttgart: Verlag W. Kohlhammer, 1978). For its history see Horst Peters, *Die Geschichte der sozialen Versicherung,* 3rd ed. (Sankt Augustin: Asgard-Verlag, 1978); Peter A. Köhler and Hans F. Zacher (eds.), *The Evolution of Social Insurance 1881-1981* (London: Frances Pinter, 1982), pp. 1-92; and Florian Tennstedt, *Soziale Selbstverwaltung: Geschichte der Selbstverwaltung in der Krankenversicherung* (Bonn: Verlag der Ortskrankenkassen, 1977).

2. For the past and recent history of the crafts sickness funds see R. G. Albrecht, "Vom Werden der Innungskrankenkassen," *Krankenversicherung,* vol. 25, no. 1 (Jan. 1973), pp. 1-8.

3. For the history and present characteristics of the miners' funds see Joseph Hoffner, *Sozialpolitik in deutschen Bergbau,* 2nd ed. (Munster: Aschendorffsche Verlagsbuchhandlung, 1956); and Nikolaus von Gellhorn, *Die Knappschaftsversicherung,* 5th ed. (Bad Godesberg: Asgard-Verlag, 1966).

4. For their history and present characteristics see Kurt Friede, *Die Betriebskrankenkassen in der Bundesrepublik Deutschland,* 2nd ed. (Essen: Fachverlag C. W. Haarfeld, 1979).

5. For their present characteristics see Horst Gerold, *Krankenversicherung der Landwirte,* 3rd ed. (Sankt Augustin: Asgard-Verlag, 1982).

6. Many present characteristics of the *Ortskrankenkassen* are described in Christa Altenstetter, *Implementation of National Health Insurance Seen from the Perspective of General Sickness Funds (AOKs) in the Federal Republic of Germany 1955-1975* and *Organizational Processes in a Three-Tiered Members Organization of Health Insurance Funds Seen from Below: Experiences from Germany* (both Berlin: Wissenschaftszentrum, 1982).

7. For the history and present characteristics of the *Ersatzkassen* see Erich Stolt and Ernest Albert Vesper, *Die Ersatzkassen der Krankenversicherung,* 7th ed. (Bonn/Bad Godesberg: Asgard-Verlag, 1973).

8. *Die private Krankenversicherung Rechenschaftsbericht* and *Die private Krankenversicherung Zahlenbericht* (both Cologne: Verband der privaten Krankenversicherung, annual).

9. For good overviews of French statutory health insurance see Jean-Jacques Dupeyroux, *Droit de la Sécurité sociale,* 10th ed. (Paris: Dalloz, 1986); Alain Foulon and others, *Comparaison des régimes de Sécurité sociale* (Paris: Documents du Centre d'Etude des Revenus et des Coûts, 1982 and 1983), 2 vols.; J. Champeix and others, *Guide pratique de Sécurité sociale à l'usage du médecin clinicien* (Paris: Masson, 1977); and Michel Trahan, *Health Insurance in France, Australia and Canada* (Ottawa: Health and Welfare Canada, 1981). The history is summarized in Köhler and Zacher, *Evolution of Social Insurance* (see note 1, above), pp. 93-149; and Henry C. Galant, *Histoire politique de la Sécurité sociale française 1945-1952* (Paris: Librairie Armand Colin, 1955).

10. Yves Saint-Jour, *La protection sociale agricole* (Paris: Librairie

Générale de Droit et de Jurisprudence, 1984); and "L'Assurance maladie des travailleurs non salariés des professions non agricoles," special issue of *Droit Social*, vol. 33, no. 3 (March 1970).

11. Summaries of the present situation are in Jean Benhamou and Aliette Levecque, *La Mutualité* (Paris: Presses Universitaires de France, 1983); *Les formes complémentaires de la protection sociale* (Paris: Inspection Générale des Affaires Sociales, Rapport annuel, 1975), pt. 3; and Michel Morisot and others, *Rapport du groupe de réflexion chargé de la réforme du Code de la Mutualité* (Paris: Ministère des Affaires Sociales, 1984). Two histories are Thierry Laurent, *La Mutualité française et le monde du travail* (Paris: Coopérative d'Information et d'Edition Mutualiste, 1973); and Bernard Gibaud, *De la Mutualité à la Sécurité sociale* (Paris: Les Editions Ouvrières, 1986).

12. Jean-Luc Volatier, *Les modes de protection sociale* (Paris: CREDES, 1990), pp. 14–38.

13. *Informations statistiques et financières sur la Mutualité* (Paris: Division des Etudes Economiques et Statistiques,, Ministère des Affaires Sociales, 1986); and Morisot and others, *Rapport* (see note 11, above), pp. 14–15.

14. *L'Assurance française* (Paris: Fédération Française des Sociétés d'Assurance, annual); and Bernard Dubois du Bellay, "L'Assurance 'maladie'" (Paris: Association Générale des Sociétés d'Assurance contra les Accidents, 1984).

15. Volatier, *Les modes de protection sociale* (see note 14, above), p. 47.

16. For the history and present characteristics of Dutch statutory health insurance see L. V. Ledeboer, *Heden en verleden* (Amsterdam: Ziekenfondsraad, 1973); Paul Juffermans, *Staat en gezondheidszorg in Nederland* (Nijmegen: Socialistiese Uitgeverij Nijmegen, 1982); and Jan Blanpain and others, *National Health Insurance and Health Resources: The European Experience* (Cambridge: Harvard University Press, 1978), chap. 5. Much information also appears in books about Dutch health care generally, such as J. M. Boot and M.H.J.M. Knapen, *De Nederlandse gezondheids* (Utrecht: Uitgeverij Het Spectrum, 1983); and E. W. Roscam Abbing (ed.), *Bouw en weking van de gezondheidszorg in Nederland*, 2nd ed. (Utrecht: Bonn, Scheltens & Hokkens, 1983).

17. For the history of Belgian statutory health insurance see *Développement et mutations de l'AMI de 1851 à 1966* (Brussels: Editions FIB, 1966); J. Engles, *L'évolution de l'assurance maladie invalidité obligatoire 1945–1970* (Brussels: Institut National d'Assurance Maladie-Invalidité, 1970); and Françoise Antoine and Jacques Lemaitre, *La mise en place de l'assurance maladie invalidité obligatoire en Belgique* (Brussels: Groupe d'Etude pour une Réforme de la Médecine, 1978). For the present characteristics see *Outline of the Belgian Compulsory Sickness and Invalidity Insurance*, 12th ed. (Brussels: Institut National d'Assurance Maladie-Invalidité, 1982); Jérome Dejardin, *Monograph on the Organisation of Medical Care Within the Framework of Social Security: Belgium* (Geneva: International Labour Office, 1968); and *Les mutualités en Belgique* (Brussels: Centre de Recherche et d'Information Socio-Politiques, 1964).

18. For the history of the health insurance laws and the sick funds see Paul

Biedermann, *Die Entwicklung der Krankenversicherung in der Schweiz* (Zurich: Buchdruckerei Davos, 1955); and Köhler and Zacher, *Evolution of Social Insurance* (see note 1, above), pp. 384-454. The current situation is described in Pierre Gygy and Heiner Henny, *Das schweizerische Gesundheitswesen*, 2nd ed. (Bern: Verlag Hans Huber, 1977), whose tables are updated periodically; and in Arnold Saxer, *Soziale Versicherung in der Schweiz*, 4th ed. (Bern: Paul Haupt Verlag, 1976). Relationships between the sickness funds and the national government are described in Markus Moser, "Zur Aufsicht des BSV über die Krankenkassen," *Schweizerische Krankenkassen Zeitung*, vol. 78, no. 3 (Feb. 1, 1986), pp. 28-29.

19. *Die privaten Versicherungseinrichtungen in der Schweiz 1987* (Bern: Bundesamt für Privatversicherungswesen, 1989).

20. For an overview of recent American private health insurance see *Health Insurance and the Uninsured: Background Data and Analysis* (Washington: Congressional Research Service, Library of Congress, 1988), chaps. 2-3; O. D. Dickerson, *Health Insurance*, 3rd ed. (Homewood, Ill.: Richard D. Irwin, 1968); and John Krizay and Andrew Wilson, *The Patient as Consumer* (Lexington, Mass.: Lexington Books, 1974).

21. The ten leading companies wrote 36 percent of the total premiums; my calculations from "Accident and Health Premiums—1988," *Best's Review: Life/Health Insurance Edition*, vol. 90, no. 8 (Dec. 1989), pp. 88-92. For an overview of the private health insurance market see Albert Woodward, "The U.S. Health Insurance Industry: An Alternative View," *International Journal of Health Services*, vol. 8, no. 3 (1978), pp. 491-507.

22. "Health Care Benefits Survey" (Princeton, N.J.: A. Foster Higgins Health Group, 1987).

23. The situation in early 1990 is described in *The InterStudy Edge* (Excelsior, Minn.: Interstudy, 1990), vol. 2, especially pp. 15-19.

24. *Abuses in the Sale of Health Insurance to the Elderly in Supplementation of Medicare: A National Scandal*, Comm. Pub. no. 95-160 (Washington: Select Committee on Aging, U.S. House of Representatives, 95th Congress, 2nd Session, 1978); and *Medigap Insurance: Law Has Increased Protection Against Substandard and Overpriced Policies* (Washington: U.S. General Accounting Office, 1986).

APPENDIX B

Research Methods

During 1986 and 1987, working alone, I collected information about social security, statutory health insurance, and private voluntary health insurance in France, West Germany, Belgium, the Netherlands, and Switzerland. I spent one or two months in each country, divided over the two years. In addition, in order to examine special topics, I spent a few weeks apiece in Italy, Spain, and Great Britain. I have done similar field research in the United States, spread over several years.

In each country, my field research has relied primarily on interviews with persons involved in social security and in health insurance. The interviews have been qualitative in their flexible style of posing and answering questions, but a definite set of topics is covered in each instance in order to elicit a systematic description of the respondent's work. Interviews lasted from one to three hours apiece. I have used these methods in all my previous research projects about comparative health services.[1]

In each country, I interviewed the following persons about their work in the following topics (where applicable to the country):

☐ Ministry officials in the national government
  • Finance and Budget
    ★ Social security payroll taxes, including those for statutory health insurance
    ★ Subsidies to the sickness funds
  • Ministry that oversees the health insurance system
    ★ Current status and future prospects of the total accounts
    ★ Proposals for payroll taxes and subsidies
    ★ Audit of sickness funds' annual accounts

      ★   Guidelines about covered persons, benefits, containment of costs
      ★   Proposals for reform

☐ Headquarters of national associations of sickness funds—both social and commercial
- Negotiations about new laws and regulations
- Strategic planning for the health insurance industry

☐ Headquarters of principal sickness funds and private insurance companies
- Setting of premiums (if done by each carrier in this country)
- Management of finances and response to difficulties
- Management of benefits
- Design and administration of policies for supplementary benefits
- Future plans

☐ Headquarters of principal social security pension fund
- Setting of premiums (if done by the fund itself)
- Management of finances and response to difficulties
- Role in financing long-term care for the elderly

☐ Programs that provide long-term care for the elderly
- Sources of finance
- Relations to sickness funds and private health insurance

☐ Scholars who have done research about health insurance, health care finance, and long-term care

Besides field notes from interviews, in each country I collected recent publications and statistics about health insurance.

The present work builds on previous efforts. I have done similar comparative studies of how statutory health insurance pays doctors (1961–1962 and 1975–1976), how statutory health insurance pays hospitals (1979–1982), and how national and provincial governments in federal systems manage health care finance (1977–1978). I have therefore observed the development of European health insurance over several decades. Several of these research projects were designed to show how the experiences of other developed countries can suggest solutions to problems in American health care finance.[2] The first stage of the present study of health insurance was such a lessons-from-abroad effort.[3]

PRINCIPAL INFORMANTS

I am deeply indebted to the following persons, who granted at least one hour in interviews. In addition, there were many others who provided invaluable information in shorter discussions.

France

Paris, Government of France. Daniel Beaune, Anne Bourjade, Monique Castets, Norbert Deville, Daniel Gautier, Jacques Lagrave, Danielle le Roux, Jacques Nougarède, Suzanne Silland, Gérard Sylvestre.

Paris, Social Security, Mutuelles, and Private Insurance. Roger Amiel, Claudine Attias-Donfut, M. Bouak, Jean Boudreau, Bernard Dubois du Bellay, Pierre-Jean Faranda, Christian Rampht, Armand Rauch, Robert Rochefort, Alain Rozenkier, Denise Schouten.

Paris, Other. Antoinette Catrice-Lorey, Claire Desserrey, Jean-Pierre Dumont, Alain Foulon, Robert Launois, Emile Lévy, Béatrice Majnoni d'Intignano, Arié Mizrahi, Gérard de Pouvourville, Simone Sandier.

West Germany

Bonn, Government. Gunnar Griesewell, Ulrich Hoffmann, Wolfgang Nusche, Lothar Seyfarth, Hans Stein, Heinz Stollenwerk, Rudolf Vollmer.

Bonn and Vicinity. Guntram Bauer, Hans Brandt, Ulrich Geissler, Werner Gerdelmann, Werner Gerlach, Dieter Paffrath, Malte Retiet, Johann-M. von Stackelberg, Friedhelm Weber.

Cologne. Günther Aumüller, Gerhard Brenner, Christian Brunjes, Christopher Gutknecht, Philipp Herder-Dorneich, Paul Müller, Sybille Sahmer, Erwin Scheuch, Erich Schneider, Jürgen Weber.

Berlin. Margret Dieck, Harald Möhlmann, Alexander Schuller, Gerd von Essen, Christine Wenk.

Elsewhere. Christa Altenstetter, Theo Giehler, Ulrich Okoniewski, Martin Pfaff, Christian von Ferber.

Belgium

Brussels, Government of Belgium. Luk Canoodt, H. Dilan, Jean Hermesse, André Maes, F. Praet, G. Van de Gaer, Jean Vandevoorde.

Brussels, Mutualités. Michel de Jaer, Jos Kesenne, Lydia Magnus-Maximus, R. Mox, Andrée Sacrez, Robert Soete, Robert Van den Heuvel, Robert Van den Oever.

Brussels and Vicinity, Other. Marie-Christine Closon, Denise Deliège, Francis Roger, Monique Van Dormael, M. Wauters, André Wynen.

Elsewhere. Jan Blanpain, Herman Deleeck, Michel Dethée, Jan Peeters, Danny C.H.M. Pieters, Jef Van Langendonck.

The Netherlands

Amsterdam and Amstelveen. Robert Berkelbach, C. Dalmeyer-Henneke, Marcel Don, Tania Geldof, H.F.A. Kerklaan, Rienk Prins, T. ten Berge, Jos van den Heuvel, J. W. van der Linden, J. H. van der Moer, J. B. van der Steur, E. van der Veen, E. H. Wierenga.

Utrecht, Zeist, and Houten. Karolien Bais, J. M. Boot, Jos G. Breit, E. H. Brouwer, J.W.M. Collaris, Rob J. M. de Jong, J.J.M. de Klein, Hugo Duvekot,

R. Scheerens, Guus Schrijvers, A. Sliedrecht, D.N.M. van de Loo, A.P.W.P. van Montfort, H. van Vliet, H.H.M. Willems.

The Hague and Vicinity. David Banta, Einte Elsinga, P. J. van de Kasteel, J.W.M. van Welzen, E. Wiebenga.

Elsewhere. W. N. Bax, Ph. J. de Koning Gans, G. W. de Wit, J.B.J. Drewes, L.M.J. Groot, Bradford Kirkman-Liff, Rudy Lapré, J.A.M. Maarse, Geert A. Tuinier, Wynand van de Ven, Bernard van Praag.

Switzerland

Bern, Government of Switzerland. Till Bandi, Danielle Bridel, Jean-François Charles, Karl Koch, Ernst Rätzer, Franz Wyss.

Bern, Other. Peter Kramer, Roland Loffel, Heinz Schmid, Pierre-M. Vallon.

Zurich. Eduard Brachetto, Ernst Menzi, Martin Peter, Andres R. Vogt, Elsbeth Wolfer, Peter Zweifel.

Elsewhere. Yvonne Bollag, Ulrich Gessner, Rudolf Gilli, Bernhard Guntert, Stephan Hill, Bruno Horisberger, Robert Leu, Josef Schurtenberger, Edwin von Büren.

Italy

Antonio Bariletti, A. M. Berardo, Giuseppe Berenzone, Carmela Caravano, Mario Alberto Coppini, Alessandro Desideri, Vincenzo-Romano Floridi, Giorgio Freddi, Franco Illuminati, Bruno Nitoglia, Aldo Piperno, G. Polettini, Ernesto Veronesi.

Spain

Manual Alonso Olea, José Maria Marco Garcia, Alfredo López Estévez, Pedro Pablo Mansilla Izquierdo, José Simón Martín.

Great Britain

Brian Abel-Smith, Brian Bricknell, Kenneth Groom, Robert Maxwell, Geof Rayner, George Teeling Smith.

International Organizations

Robert Bédard, Guy Perrin, Jean-Pierre Poullier, Vladimir Rys, Gerd Spangenberg, Franz Werle.

United States

Chicago, Blue Cross and Blue Shield Association. Naomi Aronson, Susan Barrish, Jean Broholm, Meredith Buco, Robert Cunningham, Gail David, Eileen

Doherty, Terri Gendel, James Gibbs, Lionel Graveline, James Hutchison, Peter Lopatin, Walter McNerney, Gary Mead, Lawrence Morris, Suzanne Mulstein, Douglas Peters, Theodore Raichel, William Rial, Joan Robinson, Robert Snyder, David Tennenbaum, Bruce Witkov, Stephen Wood.

New York. Seymour Bernstein, Robert Biblo, Robert Butler, Eli Ginzberg, Jack Guildroy, John Moynahan, Robert Padgug, William Rosenberg, Mal Schechter, Robert Zilg.

Washington. David Abernethy, Peter Bouxsein, Gary Christopherson, Jon Gabel, Kevin Haugh, Barbara Herzog, Frederick Hunt, Shelah Leader, David Nexon, Anita Rosen, John Rother, Susan van Gelder.

Exchange Rates

Because we are interested in the structure of financial arrangements rather than in the international equivalence of incomes and services, the text deals entirely with the local currencies. Here I present a convenient summary of the figures for the principal countries I investigated. The 1980s experienced great fluctuations in exchange rates, and doubtless the rates at the time of reading will differ from those at the time of writing.

Country	*Currency*	*Number of units equaling $US 1 in October 1990*
Belgium	Franc (FB)	32.1
France	Franc (F)	5.22
Germany	Deutsche Mark (DM)	1.55
Great Britain	Pound (£)	0.53
Italy	Lira (L or £)	1,166
Netherlands	Guilder (f. or fl)	1.76
Switzerland	Franc (FrS or SFr)	1.29

Notes

1. Such methods have become common in research about government decisions. For their use in studies of health care politics, see Frank D. Campion, *The AMA and U.S. Health Policy Since 1940* (Chicago: Chicago Review Press, 1984); and Jonas Morris, *Searching for a Cure: National Health Policy Considered* (Washington, D.C.: Berkeley Morgan, 1984). For their use in studies of comparative government, see Hugh Heclo and Aaron Wildavsky, *The Private Government of Public Money: Community and Policy Inside British Political Administration* (Berkeley: University of California Press, 1974). Only one textbook has been written about the methodology: Lewis Anthony Dexter, *Elite and Specialized Interviewing* (Evanston, Ill.: Northwestern University Press, 1970).

2. The results are published in William Glaser, *Health Insurance Bargaining: Foreign Lessons for Americans* (New York: Gardner Press and John Wiley, 1978); *Paying the Hospital: Foreign Lessons for the United States* (New York:

Center for the Social Sciences, Columbia University, 1982), a report submitted to the Health Care Financing Administration, U.S. Department of Health and Human Services; and *Federalism in Canada and West Germany: Lessons for the United States* (New York: Center for the Social Sciences, Columbia University, 1979), a report submitted to the National Center for Health Services Research, U.S. Department of Health and Human Services.

3. The results were submitted in William Glaser, *Financial Decisions in European Health Insurance: Lessons for the United States* (New York: Graduate School of Management, New School for Social Research, 1988), a report to the National Center for Health Services Research, U.S. Department of Health and Human Services.

APPENDIX C

Glossary of Abbreviations

Abbreviation	Name	Meaning
GENERAL		
CPI	consumer price index	Measure of annual change in a nation's cost of living
EEC	European Economic Community	Economic alliance of European countries
GDP	gross domestic product	GNP minus net-factor payments (interest, profits, and salary remittances) from nonresidents
GNP	gross national product	Total value of all goods and services produced each year in a nation
NHI	national health insurance	Statute requiring persons to join a sickness fund and requiring employers and workers to pay premiums
NHS	national health service	Integrated system whereby government owns, manages, and finances all health care
VAT	value-added tax	A tax on the products or services of each firm according to the value added to the product or service by that firm's work
GREAT BRITAIN		
BUPA	British United Provident Association	The United Kingdom's largest private health insurance carrier
GP	general practitioner	Dispenser of primary care; the patient's case manager
NHS	National Health Service	Hierarchy of committees and their employees who plan and manage health services

530

Abbreviation	Name	Meaning
UNITED STATES		
CPR	customary, prevailing, and reasonable charges	Method of paying physicians under Medicare Part B
DI	Disability Insurance	Social Security program of the national government that provides long-term pensions for the disabled
DRG	diagnosis-related group	A classification of patients
ERISA	Employee Retirement Income Security Act	Law of the United States government regulating private pensions granted by employers
FEHBP	Federal Employee Health Benefits Program	Health insurance for civil servants of the national government
HCFA	Health Care Financing Administration	Agency of the national government that administers Medicare and Medicaid
HI	Hospital Insurance	Social Security program that covers hospital care for the elderly (Medicare Part A)
HIAA	Health Insurance Association of America	Trade association of commercial insurers
HMO	health maintenance organization	A prepaid multispecialty group of physicians, usually with extensive facilities
IPA	independent practice association	A multispecialty association of individual office doctors who agree to care for a list of prepaid subscribers
OASI	Old Age and Survivors Insurance	Social Security program of the national government that provides pensions for the retired
PPO	preferred provider organization	Any provider list or organization that offers health care at a lower price
PRO (formerly PSRO)	Peer Review Organization	A commission created by national law to monitor utilization of hospitals under Medicare
ProPAC	Prospective Payment Assessment Commission	Agency of the national government that recommends Medicare hospital reimbursement policies
S/HMO	social health maintenance organization	A prepaid group that provides long-term care as well as acute care
SMI	Supplementary Medical Insurance	Social Security program that covers physicians' services for the elderly (Medicare Part B)
TPA	third-party administrator	An entrepreneur who administers provider relations for self-insured groups

Abbreviation	Name	Literal translation into English	Meaning
FRANCE			
ACOSS	Agence Centrale des Organismes de Sécurité Sociale	Central Office for Social Security Agencies	Collection and distribution office for all social security revenue
CNAMTS (or CNAM)	Caisse Nationale de l'Assurance Maladie des Travailleurs Salariés	National Fund for the Health Insurance of Wage Earners	Official sickness fund for the large majority of French workers
CCSMA	Caisse Centrale de Secours Mutuels Agricoles	Central Fund for Cooperative Agricultural Assistance	Official sickness fund for farmers
CANAM	Caisse Nationale d'Assurance Maladie et Maternité des Travailleurs Non Salariés des Professions Non Agricoles	National Fund for the Health Insurance and Maternity Benefits of Nonwage and Nonagricultural Workers	Official sickness fund for businessmen, professionals, artisans
CRAM	Caisse Régionale de l'Assurance Maladie	Regional Fund for Health Insurance	Regional office of CNAMTS
CPAM	Caisse Primaire de l'Assurance Maladie	Primary Fund for Health Insurance	Local office of CNAMTS that deals with subscribers and providers
CNAVTS (often CNAV)	Caisse Nationale de l'Assurance Vieillesse des Travailleurs Salariés	National Fund for the Old-Age Insurance of Wage Earners	Official retirement pension fund for the large majority of French workers
MGEN	Mutuelle Génerale de l'Education Nationale	National Mutual Aid Fund for Education	Voluntary *mutuelle* for French teachers
WEST GERMANY			
RVO	Reichsversicherungsordnung	Imperial Insurance Decree	Statute that created national health insurance
BOK	Bundesverband der Ortskrankenkassen	Federal Union of Local Sickness Funds	National leadership of the largest association of sickness funds
KA	Konzertierte Aktion im Gesundheitswesen	Coordinating Body in Health Affairs	Forum of several groups that recommends policy targets
KV	Kassenärztliche Vereinigung	Association of Physicians in Health Insurance Practice	The agency in each province that screens and pays physicians' claims
KHG	Krankenhausfinanzierungsgesetz	Hospital Finance Law	Principal law about capital grants and operating costs
BVA	Bundesversicherungsamt	Federal Insurance Office	Agency that monitors the accounts of social insurance carriers

Abbreviation	Name	Literal translation into English	Meaning
BAV	Bundesaufsichtsamt für das Versicherungswesen	Federal Inspection Office for Insurance Affairs	Agency that regulates private insurance

NETHERLANDS

Abbreviation	Name	Literal translation into English	Meaning
ZFW	Ziekenfondswet	Sickness Funds Law	Statute that created national health insurance for acute care
AWBZ	Algemene Wet Bijzondere Ziektekosten	General Law for Exceptional Medical Expenses	Statute that created national health insurance for long-term care
VNZ	Vereniging van Nederlandse Ziekenfondsen	Association of Dutch Sickness Funds	Association of social insurance carriers that administer ZFW and AWBZ
KLOZ	Kontaktorgaan Landelijke Organisaties van Ziektekostenverzekeraars	National Office for Health Insurance Carriers	Association of private health insurance companies
WVC	Ministerie van Welzijn, Volksgezondheid, en Cultuur	Ministry of Welfare, Public Health, and Culture	Ministry of the national government
COTG	Centraal Orgaan Tarieven Gesondheidszorg	Central Agency for Health Care Charges	Commission that fixes rates of hospitals and other providers
RIAGG	Regionaal Instituut voor Ambulante Geestlijke Gezondheidszorg	Regional Institute for Ambulatory Mental Health Care	Community center that provides mental health services

BELGIUM

Abbreviation	Name	Literal translation into English	Meaning
INAMI	Institut National d'Assurance Maladie-Invalidité	National Institute for Health and Disability Insurance	Autonomous national commission that monitors health insurance and sets policy targets
VIPOs	Les Veuves, les Orphelins, les Pensionnés, et les bénéficiaires d'indemnités d'Invalidité dont les revenus ne dépassent pas un montant annuel fixé par le Roi	Widows, orphans, old-age pensioners, and disability pensioners of low income defined by law	Low-income persons whose health insurance is subsidized by the national government

Index

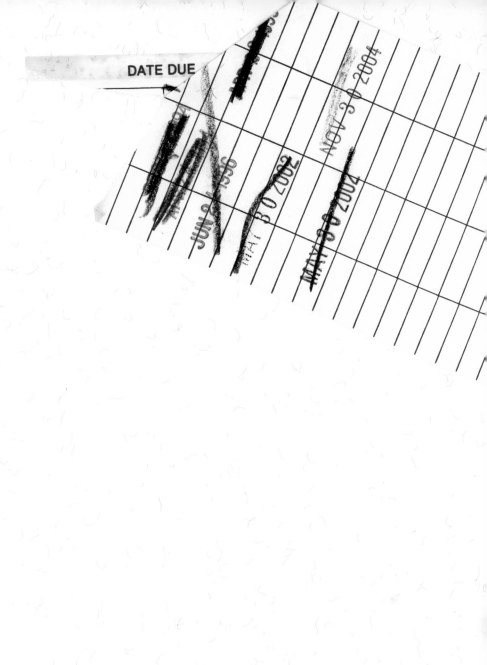

DATE DUE